hiking from here to

WOW

W9-CRM-558

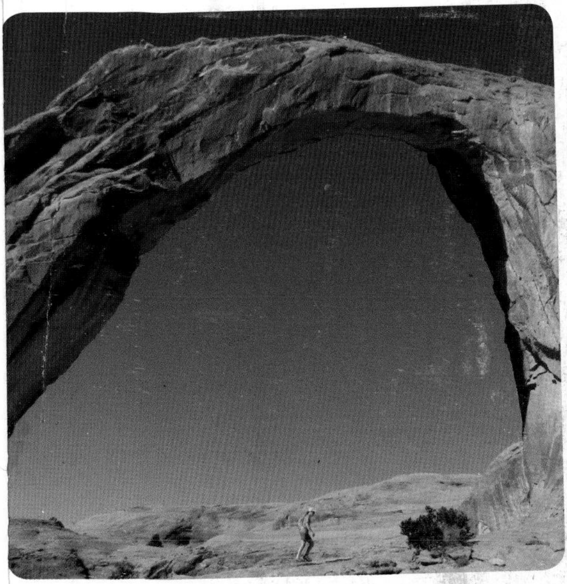

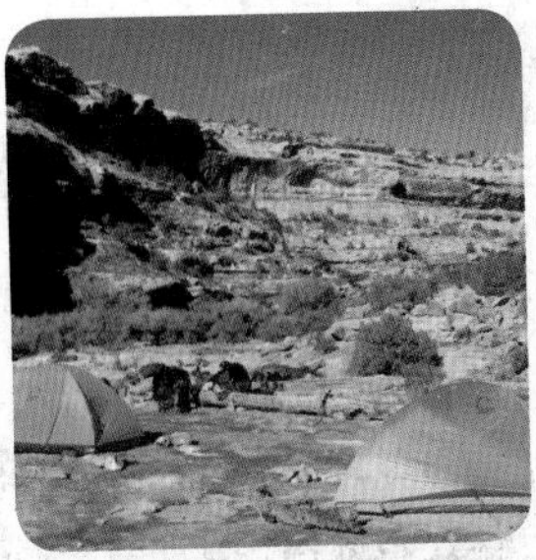

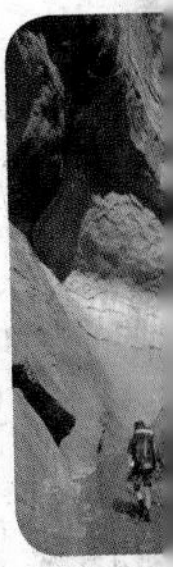

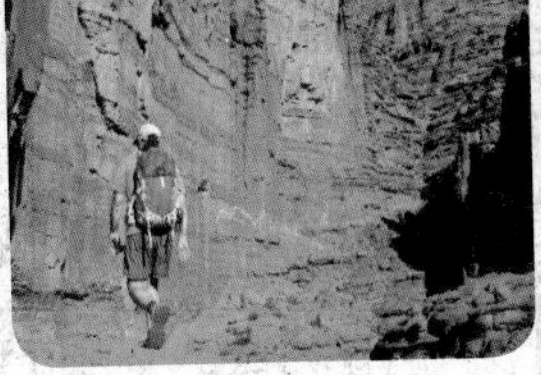

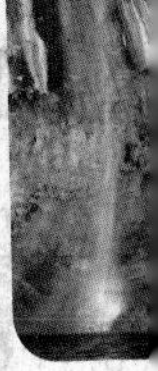

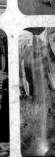

WOW GUIDES

UTAH CANYON COUNTRY

90 TRAILS TO THE WONDER OF WILDERNESS

Kathy & Craig Copeland

WILDERNESS PRESS

MEMBER 1% FOR THE PLANET®

Businesses donating 1% of their sales to the natural environment

www.onepercentfortheplanet.org

The authors are members.

Hiking from here to WOW: Utah Canyon Country

1st EDITION 2008
3rd printing 2012

Copyright © 2008 by Craig and Kathy Copeland

All photos and original maps by the authors

Book and map production by C.J. Poznansky (giddyupgraphics@mac.com)

Cover and interior design by Matthew Clark (www.subplot.com)

ISBN: 978-0-89997-452-1

Manufactured in China

Published by: **Wilderness Press**
c/o Keen Communications
PO Box 43673
Birmingham, AL 35243
(800) 443-7227; FAX (205) 326-1012
info@wildernesspress.com
www.wildernesspress.com
Visit our website for a complete listing of our titles and for ordering information.

Distributed by Publishers Group West

Authors of opinionated guidebooks always welcome readers' comments. Write them at nomads@hikingcamping.com

Cover photo: The Wave (Trip 10) *Back cover photos:* Mill Creek Canyon (Trip 53); Grand Gulch pictograph (Trip 75); Split Level Ruin (Trip 75)

Title page photos: (large one) Corona Arch (Trip 50); (top middle) Grand Gulch (Trip 75); (bottom middle) Fisher Towers (Trip 59); (top right) Fortymile Gulch (Trip 26); (bottom right) Upper Calf Creek Falls (Trip 31)

All rights reserved. No part of this book may be reproduced in any form, or by any means electronic, mechanical, recording, or otherwise, without written permission from the publisher, except for brief quotations used in reviews.

YOUR SAFETY IS YOUR RESPONSIBILITY

Hiking and camping in the wilderness can be dangerous. Experience and preparation reduce risk, but will never eliminate it. The unique details of your specific situation and the decisions you make at that time will determine the outcome. Always check the weather forecast and current trail conditions before setting out. This book is not a substitute for common sense or sound judgment. If you doubt your ability to negotiate canyon country, respond to wild animals, or handle sudden, extreme weather changes, hike only in a group led by a competent guide. The authors and the publisher disclaim liability for any loss or injury incurred by anyone using information in this book.

CONTENTS

Trip Locator Map 2

Introduction: From Here to Wow 5 / Land of Waking Dreams 5 / Trips at a Glance 6 / Taming Godzilla 8 / Ghosts in the Fog 9 / The Ancestral Puebloans 11 / Rock Art 12 / Outdoor Museum 14 / The Colorado Plateau 15 / Tough Hombres 18 / Rodentville 19 / It's Alive! 21 / Wilderness Ethics 22 / Hiking With Your Dog 24 / Maps 24 / Carry a Compass 25 / Physical Capability 26 / Leave Your Itinerary 27 / Canyon-Country Climate 27 / Flashfloods 28 / Have a Swig 29 / Thermonuclear Protection 30 / Sundown 31

The Hikes 33
Zion National Park 39
Paria Canyon – Vermilion Cliffs Wilderness 76
Kanab 100
Bryce Canyon National Park 117
Hole-in-the-Rock Road /Grand Staircase – Escalante NM 140
Capitol Reef National Park 207
San Rafael Swell 234
Arches National Park 260
Moab 272
Canyonlands National Park 314
Glen Canyon National Recreation Area 360
Cedar Mesa 368
Comb Ridge Canyons 425

Information Sources 436
Index 438
The Authors 442

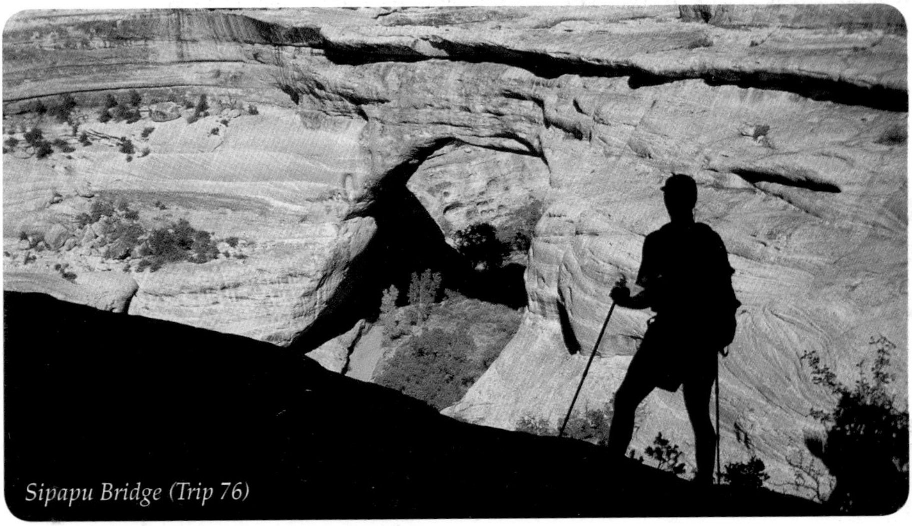

Sipapu Bridge (Trip 76)

UTAH CANYON COUNTRY TRIP LOCATIONS

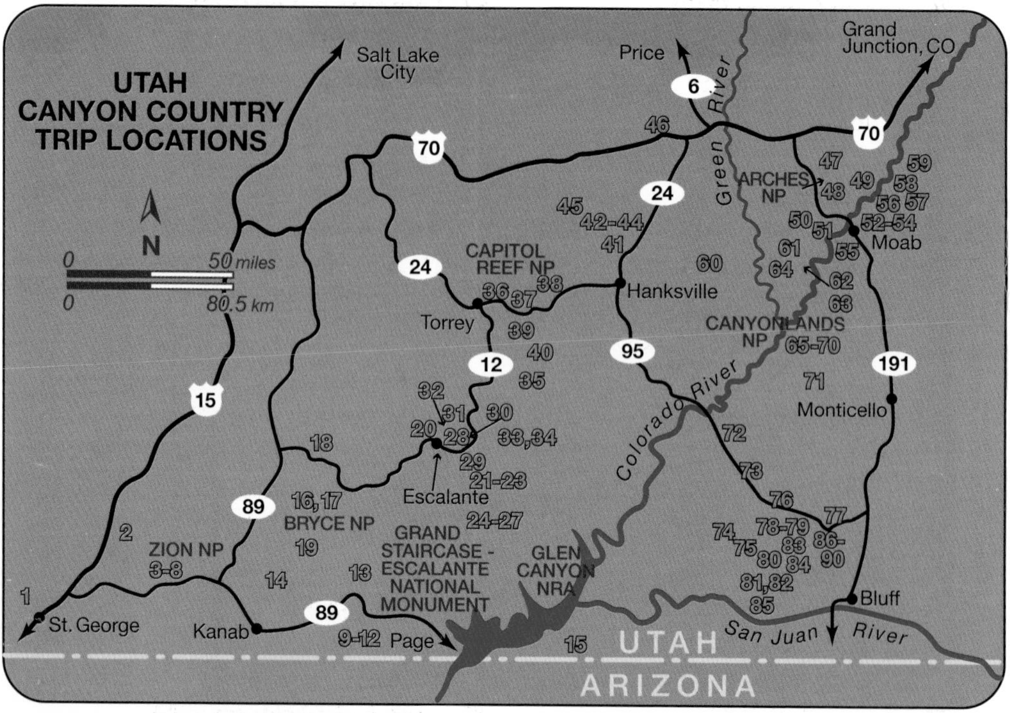

90 TRAILS TO THE WONDER OF WILDERNESS

trip number / trip name / page number

1 Snow Canyon (34)
2 LaVerkin Creek (39)
3 The Subway (46)
4 Angels Landing (51)
5 West Rim (56)
6 Observation Point (61)
7 Cable Mountain (65)
8 Zion Narrows (71)
9 The Wave (76)
10 Wire Pass (81)
11 Buckskin Gulch (84)
12 Paria River Canyon (89)
13 Yellow Rock (100)
14 Lick Wash (104)
15 Rainbow Bridge & Beyond (110)
16 Fairyland (117)
17 Peekaboo / Queens Garden (121)
18 Red Canyon (126)
19 Willis Creek Canyon (130)
20 Pine Creek (136)
21 Golden Cathedral (146)
22 Twentyfive Mile Wash (150)
23 Peek-a-boo & Spooky (154)
24 Coyote Gulch (158)
25 Crack in the Wall (162)
26 Willow & Fortymile gulches (166)
27 Davis Gulch (170)
28 Escalante River (174)
29 Phipps Arch (179)
30 Lower Calf Creek Falls (183)
31 Upper Calf Creek Falls (188)
32 Boulder Mail Trail (192)
33 Little Death Hollow (199)
34 Silver Falls Creek Canyon (203)

35 Upper Muley Twist (207)
36 Spring Canyon (212)
37 Navajo Knobs (216)
38 Cassidy Arch (221)
39 Golden Throne (227)
40 Sheets Gulch (231)
41 Goblin Valley (234)
42 Bell & Little Wild Horse (240)
43 Crack Canyon (244)
44 Chute Canyon (247)
45 Chute of Muddy Creek (250)
46 Black Dragon (256)
47 Devils Garden (260)
48 Fiery Furnace (266)
49 Delicate Arch (269)
50 Corona Arch (272)
51 Dragonfly Canyon (275)
52 Slickrock Trail (278)
53 Mill Creek Canyon (282)
54 Behind the Rocks (286)
55 Amasa Back (293)
56 Morning Glory Canyon (298)
57 Colorado River Canyon (303)
58 Professor Creek (306)
59 Fisher Towers (310)
60 Horseshoe Canyon (314)
61 Dead Horse Point (319)
62 Lathrop Canyon (322)
63 Murphy Hogback (325)
64 Upheaval Canyon (329)
65 Big Spring & Squaw (334)
66 Peekaboo (338)
67 The Needles (343)
68 Chesler Park / The Joint (344)
69 Devils Kitchen (344)
70 Druid Arch (344)
71 Salt Creek Canyon (350)
72 Dark Canyon (360)
73 Sandthrax Slickrock (365)
74 Lower Grand Gulch (373)
75 Grand Gulch: Collins to Kane (376)
76 Natural Bridges NM (383)
77 Mule Canyon South Fork (398)
78 Kane Gulch (392)
79 Fish & Owl Canyons (396)
80 Bullet Canyon (402)
81 First Fork Slickhorn (405)
82 Third Fork Slickhorn (409)
83 Road Canyon (413)
84 Lime Canyon (417)
85 Honaker Trail (421)
86-90 Comb Ridge Canyons (425)

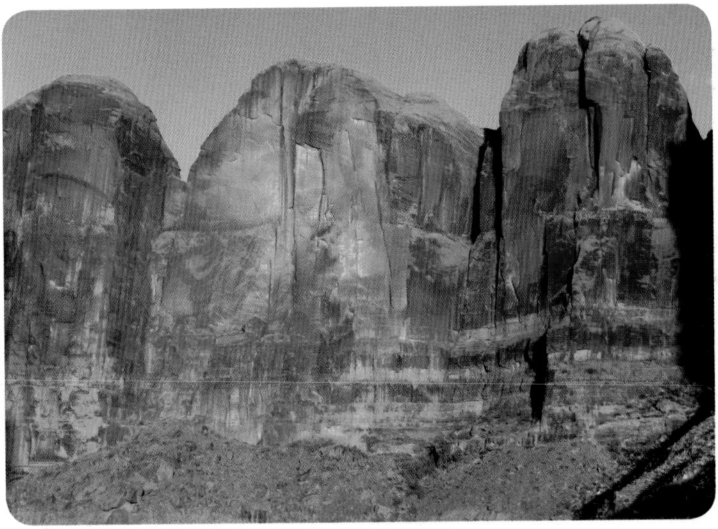

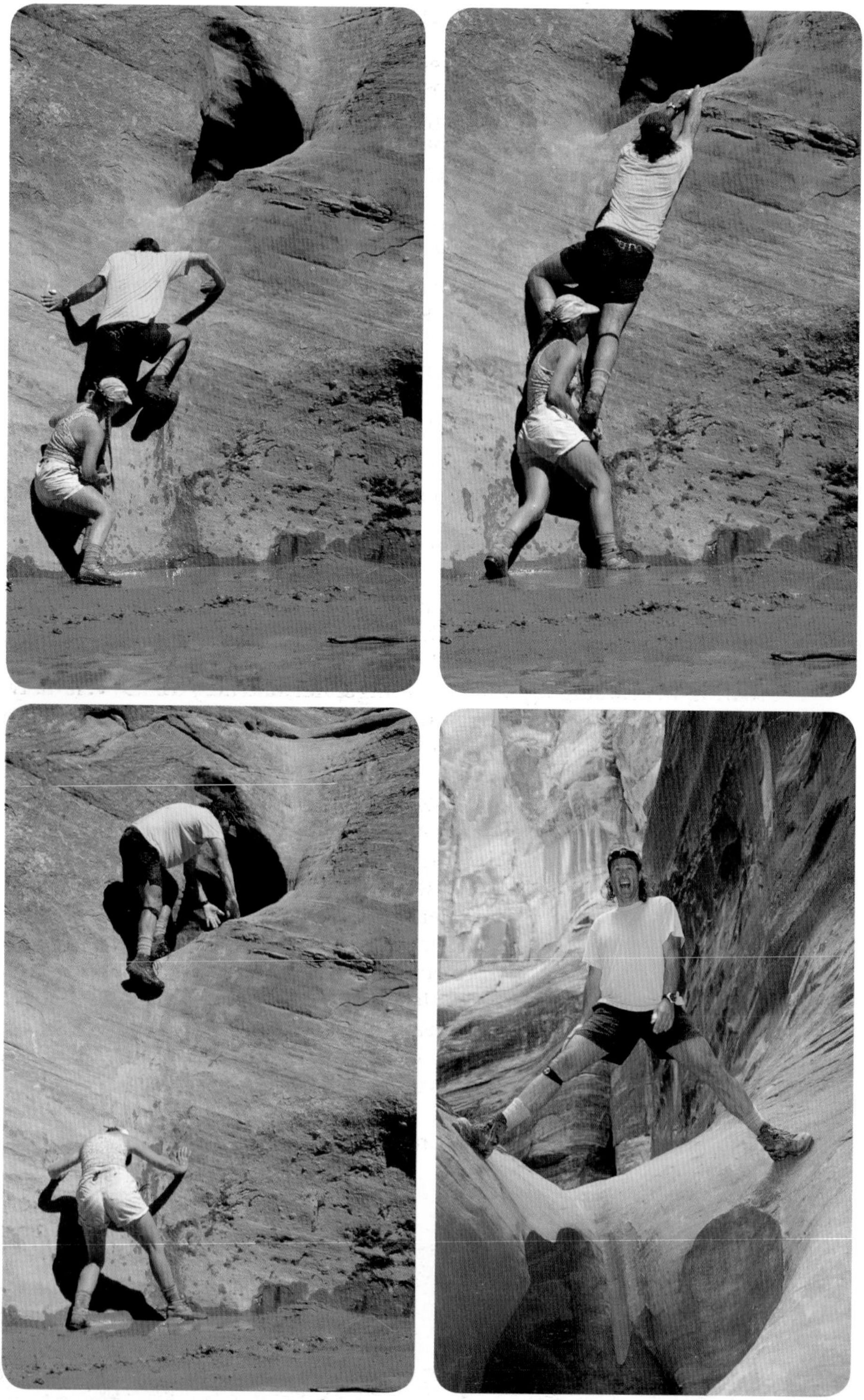

Canyon country invites play.

FROM HERE TO WOW

Your time is short, but the canyons are endless. So we've simplified the task. Here are the 90 southern-Utah trails most likely to make you say "Wow!"

No okay trails. Not even any pretty good trails. And certainly no trudgemills. Just the dayhikes and backpack trips that will get you from here to WOW—the wonder of wilderness—as swiftly as possible. Plus our boot-tested opinions: why we recommend each hike, what to expect, how to enjoy the optimal experience.

We hope our suggestions compel you to get outdoors more often and stay out longer. Do it to cultivate your wild self. It will give you perspective. Do it because the backcountry teaches simplicity and self-reliance, qualities that make life more fulfilling. Do it to remind yourself why wilderness needs and deserves your protection. A bolder conservation ethic develops naturally in the canyons. And do it to escape the cacophony that muffles the quiet, pure voice within.

LAND OF WAKING DREAMS

Humans can't survive without dreaming. Deprived of our nightly flights of imagination, our sanity disintegrates. Likewise, deprived of mystery, our soul withers.

Some think they need only answers. But the need for mystery is greater than the need for any answer.

And just as sleeping summons our dreams, hiking is an invocation to mystery. Especially if we're hiking in the most mysterious land of all: the vast, earthen sculpture known as *southern Utah.*

The soaring arches, bulging walls, towering spires, and fiery colors eventually, inexorably lull hikers into a state of contemplation in which we ponder and are strangely soothed by life's enduring mysteries.

We're aware of the scientific view. We've heard about the processes that shaped this topography. What geologists tell us makes sense. We don't question *how*. We wonder *why*. We seek a transcendent explanation.

Could aimless physics really be responsible for creating such a bizarre and sensuous wonderland? Or was there intent? The intent to inspire play and elicit joy among all creatures who wander here?

Romping like children—across slickrock, into labyrinthian canyons—we sense nature's intent. It ignites our curiosity, powers our limbs. But it remains a mystery. And it keeps us returning, to steep ourselves in it rather than solve it.

Fall asleep, plunge into the recesses of your subconscious mind, and you awaken not necessarily with answers, but refreshed. It's the same when you return from a southern-Utah sojourn, your boots covered in Navajo sandstone dust, your mind empty and clear.

Canyon country is the land of waking dreams.

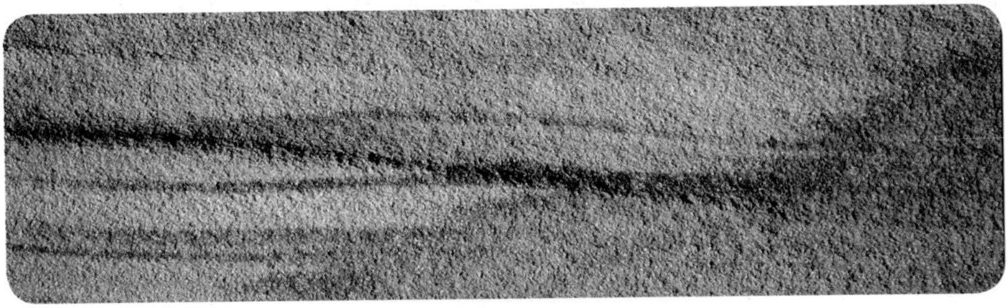

TRIPS AT A GLANCE

Trips in each category are listed according to geographic location: starting in the southwest, near St. George, moving northeast to Escalante, northeast to the San Rafael Swell, east to Moab, then south to Cedar Mesa. After the trip name is the return distance, followed by the elevation gain.

1	Snow Canyon	6 mi	(9.7 km)	460 ft	(140 m)
2	LaVerkin Creek	18.2 mi	(29.3 km)	1540 ft	(470 m)
3	The Subway	7.8 mi	(12.6 km)	1200 ft	(366 m)
4	Angels Landing	5.2 mi	(8.4 km)	1500 ft	(457 m)
5	West Rim	12.2 mi	(19.6 km)	2510 ft	(765 m)
6	Observation Point	8 mi	(12.9 km)	2147 ft	(654 m)
7	Cable Mountain	15.4 mi	(24.8 km)	2964 ft	(904 m)
8	Zion Narrows	6 mi	(9.7 km)	200 ft	(61 m)
9	The Wave	6 mi	(9.6 km)	300 ft	(91 m)
10	Wire Pass	3.4 mi	(5.5 km)	170 ft	(52 m)
11	Buckskin Gulch	20.3 mi	(32.7 km)	100 ft	(24 m)
12	Paria River Canyon	38.4 mi	(61.9 km)	1130-ft	(345-m) loss
13	Yellow Rock	4.2 mi	(6.8 km)	800 ft	(244 m)
14	Lick Wash	8 mi	(13 km)	330 ft	(100 m)
15	Rainbow Bridge & Beyond	23 mi	(27 km)	2640 ft	(805 m)
16	Fairyland	8 mi	(12.9 km)	1670 ft	(509 m)
17	Peekaboo / Queens Garden	6.4 mi	(10.3 km)	1145 ft	(349 m)
18	Red Canyon	6 mi	(9.7 km)	480 ft	(146 m)
19	Willis Creek Canyon	4.8 mi	(7.7 km)	300 ft	(91 m)
20	Pine Creek	8.5 mi	(13.7 km)	1300-ft	(396-m) loss
21	Golden Cathedral	9.2 mi	(14.8 km)	1260 ft	(384 m)
22	Twentyfive Mile Wash	15.2 mi	(24.5 km)	1030 ft	(314 m)
23	Peek-a-boo & Spooky	4.8 mi	(7.7 km)	565 ft	(172 m)
24	Coyote Gulch	18 mi	(29 km)	680 ft	(207 m)
25	Crack in the Wall	5.2 mi	(8.4 km)	880 ft	(268 m)
26	Willow & Fortymile Gulches	7.7 mi	(12.4 km)	430 ft	(131 m)
27	Davis Gulch	8 mi	(12.9 km)	755 ft	(230 m)
28	Escalante River	15.5 mi	(25 km)	760 ft	(232 m)
29	Phipps Arch	8 mi	(12.9 km)	840 ft	(256 m)
30	Lower Calf Creek Falls	6 mi	(9.7 km)	260 ft	(79 m)
31	Upper Calf Creek Falls	2.2 mi	(3.5 km)	657 ft	(200 m)
32	Boulder Mail Trail	15 mi	(24.2 km)	2500 ft	(762 m)
33	Little Death Hollow	15.2 mi	(24.5 km)	665 ft	(203 m)
34	Silver Falls Creek Canyon	12 mi	(19.3 km)	660 ft	(201 m)
35	Upper Muley Twist	14.2 mi	(22.9 km)	1060 ft	(323 m)
36	Spring Canyon	9.7 mi	(15.6 km)	1070-ft	(326-m) loss
37	Navajo Knobs	9 mi	(14.5 km)	2500 ft	(762 m)
38	Cohab Canyon / Cassidy Arch	9.2 mi	(14.8 km)	2530 ft	(771 m)
39	Golden Throne	4 mi	(6.4 km)	700 ft	(213 m)
40	Sheets Gulch	4 mi	(6.4 km)	250 ft	(76 m)
41	Goblin Valley	8 mi	(13 km)	275 ft	(84 m)
42	Bell & Little Wild Horse	8.7 mi	(14 km)	710 ft	(216 m)
43	Crack Canyon	7 mi	(11.3 km)	260 ft	(79 m)

44	Chute Canyon	4.5 mi (7.2 km)	180 ft (55 m)
45	Chute of Muddy Creek	16 mi (25.8 km)	250 ft (76 m)
46	Black Dragon	6.4 mi (10.3 km)	1400 ft (427 m)
47	Devils Garden	7.7 mi (12.4 km)	650 ft (198 m)
48	Fiery Furnace	2 mi (3.2 km)	200 ft (61 m)
49	Delicate Arch	3 mi (4.8 km)	560 ft (171 m)
50	Corona Arch	3 mi (5 km)	556 ft (170 m)
51	Dragonfly Canyon	3.2 mi (5.2 km)	887 ft (270 m)
52	Slickrock Trail	10.5 mi (16.9 km)	760 ft (232 m)
53	Mill Creek Canyon	4 mi (6.4 km)	250 ft (76 m)
54	Behind the Rocks	6.8 mi (10.9 km)	1620 ft (494 m)
55	Amasa Back	9.2 mi (14.8 km)	1644 ft (501 m)
56	Morning Glory Canyon	7.6 mi (12.2 km)	672 ft (205 m)
57	Colorado River Canyon	6.4 mi (10.3 km)	915 ft (279 m)
58	Professor Creek	8.6 mi (13.8 km)	410 ft (125 m)
59	Fisher Towers	4.6 mi (7.4 km)	1050 ft (320 m)
60	Horseshoe Canyon	7.4 mi (11.9 km)	700 ft (213 m)
61	Dead Horse Point	9.1 mi (14.7 km)	260 ft (79 m)
62	Lathrop Canyon	11 mi (17.7 km)	1815 ft (533 ft)
63	Murphy Hogback	10.8 mi (17.4 km)	1240 ft (378 m)
64	Upheaval Canyon	8 mi (12.9 km)	1480 ft (451 m)
65	Big Spring & Squaw	7.5 mi (12.1 km)	430 ft (131 m)
66	Peekaboo	10 mi (16.2 km)	940 ft (287 m)
67	The Needles	5.6 mi (9 km)	770 ft (235 m)
68	Chesler Park / The Joint	11.1 mi (17.9 km)	800 ft (244 m)
69	Devils Kitchen	10.5 mi (16.9 km)	730 ft (223 m)
70	Druid Arch	10.8 mi (17.4 km)	640 ft (195 m)
71	Salt Creek Canyon	27.5 mi (44.3 km)	940 ft (287 m)
72	Dark Canyon	8 mi (12.9 km)	1600 ft (488 m)
73	Sandthrax Slickrock	3 mi (4.8 km)	520 ft (159 m)
74	Lower Grand Gulch	13.6 mi (22 km)	400 ft (122 m)
75	Grand Gulch: Collins to Kane	38 mi (61.2 km)	1660 ft (506 m)
76	Natural Bridges Natl Mon.	8.6 mi (13.8 km)	640 ft (195 m)
77	Mule Canyon	7.5 mi (12.1 km)	400 ft (122 m)
78	Kane Gulch	8 mi (12.9 km)	520 ft (159 m)
79	Fish & Owl Creek Canyons	17 mi (27.4 km)	1360 ft (415 m)
80	Bullet Canyon	9.5 mi (15.3 km)	770 ft (235 m)
81	First Fork Slickhorn Canyon	8.8 mi (14.2 km)	670 ft (204 m)
82	Slickhorn Canyon	10.5 mi (16.9 km)	960 ft (293 m)
83	Road Canyon	8 mi (12.9 km)	800 ft (244 m)
84	Lime Canyon	4 mi (6.4 km)	500 ft (152 m)
85	Honaker Trail	8 mi (12.9 km)	1244 ft (379 m)
86-90	Comb Ridge Canyons	up to 5 mi (8 km)	up to 690 ft (210 m)

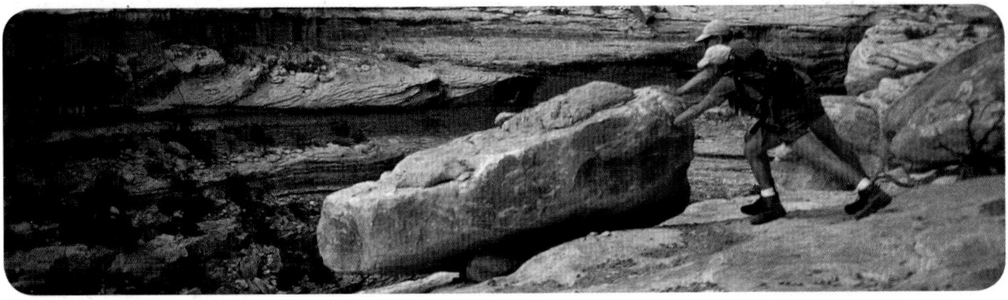

TAMING GODZILLA

The essence of hiking is appreciation of nature. As humanity's footprint on Earth continues to grow, there's less nature for hikers to appreciate. That's especially true in the redrock canyon country of southern Utah, where humanity's footprint increasingly resembles Godzilla's.

The custodian for most of Utah's public land is the Bureau of Land Management (BLM), an agency within the United States Department of the Interior. The BLM is currently deciding which canyon-country areas should be preserved in their natural state, and which should be open to energy exploration and off-road vehicle (ORV) recreation. As of this writing, the BLM intends to sacrifice nearly two-million acres of wilderness-quality land to ORV use.

You can influence the BLM, if you act now. Start by visiting the websites of the three conservation groups leading the effort to protect the fragile beauty of this spectacular region.

The Southern Utah Wilderness Alliance is the most effective group working to cure the BLM of myopia. SUWA's goal is not to ban ORVs but simply to reduce the amount of land that ORVs can legally rampage. Visit www.suwa.org to quickly voice your opinion to state officials.

Visit www.redrockheritage.org to see photos of rampaged canyon country. The website represents the Redrock Heritage Coalition, a group of southern Utah residents and organizations who created the *Redrock Heritage Plan for Sustainable Economies and Ecosystems*.

The Redrock Heritage Plan is not an extremist proposal. It acknowledges ORV recreation as well as mountain biking and hiking. But it would restrict ORVs to designated roads and trails, because the majority of canyon-country visitors prefer to hike—in tranquility.

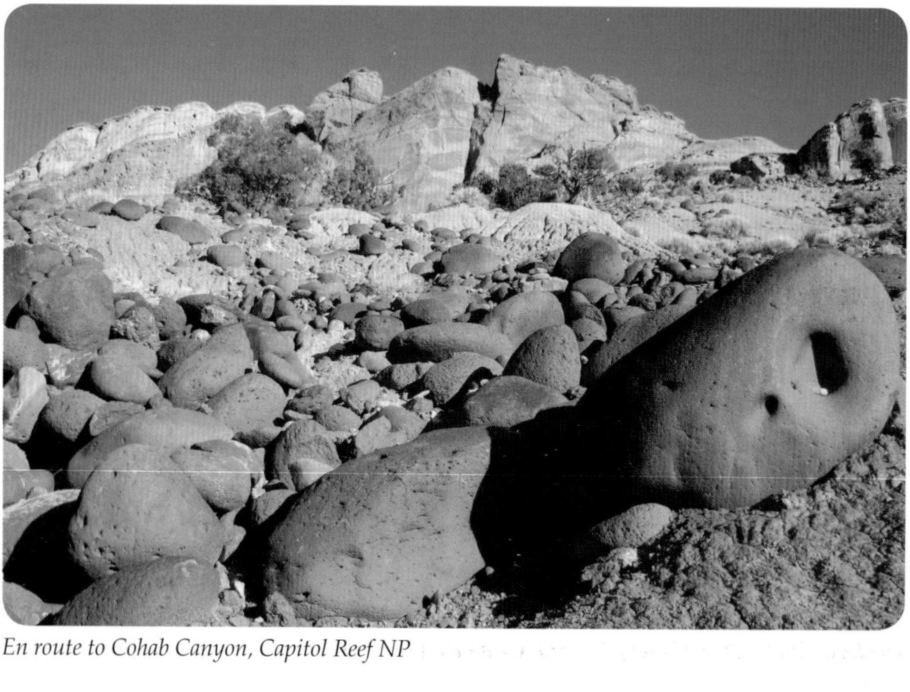

En route to Cohab Canyon, Capitol Reef NP

The plan also contends (and most geologists agree) that if all the undeveloped land in Utah were pierced with oil wells, it would extend the nation's oil supply by only three weeks and the natural gas supply by only five months, therefore oil-and-gas exploration in canyon country should be limited to existing, productive areas.

SUWA and the Redrock Heritage Coalition have a powerful ally: the Sierra Club. *America's Wild Legacy Initiative* is the their effort to protect at least one exceptional wild place in every state within ten years. In Florida, it's the Everglades. In Alaska, it's the Arctic. In Utah, it's redrock canyon country. Visit www.sierraclub.org/wildlegacy/52places/ to learn more.

GHOSTS IN THE FOG

Most accounts of canyon-country human history are brazenly ethnocentric. They make a vague, passing reference to the first people to wrest a living from this harsh land, then describe in tedious detail the relatively recent arrival of Spanish explorers (1765) and Mormon settlers (1847).

But the Paleo-Indians were here long before: roughly 14,000 years ago. And given that they roamed the region for millennia, they're the protagonists of the story. Everyone else is just a bit player.

The lack of hard information about Paleo-Indians, however, is exasperating. They're little more than ghosts in the fog. Archaeologists have nevertheless learned enough to provide us with a profile. It's only educated conjecture, much like a police artist's sketch of a suspect, but it's fascinating.

The Paleo-Indians were nomadic. Traveling on foot, carrying only a few meager possessions, they were the original ultralight backpackers. Along with their extended family—grandparents, siblings, children—they followed the seasons, always in search of food.

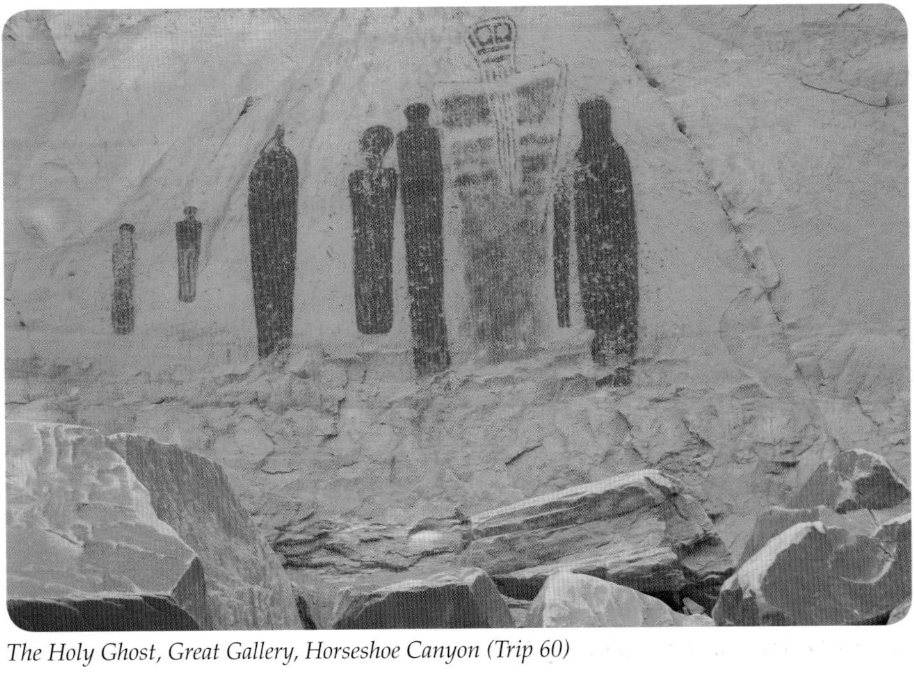

The Holy Ghost, Great Gallery, Horseshoe Canyon (Trip 60)

They wore clothing made of pelts and plant fibers. They slept in the open, took shelter in caves and canyon alcoves, or built rudimentary shelters out of brush and animal hide.

For ages, they persevered with no knowledge of how to use spearpoints for hunting. They foraged constantly, harvesting roots, seeds, fruit—whatever was edible. They cooked, but much of their diet was raw food, including larvae and insects.

Often they trapped or clubbed small game. They targeted newborn, injured, sick, and old animals, or scared away predators from fresh kills. Working together, they might have driven big-game herds over cliffs, slaughtering numerous animals at once.

By chipping stone into desired shapes, a process now known as "flint knapping," they made tools for cutting, scraping, hammering and chopping. They also made implements out of animal bones, horns or tusks, used smooth rocks to grind seeds into flour, and fashioned rudimentary equipment from plant fibers and wood.

When the Paleo-Indians began hunting with stone-pointed spears, it transformed their culture. Hunting big game (such as the wooly mammoth whose jawbone was found by palaeontologists in Arches National Park) displaced foraging as their primary means of survival.

The more they hunted, the more skilled they became at flint knapping. Today, spear points are their culture's signature artifact and are considered the most beautifully crafted stonework from all of American prehistory.

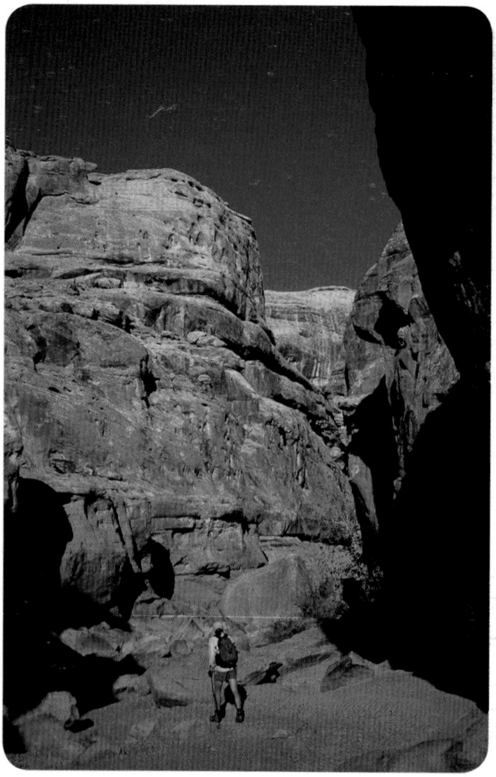

White Canyon, below milepost 55, off Highway 95

Paleo-Indian hunters threw their spears, used them as lances, or propelled them with an "atlatl" or throwing stick. They probably hid near water sources and waited for their prey to arrive. Their first spear strike was unlikely to have killed, say a mastodon, so they must have continued chasing the injured animal—for miles or even days—inflicting wounds until it collapsed.

Attacking a mammoth or mastodon with a spear makes bullfighting look like a lawn game. The potential reward, however, was immense: a feast for the entire clan, plus leftovers galore. A successful hunt must have incited an orgiastic celebration. Afterward, they'd strip the carcass. Meat, skin, ivory, bone, sinew—all were precious resources. They wasted nothing, because survival was always tenuous.

Archaeological evidence suggests Paleo-Indians did not wander aimlessly but traveled in annual circuits, following big game, seeking edible plants, mindful of the need for winter shelter. They traded and intermarried with other bands. The continent-wide distribution of similar spearpoints suggests a vast communication reach. But their precise migration vector to the present-day U.S. and into the desert southwest is unknown.

And that's just one of many questions that will remain unanswered. Who were these people, really? What kind of spirituality did they practice? What were their rituals? Did they make music? Dance? How were their small, mobile societies structured? What kind of language did they speak? The Paleo-Indians are an enigma. And a blurry one at that.

THE ANCESTRAL PUEBLOANS

By the end of the Ice Age, the earth's vegetation had changed dramatically and many big-game species were extinct. So the descendants of the Paleo-Indians—the Desert Archaic Indians—adapted to a new world. They evolved from nomads to villagers, from hunter gatherers to farmers.

It was a slow, primitive, agricultural renaissance. They formed larger bands and diversified culturally. Possibly influenced by the great Mayan civilization farther south, they created permanent settlements. Seeking more durable housing, they built pit houses (semi-subterranean lodges). They devised more complex tools, wove plant-fiber mats and baskets, made simple ceramics. And they developed new religious ideas, which they documented by painting and chiseling stone surfaces.

They built their pit houses on escarpments, knolls or mesas above drainages and arable land. Within each hamlet, they built a larger pit house for community meetings and ceremonies. They created beautiful, delicate pottery and sophisticated, ornate baskets. They cached surplus food for lean times. They began hunting—and fighting—with bows and arrows. And they were the first people in all of what is now the southwest U.S. and northern Mexico to rely more on crops (corn, beans, squash) than on hunting and gathering.

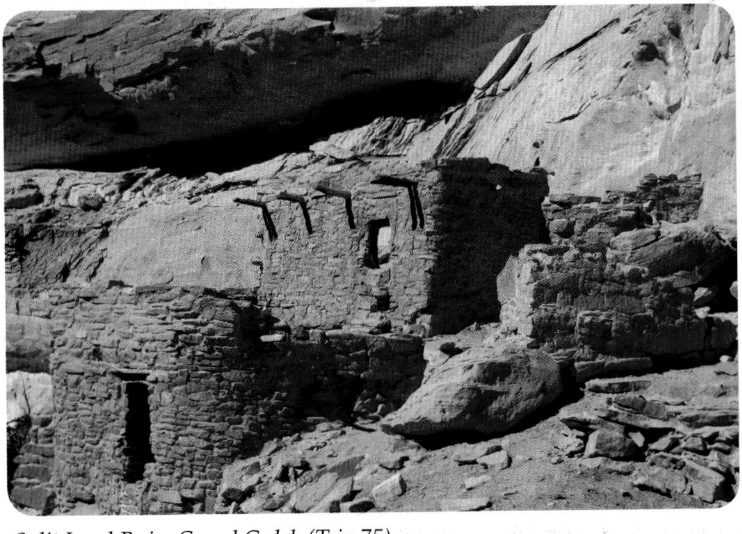

Split Level Ruin, Grand Gulch (Trip 75)

Their cultural evolution into the Ancestral Puebloans around 1200 B.C. was marked by the abandonment of pit houses in favor of contiguous and multistory stone-and-mortar structures built atop the ground but usually sheltered by canyon walls.

The Puebloan population surged after 700 A.D. They spread into less hospitable areas, planted larger fields, developed complex irrigation systems, and became master craftsmen. They celebrated rituals by drumming, chanting and dancing in their community plazas and kivas (underground ceremonial chambers). Their civilization flourished between 900 A.D. and 1130 A.D., then rapidly declined. A decades-long drought killed many of them and diminished resources so severely that survivors were constantly at war. It wasn't the scenery that inspired them to build fortress-like cliff dwellings; they were defending themselves from marauders.

Though the Puebloans seem to have simply vanished around 1240 A.D., archaeologists believe those who survived the drought and escaped conflict did so by abandoning southern Utah (in fact all of the Colorado Plateau, as well as southern New Mexico, southern Arizona, and northern Chihuahua) and migrating to other, more stable Native societies in west central New Mexico, northeast Arizona, and the upper Rio Grande River drainage.

Because the arid climate is gentle on archaeological sites, an astonishing number of Puebloan dwellings, granaries and rock-art panels are still intact today, seemingly enshrined within the canyons. This abundance of readily-visible cultural remains lends intellectual and spiritual stimulation to the experience of hiking in southern Utah.

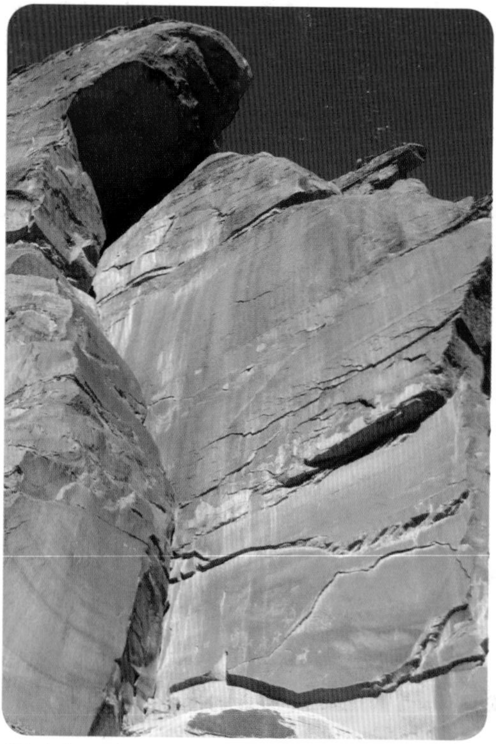
Find the rock art.

ROCK ART

Southern Utah is an immense outdoor art gallery. Natives, beginning many thousands of years ago with the Desert Archaic Indians, frequently carved and painted rock surfaces. A startling number of these rock-art sites have survived the ravages of time and are still visible today.

Archaeologists believe petroglyphs and pictographs represented spiritual visions, chronicled significant events, served as signage for passersby (advice, warnings), or were clan symbols. Though these interpretations make sense, they're merely educated conjecture. We'll never know for sure what the artists intended. Perhaps they were simply amusing each other. It will remain a mystery, adding intrigue to the allure of canyon country.

Petroglyphs were carved (pecked, scratched, incised) *into* the rock. Pictographs were painted (using mineral pigments or plant dyes) *on* the rock surface. Most people get them mixed up. But you'll remember the difference if you know the terms' origins.

"Petro" comes from the Greek "petros," which means "stone," and "glyphein," which means "carve." So a petroglyph is carved in stone.

"Picto" comes from the Latin "pictus," which means "painted." "Graph" is of Greek origin and means "record." So a pictograph is a painted record.

Petroglyphs are usually on the dark-brown or black vertical streaks called *desert varnish* that stain most canyon walls. Pictographs are usually on the smooth sandstone of the Navajo (buff colored) and Wingate (reddish) formations. The Natives created most of their art within sheltering alcoves or beneath protective overhangs where rain wouldn't harm it.

Rock art is strewn throughout canyon country. You don't even have to hike to see it. Many remarkable panels are visible from pavement, for example near Moab, along Kane Creek Road and the Potash Road. And two of the most arresting rock-art sites in the region are a short drive from downtown.

You're heading north? Visit Sego Canyon, about 45 minutes from Moab. It's not far from the junction of Hwy 191 and Interstate 70. You're heading south? Visit Newspaper Rock—on Hwy 211, which accesses the Needles District of Canyonlands National Park.

When viewing rock art, resist the urge to touch it. The oil on your skin will speed the deterioration of the paint and even the sandstone itself. Put your hand on a petroglyph or pictograph and you're defacing it. Touching = vandalism. The damage, though not immediately visible, will be irrevocable and possibly severe.

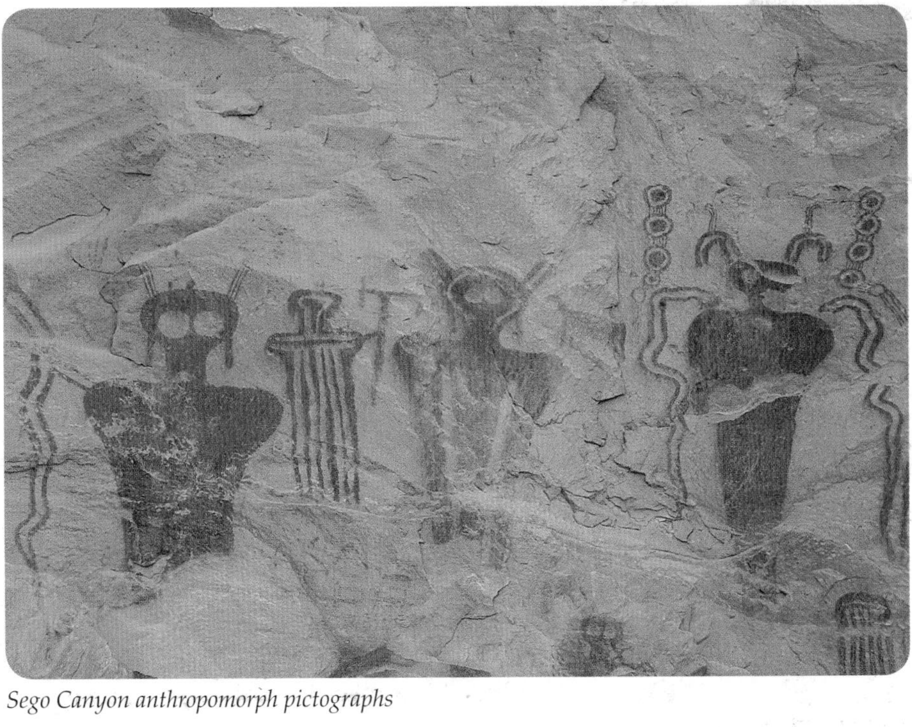

Sego Canyon anthropomorph pictographs

The way to feel rock art is not with your hands but with your heart. Remind yourself that the artists were human beings very much like you. They had desires, fears, dreams. They felt joy, sorrow, pain. They could be emotional, logical, confused. They were smart, ignorant, curious. They worked hard and got lazy. They treasured life and dreaded death. They too were perplexed by the meaning of it all. With that in mind, perhaps you can begin to fathom what they were trying to say. Empathy, after all, is the first step toward understanding.

SEGO CANYON

Rock-art panels up to 6,000 years old, from three Native American periods: Barrier Canyon, Fremont, and Ute.

The Barrier-style panel has ten nearly life-size anthropomorphic shapes. They're similar to those in the famous Great Gallery, in Horseshoe Canyon (Trip 60). Heavy trapezoidal bodies appear to float in space. Many have long, curved horns or antennae, and round, enlarged, staring eyes. Some archaeologists believe the figures were created by shamans during or after trance states in which they contacted, or felt they had become, supernatural beings. Perhaps the drawings were an attempt to communicate to others what they'd experienced.

From Moab, drive Hwy 191 north-northwest 30 mi (48 km), turn right (east) onto I-70, then proceed 5 mi (8 km) to Exit 185. Continue north 3.5 mi (5.6 km)—through the ghost town of Thompson Springs, beyond the railroad tracks—to the parking lot on the left. A path leads 165 yd (150 m) to the rock-art site. Directly across the canyon are two more panels above a corral.

NEWSPAPER ROCK

A single, spectacular panel bearing some 2,000 years of rock art from the Fremont, Ancestral Puebloan, Navajo, and Anglo cultures.

In the Navajo language, the panel is called *Tse' Hane*, which means "rock that tells a story." Though you're unlikely to decipher a story no matter how long you stare, you *will* see hundreds of figures on this 8-by-20 ft (2.4-by-6.1 m) expanse of rock. They include paw prints, hooves, elk with huge antlers, a deer herd, a migration of animals, bighorn sheep, lizards, buffalo, snakes, various symbols, shamans, even a six-toed human foot.

From Moab, drive Hwy 191 south 38.4 mi (61.8 km). Turn right (west) onto Hwy 211, which is signed for Canyonlands National Park, Needles District. Continue another 12.3 mi (19.8 km) to the parking lot on the right.

Just 1.9 mi (3 km) farther is a pullout on the left (east). From there, if you walk across dry Indian Creek and continue 110 yd (100 m) to the cliffs at the Shay Canyon confluence, you'll find two more venerable but overlooked rock-art panels.

OUTDOOR MUSEUM

Ancestral Puebloan rock art, dwellings, kivas and granaries are strewn across southern Utah like fragments from a profound cataclysm. Each time you go hiking here, you're entering the world's premier outdoor museum. It's imperative you be a deferential visitor.

Ruins are fragile despite their well-preserved appearance. It's surprisingly easy to damage them. Bump into a door frame, lean on a wall, and you could destroy a priceless, ancient relic. The collapsing rubble might seriously injure you, too.

Always pause before approaching a ruin. Consider the least impactful, most respectful way to appreciate it. Take off your pack. Set aside your trekking poles. If hiking with a dog, keep it tethered well away from the site. Then be mindful of every step.

Don't walk on the midden—the former residents' refuse pile, typically located immediately beneath the dwelling. Middens are treasure troves of archaeological evidence. Avoid the structure's foundation. Never camp near ruins. And don't eat near them. Crumbs attract rodents that might cause further damage.

Leave artifacts where you find them. That's the only place they have meaning to an archaeologist. Picking them up and placing them in a pile, as if for display, eliminates clues that help astute archaeologists learn about the ancient ones. If each of us steals just one potsherd, all will soon be gone.

THE COLORADO PLATEAU

This map shows the Colorado Plateau—130,000 sq mi (337,000 sq km) drained by the Colorado River and its major tributaries: the Green, San Juan, and Little Colorado rivers. Elevations average 4,500 to 6,500 ft (1372 to 1980 m). Elsewhere in the U.S., a mile-high tableland would be a verdant oasis. Here it's a desert.

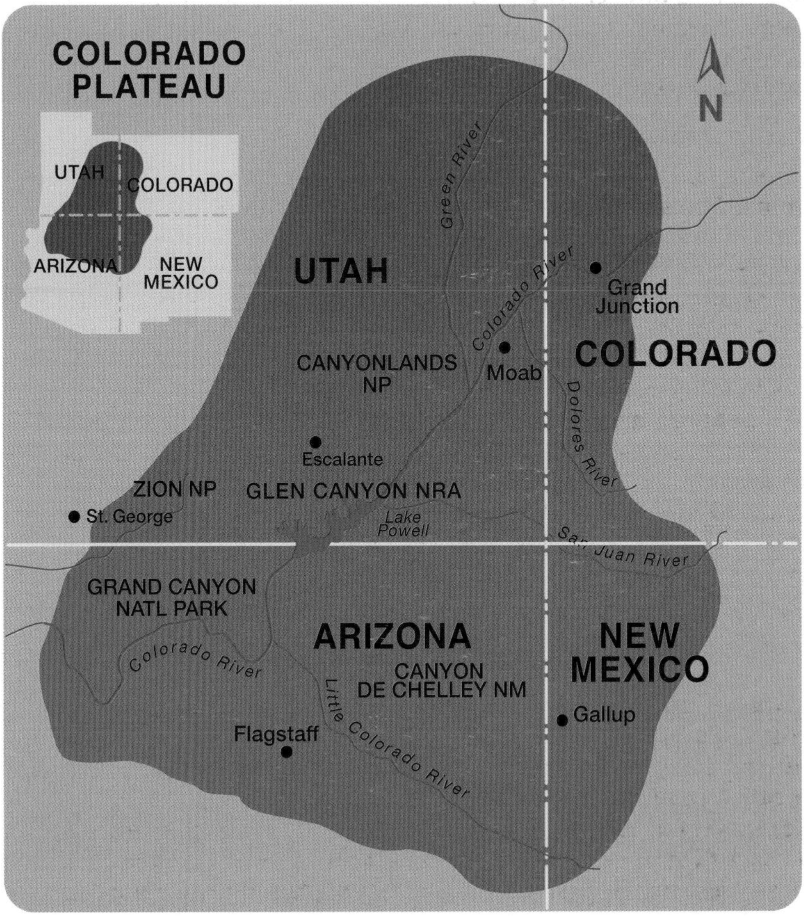

The Colorado Plateau is mostly sandstone, shale and limestone deposited in horizontal layers hundreds of millions of years ago. Much of it is deeply incised with countless canyons, valleys, gorges, chasms, gulches and arroyos. Think of the surface of the human brain. From an aerial perspective, the plateau has a similar, marvelously complex appearance created by erosion (water, wind, ice) and weathering (decomposition).

This superficial chaos, however, belies one of the Colorado Plateau's distinguishing geologic traits. It's essentially a high, thick, crustal block where relatively little rock deformation (violent uplifting, faulting, folding) has occurred within the past 600 million years. Yet the surrounding regions were dramatically deformed. The Rocky Mountains (north and east) were thrust skyward, and tremendous, earth-stretching tension created the Basin and Range (west and south).

Most of the hiking trails in this book reveal a vertical cross-section of the Colorado Plateau. The visible rock strata represent the region's geologic history from about 300 to 65 million years ago. To appreciate what you're seeing, however, you don't need to understand it. Beauty is never enhanced by explanation.

Memorizing how "the compressional impetus of the Laramide orogeny downfolded the rocks between the salt anticlines into broad synclines and reactivated the basement faults" will, unless you're a geologist, eviscerate your canyon-country experience.

Still, you might find this strange land even more captivating if you can identify its colorful, primary components. What follows is a partial list of rock strata and a brief summary of each—from top (most recent) to bottom (oldest)—so you'll be at least scantily informed.

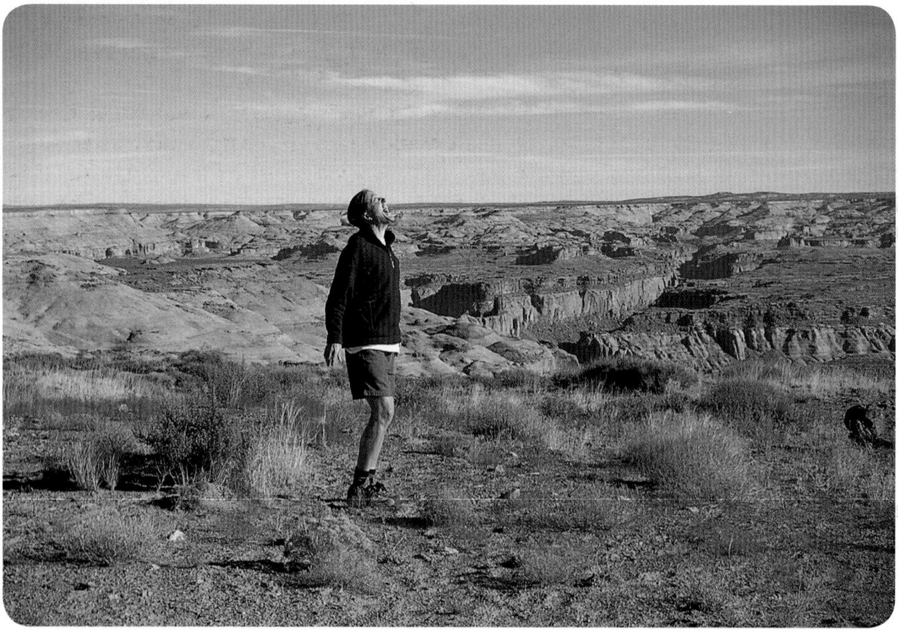

Above Dirty Devil River, south of Hanksville. Joyful to be back in canyon country after a long northern winter.

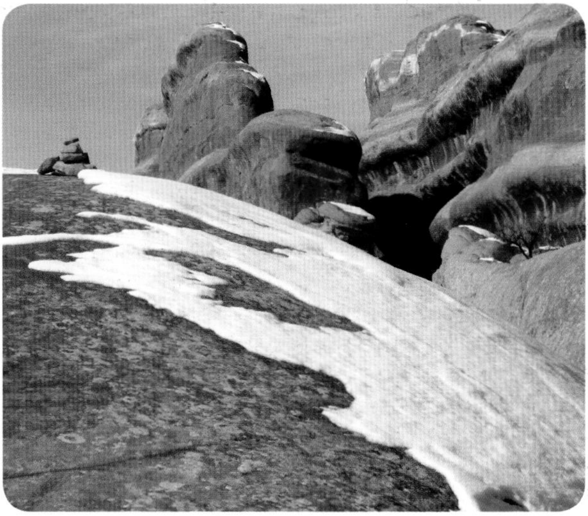

Entrada sandstone, Arches National Park

Entrada Sandstone tends to be light orange, although it ranges from cream to red. It was formed by windblown silt and sand settling in still water. Example: the celebrated arches in Arches National Park.

The Carmel Formation comprises brown to red siltstone layers mixed with limestone layers containing marine fossils. It was created by wind and stream deposits along the coast of a retreating sea. It forms unstable, sloping ledges atop Navajo sandstone in Grand Staircase-Escalante National Monument.

Navajo Sandstone is the most common yet most dramatic of southern Utah rock formations. Ranging from white to brown, it was deposited in the same environment as Wingate sandstone. Navajo sandstone forms vertical walls with smoothly rounded cliff-tops. The town of Boulder is surrounded by Navajo sandstone.

The Kayenta Formation appears as reddish-brown cliff bands and ledges. It was formed by stream-deposited sand. It provides easy-to-walk benches and sometimes contains dinosaur bones or footprints. It's usually recognizable as a distinct break, perhaps supporting shrubs or trees, between Wingate cliffs and overlying Navajo sandstone. Kayenta is visible in North Wash, where the Hog Springs slickwalk (Trip 73) begins.

Wingate Sandstone ranges from white, to red, to brown. It was deposited in vast drifting deserts during an intensely windy period. Huge amounts of sand blew down from highlands in the east and covered most of the Colorado Plateau. Sheer, Wingate cliffs, 300 to 400 ft (91 to 122 m) high, often impose a barrier to travel in southern Utah. Wingate walls line the mouth of Silver Falls Creek Canyon (Trip 34).

The Chinle Formation contains a variety of hues: red, brown, yellow, lavender, green, gray. It's the result of meandering streams depositing mud, silt and volcanic ash in alluvial plains. The gray layers are the ash, from eruptions in what is now Arizona. Chinle was the target formation during the 1950s uranium boom, so wherever it's widely exposed you'll likely see mining exploration roads. Chinle is visible near the White Rim Road, below Lathrop Canyon (Trip 62).

The Moenkopi Formation varies in color from nearly white, to red, to dark brown. It consists of stream-born silt deposited in tidal pools and mud flats. It creates vertical walls and steep slopes. Moenkopi is the most prevalent strata in the San Rafael Swell.

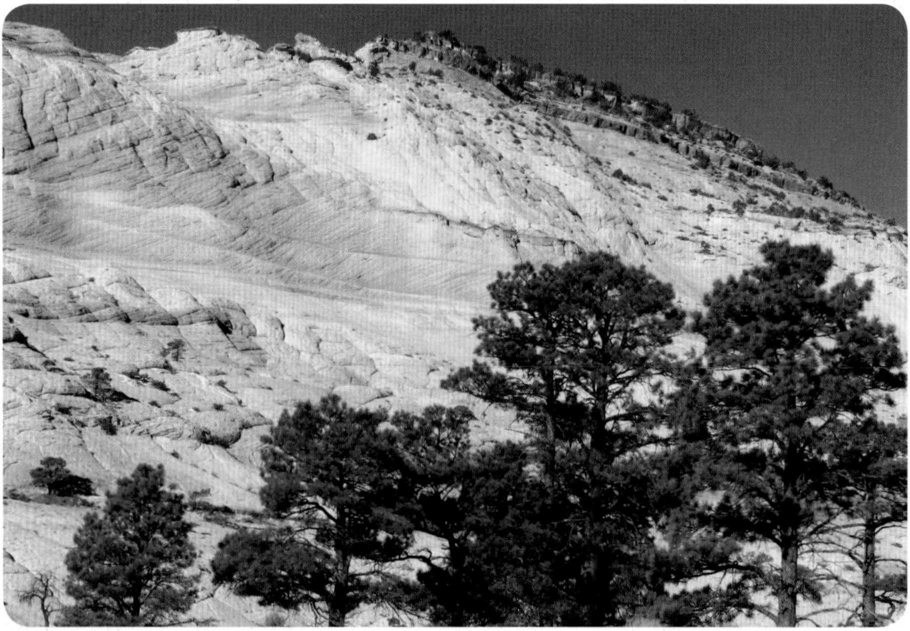

Ponderosa pines and Navajo sandstone mesa, Grand Staircase-Escalante National Monument

TOUGH HOMBRES

To survive in the Utah desert, shrubs and trees have to be tough hombres—able to withstand long periods without water, willing to split rocks with their roots in search of nutrients.

They're generally small and far apart compared to trees and shrubs in moister climes. Here, the scarcity of water limits their size and requires them to disperse. But once established, they cling obstinately to life. They're certainly hardier than most humans. Many can thrive for a century or more.

The most prolific shrubs are Mormon tea, blackbrush, rabbitbrush, saltbush, cliffrose, sage, and greasewood. Prickly-pear cactus is also common. Cottonwood and willow trees tend to grow where water is most abundant: primarily beside the watercourses on canyon and valley floors. That's also true of bamboo-like tamarisk and thorny Russian olive—aggressively invasive non-native tree species that rapidly colonize stream environments and make hiking a chore.

The predominate trees in southern Utah are piñon pine and juniper. "P-J forests," as they're known to hikers, cover millions of acres at elevations between 4,500 ft (1372 m) and 6,500 ft (1981 m).

Piñons have crooked trunks, reddish bark, and grow very slowly. A 10-ft (3-m) specimen with a 4- to 6-in (10- to 15-cm) diameter trunk might be 80 to 100 years old. Their extensive root systems mirror the size of the above-ground tree. They produce compact cones bearing tasty pinenuts, which were a vital source of protein for Natives.

Junipers are the archetypal Utah desert tree. Their gnarled, twisting branches artfully illustrate the grasping, painful effort necessary to persevere in an inhospitable environment. During a drought, junipers will prevent fluids from flowing to their peripheral branches in order to live, hence their "half flourishing, half dead" appearance. Scale-covered leaves and bluish, waxy-coated seeds help the tree conserve moisture.

Above 5700 ft (1737 m), ponderosa pines are a stately reminder that while the Colorado Plateau is mostly desert, it's higher than many mountains. Pondies are native to western North America, reach 130 ft (40 m) tall, have girthy, reddish-hued bark, and smell faintly of vanilla.

RODENTVILLE

Knowing the facts, you might think the desert itself is a mirage. How could a couple hundred species of bird, 65 species of mammal, two dozen species of reptile, nearly a dozen species of amphibian, and eight species of—get this—fish (!) exist in such a desiccated, rock-hard land? Well, they do. So rub your eyes, shake your head, look again.

Specifically, look up. Birds are the most frequently visible canyon-country creatures. Even on the hottest summer days, turkey vultures and white-throated swifts circle above. In riparian corridors, particularly along the Colorado River, birdsong is audible most mornings. The musicians include blue grosbeaks, yellow-breasted chats, spotted towhees, and canyon wrens. Great blue herons hunt the shallows for fish. Cooper's hawks flit through the dense riverside brush.

Say's phoebes, black-throated sparrows, and western meadowlarks inhabit the desert grasslands. Piñon jays, scrub jays, juniper titmice, black-throated gray warblers, and owls frequent the P-J woodlands. And it's possible to see hawks, eagles and ravens almost anywhere.

Members of the crow family, ravens are jet black, intelligent, able to solve problems, playful, and communicative. No wonder they're prescient beings in Native folklore.

As for mammals, the desert favors small ones. Diminutive size is an adaptation to the harsh environment. Smaller creatures can find shelter easier and need less water and food. So southern Utah is Rodentville. Mice and rats thrive here.

Among the most interesting desert rodents is the tiny kangaroo rat, which produces its own water by metabolizing plant matter—its only food source. It spends hot

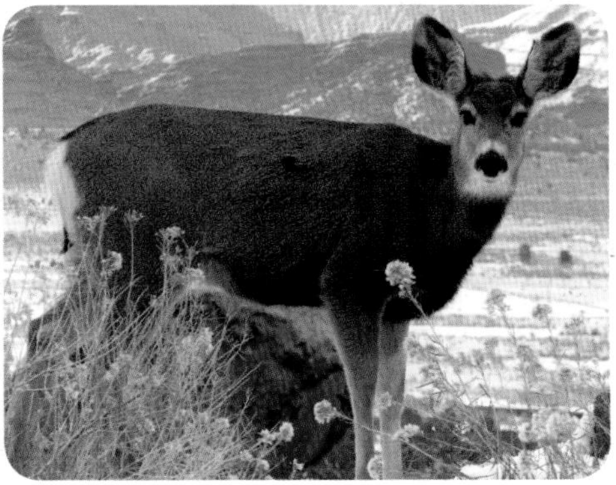

Mule deer

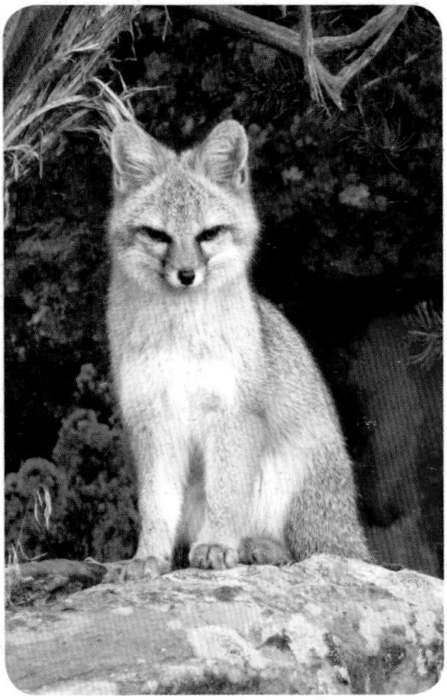

Kit fox

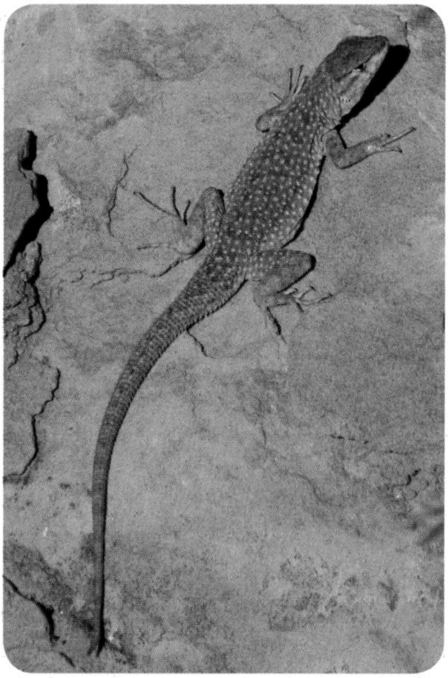
Lizard

days sleeping in a cool burrow and might even plug the opening with dirt or debris for added insulation.

Because "rodent" has negative connotations, most people don't realize squirrels, chipmunks, porcupines and beaver are rodents too. All live in southern Utah. So do skunks, which, despite their vaguely rodent-like appearance, are omnivores that help keep the desert rodent population in check. Bats are also common here but are not, as some people assume, "flying rodents." We once saw thousands of bats swoop en masse out of a crack in a canyon wall.

Other desert animals—many of which are "crepuscular" (most active at dawn and dusk) or strictly nocturnal—include cottontails, black-tailed jackrabbits, foxes, bobcats, mule deer, bighorn sheep, and mountain lions. It's rare for people to see a big cat. If you're lucky, you might see a paw print. But should you glimpse a herd of mule deer, you'll know a mountain lion is probably nearby, because deer are their primary food source.

Though coyotes range throughout Central and North America, from Panama to Alaska, they're a classic desert animal. They tend to be nocturnal or crepuscular yet can also be "diurnal" (active by day) when necessary. They're omnivorous, but their chief food in southern Utah is—hurray!—rodents.

Coyotes are wily, brave opportunists and masters of adaptability. You're as likely to see one trotting across Center Street in Moab as you are in a lonely canyon. Hearing their call-and-response yipping and howling in the desert night is a thrill. Like the raven, the coyote figures prominently in Native folklore. He's the "trickster" who scandalizes, disgusts, amuses, disrupts, chastises, or humiliates.

Reptiles, however, are the iconic desert creatures. Chances are good you'll encounter a western whiptail lizard (with a tail twice as long as its body) basking in the sun on a boulder. Or you might cross paths with a western collared lizard: bright green with a distinctive, dapper, black collar.

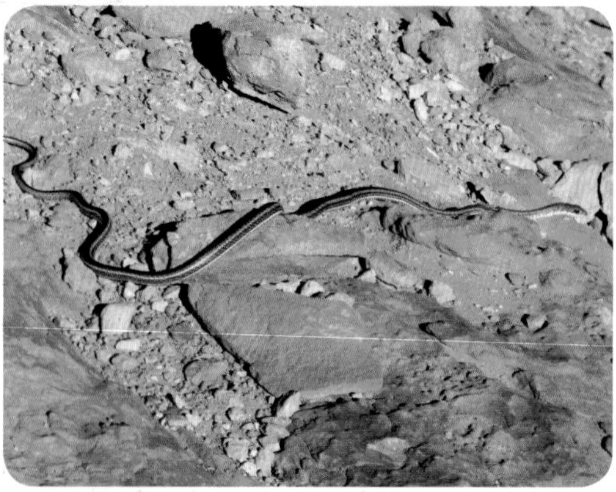
In canyon country, snakes are rare and most, like this garter snake, are harmless.

Though "desert = snakes" in most people's minds, snakes are nocturnal and therefore rarely seen. People also assume snakes are dangerous, yet most are harmless. All will escape from human confrontation given the opportunity.

A few snakes in southern Utah, of course, are venomous, for example the midget-faded rattlesnake. So are scorpions and black-widow spiders. But because they hunt only at night and will have knocked off work and be kicking back in rock crevices or under ledges during the hours you'll likely be hiking, they pose little threat. Just watch where you step, and never put your hand on a surface you can't see.

Snakes and lizards power-down to a state of torpor during the winter, are active during the day in late spring and early fall, and are crepuscular during summer. Lizards store fat in their tails—for nourishment while they're sedentary in winter. So losing a tail, even though it can grow back, is a life-threatening crisis for a lizard.

If lizards and snakes, with their scaley skin and beady eyes, make you uneasy, remember: they're on your side with regard to controlling the desert rodent population.

IT'S ALIVE!

Southern Utah's vast tracts of slickrock invite you to hike off trail, wander freely, explore at will. And as long as it's *rock* that's under foot, you can go wherever you want, as far as you like, limited only by your instinct for self preservation. But when hiking on other surfaces, there's more at stake than your own enjoyment and safety; there's the wellbeing of the desert ecosystem.

Nearly 75% of the Colorado Plateau's surface area is alive. It's covered by organisms that, though lowly in stature and humble in appearance, are critical to the survival of other desert flora, which in turn are vital to all desert fauna. These organisms are collectively known as *biological soil crust*.

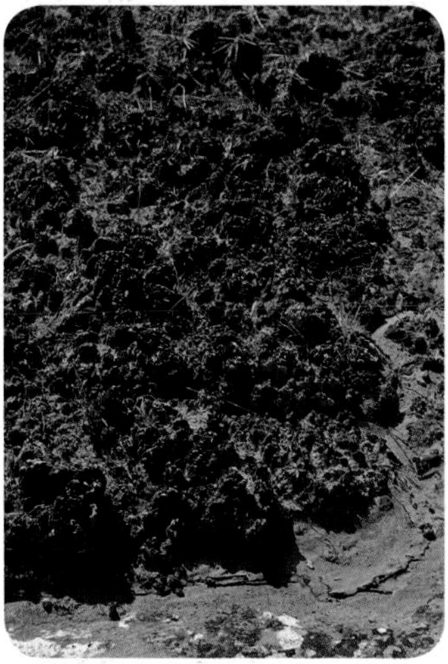

Cryptogamic soil

They're also called *microphytic, microbiotic, cryptobiotic,* or *cryptogamic soil*. The most inclusive term is probably biocrust, which distinguishes it from physical or chemical crusts while not limiting the crust components to plants. But *cryptogam* is the name you'll hear most often. To keep it simple, we'll just call it *crypto*.

Crypto comprises cyanobacteria, algae, mosses, lichens, liverworts, and fungi. On the Colorado Plateau, mature crypto is usually darker than the surrounding soil, often appears black, and can be 4 inches (10 cm) thick.

Crypto stabilizes sand and dirt, prevents erosion by water or wind, promotes moisture retention, and feeds nutrients to nearby vegetation. It even captures nitrogen from the air, converts it to a form necessary for plant growth, and assimilates it into the soil.

When wet, crypto swells and spreads, gradually creating a complex, protective, nurturing layer over the otherwise very vulnerable surface of the surrounding terrain. Without crypto, the desert would be less hospitable than it already is. Yet crypto itself is quite vulnerable. It's instantly pulverized by an errant hiker, mountain biker, or 4WD vehicle.

Each time your boot lands on a patch of crypto—crunch, crunch, crunch—you destroy it and thus jeopardize every living thing in the vicinity, all of which contribute to the beauty you came here to witness.

Crust trampled to dust can take up to 250 years to fully regenerate. Meanwhile, water runoff increases by up to 50% (think *flashflood*), soil loss increases by up to 600% (think *duststorm*), and windblown sand kills yet more crypto by burying it and preventing photosynthesis (think *Boston Strangler*).

Freeze! Step away from the crust!

Whenever you're not hiking on slickrock or established trail, be alert for crypto. Avoid it diligently. Go around. Rockhop. Opt for gravel or sand. Follow drainage paths (rivulets, washes) where crypto doesn't grow. If hiking with kids, summarize your crypto explanation with a rule they'll easily remember: "Don't bust the crust."

Stepping on a tuft of grass is preferable to stepping on crypto, because the grass will survive and rebound, the crypto won't. If you absolutely must walk on crypto, imagine it's your mother's grave. Get off asap. Minimize damage by telling companions to follow your precise steps, so your group doesn't rampage a broad swath.

WILDERNESS ETHICS

We hope you're already conscientious about respecting nature and other people. If not, here's how to pay off some of your karmic debt load.

Let wildflowers live. They blossom for only a few fleeting weeks. Uprooting them doesn't enhance your enjoyment, and it prevents others from seeing them at all. We once heard parents urge a string of children to pick as many different-coloured flowers as they could find. Great. Teach kids to entertain themselves by destroying nature, so the world continues marching toward environmental collapse.

Stay on the trail. Shortcutting causes erosion. It doesn't save time on steep ascents, because you'll soon be slowing to catch your breath. On a steep descent, it increases the likelihood of injury. When hiking cross-country in a group, soften your impact by spreading out.

Leave no trace. Be aware of your impact. Travel lightly on the land. At campgrounds, limit your activity to areas already denuded. After a rest stop, and especially after camping, take a few minutes to look for and obscure any evidence of your stay. Restore the area to its natural state. Remember: tents can leave scars. Pitch yours on an existing tentsite whenever possible. If none is available, choose a patch of dirt, sand, or slickrock.

Avoid building fires. Prohibited in many backcountry areas, they're extremely risky amid dry, desert foliage. We've seen canyons (Grand Gulch and Mill Creek, for example) where idiots burning their toilet paper set entire cottonwood groves ablaze. The blackened tree trunks and scorched earth remain an eyesore for decades. Don't risk it. Matches are for lighting your ultralight camp stove, nothing else.

Be quiet at backcountry campsites. Most of us come to canyon country in search of tranquility. If you want to party, go to a bar. Canyons, slickrock, and particularly alcoves magnify and project sound. So be quieter than you think necessary. There's no other tent in sight? Doesn't matter. Other campers still might be within earshot. And they'll rightfully be angry if your raucous banter is shattering the silence they came to enjoy.

Pack out everything you bring. Never leave a scrap of trash anywhere. This includes toilet paper, nut shells, and cigarette butts. Fruit peels are also trash. They take years to decompose, and wild animals won't eat them. And don't just pack out *your* trash. Leave nothing behind, whether you brought it or not. Keep a small plastic bag handy, so picking up trash is easy.

Poop without impact. Use the outhouses at trailheads and campgrounds whenever possible. Don't count on them being stocked with toilet paper; always pack your own in a plastic bag. If you know there's a campground ahead, try to wait until you get there.

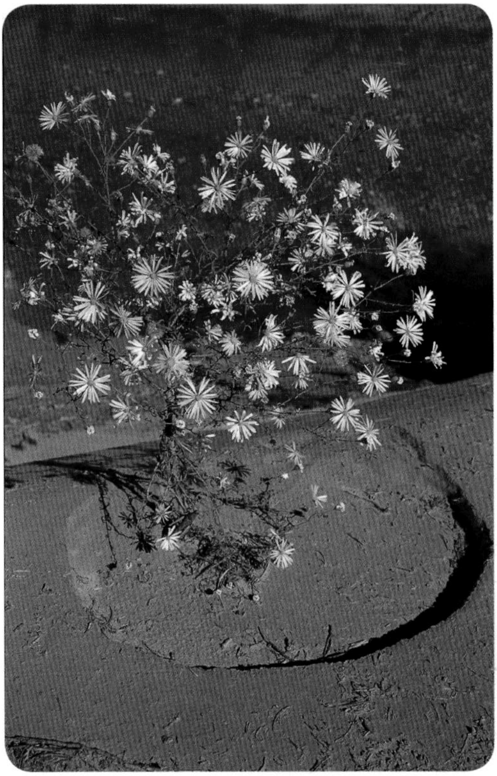

Utah daisy

In the wilds, choose a site at least 66 yd (60 m) from trails and water sources. Ground that receives sunlight part of the day is best. Use a trowel to dig a small cat-hole—4 to 8 inches (10 to 20 cm) deep, 4 to 6 inches (10 to 15 cm) wide—in soft, dark, biologically active soil. Afterward, throw a handful of dirt into the hole, stir with a stick to speed decomposition, replace your diggings, then camouflage the site. Pack out used toilet paper in a plastic bag. You can drop the paper (not the plastic) in the next outhouse you pass. Always clean your hands with a moisturizing hand sanitizer, like Purell. Sold in drugstores, it comes in conveniently small, lightweight, plastic bottles.

Urinate off trail, well away from water sources. The salt in urine attracts animals. They'll defoliate urine-soaked vegetation, so aim for sand.

Respect the reverie of other hikers. On busy trails, don't feel it's necessary to communicate with everyone you pass. Most of us are seeking solitude, not a soiree. A smile and a nod are sufficient to convey good will. Obviously, only you can judge what's appropriate at the time. But it's usually presumptuous and annoying to blurt out advice without being asked. "Boy, have you got a long way to go." "The views are much better up there." "Be careful, it gets rougher." If anyone wants to know, they'll ask. Some people are sly. They start by asking where you're going, so they can tell you all about it. Offer unsolicited information only to warn other hikers about conditions ahead that could seriously affect their trip.

HIKING WITH YOUR DOG

"Can I bring Max, my Pomeranian?" The answer depends on which trail you intend to hike.

Regulations vary widely throughout canyon country and continue to evolve. A few examples:

• In Arches, Canyonlands, Capitol Reef, Bryce Canyon, and Zion national parks, dogs are prohibited in the backcountry.

• Leashed dogs are generally allowed in Glen Canyon NRA backcountry, but dogs were banned from Coyote Gulch years ago.

• The BLM currently allows leashed dogs in most Cedar Mesa canyons but imposes a long list of restrictions and, due to numerous complaints, might ban dogs altogether.

So ask the appropriate land-management authorities about their current, specific policies regarding dogs.

Bringing your dog hiking with you, however, isn't simply a matter of "Can I or can't I?" The larger question is "Should I or shouldn't I?"

The desert is even less accommodating of dogs than it is of people. Paws are quickly abraded by slickrock and burned in scorching-hot sand. A dog's nose is vulnerable to prickly, thorny vegetation. Dogs are very susceptible to overheating and dehydration. Leave your dog in your car, and it could die surprisingly fast.

Most humane dog owners agree: do not take your dog hiking in canyon country. If you're traveling with a dog, leave it at a kennel before you drive to the trailhead.

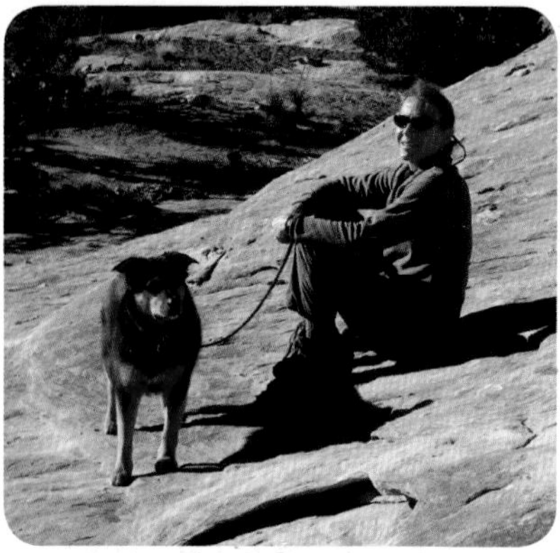

If you insist that your dog accompany you on the trail, keep it leashed at all times—for its own safety, out of respect for your fellow hikers, and to ensure your dog doesn't trample the fragile, biological soil crust.

Put protective booties on your dog's feet. Carry tweezers so you can remove spines and needles from its paws and nose. Carry lots of extra water and—so it doesn't go to waste—a bowl for your dog to drink from.

MAPS

The maps we created and that accompany each trip in this book are for general orientation only. Our *On Foot* directions are elaborate and precise—written in a way that should help you visualize the terrain without referring to a topo map.

There are many reasons, however, why you should carry a topo map. It's a safety measure. It will make it easier for you to follow our directions, particularly on a long, rough hike. And it will sharpen your ability to interpret complex canyon-country terrain, thus ensuring a richer experience. Arriving at a revelatory viewpoint is a lot more fun when you can identify what you're marveling at.

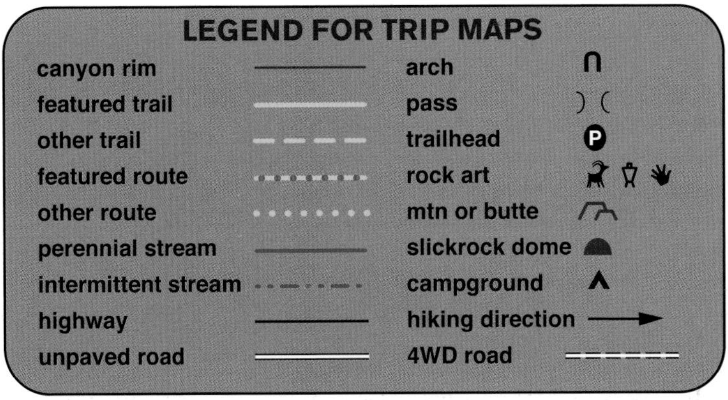
LEGEND FOR TRIP MAPS
canyon rim
featured trail
other trail
featured route
other route
perennial stream
intermittent stream
highway
unpaved road
arch
pass
trailhead
rock art
mtn or butte
slickrock dome
campground
hiking direction
4WD road

The stats box for each trip indicates which topo map to bring. The optimal maps are the 1:24 000 USGS topos, because they're highly detailed. But always having the correct one on hand is inconvenient, expensive, and therefore unlikely. So it's wise to purchase the Trails Illustrated or Latitude 40 maps. They sacrifice detail for broader coverage, but they depict numerous trails, which means you'll get your money's worth by using them repeatedly. They also contain more up-to-date information.

The USGS topos are sold at most BLM offices. Visit www.maps.nationalgeographic.com to purchase Trails Illustrated maps online. Visit www.latitude40maps.com for details about ordering Latitude 40 maps by mail. Trails Illustrated and Latitude 40 maps are also widely available in Utah outdoor shops.

CARRY A COMPASS

Left and *right* are relative. Any hiking guidebook relying solely on these inadequate and potentially misleading terms should be shredded and dropped into a recycling bin.

You'll find all the *On Foot* descriptions in this book include frequent compass directions. That's the only way to accurately, reliably guide a hiker.

What about GPS? Compared to a compass, GPS units are heavier, bulkier, more fragile, more complex, more time consuming, occasionally foiled by vegetation or topography, dependent on batteries, and way more expensive.

Keep in mind that the compass directions provided in this book are of use only if you're carrying a compass. Granted, our route descriptions are so detailed, you'll rarely have to check your compass. But bring one anyway, just in case.

A compass is required hiking equipment—anytime, anywhere, regardless of your level of experience, or your familiarity with the terrain.

Clip a small compass to the shoulder strap of your pack, so you can glance at it quickly and easily. Even if you never have to rely on your compass, occasionally checking it will strengthen your sense of direction—an enjoyable, helpful, and conceivably lifesaving asset.

Keep in mind that our stated compass directions are always in reference to true north. In Moab, that's approximately 11° left of (counterclockwise from) magnetic north. In Torrey, that's approximately 11.5° left of (counterclockwise from) magnetic north. In Kanab, that's approximately 12° left of (counterclockwise from) magnetic north. If that puzzles you, read your compass owner's manual.

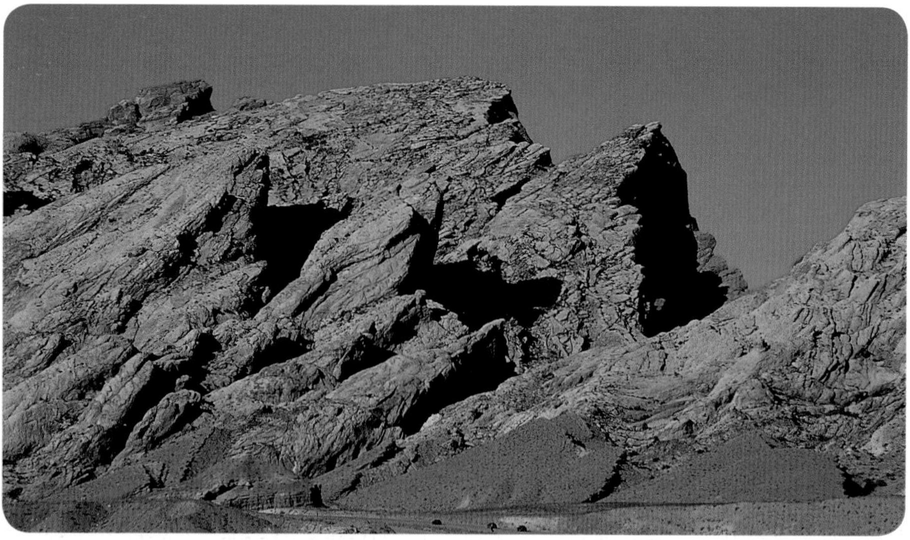

San Rafael Reef, near Spotted Wolf Canyon

PHYSICAL CAPABILITY

Until you gain experience judging your physical capability and that of your companions, these guidelines might be helpful. Anything longer than a 7-mi (11-km) round-trip dayhike can be very taxing for someone who doesn't hike regularly. A 1400-ft (425-m) elevation gain in that distance is challenging but possible for anyone in average physical condition. Very fit hikers are comfortable hiking 11 mi (18 km) and ascending 3100 ft (950 ft)—or more—in a single day.

Backpacking 11 mi (18 km) in two days is a reasonable goal for most beginners. Hikers who backpack a couple times a season can enjoyably manage 17 mi (27 km) in two days. Avid backpackers should find 24 mi (34 km) in two days no problem. On three- to five-day trips, a typical backpacker prefers not to push beyond 10 mi (16 km) a day.

Remember: it's always safer to underestimate your limits, especially in canyon country, where intense heat can be debilitating.

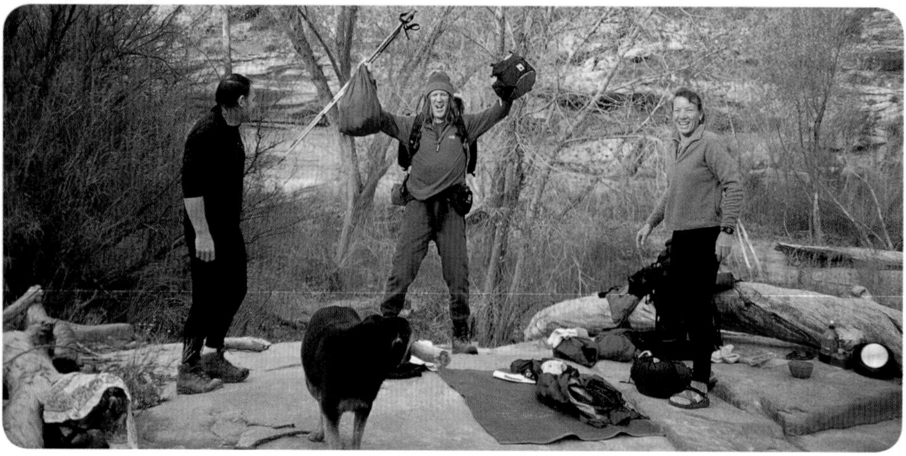

Successful hunter returns to the clan.

LEAVE YOUR ITINERARY

Even if you're hiking in a group, and especially if you're going solo, it's prudent to leave your itinerary in writing with a reliable family member or friend. Agree on precisely when they should alert the authorities if you have not returned or called. Be sure to follow through. Forgetting to tell your contact person you've safely completed your trip could result in an unnecessary, expensive search. You wouldn't want to be billed for that. Nor would you want a rescue team risking their lives, combing the wilds trying to find you, while you're actually safe, in the bosom of civilization.

CANYON-COUNTRY CLIMATE

Typically, the canyon-country climate will grant you about twelve weeks of optimal hiking-and-camping weather: mid-March through April, and mid-September through October. That's just 25% of the year. Carpe diem.

Heat? In June, July and August, hiking conditions in southern Utah range from miserable to unsafe. Intense sun exposure makes rock-walled canyons feel like ovens. Dehydration, heat exhaustion, and heatstroke are serious threats.

Rain? Afternoon thunderstorms are common during the monsoon season: mid-July through mid-September. Compare spring with fall, and you'll find it usually rains less in April than October. Remember: in canyon country, rain = flashflood danger.

Southwest Utah (Zion National Park)

Spring and fall are the ideal times to be here. Wildflowers peak in May. Autumn colors spike in late October. Winter, however, is usually mild enough for dayhiking.

During March, April, October and November, daytime highs vary from 63°to 78°F (17° to 26°C). Nighttime lows average about 45°F (4°C), except in November, when nights are much chillier.

In December and January, the daytime highs might top 50°F (10°C). Nighttime lows drop just below freezing. Trails might be icy after recent snowfall.

Northeast Utah (Canyonlands National Park)

Hiking here is usually pleasant in March, April, October and November. April and October are best for backpacking, because nighttime lows tend to stay above 40°F (4°C). In May, it gets too hot to enjoy even extended dayhikes.

In March, daytime highs average 61°F (16°C), and nighttime lows drop to freezing. In November, daytime highs average 56°F (13°C), and nighttime lows are just below freezing.

Winter can be hikeable, too, but only from mid-morning to early afternoon. Daytime highs hover around 40°F (4°C). But after 5 p.m., the temperature often plummets to 17°F (–8°C).

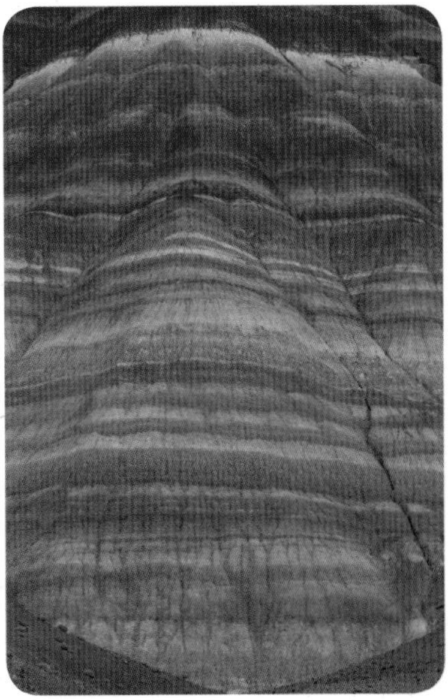

Chinle Formation

South Central Utah (Grand Staircase-Escalante National Monument)

For dayhikers, it's game on by March, when daytime highs average 55°F (13°C). The nighttime lows, however, don't stay above freezing until April, so backpackers should wait until then. In May, the daytime highs creep past 75°F (24°C) and deerflies proliferate, so hiking season wanes.

By October, the average daytime highs drop back to 67°F (19°C), and nighttime lows remain above freezing, so backpacking is again very appealing. Dayhikers will find November viable, with daytime highs averaging 53°F (12°C). But November nighttime lows averaging 24°F (–4°C) make backpacking less enjoyable.

FLASHFLOODS

A flashflood is possible any day of the year in the desert. A sudden, violent thunderstorm can—with alarming speed—send an ominous wall of water ripping through a canyon: uprooting trees, hurling boulders, sweeping hikers into a deadly maelstrom. Your chance of survival? Poor to nil.

The rain doesn't even have to fall nearby to be a threat. It's conceivable you wouldn't see the clouds, feel the rain, or hear the thunder associated with a storm that imperiled you. So always be alert for the possibility of a flashflood, regardless of how sunny it is in your immediate vicinity.

Check the weather report before hiking. Rain is likely? Alter your plans. Avoid canyons and washes, or simply don't hike. On the trail, even if the weather is fine, be observant. Watch the sky for signs of impending rain. Listen for a roar coming from up-canyon. Habitually ask yourself, "Where could I quickly escape to higher ground?"

If you're hiking in a canyon, and it starts to rain, don't continue. Assuming you'll recognize danger in time to avoid it could be your fatal mistake. Stop. Return to the trailhead. By the time you know a flashflood is imminent, you're at serious risk.

If the rain is heavy and the trailhead is too distant, seek elevation and shelter. Don't endanger yourself climbing unless you're obviously in a life-threatening

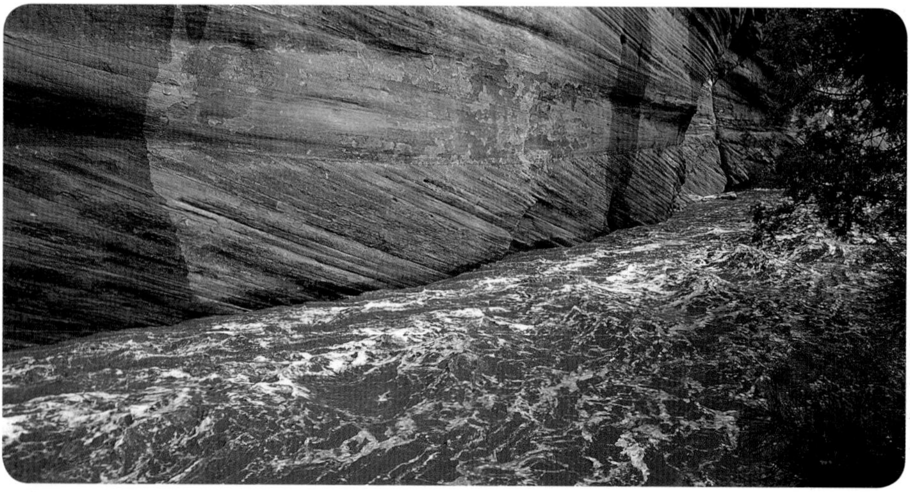

After two hours' rain, a flashflood rushes through a dry gully.

emergency. Just carefully work your way upward until you're as high above the drainage floor as you feel safe ascending.

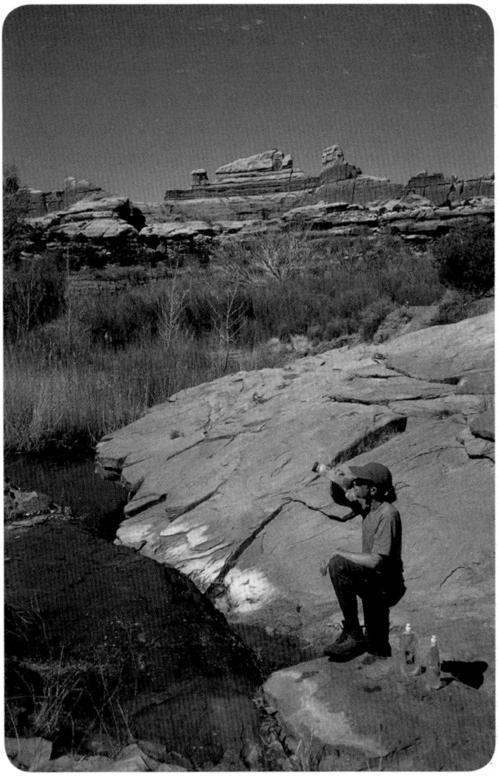
Salt Creek Canyon (Trip 71)

Try to gain about 30 to 40 ft (9 to 12 m). Ideally, find a perch beneath an overhanging ledge. But don't sacrifice elevation for shelter. Once you've reached safety, make yourself as comfortable as possible, then be patient.

Desert rainstorms, and the flashfloods they cause, tend to be shortlived. Wait until the rain stops and the water subsides before resuming your retreat to the trailhead. And don't risk getting lost by attempting an unfamiliar, cross-country return route. Stay put until you can exit via the same trail you entered.

HAVE A SWIG

Human beings are mostly water. Fully 75% of your muscles, blood and brain are H_20. In a single day, just sitting at a desk and behind the wheel of a car, you can lose up to ten cups (2.4 liters) of water.

So, thirsty or not, you must sip water frequently, especially while active, and certainly while hiking in the desert. You can be dehydrated without being thirsty. Losing a mere 2% of your body's water content will seriously impair your athletic performance. Lose 75%, and you'll collapse. In canyon country, most preventable medical emergencies are the result of dehydration.

A gallon of water is generally cited as the minimum daily requirement for a desert hiker. That's the equivalent of four, 32-ounce (one-liter) water bottles. You might need even more on a long, strenuous hike in hot weather.

Always keep a couple extra gallons of water in your vehicle while traveling in canyon country. Make sure you're fully hydrated before you depart the trailhead. Pack more water than you think you'll need for your hike.

You're dayhiking? Carry a full day's water. It will save you from searching for scarce, unreliable water sources and will prevent you from having to spend time filtering or purifying.

You're backpacking? You'll have to find water sources en route, you should top-up your supply at every opportunity, and you'll need to filter or purify whatever you consume. Carry a couple extra water bottles, or a large-but-lightweight collapsible water jug, so you can haul water from its source to your camp.

THERMONUCLEAR PROTECTION

In summer, the desert heat will bake your enchilada. So don't hike here during June, July or August. It's miserable and unsafe.

Late spring and early fall can still be hot enough to steam your tortilla, so always take these precautions:

• Pack at least two quarts (liters) of water per person on a short dayhike, and at least three per person on a long dayhike. Limit yourself to pure, fresh H_20. No pop, no juice, no alcohol. But adding electrolyte powder can help replenish what your body loses via perspiration.

• Wear sunglasses. Generously rub sunblock on all your exposed skin.

• In addition to shorts and a shortsleeve shirt, bring desert-rat clothes for when the sun is intense: a hat with a broad brim; an ultralight, longsleeve shirt; lightweight, long pants; and a bandana you can moisten and wrap around your neck.

• Be conservative when estimating the distance you intend to cover. Allow more time than you'll probably need.

• Before departing the trailhead, make sure you're completely hydrated. Leave several full water bottles in your car for a post-hike guzzle.

• Start hiking early in the morning, while it's still cool.

• Sip water throughout the day to prevent dehydration. Eat snacks frequently. Rest more often than you think necessary—in shade whenever possible. Stop for a long, relaxing, nourishing lunch.

• Pace yourself. If you feel vulnerable to the heat, shorten your hike.

Do all of the above and you'll likely experience only joy and fulfillment while hiking in the desert. But if you're able to recognize symptoms of the following ailments, and you know how to treat them, you'll be safer yet:

Heat exhaustion occurs when the body begins producing and/or absorbing more heat than it can dissipate, and when insufficient fluid intake decreases blood flow to vital organs.

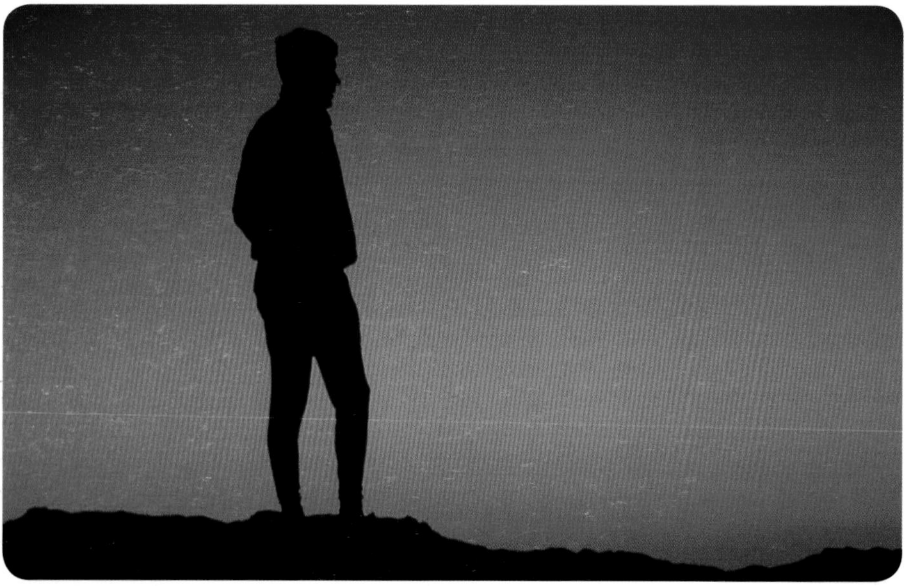

Sunrise, San Rafael Swell

initial symptoms

• no thirst • no appetite • little or no urination • cold, clammy skin

advanced symptoms

• profuse sweating • extreme fatigue • headache • loss of coordination • dizziness • fainting • nausea

treatment

• rest • drink • eat

Heatstroke (hyperthermia) is an acute form of heat exhaustion resulting from excessive exposure to extreme heat, prolonged dehydration, and dangerously elevated body temperature.

initial symptoms

• dry skin • high temperature • flushed appearance • weak, rapid pulse • erratic behavior

advanced symptoms

• headache • nausea • seizures • collapse • shock • unconsciousness

treatment

• cool the victim immediately: move him to shade, take off his excess clothing, repeatedly douse his head and torso with water, fan him to increase evaporative cooling • seek medical help asap • ideally one person should attend the victim while another initiates a rescue

Water intoxication (hyponatremia) is an abnormally low concentration of sodium in the blood caused by drinking too much water while eating little or nothing.

initial symptoms

• no thirst • no appetite • abnormally frequent, high-volume urination • clear urine

advanced symptoms

• puffy face and fingers • muscle weakness • erratic behavior • nausea • diarrhea • headache • unconsciousness

treatment

• rest • eat • swallow small amounts of electrolyte powder instead of mixing it in water • seek medical help asap

SUNDOWN

When the sun sinks in the desert, so does the temperature, perhaps by as much as 40° F (22° C). Rocks and sand don't retain heat. Neither does the dry air. Cloudless nights are especially prone to rapid cooling.

So savvy desert hikers always pack head-to-toe insulation: a fleece hat, fleece gloves, a lightweight shell, a longsleeve, midweight fleece top, and a pair of lightweight fleece tights.

In case it's necessary to hike after sundown, be sure you have a headlamp with fresh batteries. To keep yourself energized, also carry a couple extra Power Bars. Think of them as an essential item in your first-aid kit. You *do* carry a first-aid kit, right?

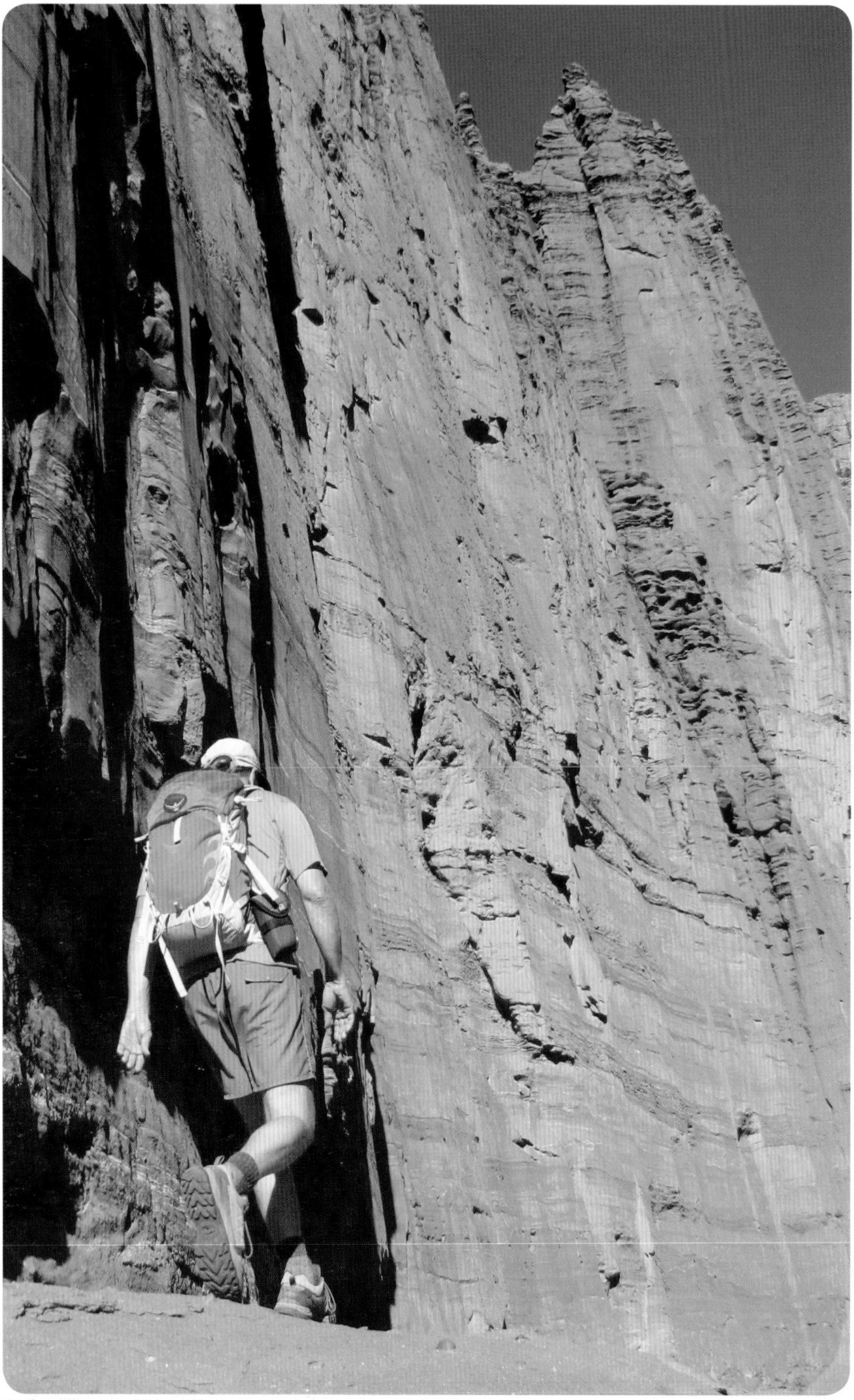

Fisher Towers (Trip 59)

WOW

THE HIKES

TRIP 1

SNOW CANYON

LOCATION	Red Cliffs Desert Reserve, northwest edge of St. George
LOOP	6 mi (9.7 km)
ELEVATION GAIN	460 ft (140 m)
KEY ELEVATIONS	trailhead 3200 ft (995 m), highpoint 3560 ft (1085 m)
HIKING TIME	3 to 4 hours
DIFFICULTY	easy
MAP	Snow Canyon State Park brochure (free, available at entry station)

OPINION

Camping is beautiful.

Travelers, strangers in a strange land, arrive from disparate paths. Seeking peace and security in the wilderness, they circle their tents, create an enclave, establish a temporary, unspoken, but genuine bond.

Whatever threat was overcome en route is forgotten. Whatever creature lurks nearby is held at bay by the glow of the campfire. Whatever future awaits beyond that night is safely distant.

It's a ritual as old as humanity. Yet one we can, in the right setting, repeat today and experience the emotions our nomadic forebears must have felt when, in ancient times, they made camp during their annual migrations.

You'll find such a setting just outside St. George, Utah, in Snow Canyon State Park. Though the city is frenetic, the park is secluded, tranquil, spacious, scenic. And the campground, despite urban amenities and penitentiary regimentation, feels like a haven. It's as frontcountry as they get, but even devoted backcountry campers love it.

Many of the campsites are beside soaring, rock walls. Most afford generous privacy. All are within a pebble's toss of a premier hiking trail. Actually it's a network of trails. Link them, and you'll stride through superlative canyon country for up to five hours.

Snow Canyon is where the Mojave and Great Basin deserts meet the Colorado Plateau. The predominant rock, Navajo sandstone, is the color of late-autumn leaves. The year-round residents include coyotes, kit foxes, quail, roadrunners, leopard lizards, gopher snakes, canyon tree-frogs, peregrine falcons, desert tortoises, and gila monsters, as well as creosote, yucca, sage, blackbrush, scrub oak, and desert willow. If conditions are right, Snow Canyon's spring wildflower bloom can be rainbowesque.

Perhaps you're wondering, does it snow here? Rarely. The canyon's name honors two esteemed Mormon leaders: Erastus Snow, a member of the Quorum of the Twelve Apostles, and Lorenzo Snow, the fifth president of the LDS Church. The Snow men, along with William J. Flake, are also immortalized in the name of a town: Snowflake, Arizona.

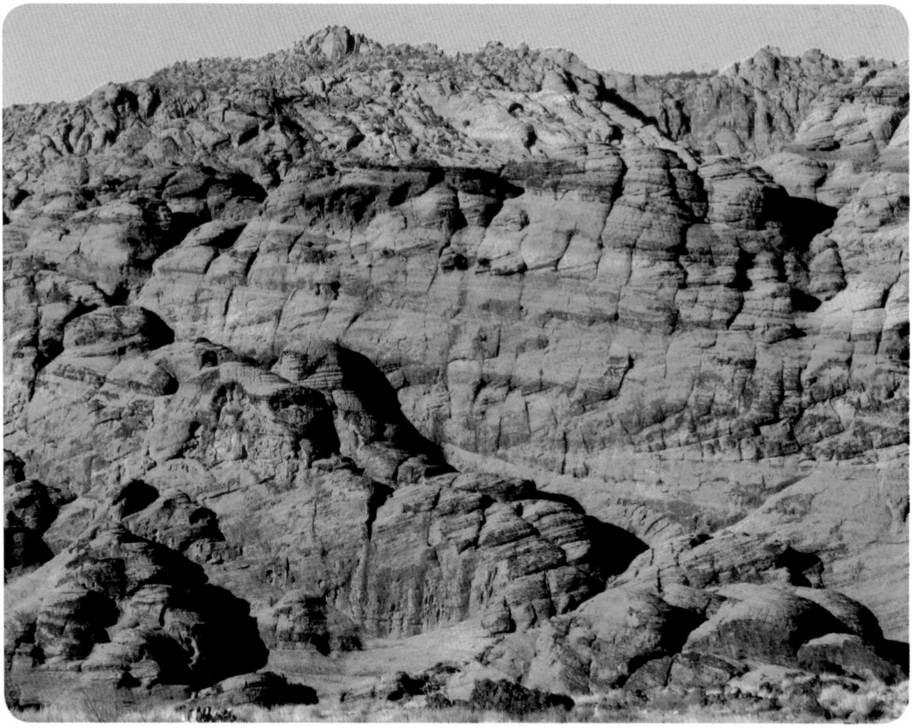

Red Cliffs Desert Reserve, from Snow Canyon

FACT

BY VEHICLE

From I-15 in St. George, take exit 6 for Hwy 18 (Bluff Street). Follow it north-northwest 5 mi (8.1 km). Turn left (west) onto Snow Canyon Parkway. Drive northwest another 3.5 mi (5.6 km). Turn right (north) onto Snow Canyon Drive. Continue past the park entry gate to the info center and campground. Elevation: 3200 ft (995 m).

ON FOOT

From the info center at the campground, go directly west to the Snow Canyon Drive pedestrian crossing. The **Hidden Piñon (HP) trail** starts on the far (west) side of the road. Follow it west-northwest toward Red Rock Mtn.

In less than a minute, go right (north) onto the paved Whiptail trail. About 30 yd/m farther, turn left onto the sandy HP trail, which is also signed for the Three Ponds (TP) trail.

The trail crosses slickrock outcroppings. Five minutes along reach a junction at 3296 ft (1005 m). Right (north) is the TP trail. Go left (northwest) to continue on the HP trail.

About ten minutes farther attain a view west to the high, sheer wall of Snow Canyon. The unpaved West Canyon Road (no public vehicle access) is visible on the canyon floor. It probes the canyon's upper reaches.

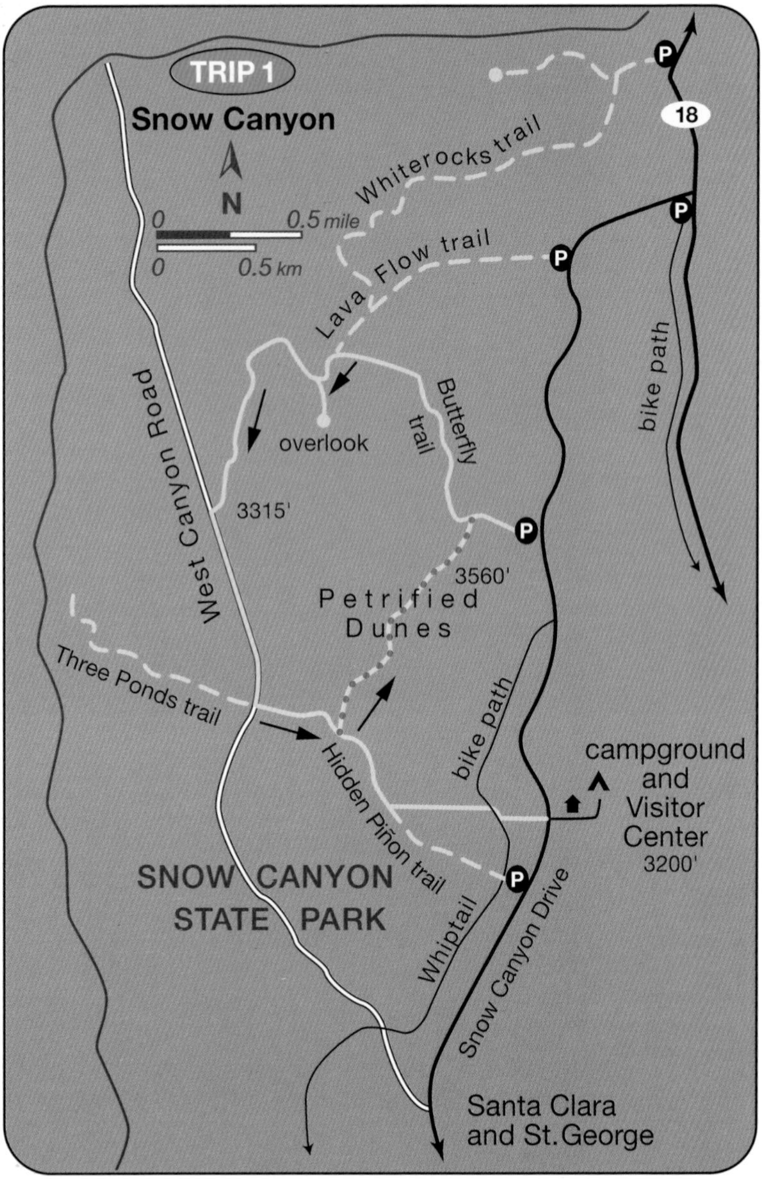

About 20 minutes along, after gentle ups and downs, reach a junction. Right (east-southeast) is another arm of the HP trail. Go left (northeast) for HP Overlook and the TP trail.

When the HP trail rejoins the TP trail, go left. One minute farther, reach a junction at 1 mi (1.6 km). Go left (southwest) and ascend the short spur to **HP Overlook**.

Upon returning to the 1-mi (1.6-km) junction, do not descend straight (northwest) on the TP trail. Instead, go right (north-northeast) and begin a 20-minute cross-country traverse of the **Petrified Dunes**—an inviting expanse of slickrock.

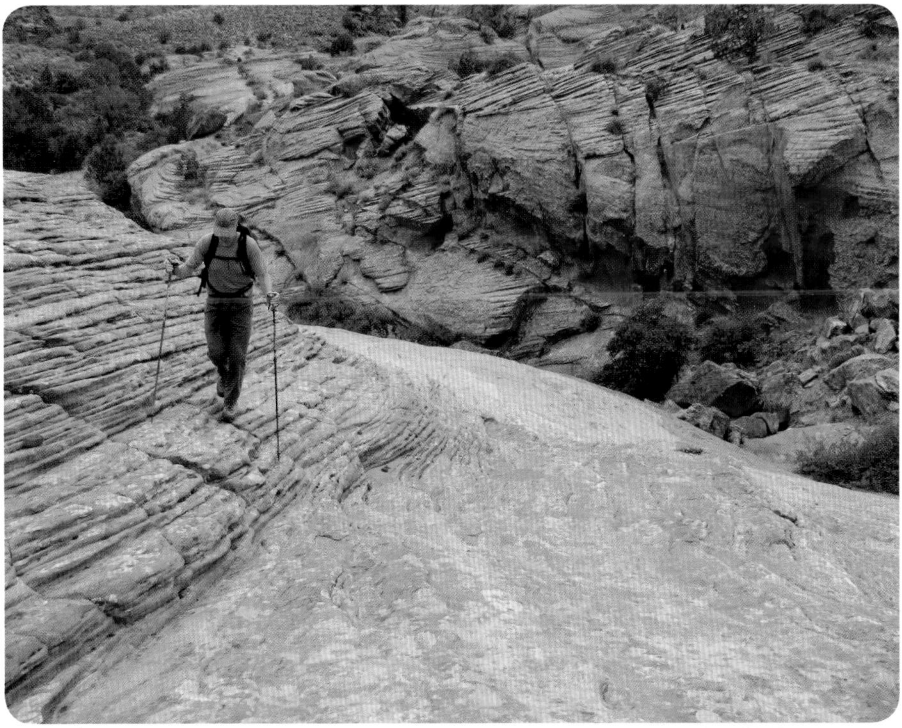

Snow Canyon slickrock near Petrified Dunes

After a short level stretch, favor the right side (next to the brushy desert floor). Bear right (east) along the edge of the slickrock (near the juniper trees), then drop into the sandy wash. Follow it north to the high, broad, slickrock mound with a swirly, terraced surface.

Heading north-northeast, work your way over the mound. Within ten minutes, top out at 3560 ft (1085 m). The view includes the campground. Descend left (west) off the mound. Scan ahead and below for the Butterfly trail running east-west through the vegetation and lava. A long finger of slickrock leads toward it.

Having hiked about 2 mi (3.2 km), intersect the **Butterfly trail** at 3485 ft (1063 m). It's sandy, lined with black, volcanic rocks. Right (east) quickly returns to Snow Canyon Drive. Go left (west).

Follow the trail north, descending on cross-hatched slickrock. After hiking the Butterfly trail for about ten minutes, intersect the **Lava Flow trail** at 3542 ft (1080 m). Right leads generally northeast to Snow Canyon Drive. Go left (southwest).

In about 50 yd/m, a short, left spur ascends south to **West Canyon Overlook**. Bear right (west) and descend past tough-spined, dark-green Mormon Tea bushes into broad West Canyon. Near the top of the descent, a sandy, right (north) spur leads to a slickrock viewpoint.

Resuming your descent on the main trail, reach the canyon floor and intersect **West Canyon Road** at 3.75 mi (6 km), 3315 ft (1011 m). Right (north) heads up canyon. Go left (south) on the unpaved road.

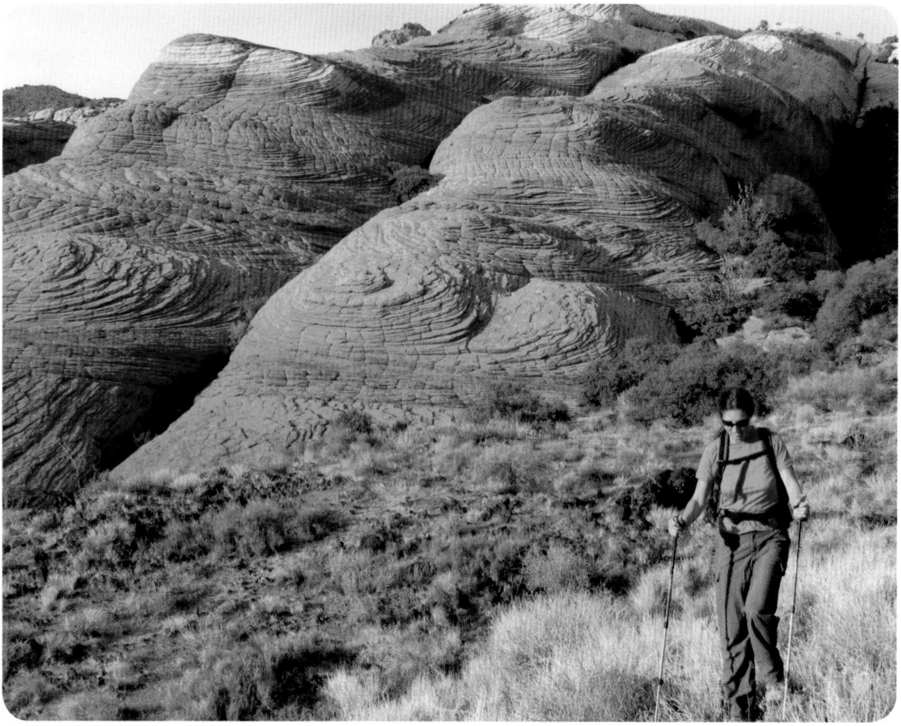

Butterfly trail, Snow Canyon

Pass a utility box on the right, an outhouse on the left, then an abandoned road on the left, all within 15 minutes. The road then intersects the TP trail. Right (west) approaches the canyon wall. The road continues straight (south). Turn left (east) onto the TP trail.

Quickly arrive at a wash. Go right, follow the wash for about 10 yd/m, then ascend left onto slickrock. About ten minutes farther, at 5 mi (8.1 km), 3345 ft (1020 m), reach the junction where you began hiking cross-country over the Petrified Dunes. You've completed a circuit and are now on **familiar terrain**.

To return to the campground, go straight (east-southeast) on the HP trail. In two minutes turn left (east-southeast) at the next junction. The campground is soon visible. Continue on the paved Whiptail trail, then turn left. Reach the **campground** a minute farther at 6 mi (9.7 km).

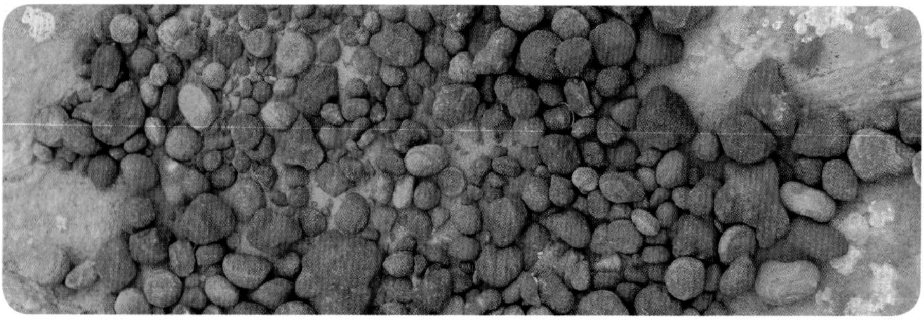

TRIP 2

HOP VALLEY / LA VERKIN CREEK / BEARTRAP CANYON / KOLOB ARCH

LOCATION	Zion National Park, Kolob Canyons section
DISTANCE	13 mi (21 km) one way plus 4 mi (6.4 km) round trip to Beartrap canyon plus 1.2 mi (1.9 km) round trip to Kolob Arch
ELEVATION GAIN	1030 ft (314 m) for one-way trip plus 510 ft (155 m) for Beartrap detour
ELEVATION LOSS	1320 ft (402 m) for one-way trip plus 510 ft (155 m) for Beartrap detour
KEY ELEVATIONS	Hop Valley trailhead 6370 ft (1942 m) Hop Valley / La Verkin junction 5346 ft (1630 m) La Verkin Creek canyon lowpoint 5050 ft (1540 m) Beartrap canyon 5760 ft (1756 m) Lee Pass trailhead 6080 ft (1854 m)
HIKING TIME	9 hours or more
DIFFICULTY	challenging dayhike, easy backpack
MAP	Trails Illustrated *Zion National Park*

OPINION

Look for smudges. That's where the earth gets interesting.

On a topo map, smudges are where the contour lines are so near one another there's no visible distance between them. Since the closer the lines the more vertical the land, smudges are your assurance of sheer canyon walls or steep mountainsides, i.e. spectacular scenery.

Look at a topo map of Zion National Park, and you'll see lots of thick, dark smudges, radiating outward like shock waves. The epicenter of this topographical eruption is Zion Canyon, in the park's south-central region. Beyond, the smudges tend to decrease in size, intensity and concentration.

But notice the cluster of smudges in the upper-left (northwest) corner of the map. See the long trail, resembling a fracture line, slicing through them? It poses an exhilarating challenge to strong, skilled hikers: a one-day, one-way traverse of Zion Park's *Kolob Canyons section.*

Ideally, set out very early from the Hop Valley trailhead, head down-valley to La Verkin Creek canyon, detour upstream to quickly probe Beartrap canyon, then head back downstream, detour north for a peek at Kolob Arch, and finally hightail it out to the Lee Pass trailhead.

The total distance is… got a Power Gel handy?…18.2 mi (29.3 km). Yet the total elevation gain is only 1540 ft (469 m)—surprisingly merciful. So the one-way dayhike is viable for athletic striders who know from experience what a

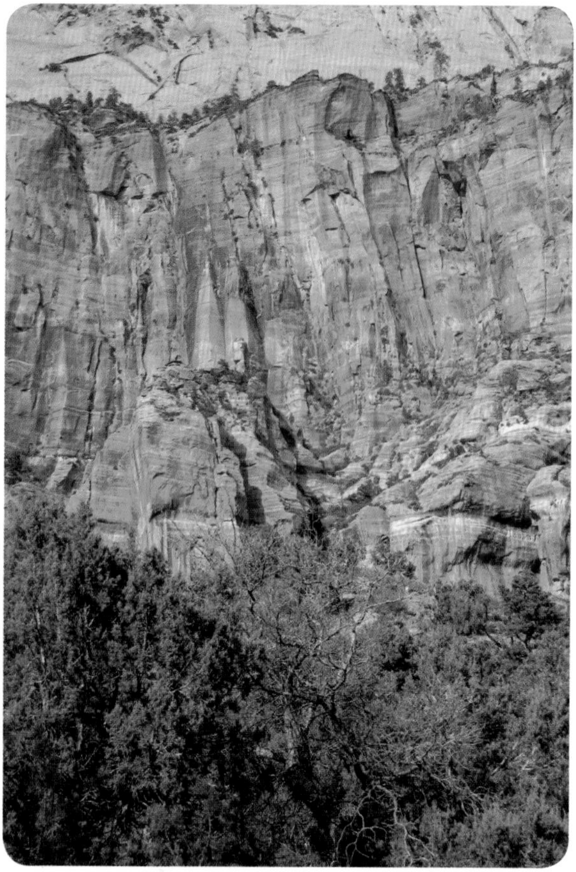
La Verkin Creek Canyon, west of Hop Valley

backcountry epic entails, and how to save their own butts if something goes wrong.

What you'll see during that nine or more hours of trekking is certainly worth the effort. After an unpromising start, the Hop Valley trail is soon intriguing. La Verkin Creek canyon—a hefty smudge on the topo map—has Navajo sandstone walls comparable to those in Zion Canyon. The creek itself is a light, playful companion. Beartrap canyon is a deep, dark, seductive slot. And Kolob Arch—spanning the length of a football field—is the second-longest natural arch in the world.

The longest is Landscape Arch (Trip 47) in Arches National Park. The two arches are so close in length, however, that ranking them is absurd. It's their appearance that distinguishes them. Landscape is so impossibly slender it looks like it will collapse any minute. Kolob, just as its name sounds, is a thick, muscular brute. You can imagine an alien monster grabbing hold of Kolob to fling our planet farther into outer space.

Don't think you can muster the entire through hike in a single day? Shorten it. Eliminate one of the detours: Beartrap or Kolob. We recommend skipping Kolob in favor of Beartrap. Not only is Beartrap itself stirring, but en route you'll probe the upper, narrower reaches of La Verkin Creek canyon, where the trail insists you get intimate with the creek by crossing it frequently.

The one-way dayhike is still too long for you? Skip both the detours. That whittles it down to 13 mi (21 km), with an elevation gain of just 1030 ft (314 m). It's still a beautiful journey and a great accomplishment.

If even the abbreviated one-way trip is more than you can hike in a day (congratulations for acknowledging your limitations), then don't dayhike. A round-trip dayhike starting at either trailhead would be monotonous, denying you sufficient scenic reward yet requiring you to hike virtually the same distance as the one-way dayhike. Instead, make this a one- or two-night backpack trip.

In lower Hop Valley, you can pitch your tent beneath impressive cliffs, among Ponderosa pines. The creekside campsites in La Verkin canyon are idyllic.

Backpacking might also allow you to explore beyond Beartrap, perhaps into Willis Creek canyon. You'll forego the thrill of a high-speed assault, but you'll have time for greater depth of appreciation.

Whether dayhiking or backpacking, follow our directions from south (Hop Valley) to north (Lee Pass). You'll gain less elevation, and the scenery improves in that direction. Entering via Hop Valley will slowly pique your interest, but exiting that way would be tedious and anticlimactic.

And now, the answer to a question most of us would never think to ask. What does the name *La Verkin* mean? It's an anglo derivative of the Spanish *la virgen*. Therefore the centerpiece of this hike is the Virgin Creek, whereas Zion Canyon is cleaved by the Virgin River.

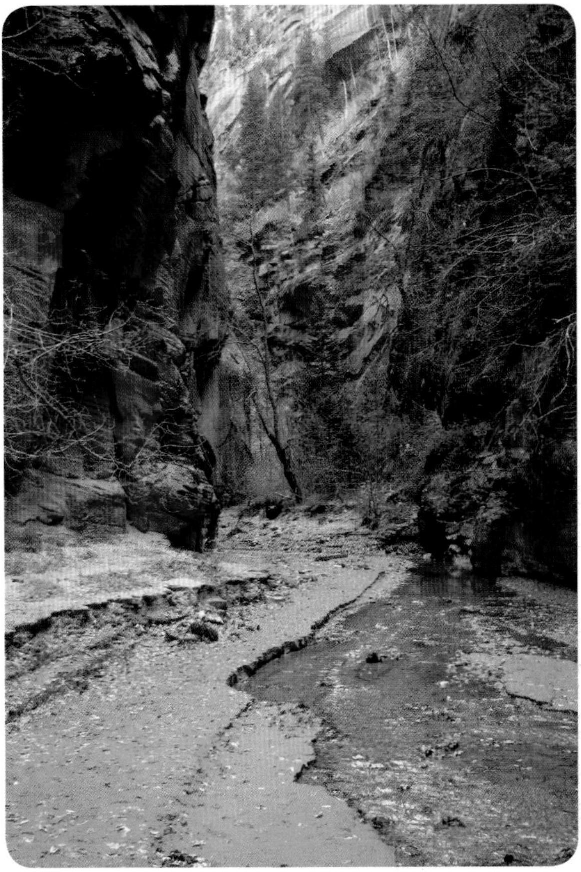

Beartrap Canyon

FACT

BEFORE YOUR TRIP

If you're backpacking, you must get a backcountry camping permit in person at the Zion Canyon visitor center in Springdale, or the Kolob Canyons visitor center en route to Lee Pass trailhead (see *Information Sources*). For permit details, visit www.nps.gov/zion, click on "Backcountry Information," then click on and read "Reservations and Permits" and "Other Backcountry Reservations."

If you want to hike one-way but lack a shuttle slave or compadres with a second vehicle, make arrangements with the Zion Canyon Transportation Company in Springdale (435-635-5993).

BY VEHICLE

Lee Pass trailhead

From Cedar City, drive Interstate 15 south 18 mi (29 km) to Exit 40. Or, from the Hwy 17 junction, drive Interstate 15 north 13 mi (21 km) to Exit 40.

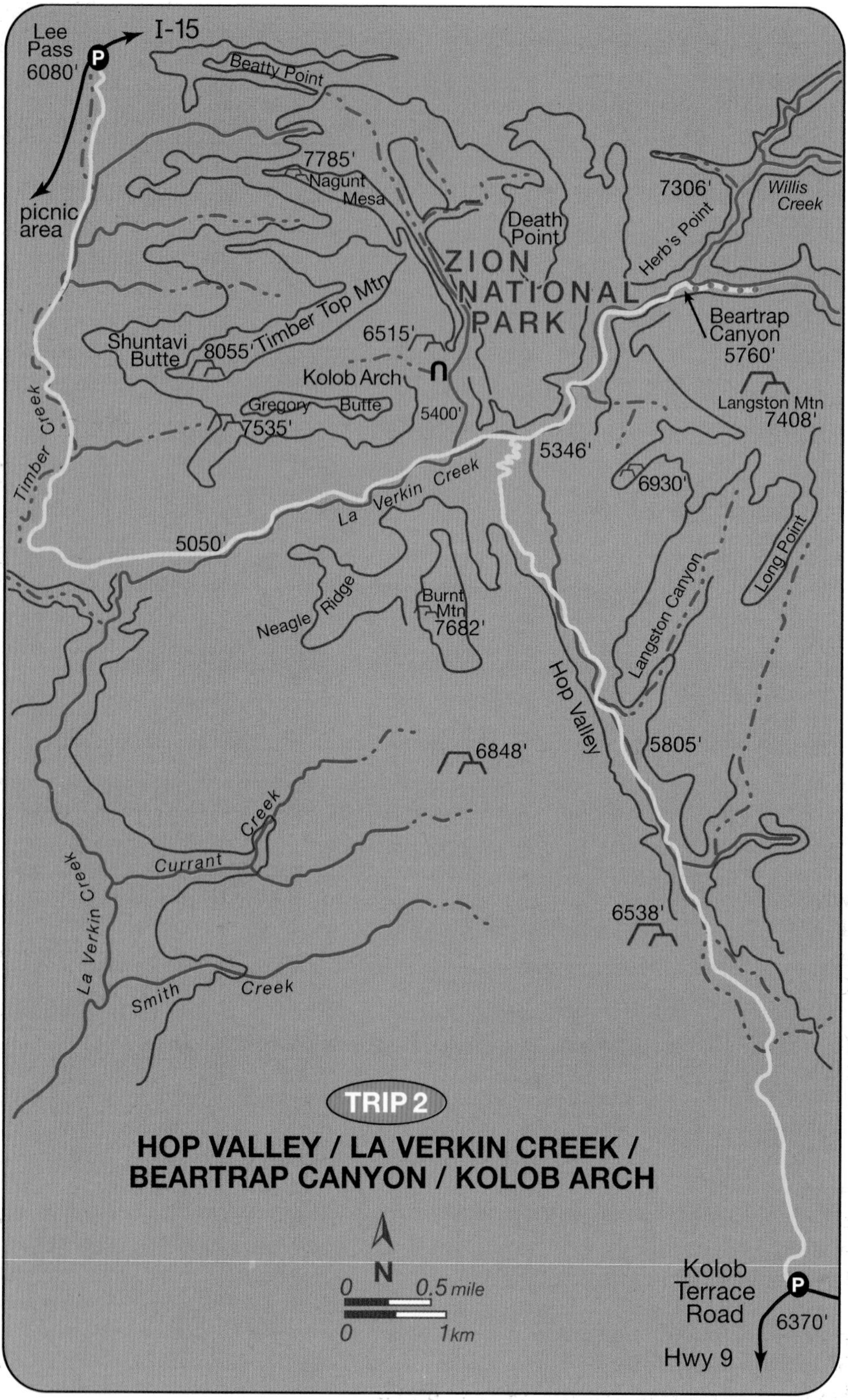

HOP VALLEY / LA VERKIN CREEK / BEARTRAP CANYON / KOLOB ARCH

From either approach, reset your trip odometer to 0 and follow paved Kolob Canyons Road east into Zion Park. Pass the Kolob Canyons visitor center at 0.5 mi (0.8 km). Reach the Lee Pass trailhead at 4.2 mi (6.8 km), 6080 ft (1854 m). Leave your shuttle vehicle here, where the one-way hike ends.

Hop Valley trailhead

From the Kolob Canyons visitor center, return to Interstate 15 and drive south 13 mi (21 km). Exit onto Hwy 17. Follow Hwy 17 south toward La Verkin, then turn left (east) onto Hwy 9. On the east side of Virgin, turn left (north) onto paved Kolob Reservoir Road (*Kolob Terrace Road* on some maps). Reset your trip odometer to 0 and proceed 13.4 mi (21.6 km) to the Hop Valley trailhead at 6370 ft (1942 m). Begin hiking here.

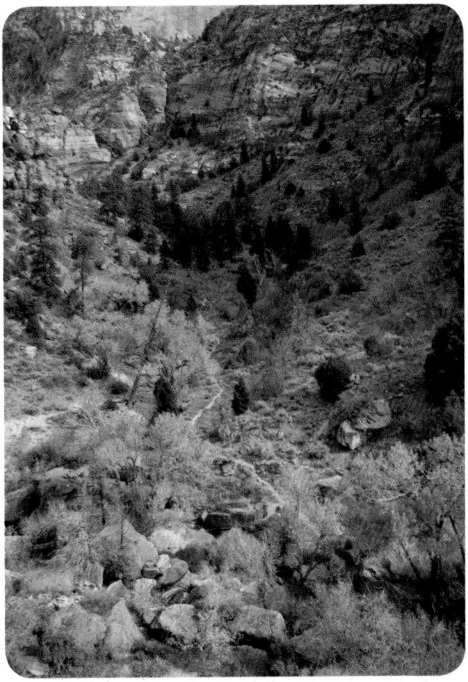

The heart of La Verkin Creek Canyon

ON FOOT

Follow the signed Hop Valley trail north through open P-J forest (piñon pine and juniper). In 1.3 mi (2.1 km) arrive at a fence. Pass through the gate onto private land—an inholding within the national park. Here the trail angles right (northeast) toward sandstone walls, descends into a draw, then curves north again.

Approaching the south end of **Hop Valley**, the trail crosses grazing land where, even if you don't see cattle, their presence will be obvious. About 45 minutes along, at 2 mi (3.2 km), 6050 ft (1845 m), the valley's embrace is evident and the scenery is more engaging. Red sandstone cliffs enclose the wash. Canyon walls are visible ahead, on the north horizon.

About one hour along, reach the **wash bottom** in Hop Valley at 3 mi (4.8 km), 5860 ft (1787 m). Soon pass a substantial tributary canyon (right / east) issuing a perennial stream. Beyond, you'll have to cross the water several times. It's broad but very shallow, so a little scouting and some athletic leaps might enable you to keep your boots on and your feet dry.

At 5 mi (8 km), 5700 ft (1738 m), about 1¾ hours from the trailhead, arrive at another fence. Pass through the gate, close it securely, leave the ranchland behind, and re-enter the national park. The valley's west wall is now sheer. Just ahead, on a bench above the creek's right (east) bank, are three **campsites** beneath ponderosa pines.

From the bench, drop to the creek, cross to the left (west) bank, and resume north-northwest. The trail gradually ascends among pine and gambel oak to 5800 ft (1768 m). Attain an aerial view of La Verkin Creek canyon (north), then begin a sharp, switchbacking descent into it.

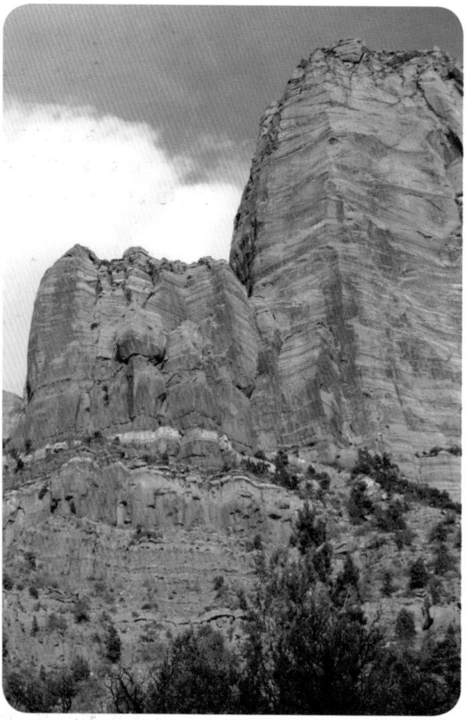

Above Kolob Canyons, northwest corner of Zion Park

Reach a T-junction at 6.3 mi (10.1 km), 5346 ft (1630 m), still above the south bank of **La Verkin Creek**. Total hiking time: about 2½ hours.

Right (east-southeast) descends past a deep pool at the mouth of Hop Valley, drops to the canyon floor, then leads upstream, generally northeast. It passes several campsites en route to Beartrap canyon then continues to Willis Creek canyon. If detouring to Beartrap or Willis, skip below for directions.

Left (west-northwest) gradually descends to the creek, then leads down-canyon, generally west-southwest, passing numerous campsites en route. It quickly reaches the mouth of Kolob Canyon, eventually curves north, then ascends to Lee Pass trailhead. If continuing this one-way trip, keep reading.

Lower La Verkin Canyon

From the **T-junction** at 6.3 mi (10.1 km), still above La Verkin Creek, turn left to resume the one-way trip. Begin a gentle, west-southwest descent of lower La Verkin Creek canyon. The trail soon passes the first of many campsites and crosses to the creek's north bank. Reach a junction at 6.6 mi (10.6 km). Right (north) is a 0.6-mi (1-km) spur ending near **Kolob Arch** (described above, in *Opinion*). The main trail continues following La Verkin Creek downstream, generally west-southwest, beneath the massive south wall of 7535-ft (2297-m) Gregory Butte (right / north).

At 8.4 mi (13.5 km) reach the one-way trip's 5050-ft (1540-m) **lowpoint**. The trail pulls away from the creek, passes campsite #3, and begins a westward traverse of gentle, P-J covered slopes.

After curving north to ascend the **Timber Creek** drainage, pass campsite #2 at 5380 ft (1640 m), then cross the creek in a ravine. Firm ground soon gives way to sand, but the trail remains distinct. Cross the ravine again and pass campsite #1. Shuntavi Butte is right (east) above you.

In the next hour, the trail ascends north on a narrow spine between the highway (visible and audible, left / west) and the steep fingertips of Timber Top Mtn and Nagunt Mesa (right / east).

Finally, curve left (east) and arrive at **Lee Pass trailhead** on the paved Kolob Canyons Road. Elevation: 6080 ft (1854 m). Total one-way distance: 13 mi (21 km). The parking lot is 110 yd (100 m) left (south-southwest).

Beartrap, Willis, and Upper La Verkin Canyons

From the **T-junction** at 6.3 mi (10.1 km), still above La Verkin Creek, turn right to begin your up-canyon detour. The trail drops to the canyon floor and follows the south bank upstream, generally northeast.

Quickly arrive at the first of a dozen creek crossings, all of which are easy, boots-on, hopscotch affairs. Soon begin passing campsites—each one an inviting creekside haven. About 1.5 mi (2.4 km) from the T-junction, the left (northwest) canyon wall towers 1000-ft (305-m) overhead.

At 2 mi (3.2 km), 5760 ft (1756 m), the trail bisects a campsite beside the mouth of **Beartrap canyon** (right / east). Probing this dark, tributary slot canyon is easy until a 12-ft (3.7-m) cascade at 0.3 mi (0.5 km) blocks passage for most hikers.

If you're camping, you'll have time to explore farther up La Verkin Creek canyon. Shortly after passing an obvious tributary (left / northwest), reach the **confluence** of upper La Verkin Creek canyon (left / north) and Willis Creek canyon (right / east), beneath a massive, pyramidal monolith. This is the only feasible campsite since Beartrap.

Willis Creek canyon, which conveys only an intermittent stream, is intriguingly narrow for another 1 mi (1.6 km). The hiking route continues up the widening canyon, exits the national park, and connects with a 4WD road leading to Kolob Reservoir.

Upper La Verkin Creek canyon, which conveys a perennial stream, is also intriguingly narrow for another 1 mi (1.6 km) even though it quickly exits the national park and enters a BLM wilderness study area. There's no hiking route here, but that won't deter hardy explorers.

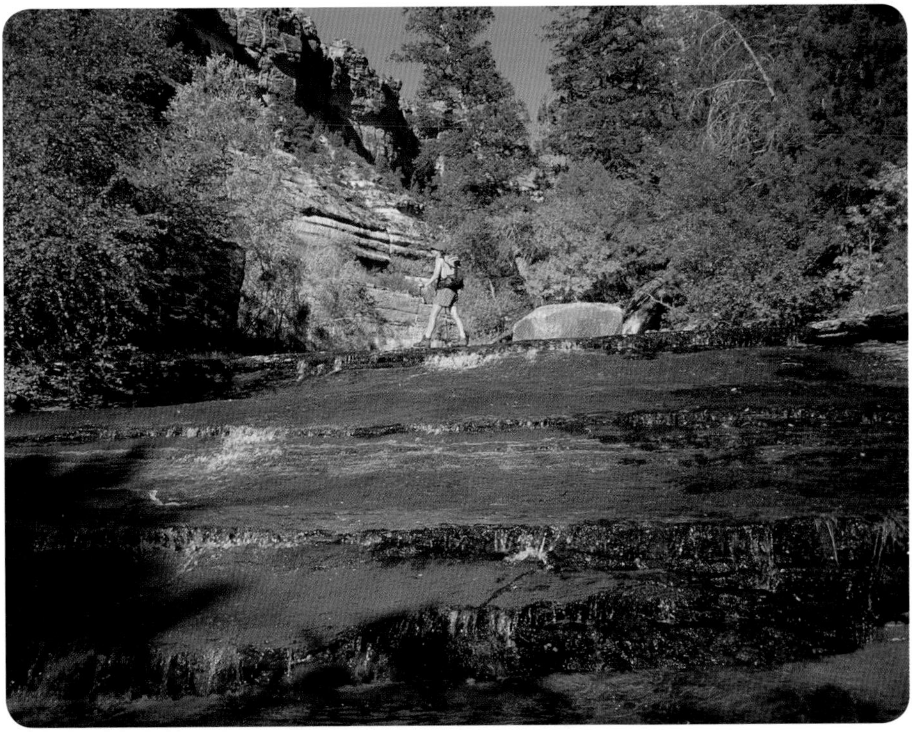

En route to the Subway (Trip 3)

TRIP 3

THE SUBWAY

LOCATION	Kolob Terrace Road, Zion National Park
ROUND TRIP	7.8 mi (12.6 km)
ELEVATION GAIN	1200 ft (366 m)
KEY ELEVATIONS	trailhead 5100 ft (1555 m) Left Fork North Creek 4630 ft (1412 m) The Subway 5360 ft (1634 m)
HIKING TIME	5 to 6 hours
DIFFICULTY	moderate
MAP	Trails Illustrated *Zion National Park*

OPINION

Imagine a keyhole: a circle atop an elongated triangle. Flip it upside down. That's roughly the shape of Great West Canyon at its narrowest point, known as *the Subway*.

Canyons don't come much narrower and darker than this. If they did, they'd be tunnels. So if hiking into a tubular, virtually subterranean passage quickens your pulse, this is the destination for you.

You likely won't be in the Subway for long, however. You'll spend most of your time hiking to and from via the Left Fork of North Creek—enjoyable, but unremarkable compared to other trails in Zion National Park. Upon reaching the Subway, you'll probe it only a short distance before a waterfall halts up-canyon progress. At that point, you must retrace your steps to the trailhead.

Why then is the Subway so famous that the park limits the number of hikers per day and requires you to get a permit before setting foot on the trail—even if you're merely dayhiking? Because canyoneers start at the top of the canyon and navigate the entire length of the Subway. Now *that's* a thrilling exploit, but it requires technical climbing proficiency most hikers lack.

Clearing administrative hurdles just to go on a dayhike is a pain. Knowing you almost certainly will not find solitude here is a drawback. Hiking to the Subway, only to peek into it then leave, is disappointing. It's a worthwhile hike, too popular to exclude from this book, but its inflated reputation among hikers is undeserved.

If your time in Zion is severely limited, hike elsewhere. We recommend La Verkin Creek canyon (Trip 2) for a long trek, Observation Point (Trip 6) or Angels Landing (Trip 4) for a scenic ascent, Zion Narrows (Trip 8) for a wet adventure.

If you're intent on seeing the Subway, start hiking in boots but pack a pair of sandals and, ideally, neoprene socks. You'll want boots for ascending, descending, and boulder hopping. You'll want sandals for splashing through the creek, which is cold, hence the insulating socks. Also carry trekking poles. They'll help you stay upright while walking the slick creekbed near the mouth of this geologic anomaly.

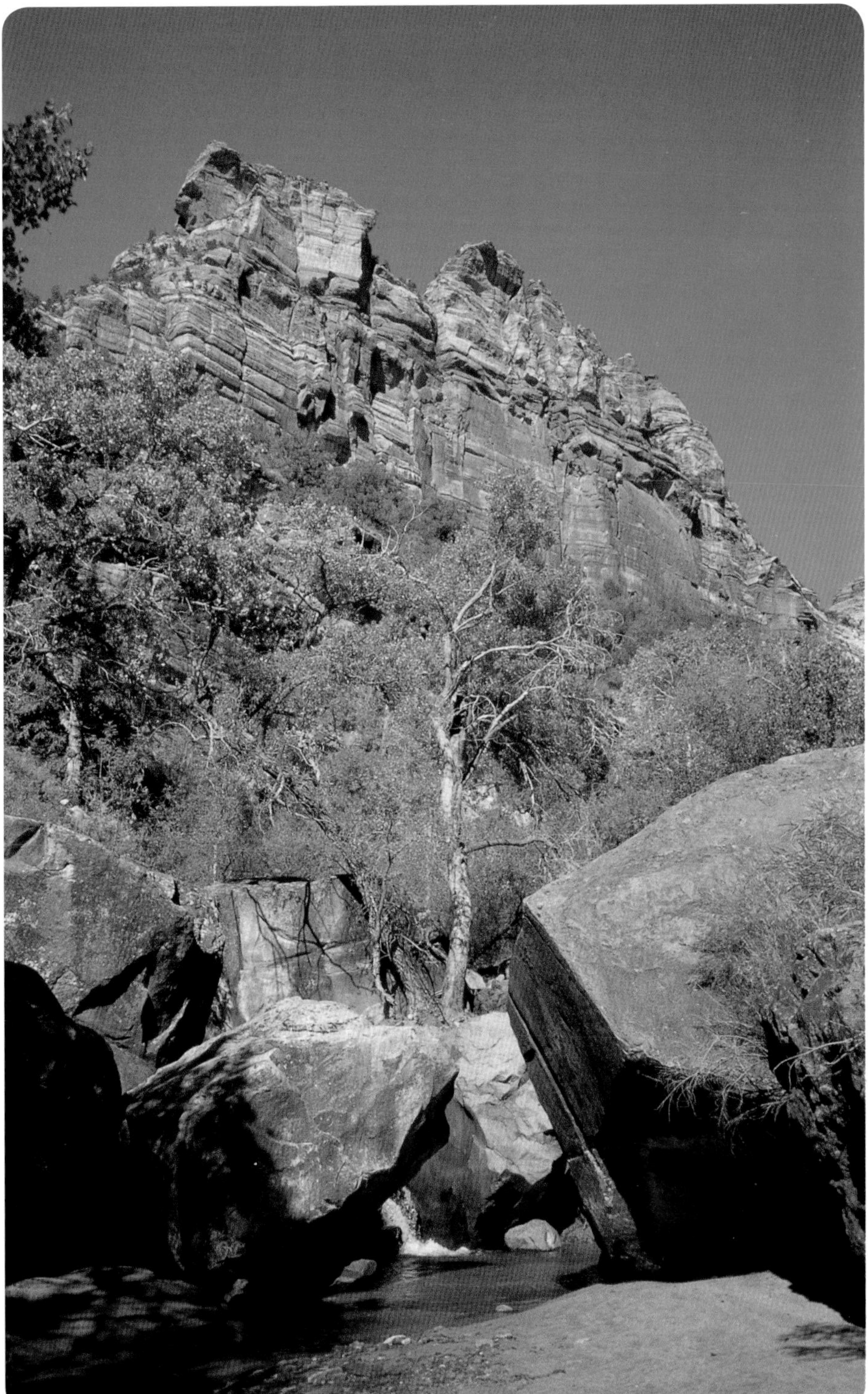

Left Fork of North Creek

FACT

BEFORE YOUR TRIP

Even for the round-trip dayhike described here—from the Left Fork trailhead to the Subway mouth (not a through trip, not an overnighter)—you must get a backcountry permit in person at the Zion Canyon visitor center in Springdale, or the Kolob Canyons visitor center off Hwy 15 at Exit 40 (see *Information Sources*). For permit details, visit www.nps.gov/zion, click on "Backcountry Information," then click on and read "Reservations and Permits," "Subway and Mystery Canyons Reservations," and "Subway/Mystery Canyon Lottery and Reservations."

BY VEHICLE

From Hurricane, drive Hwy 9 north to La Verkin, then east to Virgin. From Springdale, drive Hwy 9 southwest to Rockville, then northwest to Virgin. From either approach, on the east side of Virgin, turn north onto paved Kolob Reservoir Road (*Kolob Terrace Road* on some maps). Reset your trip odometer to 0 and proceed 8 mi (13 km) to the Left Fork trailhead parking lot, on the right (east), at 5100 ft (1555 m).

ON FOOT

The trail departs the northeast corner of the parking lot. Follow it generally east across a **wooded bench** dominated by P-J forest (piñon pine and juniper). Soon cross two dry forks of Grapevine Wash.

Reach the **rim** at 0.6 mi (1 km) and begin descending the **talus slope**. Visible below is North Creek's Left Fork canyon, which you'll follow upstream (northeast) to the Subway. Turn around and note your surroundings, so the return route will be easy to recognize.

After hiking 1 mi (1.6 km) in about 30 minutes, arrive at the canyon floor, among cottonwoods, beside the **Left Fork of North Creek**. Elevation: 4630 ft (1412 m). Pause again and note your surroundings, so you'll recognize where to leave the creek and ascend to the trailhead. Then turn left and hike up-canyon, generally northeast.

Soon rockhop to the creek's right (southeast) bank. Follow cairns and fragments of bootbeaten path. Ragged cliffs are above. Watch the creek for cutthroat trout and the trailside vegetation for agave.

At 1.3 mi (2.1 km), about 45 minutes from the trailhead, pass **Pine Spring Wash** (left / north-northwest). Ten minutes later, at 1.5 mi (2.4 km), pass **Little Creek** (left / north). Attention aquanauts: between these two tributary drainages is a pool in North Creek that's deep enough for a dip.

Be alert for a row of pinnacles on the north skyline. Beneath them, above the left (northwest) bank, are large, titled slabs of grey mudstone bearing three-toed dinosaur tracks from the early Jurassic Period.

After the bootbeaten path disappears in the rocks, continue boulder hopping upstream, switching banks as necessary. Pass another pool: deep, sandy, between huge boulders.

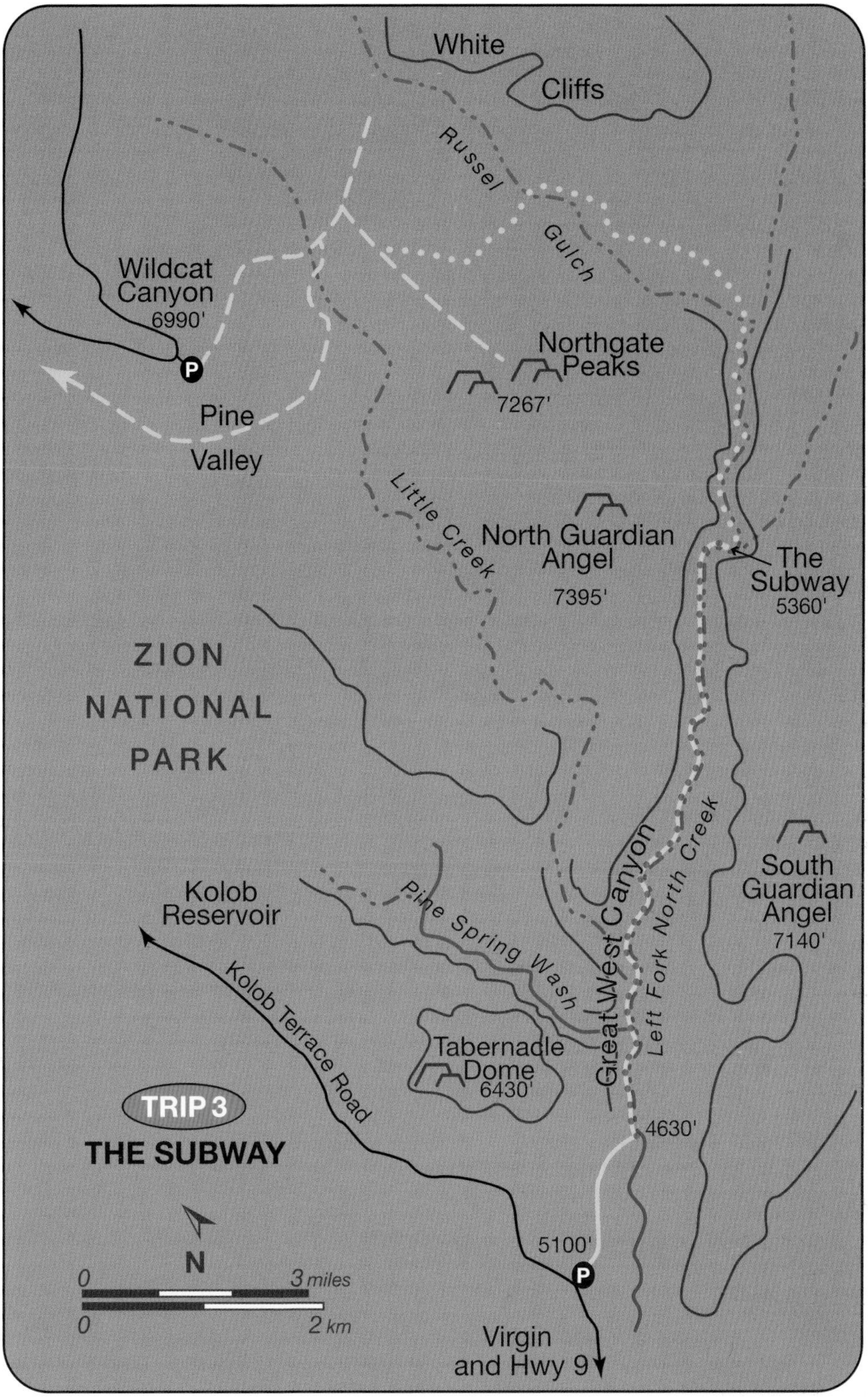
White
Cliffs
Russel
Gulch
Wildcat
Canyon
6990'
Northgate
Peaks
7267'
Pine
Valley
Little Creek
North Guardian
Angel
7395'
The
Subway
5360'
ZION
NATIONAL
PARK
Great West Canyon
Left Fork North Creek
South
Guardian
Angel
7140'
Kolob
Reservoir
Pine Spring Wash
Kolob Terrace Road
Tabernacle
Dome
6430'
TRIP 3
THE SUBWAY
4630'
N
0
3 miles
0
2 km
5100'
Virgin
and Hwy 9

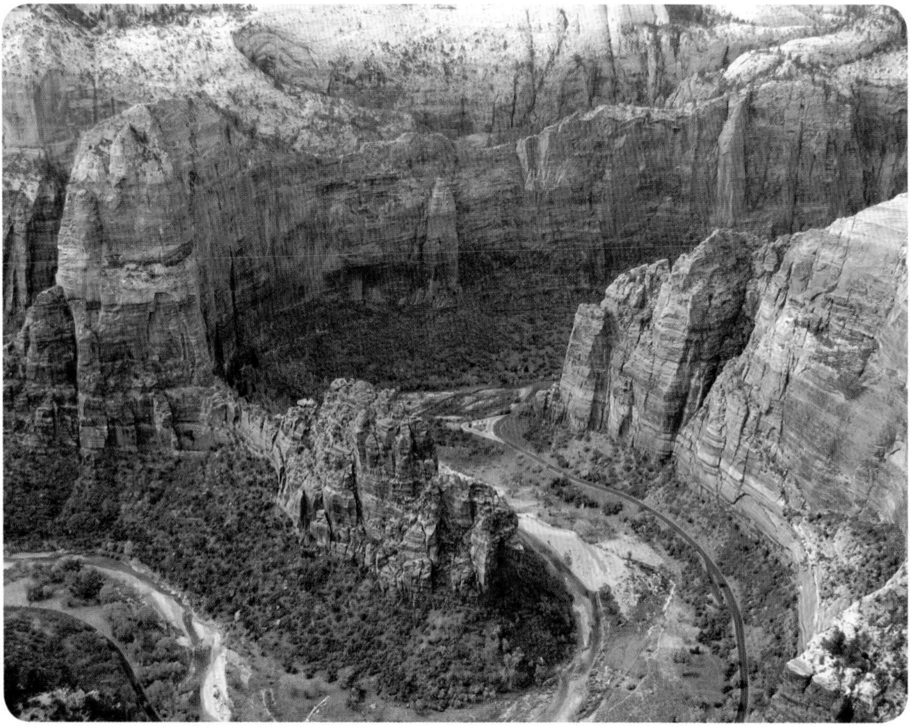

Virgin River North Fork at Big Bend, beneath ridgecrest route to Angels Landing (Trip 4)

At 3.4 mi (5.5 km), 5250 ft (1600 m), reach a **waterfall**. Bypass it, and a second cascade just beyond, following a route on the canyon's right (southeast) wall. Resume along the creekbed.

The way forward is now *in* the shallow creek, which flows over moss-covered bedrock. It's slippery. To prevent falling, take smaller strides, step flat-footed, keep your weight directly over your boots or sandals.

Finally, at 3.9 mi (6.3 km), 5360 ft (1634 m), the canyon curves southeast and approaches the mouth of the **Subway**: a narrow, tunnel-like groove in the canyon floor. Along the "roof" of the tunnel is a slit, above which the canyon widens but continues soaring 800 ft (2440 m) higher.

Hikers can probe the Subway only a short distance before a waterfall bars easy passage, forcing them to turn around and retrace their steps to the trailhead. A through-trip is possible for those with canyoneering skills and equipment, but the optimal route is *down*stream, not up.

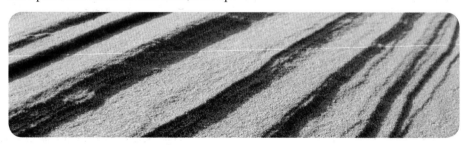

TRIP 4

ANGELS LANDING

LOCATION	Zion Canyon, Zion National Park
ROUND TRIP	5.2 mi (8.4 km)
ELEVATION GAIN	1500 ft (457 m)
KEY ELEVATIONS	trailhead 4290 ft (1308 m)
	summit 5790 ft (1765 m)
HIKING TIME	2 to 3 hours
DIFFICULTY	moderate
MAP	Trails Illustrated *Zion National Park*

OPINION

Looking upward from our humble perspective, it's easy to imagine that if angels do indeed visit us, and they need a majestic place to land—someplace near to earth yet close to heaven—this would be it.

Angels Landing thrusts into Zion Canyon from the West Rim, forcing the south-flowing Virgin River to make a deferential, briefly northward detour around this slender, monolithic peninsula and its lower satellite rock, The Organ.

The short, steep trail ascending this Zion National Park icon is, depending on how comfortable you are with exposure, either thrilling or terrifying. The final approach is along the crest of the peninsula, where there's nothing but air a few feet beyond your shoulders, and it's an alarmingly long way down both sides.

Actually, there's only a *sense* of exposure here. A sharp sense, to be sure, but only a sense. You wouldn't fall if you stumbled. To go over the edge, you'd have to jump off. The trail is remarkably safe given the terrain. Thousands of people hike it every year without incident. But acrophobes are deaf to reassuring facts and should stay away.

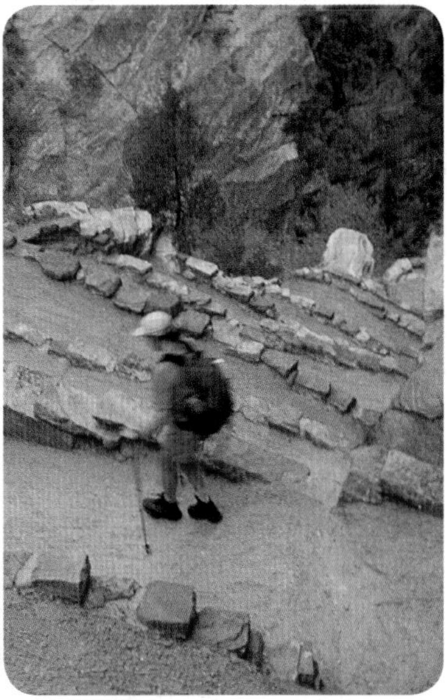

21 switchbacks, known as Walter's Wiggles, lead to the rim of Zion Canyon

Atop the summit of Angels Landing, you'll be high above Zion Canyon's upper reaches, overlooking the very heart of this great park. It ranks among our planet's most dramatic viewpoints. And that's why hikers throng this trail.

The earlier or later you start the fewer you'll see, of course. But during prime hiking season, the trailhead is accessible only by shuttle bus, which runs 8 a.m. to 6 p.m., so your options for achieving tranquility are limited. Expect a crowd. Wear a smile. Post a sentry before you stop to pee.

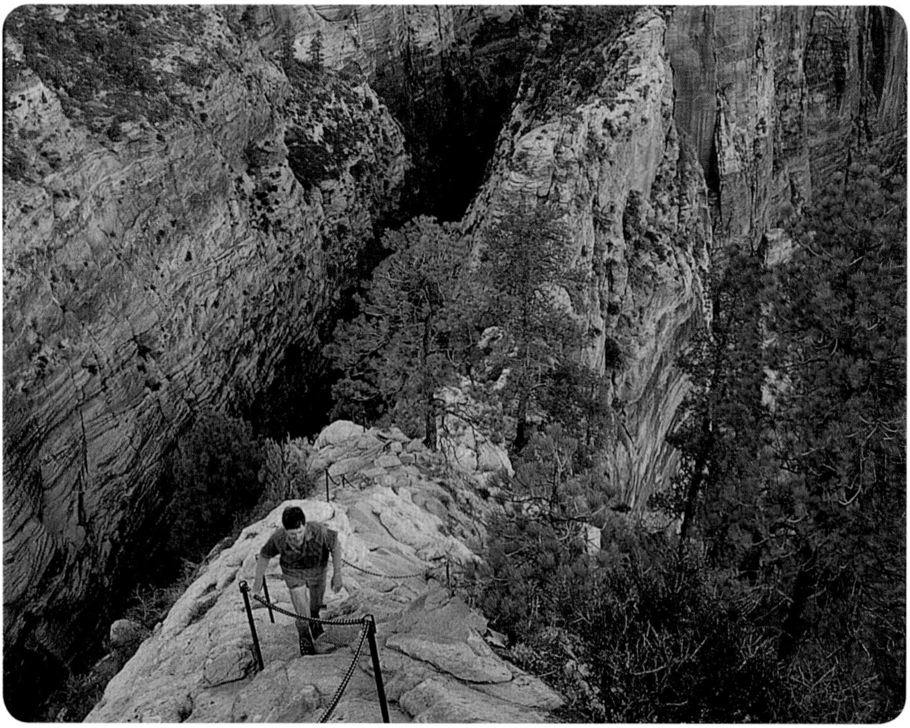

The sandstone peninsula leading to Angel's Landing

Many park visitors who rarely hike attempt to surmount Angels Landing. Some attain only a harsh self-assessment of their fitness level. If you're among them, you'll be encouraged to learn this isn't an all-or-nothing venture. Scout Lookout, though shy of Angels Landing, is a grand viewpoint and a rewarding destination.

Nobody should hike here if there's any chance of a thunder storm or if the trail might be snowy or icy. But if the weather's fine, you're strong, and you start striding early, consider Angels Landing the first stop on a longer trek up the West Rim trail (Trip 5).

The passage to Scout Lookout is an engineering marvel, a gift of the Civilian Conservation Corps (see pages 56-7). Completed in the 1930s, it was one of the first trails in Zion, then a national monument. Beyond the lookout, farther up the West Rim, the CCC blasted the trail out of sandstone cliffs.

FACT

BY VEHICLE

Early April through Late October

Private vehicles are *not* allowed north of Canyon Junction on Zion Canyon Scenic Drive. Access is by shuttle bus only, but you can ride it free of charge. So, after driving Hwy 9 through Zion's south or east entrances, continue to the visitor center near the south entrance. Park here and catch the shuttle bus that

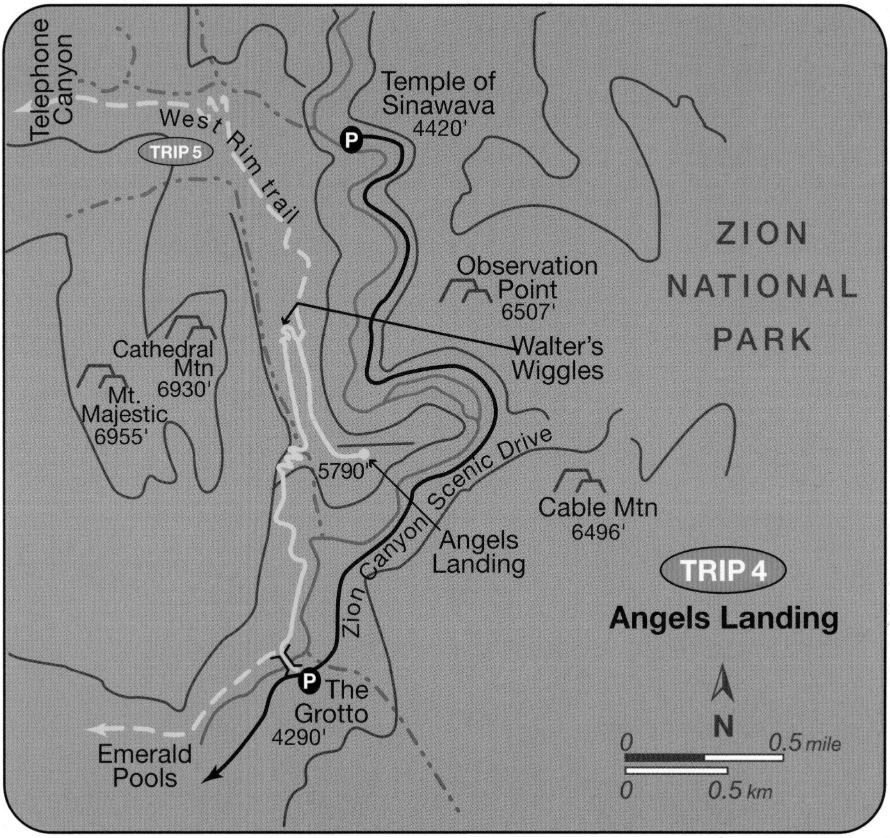

stops at all the Zion Canyon trailheads. It runs daily, 8 a.m. to 6 p.m. Get off at the Grotto trailhead parking lot, on the left, at 4290 ft (1308 m).

Late October through Early April

Private vehicles *are* allowed north of Canyon Junction on Zion Canyon Scenic Drive. So, after driving Hwy 9 through Zion's south or east entrances, proceed to Canyon Junction. Turn north here and continue 3.4 mi (5.5 km) to the Grotto trailhead parking lot, on the left, at 4290 ft (1308 m).

ON FOOT

Follow the trail to the bridge spanning the Virgin River. Cross to the northwest bank and intersect the West Rim trail at a signed T-junction. Left (southwest) leads downstream to the Emerald Pools. Turn right (northeast) and hike upstream.

After curving north, the trail pulls away from the river and begins ascending among the boulders of a Cathedral Mtn rockslide. Soon reach **paved switchbacks** climbing the Navajo sandstone canyon wall.

At 1.5 mi (2.4 km), 4930 ft (1503 m), about 20 minutes from the trailhead, enter **Refrigerator Canyon.** The grade eases in this cool, shady, hanging chasm.

The trail then resumes ascending north via 21 switchbacks known as **Walter's Wiggles**. Fit hikers dispatch this 250-ft (76-m) pitch within ten minutes.

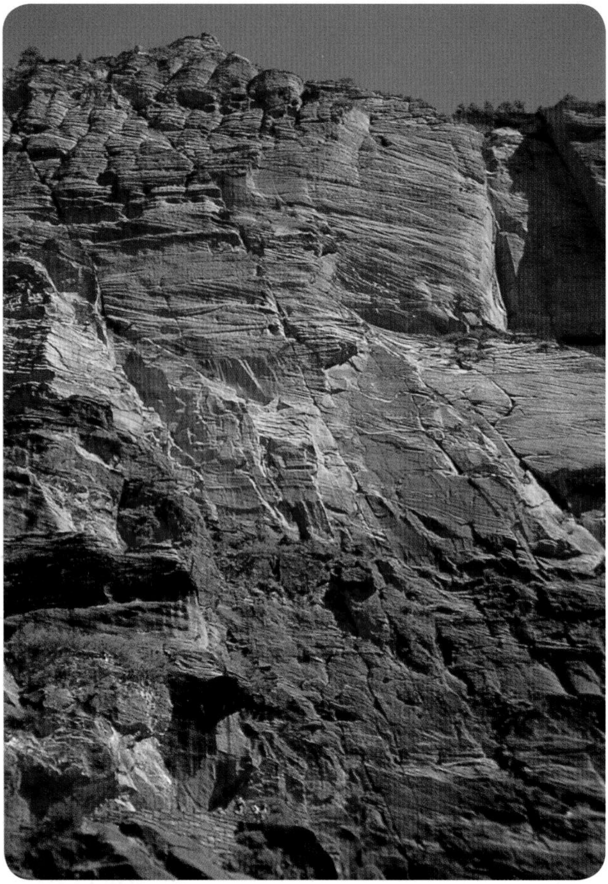

Ascending from Zion Canyon to Angels Landing

Above the wiggles, crest the rim of Zion Canyon amid scattered ponderosa pines. Reach a signed junction at 2.2 mi (3.5 km), 5270 ft (1607 m), immediately below **Scout Lookout**. Total hiking time: about 45 minutes. Left (southeast), the West Rim trail (Trip 5) continues generally north. Go right (south) for Angels Landing.

Ascend the steps cut into the narrow, sheer-sided sandstone rib. Short segments of chain, bolted to the rock, offer handholds. Proceed along the crest among scattered pines to the **Angels Landing** summit at 2.6 mi (4.2 km), 5790 ft (1765 m).

The Virgin River is 1450 ft (442 m) directly below. Southeast, across the river, is the 6744-ft (2056-m) Great White Throne, whose vertical face rises 2300 ft (701 m). East, on Cable Mtn (Trip 7), is the headframe of an ingenious cable structure Mormon pioneers devised to transport lumber from the rim to the canyon floor. Below (north of) Cable Mtn is Weeping Rock alcove, where the East Rim trail ascends to Echo Canyon and provides access to Cable Mtn (Trip 7) and Observation Point (Trip 6), which is northeast.

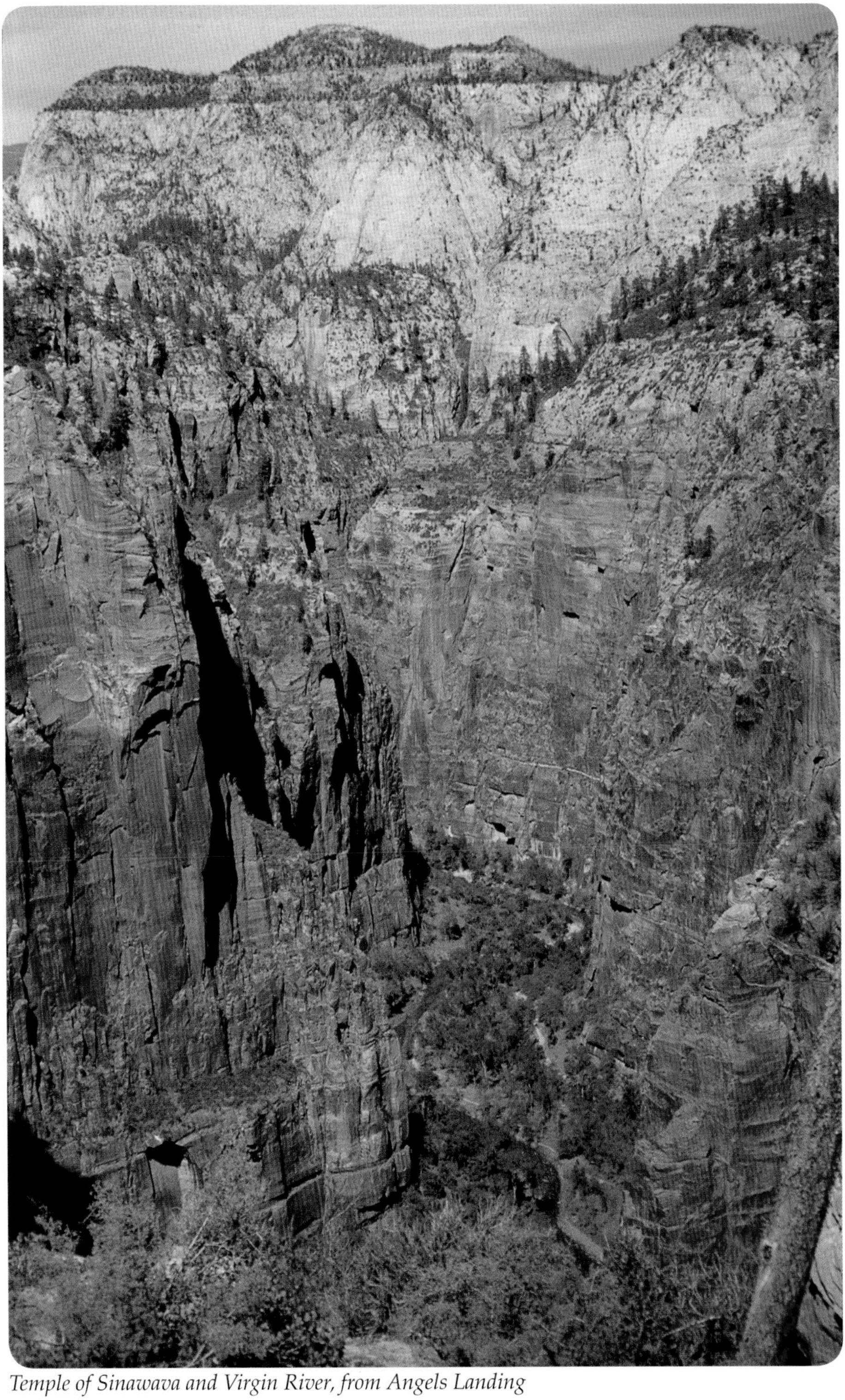

Temple of Sinawava and Virgin River, from Angels Landing

TRIP 5

WEST RIM

LOCATION	Zion Canyon, Zion National Park
DISTANCE	12.2-mi (19.6-km) round trip, 15.2-mi (24.5-km) circuit
ELEVATION GAIN	2510 ft (765 m) for round trip, 2995 ft (913 m) for circuit
KEY ELEVATIONS	trailhead 4290 ft (1308 m), Scout Lookout 5270 ft (1607 m), West Rim 6800 ft (2073 m), circuit highpoint 7285 ft (2220 m)
HIKING TIME	5 to 6 hours for round trip, 7 to 8 hours for circuit
DIFFICULTY	moderate
MAP	Trails Illustrated *Zion National Park*

OPINION

The men who constructed this trail were paid just $1 a day.

It was the 1930s. The Great Depression had ravaged the U.S. economy. Desperate for jobs—any work at any wage—they'd joined the Civilian Conservation Corps*.

But what they accomplished bears no trace of the despair that was then gripping the nation. Just the opposite. And this trail ascending the West Rim of Zion Canyon is a prime example. It's a marvel. A triumph. A magnum opus among trails.

It climbs sheer sandstone, ventures out to Angels Landing (Trip 4), then continues scaling yet more vertical walls to a stunning, rim-crest vantage high above the Virgin River.

By blasting the trail out of solid rock, the CCC allowed subsequent generations of hikers to enjoy a fascinating ascent, pierce the canyon's seemingly impregnable ramparts, and overlook the very heart of this great national park.

To fully appreciate the scenery and the trail itself, dayhikers should follow the West Rim trail at least 1 mi (1.6 km) past the first junction with the Telephone Canyon trail. Turn back there and your round-trip distance will be 12.2 mi (19.6 km).

Ideally, proceed farther along the West Rim trail, contour above Phantom Valley, continue gazing across Zion Park's nether regions, then loop back via the Telephone Canyon trail to complete a 15.2-mi (24.5-km) circuit. Strong hikers do this in a day, but breaking it into a two-day, one-night backpack trip is viable.

Beyond (north-northwest) of where the West Rim and Telephone Canyon trails rejoin, the West Rim trail undulates across Horse Pasture Plateau, which is no more exciting than its name implies. There's nothing Zionesque about it. Instead, invest your time on the park's premier trails, all of which this book describes.

*The Civilian Conservation Corps (CCC) was a work relief program for young men from unemployed families. Established in 1933 by President Franklin Roosevelt, it was part of the New Deal legislation intended to combat poverty caused by the Great Depression. It earned enthusiastic public support and operated in every state and several territories.

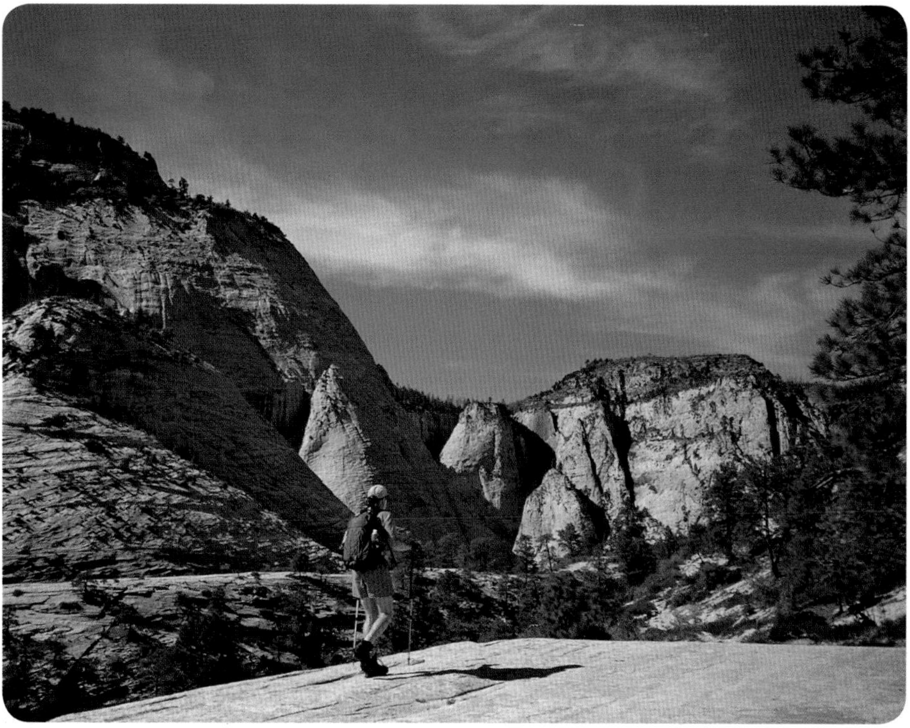

West Rim trail

The corps was essentially an outdoor-construction-project army. Workers lived in quasi-military camps of about 200 men each for six-month periods. There was also a separate Indian Division that became an effective relief force for Native American reservations.

CCC workers were 18 to 25 years old. When they entered the program, most were malnourished and poorly clothed. Few had more than a year of high school education or any work experience beyond occasional odd jobs. By 1935 there were 505,000 workers in 2,650 CCC camps. Ultimately, three million men participated in the program.

Many of the structures and trails still used today in national, state and city parks throughout the U.S. were built by the CCC. The corps established the nation's first organized wildland fire suppression crews. CCC workers installed power and phone lines, constructed roads, checked soil erosion, and planted 5 billion trees.

When the U.S. economy began to rebound in about 1940, the CCC declined. Organized labor opposed it, but the need for the CCC simply decreased as employment increased. After Japan bombed Pearl Harbor in 1941, national attention shifted away from domestic issues toward the war effort. CCC operations ceased in 1942 when Congress stopped funding it.

FACT

BEFORE YOUR TRIP

If you're backpacking, you must get a backcountry camping permit in person at the Zion Canyon visitor center in Springdale (see *Information Sources*). For permit details, visit www.nps.gov/zion, click on "Backcountry Information," then click on and read "Reservations and Permits" and "Other Backcountry Reservations."

BY VEHICLE

Early April through Late October

Private vehicles are *not* allowed north of Canyon Junction on Zion Canyon Scenic Drive. Access is by shuttle bus only, but you can ride it free of charge. So, after driving Hwy 9 through Zion's south or east entrances, continue to the visitor center near the south entrance. Park here and catch the shuttle bus that stops at all the Zion Canyon trailheads. It runs daily, 8 a.m. to 6 p.m. Get off at the Grotto trailhead parking lot, on the left, at 4290 ft (1308 m).

Late October through Early April

Private vehicles *are* allowed north of Canyon Junction on Zion Canyon Scenic Drive. So, after driving Hwy 9 through Zion's south or east entrances, proceed to Canyon Junction. Turn north here and continue 3.4 mi (5.5 km) to the Grotto trailhead parking lot, on the left, at 4290 ft (1308 m).

ON FOOT

Follow the trail to the bridge spanning the Virgin River. Cross to the northwest bank and intersect the West Rim trail at a signed T-junction. Left (southwest) leads downstream to the Emerald Pools. Turn right (northeast) and hike upstream.

After curving north, the trail pulls away from the river and begins ascending among the boulders of a Cathedral Mtn rockslide. Soon reach **paved switchbacks** climbing the Navajo sandstone canyon wall.

At 1.5 mi (2.4 km), 4930 ft (1503 m), about 20 minutes from the trailhead, enter **Refrigerator Canyon.** The grade eases in this cool, shady, hanging chasm.

The trail then resumes ascending north via 21 switchbacks known as **Walter's Wiggles**. Fit hikers dispatch this 250-ft (76-m) pitch within ten minutes.

Above the wiggles, crest the rim of Zion Canyon amid scattered ponderosa pines. Reach a signed junction at 2.2 mi (3.5 km), 5270 ft (1607 m), immediately below **Scout Lookout**. Total hiking time: about 45 minutes. Right (south) leads 0.4 mi (0.7 km) to the summit of Angels Landing (Trip 4). Go left (southeast), to continue following the West Rim trail generally north.

The West Rim trail ascends slickrock and sections of cement path to 5780 ft (1762 m), then descends north-northwest beneath Cathedral Mtn (left / west). About 30 minutes from Scout Lookout (1¼ hours total), cross a bridge to the west side of a **chasm** at 5200 ft (1585 m). A gentle ascent ensues on paved path.

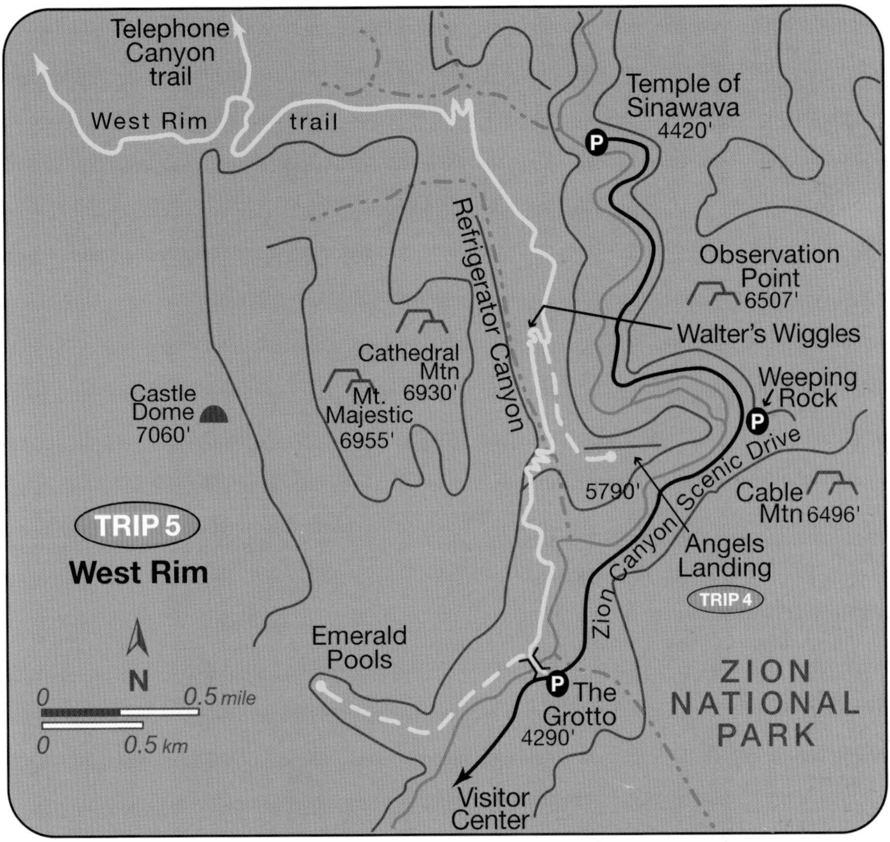

Nearly an hour from Scout Lookout (1¾ hours total), traverse Navajo sandstone above the head of **Telephone Canyon** (right / north). Then begin ascending a cunningly engineered trail blasted out of the cliffs by the Civilian Conservation Corps in the 1930s. To prevent erosion, the path has since been reinforced with concrete. White fir, Douglas fir, and ponderosa pine adorn the canyon walls.

After gaining 1530 ft (466 m) in about 1½ hours from Scout Lookout, reach a **junction atop the West Rim** at 6800 ft (2073 m). Since departing the trailhead, you've hiked 5.1 mi (8.2 km) in about 2¼ hours. The Telephone Canyon (TC) trail forks right (north-northeast). The West Rim trail proceeds left (northwest).

Stay on the West Rim trail for the most impressive views. For a sample, go 1 mi (0.6 km) in that direction then retrace your steps to complete a 12.2-mi (19.6-km) round trip. Otherwise, continue along the West Rim trail to where it rejoins the TC trail farther northwest, then return via the TC trail to complete a 15.2-mi (24.5-km) circuit.

For the optimal rest stop, briefly detour along the TC trail. Descend past **Cabin Spring** and within five minutes reach a campsite where you'll find an inviting log to sit on beneath giant ponderosa pines. The pink sandstone of Bryce Canyon National Park is visible on the northeast horizon. The Temple of Sinawava is east, across Zion Canyon.

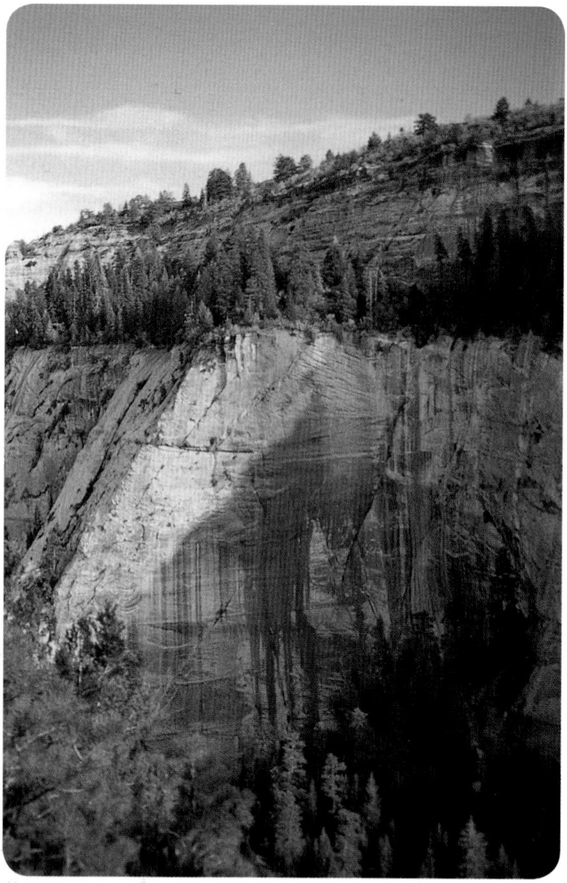

West Rim

So, from the 5.1-mi (8.2-km) junction, go left (northwest) on the West Rim trail. Behunin Canyon is soon visible south. Beyond it and slightly right (west) are the Three Patriarchs. On the east-southeast horizon are the Vermilion Cliffs above Kanab. Later, Phantom Valley is below you (west-southwest).

After contouring southwest, the trail curves northwest. Pass several campsites perched along the rim. Then curve northeast, away from the rim, pass another campsite, and reach the second **junction** with the TC trail at 8.3 mi (13.4 km), 7285 ft (2220 m).

The West Rim trail turns left, heading 6.7 mi (10.8 km) generally north-northwest across Horse Pasture Plateau to the West Rim trailhead at 7460 ft (2274 m), just shy of Lava Point. Go right and follow the TC trail generally southeast.

At 10.1 mi (16.3 km) reach the **junction** where the TC and West Rim trails originally split. Having looped around the south end of the plateau, you're now on familiar ground. Turn left and descend the West Rim trail. Retrace your steps past **Scout Lookout** to the **Grotto trailhead**, where your total circuit distance will be 15.2 mi (24.5 km).

TRIP 6

OBSERVATION POINT

LOCATION	Zion Canyon, Zion National Park
ROUND TRIP	8 mi (12.9 km)
ELEVATION GAIN	2147 ft (654 m)
KEY ELEVATIONS	trailhead 4360 ft (1330 m) Echo Canyon fork 5592 ft (1705 m) Observation Point 6507 ft (1983 m)
HIKING TIME	4 hours
DIFFICULTY	moderate
MAP	Trails Illustrated *Zion National Park*

OPINION

Natives, on hunting and gathering forays, devised this clever route to the rim of Zion Canyon. Mormon pioneers later improved it so they could drive cattle to summer pasture. Today, hikers follow it to the quintessential view of a celebrated national park.

The panorama at trail's end is transfixing. It includes the luxuriant green ribbons of vegetation lining the banks of the Virgin River 2147 ft (654 m) below; Angels Landing (Trip 4) atop a massive, sheer rampart where you might see rock climbers; the Yosemite-like walls of nearby Cable Mtn and the Great White Throne; and, beyond the West Rim, a horizon crowded with domes, mountains and mesas.

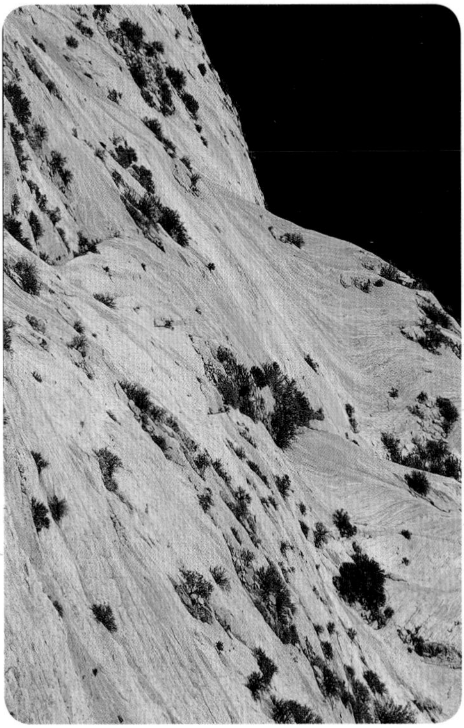

Navajo sandstone near Observation Point

But the climactic view isn't the only reward here. The trail itself is miraculous—a steep, intriguing ascent that pierces the sheer, Zion Canyon wall. You'll also probe the recesses of Echo Canyon, which narrows to just 20 ft (6 m).

Most park visitors, upon arriving at the trailhead, tilt their heads back, see the trail's skyward trajectory, and think "I could never do that." But it's less challenging than it appears from below. Frequent switchbacks moderate the grade, allowing mere mortals to vanquish the substantial elevation gain. And this isn't a rocky,

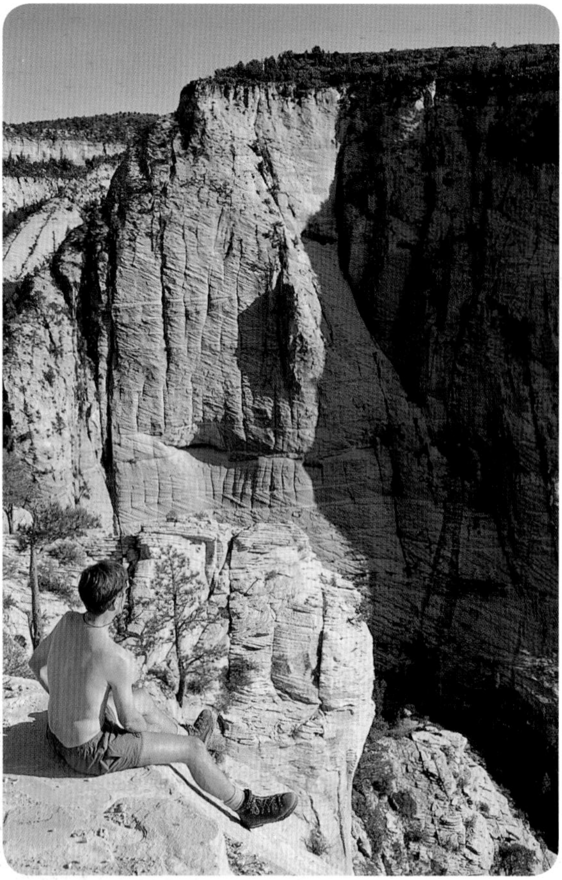

Zion Canyon, from Observation Point

precarious, mountain-goat passage. Much of the way is paved (!) to prevent the trail from eroding.

Whether you're hiking to Observation Point or Cable Mtn (Trip 7), you'll start at the same trailhead and follow the same trail until reaching a fork at 2.1 mi (3.4 km). So before setting out, compare these two options and decide which you prefer.

The culminating vistas at Cable Mtn and Observation Point are similarly spectacular, although Observation's down-canyon orientation allows you to see farther. Also, the Observation Point trail contours near the canyon rim for about 1 mi (1.6 km), whereas the Cable Mtn trail leads *to* the rim but never follows it.

The primary difference is that the Cable Mtn round trip is 7.4 mi (11.9 km) longer and climbs 817 ft (249 m) higher, so it's more difficult and less popular. You're hungry for challenge and solitude? Go to Cable Mtn. The majority of hikers happily head for Observation Point.

FACT

BY VEHICLE

Early April through Late October

Private vehicles are *not* allowed north of Canyon Junction on Zion Canyon Scenic Drive. Access is by shuttle bus only, but you can ride it free of charge. So, after driving Hwy 9 through Zion's south or east entrances, continue to the visitor center near the south entrance. Park here and catch the shuttle bus that stops at all the Zion Canyon trailheads. It runs daily, 8 a.m. to 6 p.m. Get off at the Weeping Rock parking lot, on the right, at 4360 ft (1330 m).

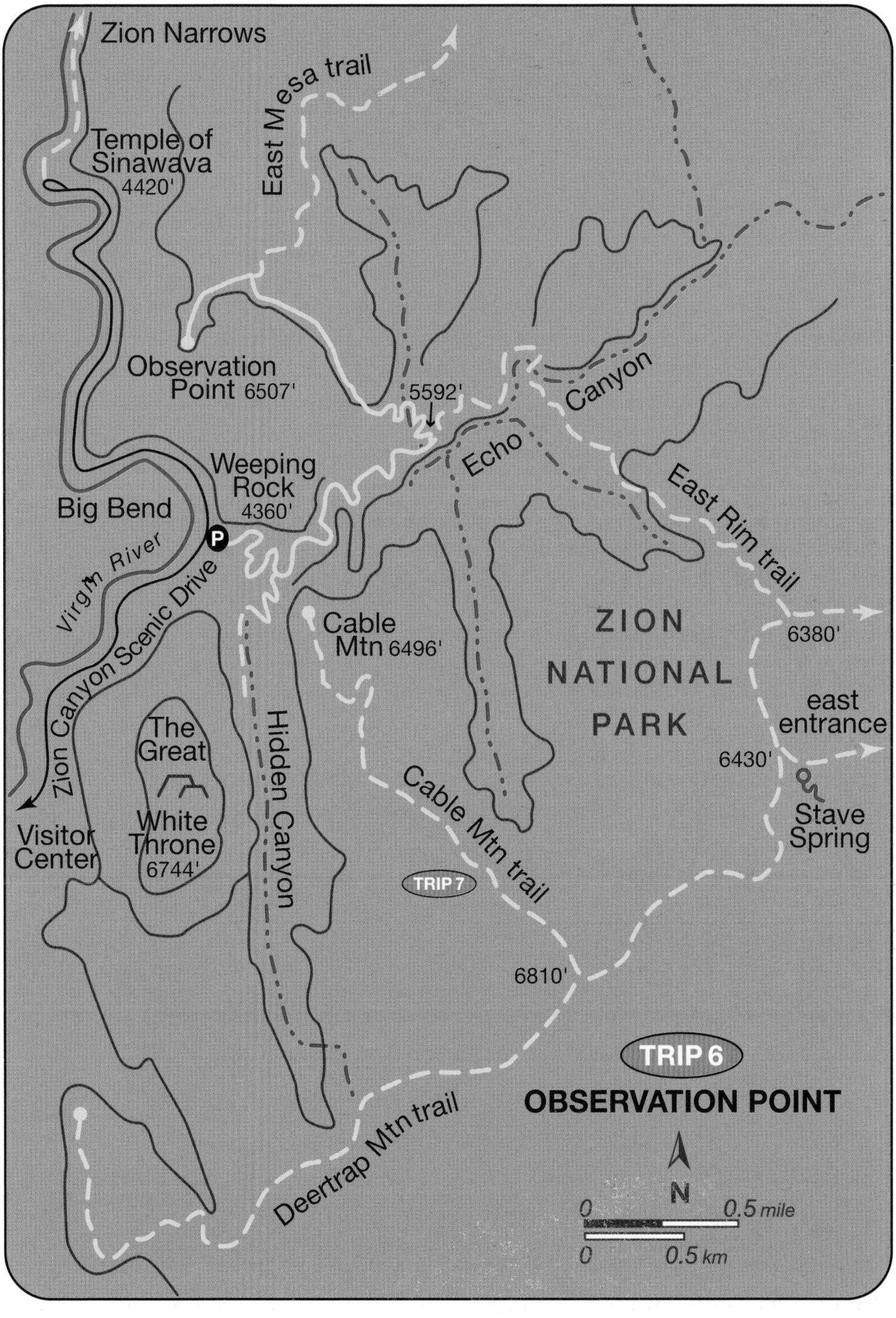
Zion Narrows
East Mesa trail
Temple of Sinawava
4420'
Observation Point 6507'
5592'
Echo Canyon
Weeping Rock
4360'
Big Bend
Virgin River
Zion Canyon Scenic Drive
East Rim trail
Cable Mtn 6496'
ZION NATIONAL PARK
6380'
east entrance
6430'
Stave Spring
The Great White Throne
6744'
Hidden Canyon
Cable Mtn trail
Visitor Center
TRIP 7
6810'
TRIP 6
OBSERVATION POINT
N
Deertrap Mtn trail
0
0.5 mile
0
0.5 km

Late October through Early April

Private vehicles *are* allowed north of Canyon Junction on Zion Canyon Scenic Drive. So, after driving Hwy 9 through Zion's south or east entrances, proceed to Canyon Junction. Turn north here and continue 4.6 mi (7.4 km) to the Weeping Rock parking lot, on the right, at 4360 ft (1330 m).

ON FOOT

Depart the southwest corner of the paved parking lot. Follow the trail south across the bridged creek. Ignore the left spur to weeping rock; you'll see it soon, from above. Proceed straight.

The **East Rim trail**, actually a broad path, remains paved for a surprising distance. It curves left (east) and ascends steeply. The weeping rock is visible left. Switchbacks convey you up the canyon wall.

Within 20 minutes, at 4855 ft (1480 m), a right (west) spur leads 0.5 mi (0.8 km) into Hidden Canyon—a worthwhile detour. For Observation Point, proceed straight (east) on the main trail, ascending through **Echo Canyon** beneath Cable Mtn (right/south).

About 40 minutes along, at 5205 ft (1587 m), the trail curves right (southeast) into a narrow, sheer-walled defile. Pavement briefly ends here. Proceed on sand, then slickrock, then on a rocky wash bottom. Ascend the slickrock ledge on the left. Pavement soon resumes.

At 2.1 mi (3.4 km), 5592 ft (1705 m), about an hour from the trailhead, reach a **signed fork**. Go straight (northeast) on the paved path to ascend out of Echo Canyon and continue to Observation Point, farther northwest. The narrow, rocky trail descending right (east-southeast) leads to Cable Mtn (Trip 7), Zion Park's east entrance, and Deertrap Mtn.

Begin a vigorous, switchbacking ascent of Echo Canyon's 800-ft (244-m) **north wall**. The trail negotiating this steep Navajo sandstone is airy—thrilling to some, alarming to others—but safe. Tenacious shrubs and trees cling to life on small ledges where tiny pockets of soil have collected over the ages.

Above the switchbacks, the ascent eases into P-J forest (piñon pine and juniper). Having surmounted the cliffs and delivered you to the brush-clad plateau, the trail is now unpaved.

Reach a **junction** at 3.7 mi (6 km). Right is the East Mesa trail, heading northeast to nowhere you want to go. Turn left, continue generally west, then curve left (south) onto a promontory where gambel oak and manzanita are profuse.

The trail soon ends at 6507-ft (1983-m) **Observation Point**, where your total distance is 4 mi (6.4 km).

Echo Canyon trail, from Cable Mountain

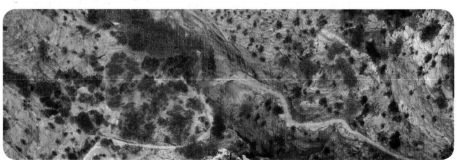

TRIP 7

CABLE MOUNTAIN

LOCATION	Zion Canyon, Zion National Park
ROUND TRIP	15.4 mi (24.8 km)
ELEVATION GAIN	2964 ft (904 m)
KEY ELEVATIONS	trailhead 4360 ft (1330 m) Echo Canyon 5656 ft (1724 m) highpoint 6910 ft (2107 m), Cable Mtn 6496 ft (1980 m)
HIKING TIME	6 to 7½ hours
DIFFICULTY	challenging
MAP	Trails Illustrated *Zion National Park*

OPINION

Depending on your viewpoint, prophecy is the sand or bedrock on which Joseph Smith founded the Church of Jesus Christ of Latter-day Saints. His successor, Brigham Young, was a prophet as well. And if you hike to Cable Mountain, you'll see physical evidence of a prophecy Brigham nailed.

Mormon pioneers were quickly settling along the Virgin River, from Springdale (next to present-day Zion Park), downstream to St. George. But sizeable hardwood trees—necessary for construction—were scarce in the desert canyon. So the question was how to retrieve lumber from the forests on the East Rim Plateau, high above the towering canyon walls.

"Like a hawk flies," said Brigham Young, the settlers would transport wood to their growing communities below. And they did, by constructing a fantastic cable system that sent each load of milled lumber soaring from mesa-top to canyon-floor in just 2½ minutes. In 1920 it conveyed the ponderosa pine used to build the original Zion Lodge.

The headframe of the cableworks still stands on the canyon rim. It's listed in the National Register of Historic Places. You'll find it at trail's end, where you can creep out to the edge, look down at the Virgin River 2140 ft (652 m) below, and marvel not only at a prophecy fulfilled but at the industrious beehive spirit that built the state of Utah.

But there's much more to this hike than the cableworks and the climactic panorama. There's the trail itself—a steep, intriguing ascent that pierces the sheer, Zion Canyon wall via Echo Canyon, which narrows to just 20 ft (6 m). Plus there's the solitude you'll likely find.

Angels Landing (Trip 4) and Zion Narrows (Trip 8), both widely known, attract far more hikers. And most park visitors, upon arriving at the Cable Mtn trailhead, tilt their heads back, see the trail's skyward trajectory, and think "I could never do that."

Actually, it's less challenging than it appears from below. It gains substantial elevation but at a moderate grade due to frequent switchbacks. And it's not a

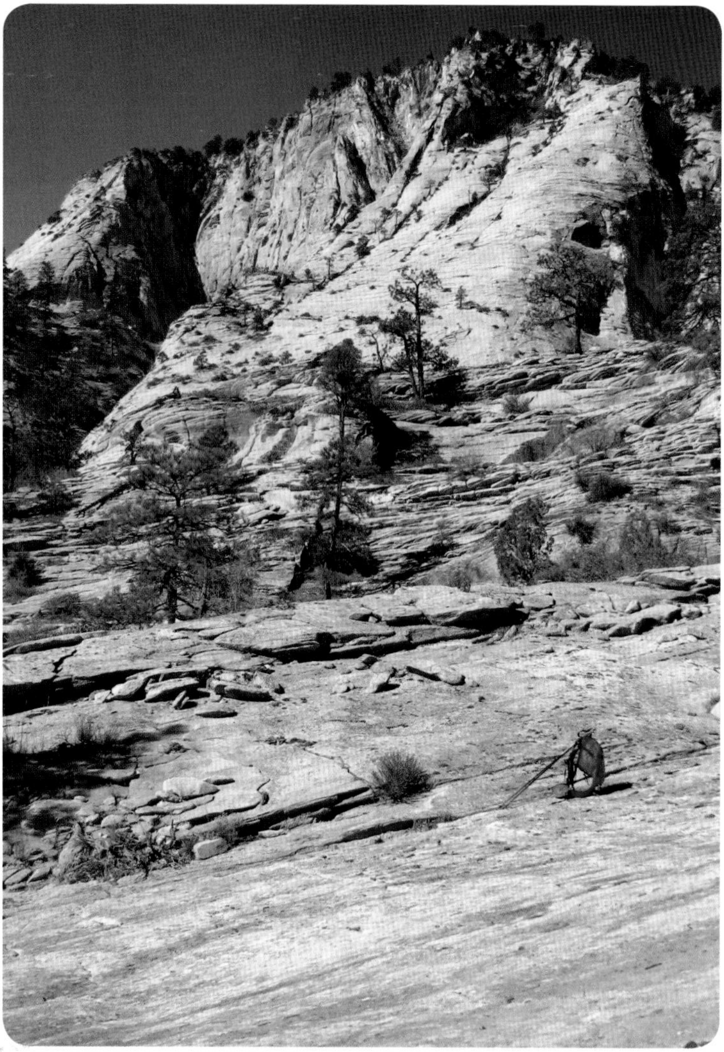

Slickrock route between Echo Canyon and Cable Mountain

rocky, precarious, mountain-goat passage. Much of the way is paved (!) to prevent the trail from eroding. Nevertheless, you won't have to head-butt your way through a crowd. Our most recent trip to Cable Mtn was on a perfect October weekend, and we encountered just one other hiker.

Even if you do find yourself sharing the trail with others, they'll probably stop at Hidden Canyon or will, midway along, veer off to Observation Point (Trip 6). The culminating vistas at Cable Mtn and Observation Point are similar. The Virgin River, Big Bend, Angel's Landing, and the West Rim are visible from both vantages. The primary difference is that the Cable Mtn round trip is 7.4 mi (11.9 km) longer and climbs 817 ft (249 m) higher. Also, the Observation Point trail contours near the canyon rim for about 1 mi (1.6 km), whereas the Cable Mtn trail leads *to* the rim but never follows it.

Hardened athletes who start early might consider detouring to Observation Point while returning from Cable Mtn. Doing so would add 3.8 mi (6.1 km) to the day, upping the total round-trip mileage to 19.2 mi (30.9 m)—a strenuous endeavor.

Most hikers, however, should simply aim for Observation Point. From there, they can still gaze across the canyon at Cable Mtn and imagine the lumber swooping earthward via the miraculous cable.

Other Options

The Hidden Canyon detour, about 20 minutes from the trailhead, is worthwhile, but leave it for the return, to make sure you have time to lengthen your round trip by 1 mi (1.6 km).

The Deertrap Mtn detour, which begins at the final Cable Mtn junction, is not worthwhile. It too ends at a canyon-rim viewpoint, but adds 5.4 mi (8.7 km) to your round trip and traverses monotonous terrain made downright dispiriting by a recent fire.

Continuing from Stave Spring junction, across the mesa 5.7 mi (9.2 km) to the park's east entrance on Hwy 9, is not the adventure it might seem. It's astonishing in only one respect: how boring it is. You'll see nothing even remotely Zionesque. And you'd have to arrange a shuttle, or hitchhike, back to Zion Canyon. Your Cable Mtn dayhike will be much more memorable if you make it a round trip returning via magnificent Echo Canyon.

FACT

BY VEHICLE

Early April through Late October

Private vehicles are *not* allowed north of Canyon Junction on Zion Canyon Scenic Drive. Access is by shuttle bus only, but you can ride it free of charge. So, after driving Hwy 9 through Zion's south or east entrances, continue to the visitor center near the south entrance. Park here and catch the shuttle bus that stops at all the Zion Canyon trailheads. It runs daily, 8 a.m. to 6 p.m. Get off at the Weeping Rock parking lot, on the right, at 4360 ft (1330 m).

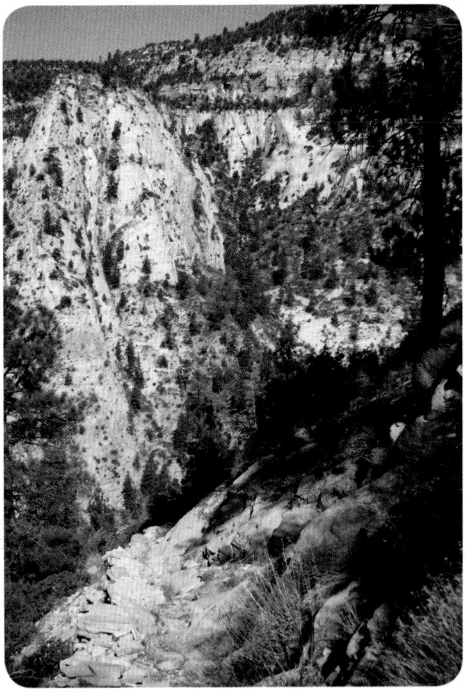

Cable Mountain trail

Late October through Early April

Private vehicles *are* allowed north of Canyon Junction on Zion Canyon Scenic Drive. So, after driving Hwy 9 through Zion's south or east entrances, proceed to Canyon

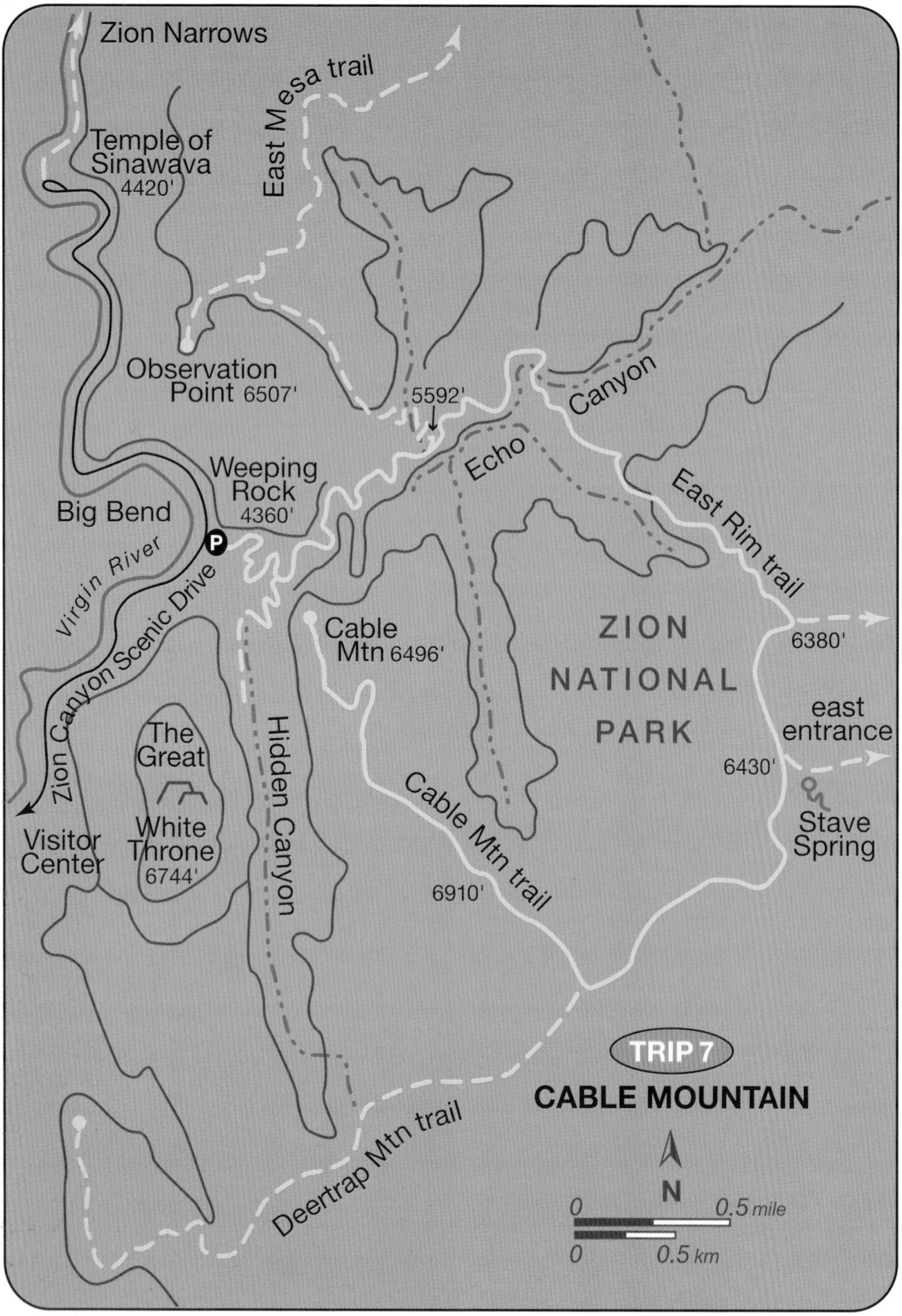
Zion Narrows
East Mesa trail
Temple of Sinawava 4420'
Observation Point 6507'
5592'
Canyon
Echo
Weeping Rock 4360'
Big Bend
Virgin River
Zion Canyon Scenic Drive
East Rim trail
Cable Mtn 6496'
ZION NATIONAL PARK
6380'
east entrance
6430'
Stave Spring
The Great White Throne 6744'
Visitor Center
Hidden Canyon
Cable Mtn trail
6910'
TRIP 7
CABLE MOUNTAIN
N
0
0.5 mile
0
0.5 km
Deertrap Mtn trail

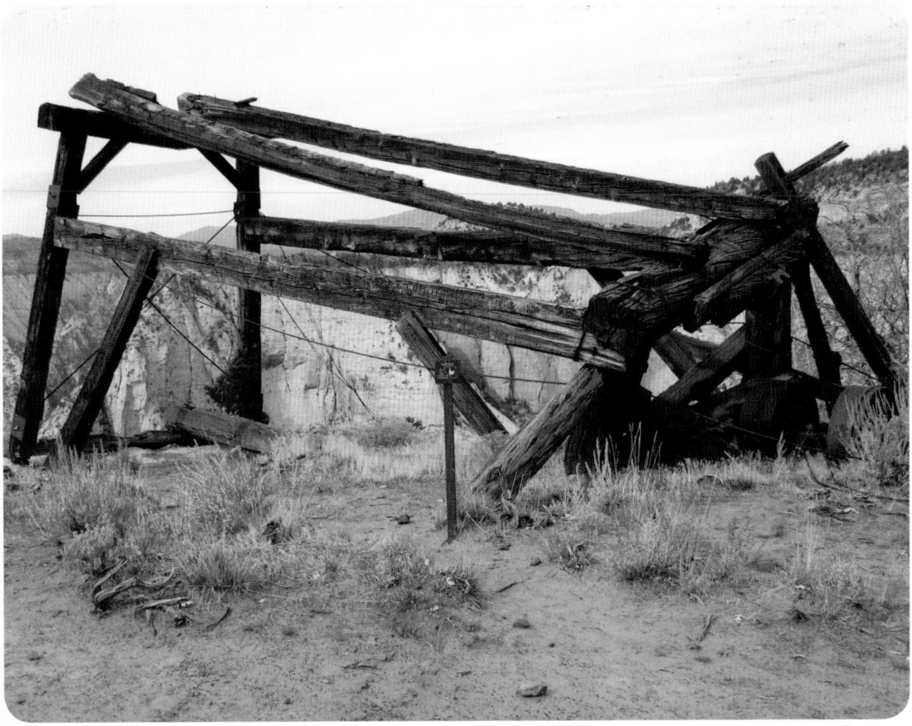

The headframe of the cableworks that once transported lumber from the East Rim Plateau to the floor of Zion Canyon

Junction. Turn north here and continue 4.6 mi (7.4 km) to the Weeping Rock parking lot, on the right, at 4360 ft (1330 m).

ON FOOT

Depart the southwest corner of the paved parking lot. Follow the trail south across the bridged creek. Ignore the left spur to weeping rock; you'll see it soon, from above. Proceed straight.

The **East Rim trail**, actually a broad path, remains paved for a surprising distance. It curves left (east) and ascends steeply. The weeping rock is visible left. Switchbacks convey you up the canyon wall.

Within 20 minutes, at 4855 ft (1480 m), a right (west) spur leads 0.5 mi (0.8 km) into Hidden Canyon. Proceed straight (east) on the main trail, ascending through **Echo Canyon** beneath Cable Mtn (right/south).

About 40 minutes along, at 5205 ft (1587 m), the trail curves right (southeast) into a narrow, sheer-walled defile. Pavement briefly ends here. Proceed on sand, then slickrock, then on a rocky wash bottom. Ascend the slickrock ledge on the left. Pavement soon resumes.

At 2.1 mi (3.4 km), 5592 ft (1705 m), about an hour from the trailhead, reach a **signed fork**. The paved path straight (northeast) ascends out of Echo Canyon to Observation Point, farther northwest. The narrow, rocky trail descending right (east-southeast) leads to Cable Mtn, Zion Park's east entrance, and Deertrap Mtn. Go right.

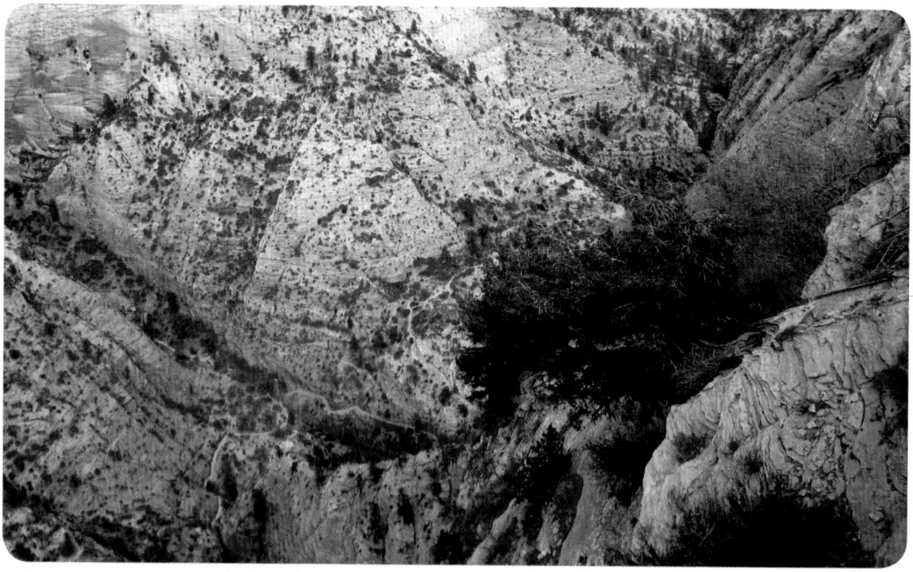

Echo Canyon trail, from Cable Mountain

For the next ten minutes, the way forward is obscure. This section is a **slickrock route**, not a trail. And it's loopy—winding in all directions, even north, as it skirts washes. So concentration is necessary here. Watch for the infrequent cairns and perhaps bootprints in the few patches of dirt.

Defined trail soon resumes, ascending steeply south. Attain views right (east) into the canyon you've ascended, and beyond to the west rim.

About 1¼ hours along, at 6350 ft (1936 m), the trail levels. This sandy stretch among P-J (piñon and juniper) is near the edge of an Echo Canyon tributary drainage. It's apparent you've arrived atop a **mesa**. After the canyon pinches out, proceed across a sage-covered flat.

Twenty minutes farther, reach a **signed T-junction** at 4.4 mi (7.1 mi), 6380 ft (1945 m). Left (northeast) ends in 0.3 mi (0.5 km) at a dirt road. Go right (south) on the trail signed for the park's east entrance (5.5 mi) and Cable Mtn (3.3 mi).

Five minutes farther, or about 1¾ hours from the trailhead, reach a **fork** at 4.8 mi (7.8 mi), 6430 ft (1960 m). Left (southeast), the East Rim trail continues 150 yd (137 m) to Stave Spring and 5.7 mi (9.2 km) across the mesa to the park's east entrance on Hwy 9. Go right (south-southwest) for Cable Mtn.

The hiking is now easy, the grade gentle, the trail well defined. Take advantage of it, and speed through this dull stretch made grim by a recent fire. The only scenery—the pink sandstone of Bryce Canyon National Park on the north horizon—is too distant to be compelling.

About 20 minutes farther, reach a **junction** at 5.9 mi (9.5 km), 6810 ft (2076 m). Left (southwest) leads to Deertrap Mtn. Go right (west-northwest) for Cable Mtn.

Within 15 minutes, top out at 6910 ft (2107 m). The view extends across Zion Canyon but remains unimpressive. A gradual descent ends at 7.7 mi (12.4 km), 6496 ft (1980 m), on the **canyon rim**. Suddenly, the view *is* impressive, indeed heart-stopping if you peer over edge. The wooden structure that stands here is, of course, the headframe of the cableworks that once transported lumber down to the Virgin River below.

TRIP 8

ZION NARROWS

LOCATION	North Fork Virgin River, upper Zion Canyon, Zion National Park
ROUND TRIP	6 mi (9.7 km) to Orderville Canyon 10 mi (16 km) to Big Spring
ELEVATION GAIN	200 ft (61 m) to Orderville Canyon 480 ft (146 m) to Big Spring
KEY ELEVATIONS	trailhead 4420 ft (1348 m) Orderville Canyon 4620 ft (1409 m) Big Spring 4900 ft (1494 m)
HIKING TIME	4 to 8 hours
DIFFICULTY	challenging
MAP	Trails Illustrated *Zion National Park*

OPINION

Zion National Park has the densest concentration of slot canyons in the world. If the park's topography were flattened, the surface area would blanket a third of Utah. And the most famous slot in this slot-haven is upper Zion Canyon, where the Virgin River's north fork has slashed an especially long, penetrating defile whose crux—known as the *Zion Narrows*—is the state's most famous hiking destination.

What it's best known as, however, is either a backpack trip or a brief stroll. We recommend neither.

Backpackers start at Chamberlain's Ranch, hike downstream, spend one night in the canyon, then exit at Temple of Sinawava. The trip requires you to make reservations, obtain a permit, and arrange a shuttle. And because the hike is largely *in* the river—wading on slippery rocks you can't see, and occasionally swimming across deep pools—a full pack is more burden than usual.

Strollers start at Temple of Sinawava, follow a short, paved path upstream, then about face. They see little of the canyon but gain new insight into mass human migrations because the strollers can number a thousand a day.

Instead of backpacking or strolling, we suggest an ambitious dayhike. Start at Temple of Sinawava, surge past the strollers, splash into the river, hike all the way through the narrows, then return, ultimately spending more time in the canyon's most spectacular hallways than the backpackers do, and concentrating on the magnificence of it all rather than on transporting your cargo through it.

Those words—*spectacular* and *magnificent*—tend to be overkill, but here they're inadequate. In Zion Canyon's upper reaches, the sandstone walls are red, buff, gold, black, streaked with charcoal desert varnish, and tall as skyscrapers. They rise 1000 to 1700 ft (305 to 518 m) above the river but are so vertical, no matter how long you crane your neck and how intently you stare, you can only guess where they meet the sky.

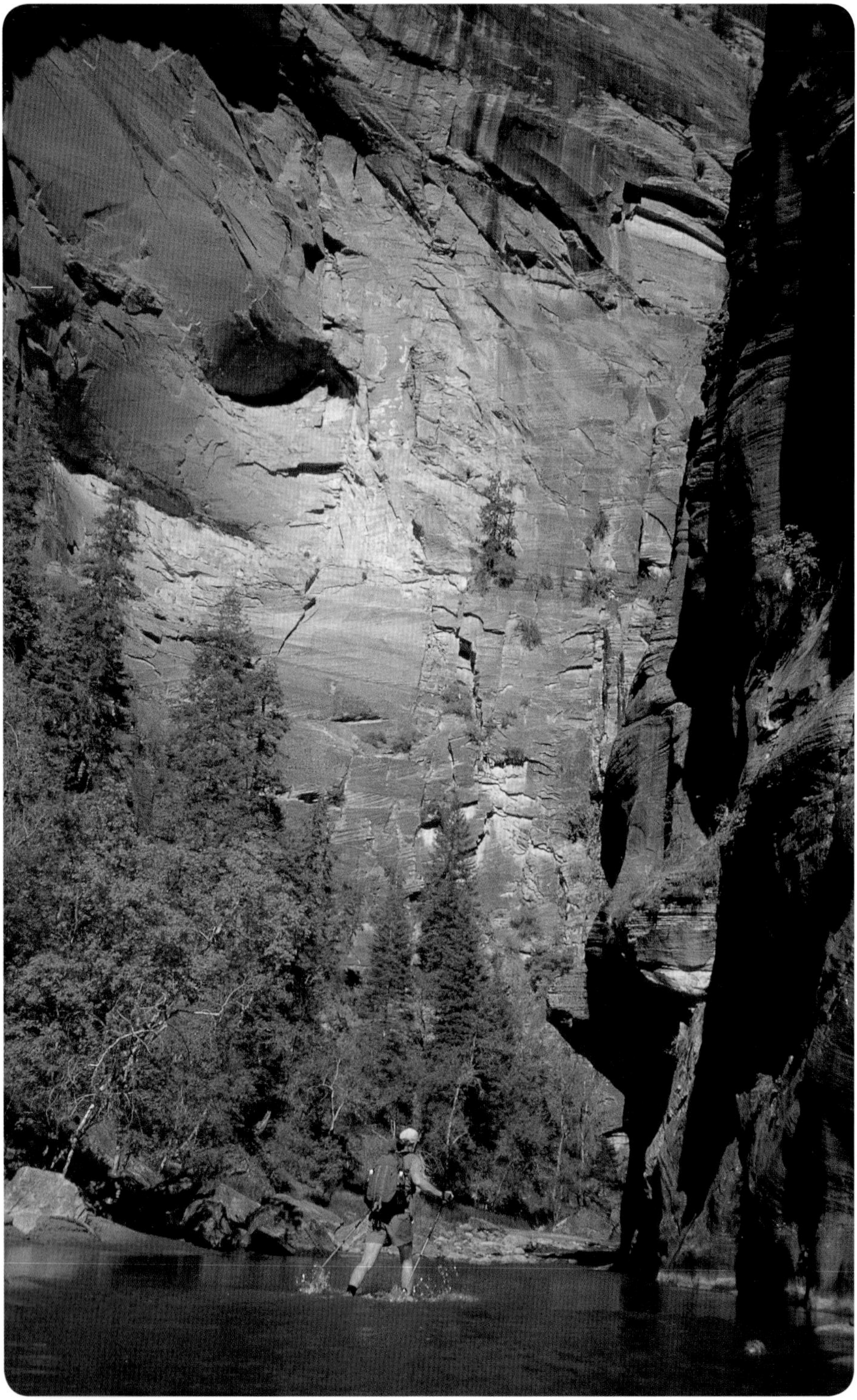

Zion Canyon Narrows

At Temple of Sinawava, the canyon is already quite narrow: a mere 200 yd (183 m) wide. A mile upstream, the walls are so close that the river covers the canyon floor. Two miles farther, the canyon narrows to just 20 ft (6 m).

The depth and slenderness of the Zion Narrows keeps sunlight a stranger. Dark + wet = cold. It's as if you're hiking through the veins of the earth, and she's not maternal after all. She's not even warm blooded. It might be discomfiting, but it's certainly fascinating.

Though you'll soon leave the tourist hordes behind, you'll likely be among dayhikers until you pass Orderville Canyon, where the majority turn around. Instead of solitude, you get to see others relishing the unique experience. Enjoy it. Sharing the canyon can be a hoot.

At 3 mi (4.8 km), Orderville Canyon is a reasonable, rewarding goal for intermediate dayhikers. But if you're fit, keen and experienced, aim for Big Spring, at 5 mi (8 km). It's at the far end of the narrows, so you'll see the climactic section of the canyon twice and will almost certainly be alone some of the time.

Trudging upstream, however, is slower and more tiring than walking a trail. When the river's low (which is the only time you should hike here) it's about 6 inches (2.4 cm) deep for much of its length. Some sections might be knee deep. The occasional hole is waist deep. A few chest-deep pools require you to swim 50 ft (15 m).

So be flexible. The time to turn around is whenever you feel you've had enough yet it's still fun.

FACT

BEFORE YOUR TRIP

Be aware that the Virgin River's north fork drains several hundred square miles of canyon country. Rain can raise the water level several feet within minutes. Hike here only during a period of sunny weather, when there's little risk of a flashflood.

Plan your Zion Narrows hike for late June, or between late September and early October. That's when the river tends to be lowest, the water temperature reasonably warm, and thunderstorms least likely.

A backcountry permit is not required to dayhike upstream from Temple of Sinawava into the Zion Narrows and back. But it's wise to visit the Zion Canyon visitor center, ask about the river's current depth, and check the weather forecast.

You'll be in the river constantly, so wear amphibious boots. Those designed specifically for hiking in water are ideal, but a sturdy pair of fabric hiking boots you don't mind dunking are fine too. Wear insulating neoprene socks to keep your feet warm. Leave your sandals behind; they lack sufficient ankle support and allow pebbles to lodge beneath your feet.

Pack extra layers of warm clothing (tights, pullover, gloves, hat) that insulate even when wet. But try to keep them dry by putting them in plastic bags or a waterproof stuffsack. An ultralight towel is handy for drying off at rest stops.

Carry trekking poles. They'll help you stay upright when entering and

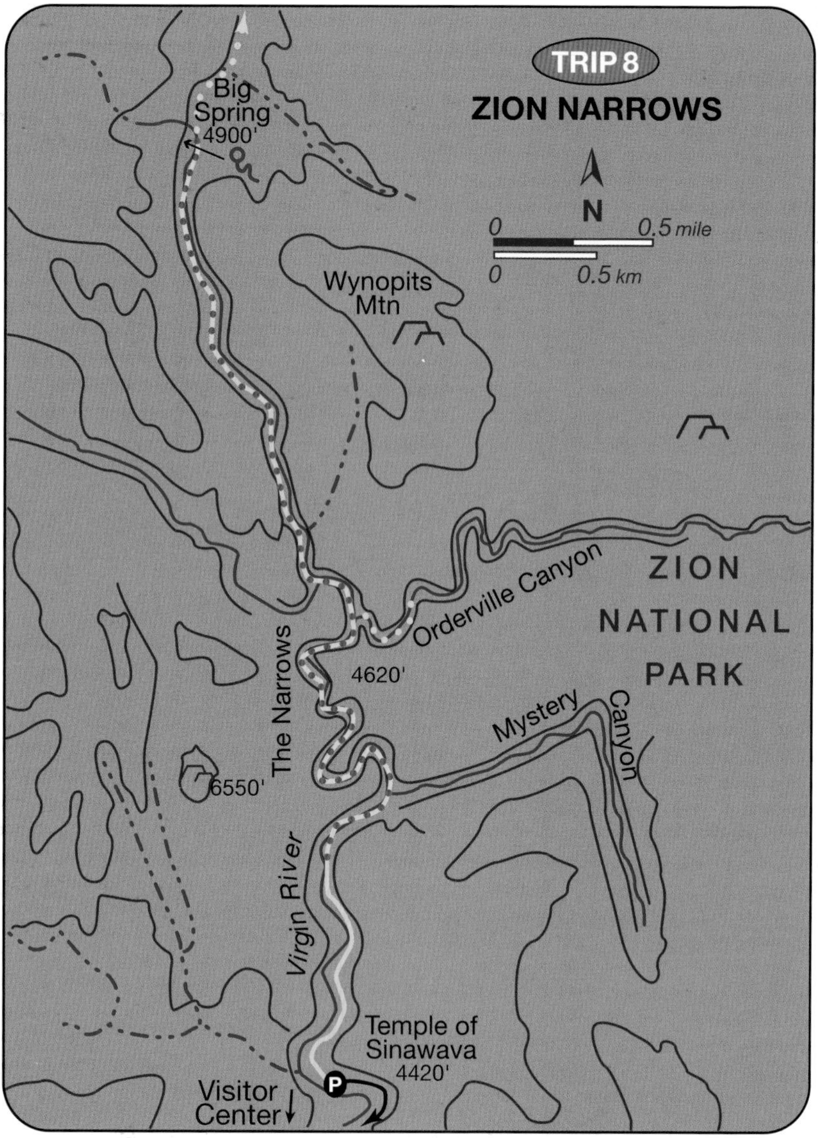

exiting the water, wading along the rocky riverbed, or fighting the current.

Bring a means of purifying or filtering water. The Virgin River is not safe to drink.

BY VEHICLE

Early April through Late October

Private vehicles are *not* allowed north of Canyon Junction on Zion Canyon Scenic Drive. Access is by shuttle bus only, but you can ride it free of charge. So, after driving Hwy 9 through Zion's south or east entrances, continue to the visitor center near the south entrance. Park here and catch the shuttle bus that stops at all the Zion Canyon trailheads. It runs daily, 8 a.m. to 6 p.m. Get off at road's end, in

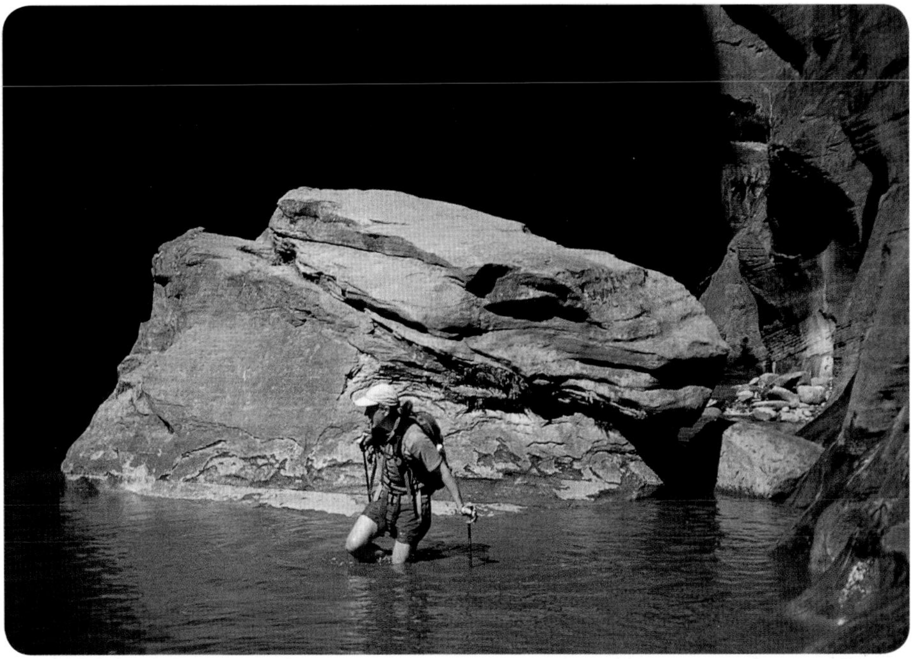

Zion Canyon's deepest, narrowest section, north of Orderville Canyon

the Temple of Sinawava trailhead parking lot. Elevation: 4420 ft (1348 m).

Late October through Early April

Private vehicles *are* allowed north of Canyon Junction on Zion Canyon Scenic Drive. So, after driving Hwy 9 through Zion's south or east entrances, proceed to Canyon Junction. Turn north here and continue 6.2 mi (10 km) to the Temple of Sinawava trailhead parking lot at road's end. Elevation: 4420 ft (1348 m).

ON FOOT

Follow the paved path upstream, generally north, along the right (east) bank of the Virgin River's north fork.

At 1 mi (1.6 km) the **paved path ends**. Enter the river and proceed upstream.

Where benches allow, it's possible to speed your progress by walking on dry ground, but these opportunities diminish the farther north you go.

Pass 100-ft (305-m) **Mystery Falls** (right / east) at 1.5 mi (2.4 km).

At 3 mi (4.8 km), 4620 ft (1409 m), reach **Orderville Canyon** (right / east), which is often dry.

Ahead is Zion Canyon's deepest, narrowest section. It remains constricted for nearly 2 mi (3.2 mi), then relents and occasionally broadens.

If you're comfortable and have sufficient time, continue at least another 0.5 mi (0.9 km) into the narrows. But expect to swim through a few chest-deep pools.

At 3.4 mi (5.5 km) pass **Imlay Canyon** (left / southwest).

Reach **Big Spring** at 5 mi (8 km), 4900 ft (1494 m). It gushes out of the left (west) canyon wall about 10 ft (3 m) above the river. All dayhikers should turn around here, at the end of the narrows.

TRIP 9

THE WAVE

LOCATION	Coyote Buttes North, Paria Canyon / Vermilion Cliffs Wilderness, between Kanab UT and Page AZ
ROUND TRIP	6 mi (9.6 km)
ELEVATION GAIN	300 ft (91 m)
KEY ELEVATIONS	trailhead 4900 ft (1494 m), the Wave 5200 ft (1585 m)
HIKING TIME	2 to 3 hours
DIFFICULTY	moderate (due only to navigation)
MAP	*Coyote Buttes* (free, available at BLM Kanab field office and BLM Paria River contact station)

OPINION

Long ago near Escalante we met a desert rat—a man who'd spent much of his life exploring Utah canyon country. We were headed in the same direction, so we hiked together. Near day's end he tantalized us with a secret.

"I know a magical place in the desert that I bet you haven't been to," he said.

"Where?" we asked.

"I'd tell you..." he hesitated, "but I don't know if you're strong enough for it."

We glanced at each other in disbelief. We were fleet, tireless. Surely he'd noticed. We'd just spent the day hiking cross-country with him. If he thought we were wimps...

"You mean physically?" we asked.

"No," he said. "I mean deeper strength. It's a powerful place. A spiritual place."

Instantly we were compelled to go there, wherever it was, and determined to prove ourselves strong enough, whatever that meant. But apparently we wouldn't get the chance, because he thought us unworthy.

We'd enjoyed a vigorous, harmonious day together, but it seemed to be ending in a strange and disappointing way.

It was nearly dark when we reached our vehicles. That's when he turned to us, smiled, and quietly said "Coyote Buttes."

"Coyote Buttes?" we asked. "That's the place?"

"Yup," he said.

"But why didn't you think we were strong enough for it?" we asked.

"Strong enough to leave once you've seen it," he clarified. "Because it's so beautiful. Getting there isn't hard, if you know how to find it. But leaving? That's tough."

Brief, sketchy, verbal directions to Coyote Buttes were his parting gift to us.

It truly was a gift, we soon discovered, because Coyote Buttes was sublime yet remained a secret: slowly passed along by word of mouth between canyon-country aficionados.

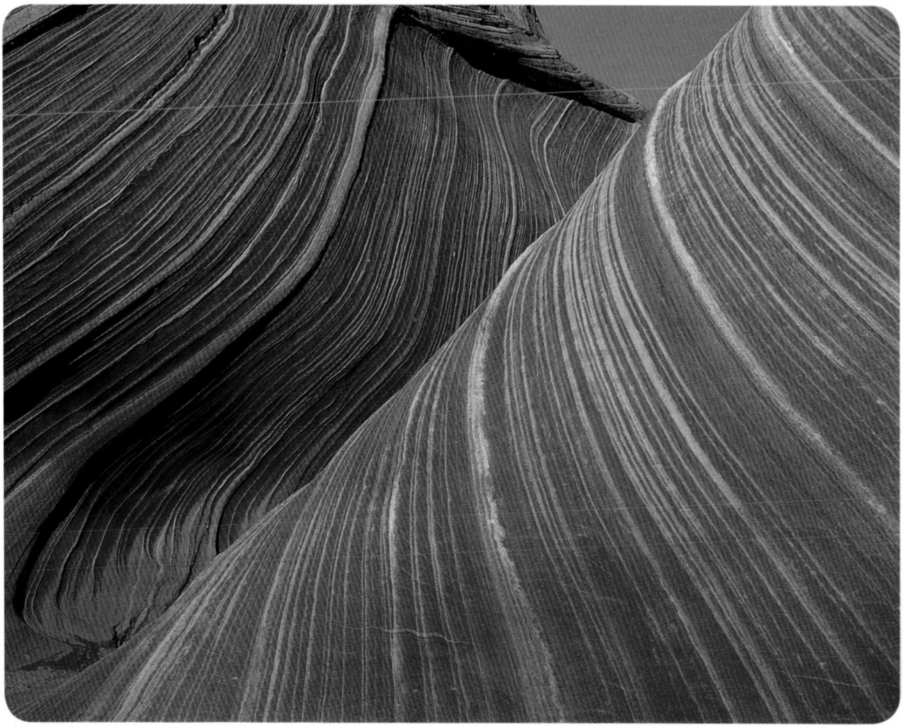

The Wave

Coyote Buttes is still sublime. But no longer is it a secret. Soon after we learned about it, a photograph of the Wave—the most visually distinct feature in the Coyote Buttes area—was published in a German calendar.

That single image inspired thousands of Europeans to seek out the previously little-known landmark. The Wave became world famous. Hundreds of photos of it have been published. Countless pilgrims have journeyed to see it, starting in Utah then nipping over the border into Arizona.

The Wave's immense popularity forced the Bureau of Land Management (BLM) to restrict access. Only 20 hikers per day are now allowed to visit the Wave, and each must have a permit.

The process of obtaining a permit is described below. It's discouraging, but don't let it prevent you from hiking here. Restricted access has proven to be a necessary and effective means of protecting Coyote Buttes from overuse and ensuring hikers can appreciate the Wave in relative serenity.

You are, after all, coming here to admire art. The purpose of art, whether created by man or nature, is to open a door to the unknown. And it's difficult, perhaps impossible, to step through that door—to contemplate the unknown—in a clamorous atmosphere.

Because you won't be pushed by a crowd, and because the hike itself is fairly short, you'll have opportunity to sit, gaze and absorb the essence of this unique, Navajo sandstone masterwork. Not the geological explanation, which would be like analyzing Monet's brush technique, but the overall effect, the inspiration it holds for you.

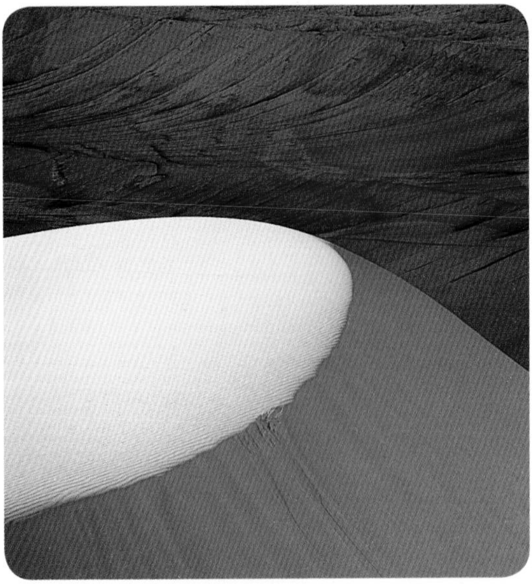

Sand dune in North Coyote Buttes

Be patient. Relax. Let go of judgment. Empty yourself of thought. Observe without question or conclusion. Surrounding you is sacred art sculpted over eons by creation itself. Commune with it rather than critique it.

Then move on. Don't limit yourself to this arresting sight. Keep exploring. The Wave is but one aspect of Coyote Buttes. Wandering beyond the Wave will reveal marvels few Wave worshippers ever see.

FACT

BEFORE YOUR TRIP

You must get a permit to dayhike to the Wave. The Bureau of Land Management (BLM) issues only 20 permits per day. Each permit allows just one person to enter the area, so you'll need a permit for each member of your group. Of course there's also a per-person, per-day, permit fee.

Half the permits (ten per day) are available for reservation. Visit www.blm.gov/az/asfo/paria/coyote_buttes/trails.htm to check availability and make reservations up to four months in advance. Reserving a permit for spring (April, May) or fall (September, October) is difficult because demand is high.

The rest of the permits (ten per day) are assigned by lottery, one day in advance, to hikers who show up in person by 8:30 a.m. Between mid-March and mid-November, go to the BLM Paria River contact station on Hwy 89. Open daily, it's 42.2 mi (68 km) east of Kanab, or 13.5 mi (21.7 km) west of Big Water. Between mid-November and mid-March, go to the BLM Kanab field office (435-644-1200), at 318 North First East. Open weekdays only, it issues permits for Saturday, Sunday and Monday on the previous Friday.

Only one person per group may enter the lottery. If your name is chosen in the draw, you'll get permits for your entire group—assuming that many permits remain available.

If you win a permit in the lottery, it will allow you to hike to the Wave the following day. So you'll have to wait one day. Spend it hiking to Buckskin Gulch via Wire Pass (Trip 10), which begins at the same trailhead. The optimal place to stay the night before hiking to the Wave is Stateline campground, just south of the trailhead.

The self-registration day-use permits available at the trailhead are valid only for Wire Pass, Buckskin Gulch, and Paria Canyon. The only way to obtain a permit for the Wave is by advance reservation or in the daily lottery.

The BLM allows you to bring your dog to the Wave but charges an additional day-use fee for the privilege and requires you to keep your pet leashed.

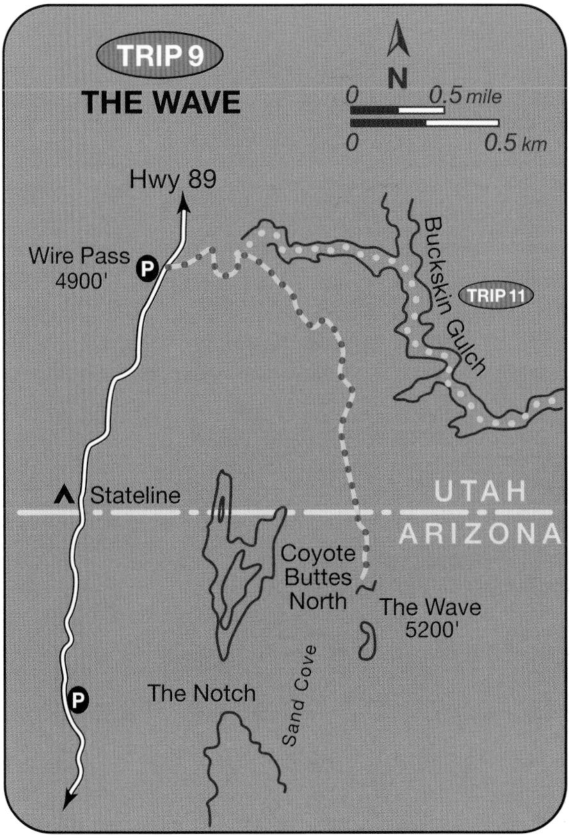

If rain is imminent, alter your plans. The road to Wire Pass trailhead can become impassable when wet, making a mockery of your 4WD vehicle's vaunted capabilities.

BY VEHICLE

From the Grand Staircase-Escalante National Monument visitor center at the east edge of Kanab, drive Hwy 89 east 37.4 mi (60.2 km).

From the Grand Staircase-Escalante National Monument visitor center in Big Water, drive Hwy 89 west 18.3 mi (29.5 km).

From either approach, turn south onto unpaved **House Rock Valley Road**. It's at a hairpin turn, immediately west of the Cockscomb, between mileposts 25 and 26. Reset your trip odometer to 0.

At 4.3 mi (6.9 km) pass Buckskin wash. At 8.3 mi (13.4 km) reach **Wire Pass trailhead**. Park here, on the right (west), at 4900 ft (1494 m). Stateline campground is at 9.3 mi (15 km). If it's full, camping is allowed at Wire Pass trailhead.

ON FOOT

Go northeast across the road to the trailhead register. Proceed through a hiker's maze, which allows people but not cows to pass through the fence.

Follow the signed trail into the **wash**. In ten minutes reach a signed fork. Left (north) continues in the wash, through Wire Pass (Trip 10) to Buckskin

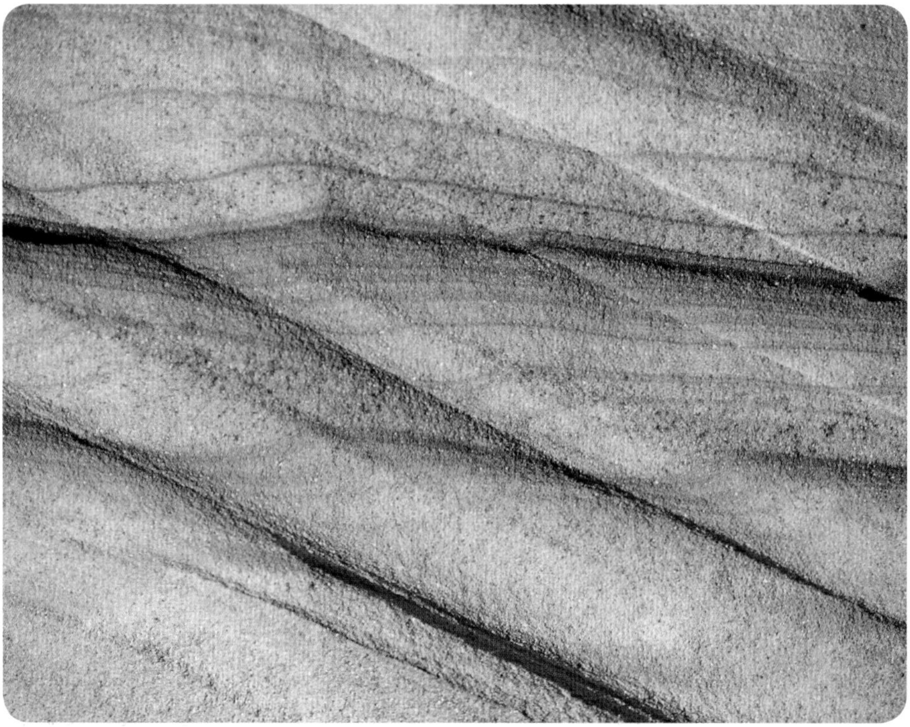

Navajo sandstone

Gulch. For Coyote Buttes, ascend right (east) onto a sandy, former road now serving as a trail.

Follow the road/trail to dry **Bull Pasture Reservoir** at 1.2 mi (1.9 km). Go left (east) on a bootbeaten path. About 50 yd/m farther ascend on slickrock through a shallow V.

From this point on, there is no trail. You're navigating cross-country. Turn right and begin contouring due south near 5000 ft (1524 m). Your general direction of travel will remain south to the Wave.

Don't drift left (downslope). Don't wander southeast toward the buttes on the distinctly smoother ridge. Upon broaching the next ridge, proceed south toward the two conical buttes.

A **vertical crack** is visible in the dominant sandstone massif directly south. Aim for it. Traverse left of and just beneath a swirled, multi-hued knob (yellow, salmon, beige, mauve).

Drop onto sand. Ten minutes farther, cross a wash. Ascend a steep slickrock gully toward the vertical crack. Don't veer left (east-southeast) toward the chocolate drops.

See the saddle left of the ridge? Cross it on the north side. Don't descend. Stay on the back of the ridge, contouring south. Don't drift southeast toward the Teepees.

Two slickrock cones, known as *the Center of the Universe*, are visible ahead. Cross the base of these cones. Enter **the Wave** at 3 mi (4.8 km), 5200 ft (1585 m). Freelance exploration is fruitful beyond.

TRIP 10

WIRE PASS

LOCATION	Paria Canyon / Vermilion Cliffs Wilderness between Kanab UT and Page AZ
ROUND TRIP	3.4 mi (5.5 km) to Wire Pass / Buckskin Gulch confluence
ELEVATION CHANGE	170-ft (52-m) loss and gain
KEY ELEVATIONS	Wire Pass trailhead 4900 ft (1494 m) confluence 4730 ft (1442 m)
HIKING TIME	1½ to 2 hours, or more for Buckskin
DIFFICULTY	easy
MAP	*Hiker's Guide to Paria Canyon* (free, available at BLM Paria River contact station)

OPINION

Americans are habitual drivers. Many don't even think of walking as an alternative, unless forced to do so by a dead battery or flat tire. Walking might be safer, healthier, cleaner, more enjoyable, even faster, yet they'll drive instead. Fifty percent of the time they get behind the wheel, they travel less than three miles.

That's about the distance you'll hike on a round trip from Wire Pass to Buckskin Gulch, where you'll peek into the longest, narrowest canyon on earth and glimpse the abyss separating you from those who flaunt "America, love it or leave it" bumper stickers yet will never truly know or appreciate their country because doing so would require them to walk.

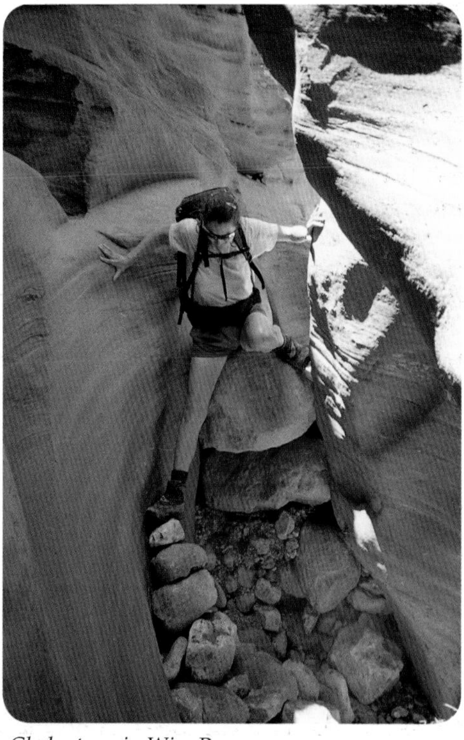

Chokestone in Wire Pass

Typically, a *pass* is a cleft among mountains. Wire Pass, however, is a gorge cut by Coyote Wash through the Cockscomb—the ridge of steeply tilted Navajo sandstone bisecting Hwy 89.

Initially unpromising—broad, shallow—Wire Pass quickly slots up. In places, the walls are shoulder width apart. Log jams high overhead attest to the power and volume of flash floods, though the wash bottom remains dry except during or immediately after a rain.

Slither through Wire Pass and you'll soon arrive at its confluence with Buckskin Gulch (Trip 11)—the most famous slot in slot-canyon

Buckskin Gulch, near Wire Pass confluence

country. Though Buckskin never constricts quite like Wire Pass, it's astonishingly narrow, much deeper, and far longer.

Hiking the length of Buckskin is a demanding backpack trip (skip below for details) but probing it on a dayhike, either upstream or down, is easy—*if* you bring sandals or wear boots you don't mind getting wet, because you'll soon encounter pools that require wading.

If you're in the Kanab area with a day at your disposal before hiking to the Wave (Trip 9) or down Paria Canyon (Trip 12), Wire Pass is a convenient place to invest your anticipatory energy.

FACT

BEFORE YOUR TRIP

Get a current weather report in Kanab, either at the BLM field office (318 North First East) or the Grand Staircase-Escalante National Monument visitor center (east edge of town). If driving Hwy 89 northwest from Page, Arizona, get a current weather report at the Grand Staircase-Escalante National Monument visitor center in Big Water, or 13.5 mi (21.7 km) farther at the BLM Paria River contact station.

If rain is imminent, alter your plans. The road to the trailhead can become impassable when wet, making a mockery of your 4WD vehicle's vaunted capabilities. Even distant rain can cause a dangerous volume of water to suddenly rush through the drainage. Hike here only during a period of sunny weather, when there's little risk of a flash flood.

A day-use permit is necessary for each person hiking to Buckskin Gulch via Wire Pass. Register and pay at the trailhead.

BY VEHICLE

From the Grand Staircase-Escalante National Monument visitor center at the east edge of Kanab, drive Hwy 89 east 37.4 mi (60.2 km).

From the Grand Staircase-Escalante National Monument visitor center in Big Water, drive Hwy 89 west 18.3 mi (29.5 km).

From either approach, turn south onto unpaved **House Rock Valley Road**. It's at a hairpin turn, immediately west of the Cockscomb, between mileposts 25 and 26. Reset your trip odometer to 0.

Pass Buckskin wash at 4.3 mi (6.9 km). Reach **Wire Pass trailhead**, on the right (west), at 8.3 mi (13.4 km), 4900 ft (1494 m). Stateline campground is at 9.3 mi (15 km). If it's full, camping is allowed at Wire Pass trailhead.

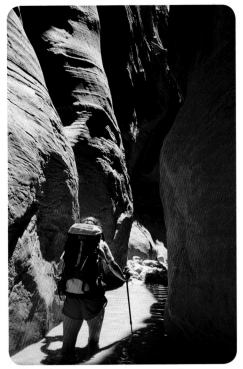

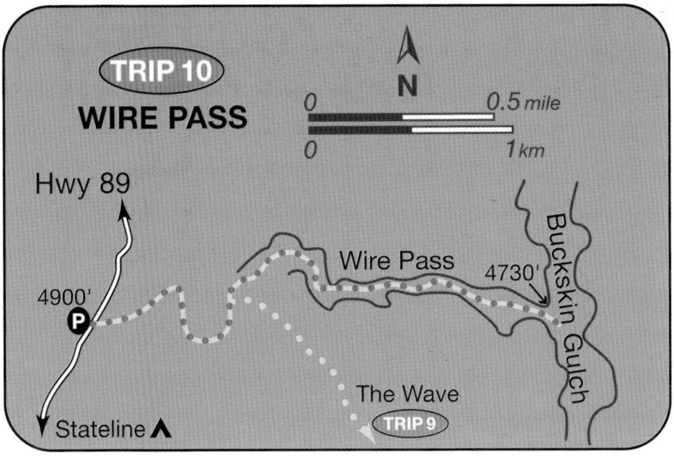

ON FOOT

Go northeast across the road to the trailhead register. Proceed through a hiker's maze, which allows people but not cows to pass through the fence.

Follow the signed trail into the **wash**. In ten minutes reach a signed fork. Right (east) ascends onto a sandy, former road and leads to The Wave (Trip 9) in Coyote Buttes. Go left (north) and continue down the wash. The crest of Coyote Buttes is soon visible right (south).

The wash drains generally east. Bound by sandy slopes and slickrock bluffs, it remains wide and shallow for 1.2 mi (1.9 km). Then, about 30 minutes from the trailhead, it narrows and deepens into a **slot**.

In the recent past, a chokestone required hikers to negotiate an 8-ft (2.5-m) drop, but like all canyon-country drainages this one is constantly changing. Precisely what you'll encounter depends on the severity of the last deluge and is therefore unpredictable.

After hiking about 45 minutes, intersect **Buckskin Gulch** at 1.7 mi (2.7 km), 4730 ft (1442 m). Immediately before the confluence, examine the right (south) wall for a petroglyph panel bearing several bighorn sheep.

Right (downstream), Buckskin Gulch leads 11.4 mi (18.4 km) generally southeast to Paria River Canyon, at 4180 ft (1274 m). Buckskin—the world's longest slot canyon—quickly narrows and deepens. The distance between the walls is often 12 to 15 ft (4 to 5 m) but occasionally constricts to just 3 ft (1 m). The depth of the gulch averages 100 to 200 ft (31 to 60 m) but is 300 to 500 ft (91 to 152 m) near the Paria confluence.

Fit, experienced backpackers hike the length of Buckskin Gulch in a single day, camp near the Paria confluence, then hike 7.2 mi (11.6 km) generally north to the White House trailhead, at 4280 ft (1305 m). It's an arduous journey. Class 4 downclimbing is necessary in one place, and numerous stagnant pools require wading or swimming. Pitching a tent in the gulch is difficult due to the rocky floor, and dangerous due to the constant threat of a flash flood. There's only one escape route—easily overlooked—on the left (northwest) at 8 mi (12.9 km).

Dayhikers, however, can venture downstream from the Wire Pass / Buckskin Gulch confluence, turning back as time dictates or when their energy or curiosity diminish. If you're soon deterred by a stagnant pool, try probing the gulch upstream instead; you'll find intriguing narrows there as well. After forays in either or both directions, retrace your steps to the trailhead through Wire Pass.

TRIP 11

BUCKSKIN GULCH

LOCATION	Paria Canyon / Vermilion Cliffs Wilderness between Kanab UT and Page AZ
DISTANCE	20.3 mi (32.7 km) one way
ELEVATION CHANGE	720-ft (219-m) loss, 100-ft (30-m) gain
KEY ELEVATIONS	Wire Pass trailhead 4900 ft (1494 m) Wire Pass / Buckskin Gulch confluence 4730 ft (1442 m) Buckskin Gulch / Paria Canyon confluence 4180 ft (1274 m) White House trailhead 4280 ft (1305 m)
HIKING TIME	11 hours or 2 days
DIFFICULTY	challenging
MAP	*Hiker's Guide to Paria Canyon* (free, available at BLM Paria River contact station)

OPINION

Canyons are like people. Both are more interesting when scoured to their essence. And the most thoroughly scoured canyon on our planet is Buckskin Gulch.

It's a slot. The longest, narrowest slot of all. A serpentine hallway with walls of solid stone and a floor strewn with boulders. In places, not even a sliver of sky is visible above.

Little sun penetrates, so as flashfoods continue sculpting this unique passage, they leave stagnant pools that rarely evaporate. They're frigid, putrid, and hikers must wade or swim through them.

A thunderstorm as far away as Bryce can quickly fill Buckskin with a torrent 50 ft (15 m) deep, so camping inside the gulch is suicidal. You must either barrel through it *and* Paria Canyon Narrows in a single day, or carry a full pack and pitch your tent at the east end of the gulch, near the Buckskin/Paria confluence.

Both options are challenging because the distance is long, the terrain rough, and, despite all this talk of water, you'll find none that's potable in Buckskin.

Yet both options are desirable, too. Flash Buckskin in a single push and you'll be exhilarated for days. Backpack it, and you'll sacrifice the thrill of traveling fast and working without a net, but you'll enjoy the heady experience of sleeping in the tight embrace of mother Earth.

Wondering if Buckskin Gulch will be to your liking? Probe its west end on a short dayhike through Wire Pass (Trip 10). Wishing you could hike Buckskin without enduring those creature-from-the-black-lagoon pools? It's possible.

In the spring of 2002, we hiked Buckskin Gulch when it was completely dry. We were lucky. We drove there assuming the conditions would be typical. Only when we picked up our permits did we learn we wouldn't be getting wet.

Either way, dry or wet, expect friction between you and the walls of Buckskin Gulch as you pass between them. It probably won't be evident at the time. You might not be aware of it until much later. But adventures like this are the kind that scour you down to your essence.

FACT

BEFORE YOUR TRIP

Get a current weather report in Kanab, either at the BLM field office (318 North First East) or the Grand Staircase-Escalante National Monument visitor center (east edge of town). If driving Hwy 89 northwest from Page, Arizona, get a current weather report at the Grand Staircase-Escalante National Monument visitor center in Big Water, or 13.5 mi (21.7 km) farther at the BLM Paria River contact station.

If rain is imminent, alter your plans. The road to Wire Pass trailhead can become impassable when wet, making a mockery of your 4WD vehicle's vaunted capabilities. Even distant rain can cause a dangerous volume of water to suddenly rush through Buckskin Gulch. Hike here only during a period of sunny weather, when there's little risk of a flashflood.

You're dayhiking through Buckskin Gulch? Each person in your group must have a day-use permit. Register and pay at Wire Pass trailhead.

You're backpacking through Buckskin Gulch? Each person in your group must have an overnight permit in advance. The BLM allows only 20 backpackers per day to enter Paria Canyon. Visit www.blm.gov/az/asfo/paria/wilderness.htm to check availability, make reservations, or learn about obtaining a permit in person at the BLM Paria River contact station (see *By Vehicle / White House trailhead* below).

Complete all your trip preparations the day before you begin hiking. An early start is essential to ensure you reach your goal by nightfall: White House trailhead if dayhiking, the Paria confluence if backpacking. Pitching a tent in the gulch is difficult due to the rocky floor, and dangerous due to the constant threat of a flashflood. There's only one escape route—easily overlooked—on the left (northwest) at 8 mi (12.9 km).

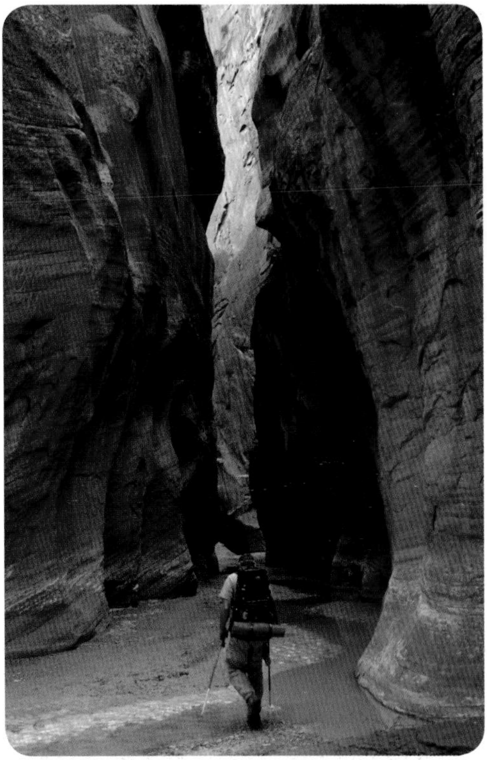

Buckskin Gulch, near Paria River confluence

Pack all the water you'll need for the long, arduous hike through Buckskin Gulch, because you'll find no fresh-water source until reaching the perennial stream within 0.5 mi (0.8 km) of Paria Canyon. The stagnant pools en route are a health hazard. Even the stream water is unsafe unless filtered or purified. Because the Paria River is turbid and mineral-laden, fill your water bottles from the stream before hiking out to White House trailhead.

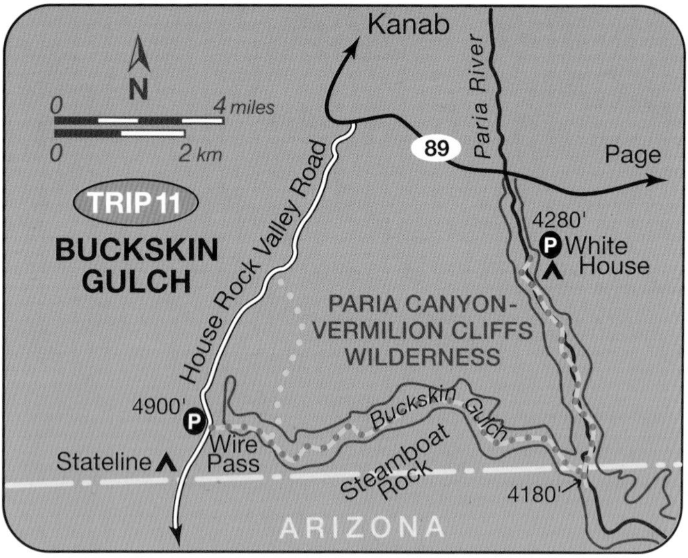

Buckskin Gulch is a bouldery morass. For stability, wear sturdy boots, not sandals, and carry two trekking poles. Bring a reliable rope for negotiating the 18-ft (5.5-m) Class 4 downclimb. Neoprene socks will insulate your feet when wading the frigid pools. If they're deep enough to require swimming, you'll appreciate having a means of floating your pack.

Bear in mind that Buckskin Gulch, like all canyon-country drainages, is constantly changing. Precisely what you'll encounter depends on the severity of the last deluge and is therefore unpredictable.

BY VEHICLE

White House trailhead

From the Grand Staircase-Escalante National Monument visitor center at the east edge of Kanab, drive Hwy 89 east 42.2 mi (68 km).

From the Grand Staircase-Escalante National Monument visitor center in Big Water, drive Hwy 89 west 13.5 mi (21.7 km).

From either approach, turn south onto unpaved **White House Road**, between mileposts 20 and 21.

Stop just ahead at the **BLM Paria River contact station** to get your permit. Then proceed south 1.8 mi (2.9 km) to **White House trailhead** and campground at road's end. Elevation: 4280 ft (1305 m). Leave your shuttle vehicle here, where the one-way hike ends.

Wire Pass trailhead

From the Grand Staircase-Escalante National Monument visitor center at the east edge of Kanab, drive Hwy 89 east 37.4 mi (60.2 km).

From the Grand Staircase-Escalante National Monument visitor center in Big Water, drive Hwy 89 west 18.3 mi (29.5 km).

From either approach, turn south onto unpaved **House Rock Valley Road**. It's at a hairpin turn, immediately west of the Cockscomb, between mileposts 25 and 26. Reset your trip odometer to 0.

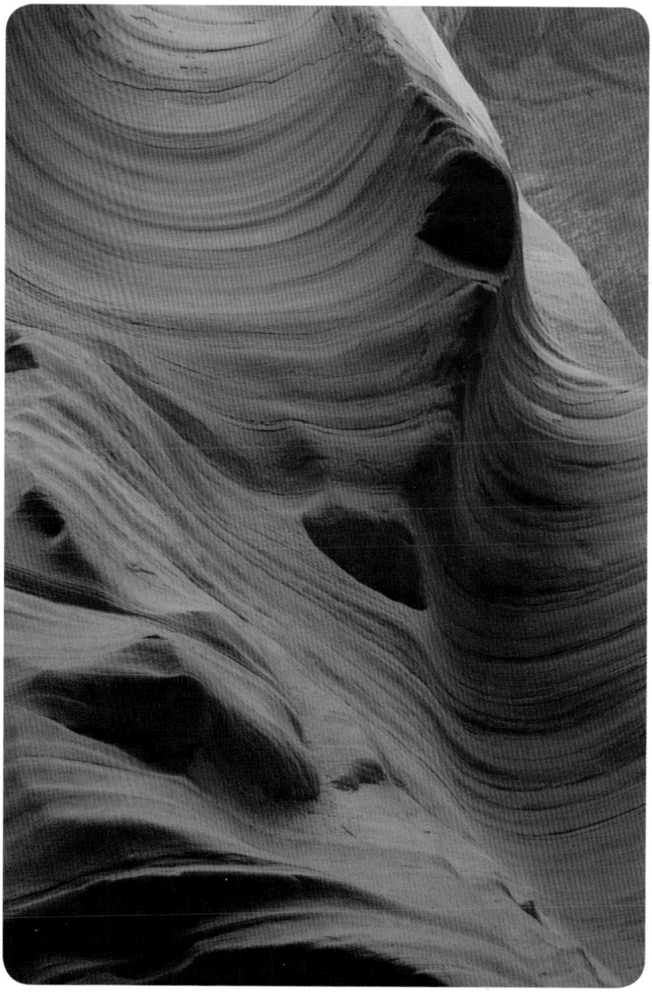

Buckskin Gulch

Pass Buckskin wash at 4.3 mi (6.9 km). Reach **Wire Pass trailhead**, on the right (west), at 8.3 mi (13.4 km), 4900 ft (1494 m). Begin hiking here.

Stateline campground is at 9.3 mi (15 km). If it's full, camping is allowed at Wire Pass trailhead.

ON FOOT

Go northeast across the road to the trailhead register. Proceed through a hiker's maze, which allows people but not cows to pass through the fence.

Follow the signed trail into the **wash**. In ten minutes reach a signed fork. Right (east) ascends onto a sandy, former road and leads to The Wave (Trip 9) in Coyote Buttes. Go left (north) and continue down the wash. The crest of Coyote Buttes is soon visible right (south).

The wash drains generally east. Bound by sandy slopes and slickrock bluffs, it remains wide and shallow for 1.2 mi (1.9 km). Then, about 30 minutes from the trailhead, it narrows and deepens into a **slot**.

In the recent past, a chokestone required hikers to negotiate an 8-ft (2.5-m) drop, but slot canyons can change dramatically with each flood. You can hope conditions have improved, but it's wise to assume they've worsened.

After hiking about 45 minutes, intersect **Buckskin Gulch** at 1.7 mi (2.7 km), 4730 ft (1442 m). Immediately before the confluence, examine the right (south) wall for a petroglyph panel bearing several bighorn sheep.

Right (downstream), Buckskin Gulch leads 11.4 mi (18.4 km) generally southeast to Paria River Canyon, at 4180 ft (1274 m). Buckskin quickly narrows and deepens below the Wire Pass confluence. The distance between the walls is often 12 to 15 ft (4 to 5 m) but occasionally constricts to just 3 ft (1 m). The depth of the gulch averages 100 to 200 ft (31 to 60 m) but is 300 to 500 ft (91 to 152 m) near the Paria confluence.

There are no routefinding challenges in the Gulch. Just follow the tortuous hallway down-canyon, generally east.

After hiking 8 mi (12.9 km) from Wire Pass trailhead, watch left (northwest) for **Middle Route**—a sandy crack, 30 ft (9 m) wide, where it's possible to scramble out of the gulch in case of emergency. Other than the two ends of the gulch, this is the only exit, and unless you're a skillful scrambler or high on adrenaline you'll find it hazardous.

About 11.5 mi (18.5 km) from the trailhead, reach a **boulder jam**. Expect an 18-ft (5.5-m) Class 4 downclimb here. Take time to evaluate the options before choosing the route you're most comfortable with.

At 12.5 mi (20.1 km) sandy benches on both walls used to offer campsites. Flooding washed them away. Trees and vegetation welcome you to habitable terrain. A perennial stream appears near here. Finally, you can refill your bottles and, after filtering or purifying the water, slake your thirst.

Intersect Paria River Canyon at 13.1 mi (21.1 km), 4180 ft (1274 m). If dayhiking, turn left (north) and proceed upstream. If backpacking, turn right (south) and proceed downstream. You might have to hike a couple miles to find a campsite. Next day, return upstream.

Expect to splash through ankle-deep water in the **Paria Narrows**. Near 16 mi (25.8 km) the sheer canyon walls begin to relax and recede.

Pass beneath powerlines at 17.8 mi (28.7 km). You're now hiking on sandy benches between river crossings. Watch for a sign indicating where to exit the wash. Follow a short trail right (east) to **White House trailhead** and campground at 20.3 mi (32.7 km), 4280 ft (1305 m).

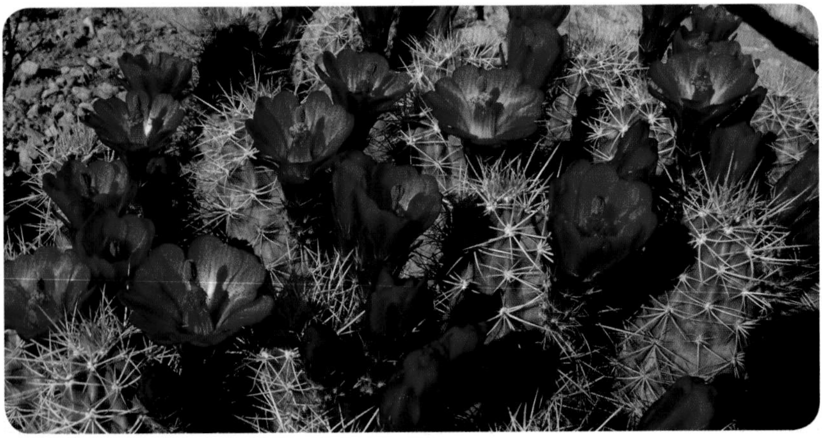

Claret Cup

TRIP 12

PARIA RIVER CANYON

LOCATION	Paria Canyon / Vermilion Cliffs Wilderness between Kanab UT and Page AZ
DISTANCE	38.4 mi (61.9 km) one way
ELEVATION LOSS	1130 ft (345 m)
KEY ELEVATIONS	White House trailhead 4280 ft (1305 m) Buckskin / Paria confluence 4180 ft (1274 m) Lee's Ferry trailhead 3150 ft (960 m)
HIKING TIME	3 to 5 days
DIFFICULTY	moderate
MAP	*Hiker's Guide to Paria Canyon* (free, available at BLM Paria River contact station)

OPINION

She was 16 when her high-school outing club announced a five day, spring-break backpack trip through Paria River Canyon. She'd never done anything like it.

Two nights before the group left, she stayed up late, frantically preparing and packing for a journey she didn't yet comprehend. The night before, she was still awake at 3 a.m., writing a term paper on James Joyce's *Portrait of an Artist as a Young Man* for her literature class. By departure time, she was exhausted, coming down with a cold.

Unfit, ill, burdened with a heavy, creaky, overloaded, antiquated Camp Trails backpack, wearing Tretorn tennis shoes floppy as house slippers, she slogged down the sandy riverbed into the canyon. Her hips hurt, so she stuffed socks beneath the hipbelt to reduce the pain. Her Achilles tendons ached, so she limped. Each night, coughing and sneezing, she collapsed in her tent after dinner while her friends revelled beneath the star-filled sky.

By the time she rode the bus home, she hadn't bathed for six days—yet another new experience—and felt wretched. But what she remembers feeling most is awe. The sheer, soaring, canyon walls were the most spectacular sight she'd ever seen. Meandering through the serpentine narrows—so constricted she tried to touch both sides at once—had been wondrous. Surrendering to the embrace of wilderness left her yearning to do it again.

And she did. Repeatedly. Throughout the world. Until hiking, and inspiring others to hike, became her career. She's the co-author of this book. And the story of how that first backpack trip aroused her true self is the most compelling testament we can offer to the beauty and power awaiting you in Paria River Canyon.

It ranks among the world's great treks. No matter how far you must travel to get there or how difficult it is to arrange the time off, Paria Canyon is worth it.

Many hikers prefer it to the Grand Canyon, because Paria is intimate and mysterious rather than overwhelming, and because you can complete it rather

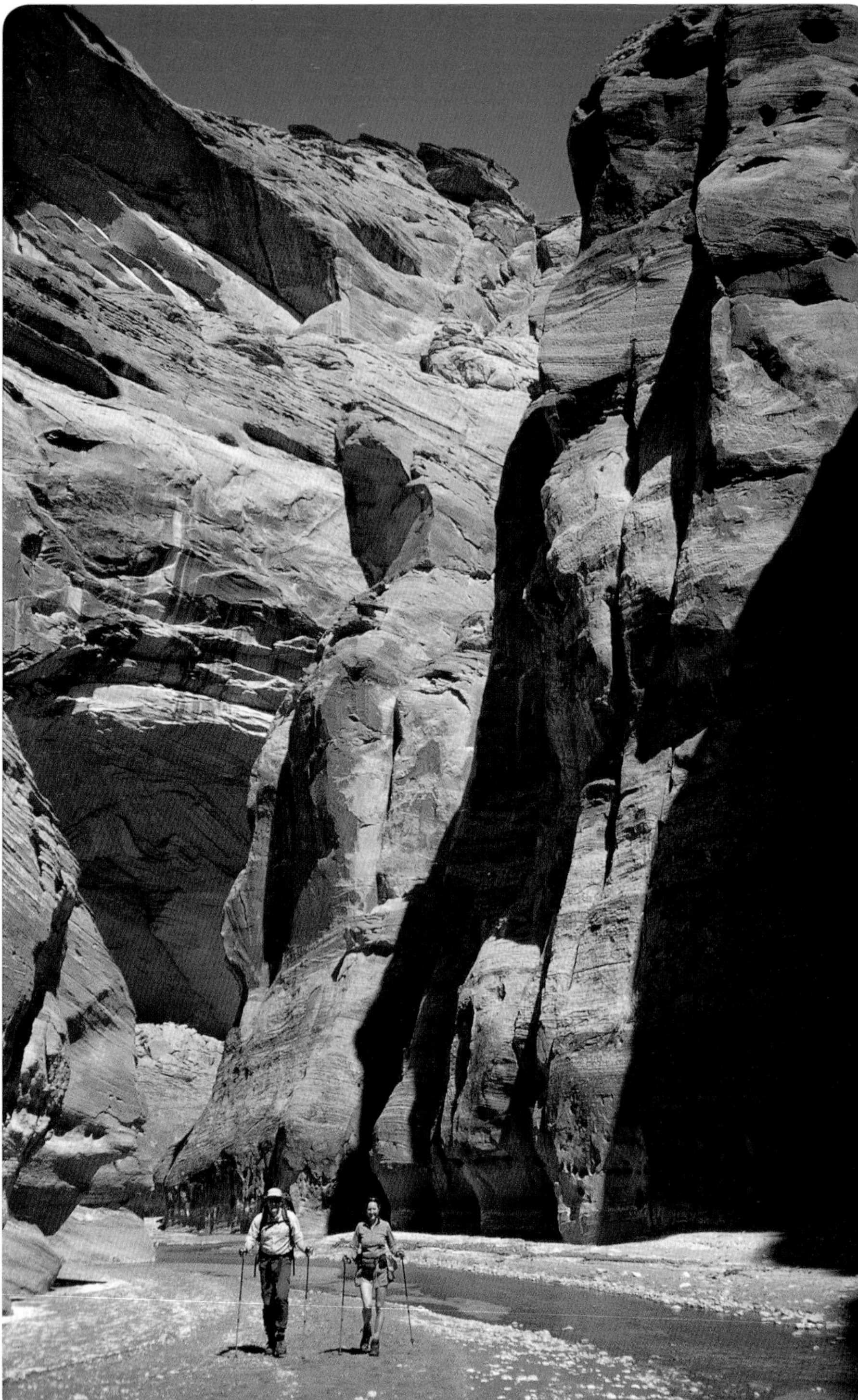

Paria Canyon

than merely sample it. Most hikers prefer it to Escalante Canyon, because you'll generally be splashing through ankle-deep water rather than wading up to your thighs. Since Kathy's first adventure, we've hiked the Paria three times and are convinced it's the premier canyon-country backpack trip.

The Paria River flows intermittently from its headwaters in Bryce Canyon National Park, through south-central Utah, into Arizona where it joins the Colorado River at Lees Ferry, southwest of Page. The three- to five-day journey described here weaves through the most captivating, 38.4-mi (61.9-km) stretch, starting near Hwy 89, east of Kanab.

For most of the first half of the hike, the canyon is extremely narrow, a mere 2 yd/m wide at one point, with monolithic, nearly vertical walls 500 to 800 ft (152 to 244 m) high. Shade is frequent, because the sun beams directly into the gorge only a few hours each day.

The lower reaches of the canyon are magnificent too, but quite different. Here, the Paria is a classic desert chasm: broad, deep, sun baked. More than 35 million years of geologic history are visible between the bouldery riverbed and the colorful, broken walls soaring 2700 ft (823 m) to the canyon rims.

Most of the way, the riverbed will be your trail. Flashfloods occasionally scour the canyon, so you won't encounter the thick riparian webs of tamarisk, willow and Russian olive that make hiking many canyon floors a thrash-and-bash chore. Nor will you encounter deep pools that require swimming. You'll often walk on sand, occasionally on rock, frequently in shallow water. In the lower canyon, you'll follow stretches of rocky trail or bootbeaten path between river crossings. Overall, you'll be cruising downhill. Assuming you have good weather and there's no threat of a flood, you'll face only the minor challenge of carrying sufficient fresh water between the widely scattered springs.

We strongly recommend the one way, north-to-south trip described here. Hiking south to north, the first reliable spring would be 12.4 mi (20 km) distant, so you'd be carrying maximum water when your pack is heaviest and sun exposure constant. A popular alternative is to start in the north, enter the narrows, establish camp, then dayhike farther down-canyon or up Buckskin Gulch, but a through-trip is much more fulfilling. Read Trip 11 to learn about the exciting but arduous option of entering Paria Canyon via Buckskin Gulch.

HISTORY

The ancient ones explored Paria Canyon 10,000 years before the first Europeans wandered past. Natives lived in the region for vastly longer periods than anyone has since, and they certainly knew the canyon far more intimately.

Yet little is known about Paria's Native history. Other than a small rock-art site near the south end of Paria Canyon, most hikers will see no evidence of Native habitation.

The explorers and pioneers who arrived at Paria Canyon in recent history were mere visitors, tourists actually, compared to the previous residents. Yet far more is known about the newcomers because their exploits are documented.

Two missionaries, Fathers Dominguez and Escalante, were the first Europeans to see Paria Canyon. After surviving starvation, dehydration, and severely cold weather during an attempt to establish a route from Santa Fe, New Mexico, to the California missions, they turned back 500 mi (805 km) from the coast. They camped at the mouth of Paria Canyon for several days in 1776.

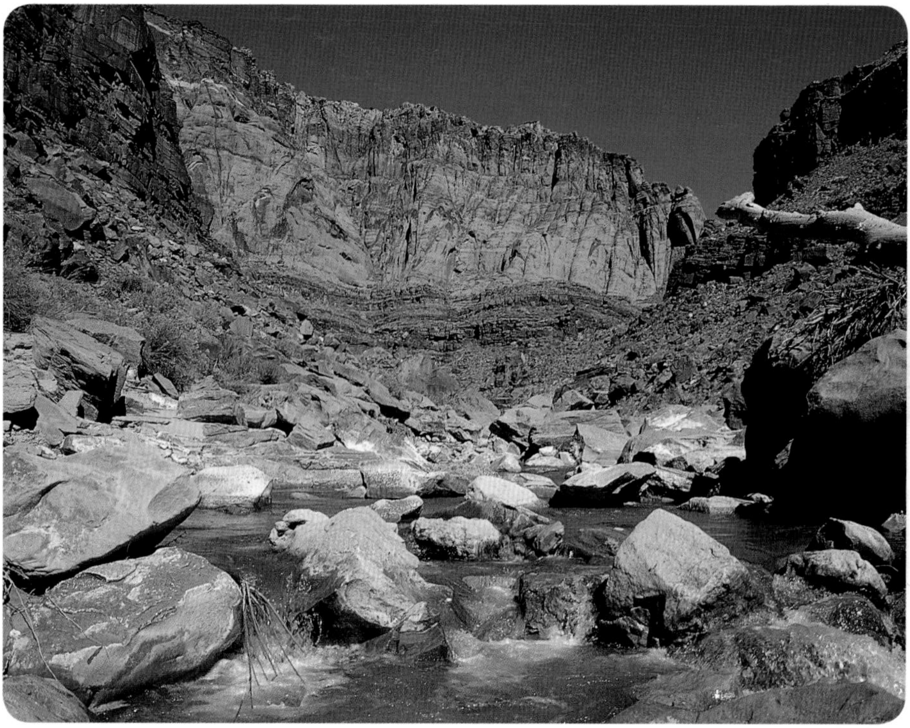

Lower reaches of Paria Canyon

In the winter of 1858, John Lee herded livestock, two of his nineteen wives, and who knows how many of his 65 children down the frigid Paria River. He and his family were the first white people known to travel the length of the canyon. But theirs was hardly a recreational adventure. They were fugitives.

Lee was a Mormon polygamist, and polygamy was a felony. The previous autumn, Lee had also led the Mountain Meadows Massacre, in which his Mormon militia killed innocent non-Mormon immigrants whom they mistakenly suspected might persecute them. The immigrants surrendered, but the Mormons executed 120 men, women and children, then buried them in a mass grave.

Lee had served as Joseph Smith's bodyguard. He'd been a leader in the Mormon migration to Zion. He was one of Brigham Young's lieutenants, the one selected for difficult, dangerous tasks. So instead of remanding him to the authorities, Young ordered him to steal away from society, vanish into the wilderness via Paria Canyon, and establish a ferry across the Colorado River.

Lee obeyed. He founded a farm, *Lonely Dell*, near the confluence of the Paria and Colorado rivers. And in 1871, he fulfilled his mission to build the ferry. In the early 1900s, Lee's was still the only ferry operating on the Colorado between Moab, Utah, and Needles, California.

Trekking through Paria Canyon, your trail's end goal is Lonely Dell and Lees Ferry. So you'll be following in the footsteps of John Lee—outlaw, butcher, harem master, farmer, ferryman.

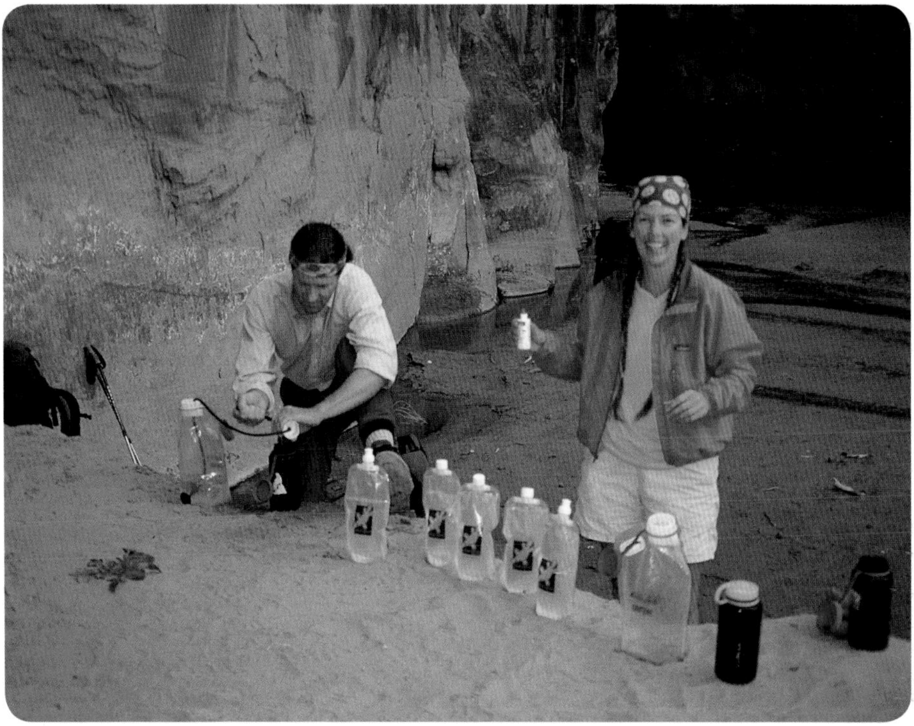

Tanking up near the confluence of Buckskin Gulch and Paria Canyon

BEFORE YOUR TRIP

Each person in your group must have an overnight permit in advance. The BLM allows only 20 backpackers per day to enter Paria Canyon. Visit www.blm.gov/az/asfo/paria/wilderness.htm to check availability, make reservations, or learn about obtaining a permit in person at the BLM Paria River contact station (see *By Vehicle / White House trailhead* below).

Get a current weather report in Kanab, either at the BLM field office (318 North First East) or the Grand Staircase-Escalante National Monument visitor center (east edge of town). If driving Hwy 89 northwest from Page, Arizona, get a current weather report at the Grand Staircase-Escalante National Monument visitor center in Big Water, or 13.5 mi (21.7 km) farther at the BLM Paria River contact station.

If rain is imminent, cancel your trip. The BLM will allow you to reschedule for up to one year. Even distant rain can cause a dangerous volume of water to suddenly rush through Paria Canyon. Hike here only during a period of sunny weather, when there's little risk of a flashflood.

You'll be in the river frequently, so wear amphibious boots. Those designed specifically for hiking in water are ideal, but a sturdy pair of fabric hiking boots you're willing to dunk are fine too. Don't hike in sandals; they lack sufficient ankle support and allow pebbles to lodge beneath your feet. And don't hike in runners; they're too flexible, causing your feet to quickly tire. Under the weight of a full pack, especially when walking in sand, you need boots that provide lateral support and have a stiff shank. You'll also find trekking poles invaluable here.

The Paria River flows year-round below the Buckskin Gulch confluence. But the water is contaminated, extremely silty, and laden with minerals. Drink it only as a last resort, and then only after you've filtered or purified it. Filters clog less often if you first let the water sit overnight, so the sediment will settle. A large collapsible water container is helpful for this purpose. Ideally, all your water for drinking and cooking should come from springs, although you should still filter or purify it.

There are numerous seasonal springs in Paria Canyon. You'll also find perennial springs at 9.9 mi (15.9 km), 12.2 mi (19.6 km), 22 mi (35.4 km), 25.2 mi (40.6 km), and 0.4 mi (0.6 km) up Bush Head Canyon at 26.4 mi (42.5 km). There are no reliable springs between Bush Head Canyon and Lees Ferry trailhead at 38.4 mi (61.9 km). Each person in your group should pack enough containers to carry at least one gallon (four liters) of water and should top them up at every spring.

BY VEHICLE

A through-hike of Paria River Canyon necessitates a vehicle shuttle. The White House trailhead, where the trip begins, is a 2½ hour drive from the Lees Ferry trailhead, where the trip ends. The logical plan is to leave a vehicle at Lees Ferry the evening before you start hiking, and camp that night at White House. If you're not hiking with friends who have a second vehicle, visit www.blm.gov/az/asfo/paria/wilderness.htm for a list of authorized shuttle providers.

Lees Ferry trailhead

From Kanab, drive Hwy 89 east, past Big Water, then southeast to Page. Continue on Hwy 89 south-southwest 23 mi (37 km), then turn right (north) onto Hwy 89A. Follow it 14.3 mi (23 km), then turn right (north) for Less Ferry. In 4.4 mi (7.1 km) reach a junction near the campground. Proceed straight. At 4.7 mi (7.6 km) pass the ranger station and a pay phone. Bear left at the next junction. At 5.1 mi (8.2 km) pass the spur to Lonely Dell Ranch. At 5.5 mi (8.9 km) reach the Lees Ferry trailhead parking lot at 3150 ft (960 m). Leave your shuttle vehicle here, where the one-way hike ends.

White House trailhead

From the Grand Staircase-Escalante National Monument visitor center at the east edge of Kanab, drive Hwy 89 east 42.2 mi (68 km). From the Grand Staircase-Escalante National Monument visitor center in Big Water, drive Hwy 89 west 13.5 mi (21.7 km). From either approach, turn south onto unpaved White House Road, between mileposts 20 and 21. Stop just ahead at the BLM Paria River contact station to get your permit. Then proceed south 1.8 mi (2.9 km) to White House trailhead and campground at road's end. Elevation: 4280 ft (1305 m). Begin hiking here.

ON FOOT

The riverbed is the trail through most of Paria Canyon. In May and June, the first 7 mi (11.3 km)—as far as the Buckskin confluence—can be dry. At other times you'll soon be hiking in water a couple inches deep. Beyond Buckskin, the river usually varies from ankle- to knee-deep. At 28 mi (45 km) boulders in the riverbed shunt hikers above the south bank. In the lower canyon, expect to cross the river occasionally and follow long stretches of bootbeaten path on sandy benches.

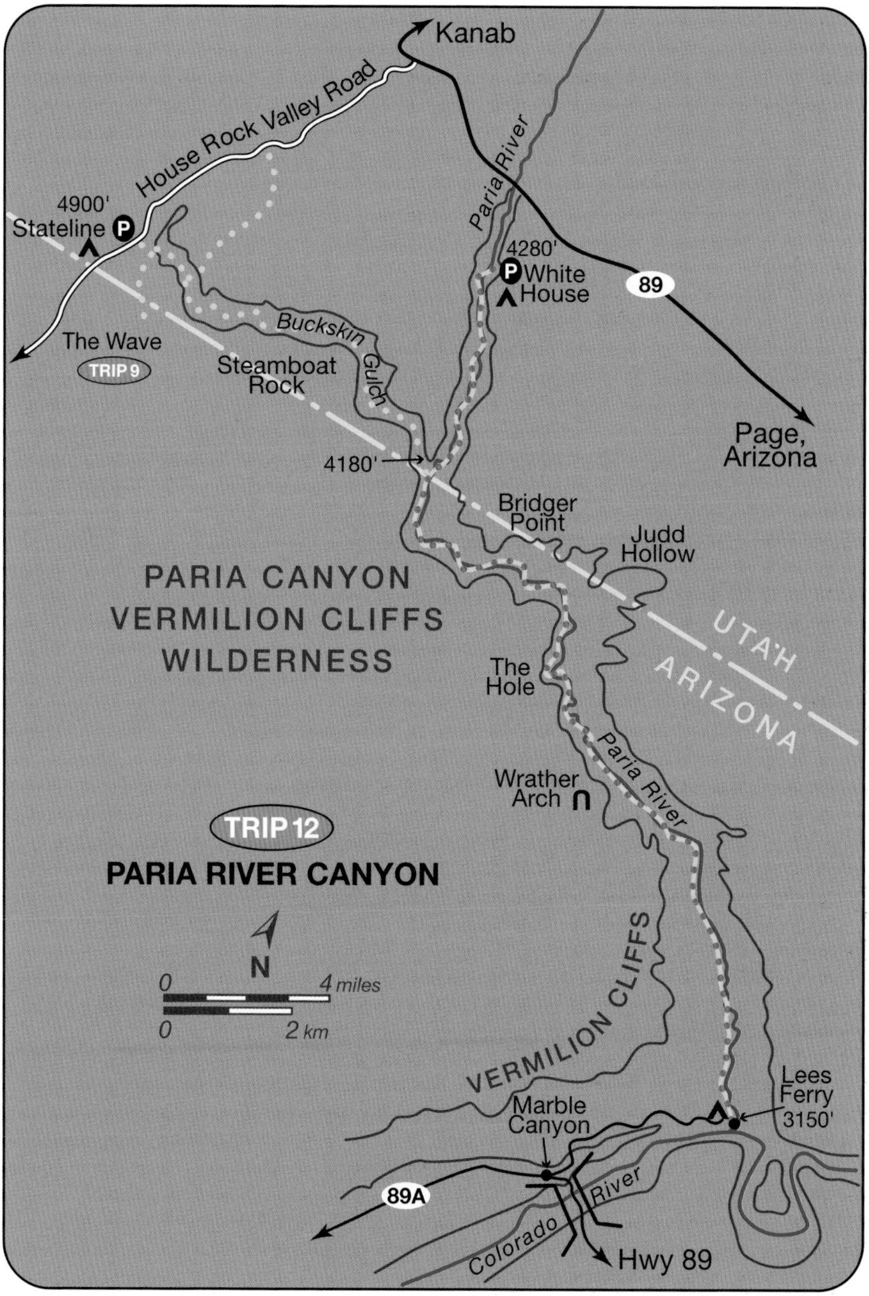

The following route description is abbreviated and states compass directions infrequently. Detailed directions are unnecessary here and would only be dizzying. The way forward is constant: hike down-canyon, following the Paria River downstream. From the White House trailhead, your general direction of travel will be south to about 8.2 mi (13.2 km), or roughly 1 mi (1.6 km) past Buckskin confluence. You'll then hike generally east past Big Spring to about 17.5 mi (28.2 km). From there, you'll hike generally southeast to the Lees Ferry trailhead.

Though viable campsites are limited in some stretches of Paria Canyon, overall there are more than we've cited. Some will no doubt be occupied when you arrive. To claim a campsite that appeals to you, be prepared to hike farther or stop sooner than you'd prefer. Also be aware that recent flooding might have dramatically rearranged the canyon floor, washing away some camping sites and creating others.

0 mi (0 km)
Depart the White House trailhead between the walk-in campsites and the toilets. Beyond the **trail register**, proceed through a hiker's maze, which allows people but not cows to pass through the fence. Drop into the broad **riverbed**. Bear left (south) and hike downstream. Within 15 minutes, Paria Canyon is apparent ahead.

4 mi (6.4 km)
Enter the **Paria Narrows**. The sheer Navajo sandstone walls are 500 to 800 ft (152 to 244 m) high and, at one point, just 2 yd/m apart. Mud on the walls indicates the height of recent floodwaters. Expect to splash through the river, which will likely be ankle deep.

6.7 mi (10.8 km)
Pass **Slide Rock Arch**. The canyon is 35 to 50 ft (10.5 to 15 m) wide here.

7.2 mi (11.6 km)
Intersect **Buckskin Gulch** (right / west) at 4180 ft (1274 m). It's worthwhile dropping packs beside the confluence and detouring up Buckskin (Trip 11). Sandy benches on both walls used to offer campsites. Flooding washed them away. Resume following the Paria River downstream (south-southeast) and cross the Utah / Arizona border.

7.7 mi (12.4 km)
Reach a **campsite** on a sandy bench (right / south).

9.4 mi (15.1 km) and
Reach a **campsite** (right / west) just before a **seasonal spring** (right / southwest).

9.9 mi (15.9 km)
Reach a **campsite** (left / north) opposite a **perennial spring** (right / south).

10 mi (16.1 km)
The canyon, 400 to 500 ft (122 to 152 m) deep here, is particularly sinuous for the next 8 mi (12.9 km).

12.2 mi (19.6 km)
Arrive at **Big Spring**. This reliable gusher is on the right (south) wall amid lush, hanging gardens. Campsites are on the left (north) bench.

12.8 mi (20.6 km)
Reach another **campsite** (right / south).

14.7 mi (23.7 km)
A grand **amphitheater** (right / west) rises 650 ft (198 m) from the riverbed. It harbors a seasonal seep. There's a campsite opposite the amphitheater. If it's occupied, the canyon soon widens, affording campsites among cottonwoods on terraces.

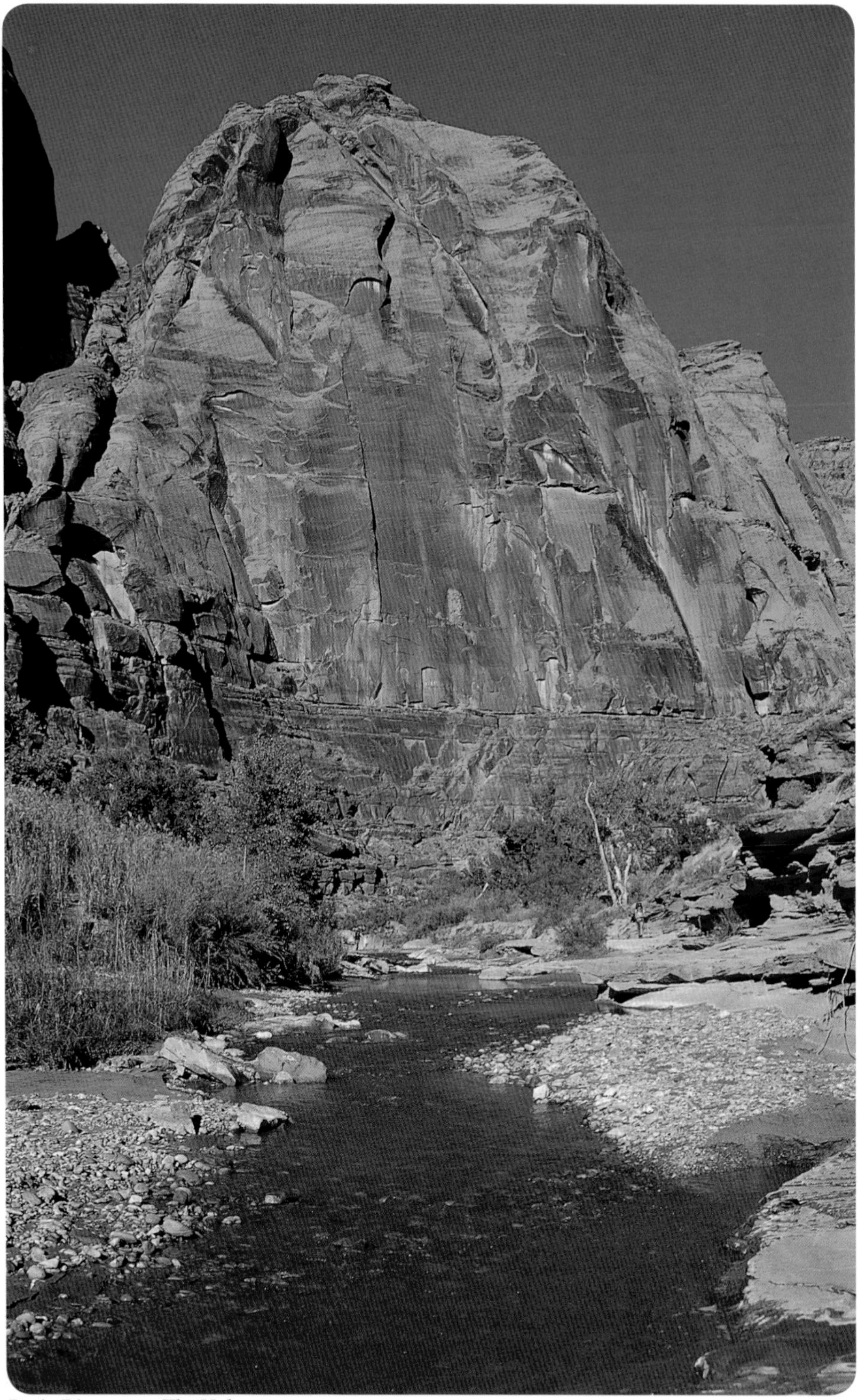

Paria River, near The Hole

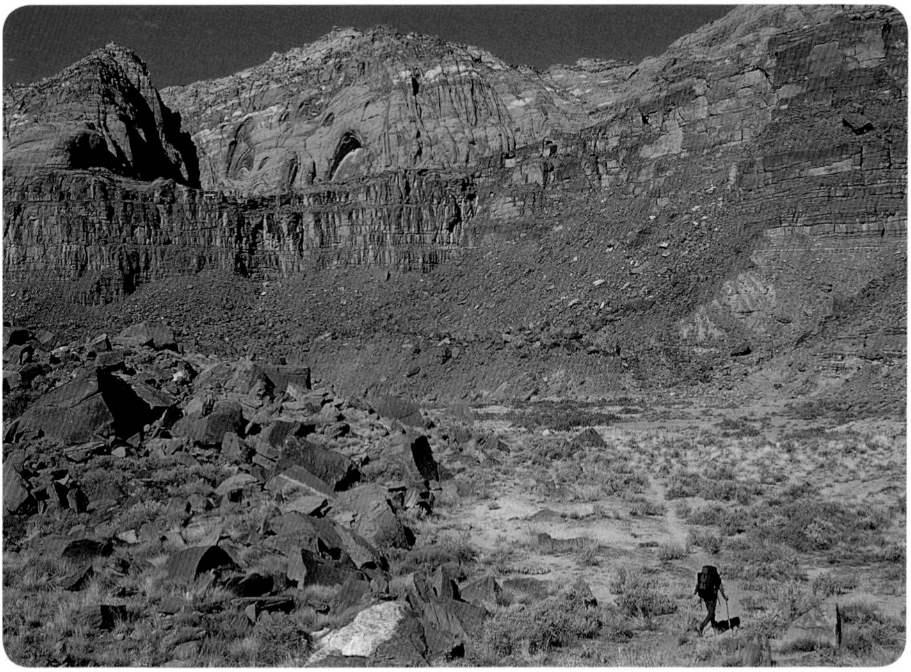

The Vermilion Cliffs, from the lower reaches of Paria Canyon

16 mi (25.8 km)
Negotiate a **boulder jam** in the riverbed.

17.4 mi (28 km)
Pass **Judd Hollow Pump**—transported to the canyon in 1939 by ranchers seeking to water livestock on the canyon rim. They tested and immediately abandoned the pump in 1949.

18 mi (29 km)
Reach the first of several **campsites**.

18.3 mi (29.5 km)
Arrive at a **reliable spring** and **campsite** (right / west).

19 mi (30.1 km)
The Hole (right / northwest) is a huge slickrock bay offering campsites and seasonal water. Ahead, the hiking entails less wading. Ford the river occasionally between stretches of trail across sandy benches.

20.5 mi (33 km)
Wrather Canyon opens on the right (west). Here, a 25-minute detour entailing a short ascent leads to impressive **Wrather Arch**. Camping is prohibited in the treed, bushy canyon, which has an intermittent stream.

21.5 mi (34.6 km)
Paria Canyon's sheer Navajo sandstone walls gradually begin giving way to terraces and scree slopes of Red Kayenta sandstone. Though the canyon ahead is 1400 ft (427 m) deep, it broadens dramatically, so sun exposure is constant. Expect to encounter an increasingly boulder-strewn riverbed. The river itself becomes more precisely channeled: narrower and deeper.

22 mi (35.4 km)
Listen for **Shower Spring**. It's hidden behind a curtain of vegetation on the left (east) wall. There's a **campsite** opposite the spring.

25.2 mi (40.6 km)
Pass the **last, convenient, reliable spring** (left / east).

26 mi (41.9 km)
Follow a path paralleling the river's right (south) bank for about 5 mi (8.1 km)—the canyon's longest stretch where crossing the river or hiking in it are unnecessary.

26.4 mi (42.5 km)
Pass **Bush Head Canyon** (right / west). The fire that charred the foliage at the canyon mouth was started by a careless camper burning toilet paper. If in need of water, detour 0.4 mi (0.7 km) up the canyon to a **reliable spring**. Ahead, Paria Canyon widens further and deepens to 2000 ft (610 m).

28 mi (45 km)
The river is riddled with deep holes and crowded with boulders. Follow the rocky trail traversing talus slopes above the south bank.

30.2 mi (48.6 km)
Pass a lone, ancient cottonwood on a sandy bench. The tree offers enough shade to make this an inviting rest stop on a hot day. This is also a reasonable **campsite** if you can't make Lees Ferry by nightfall. Ahead, you'll ford the river between long stretches of trail traversing silty benches.

31.5 mi (50.7 km)
Petroglyphs adorn several boulders on a barren Chinle bench above the river's left (north) bank. The small grove of cottonwoods just past the next river crossing is the **last good campsite.**

33.4 mi (53.8 km)
Pass the remains of the 1918 **Wilson Ranch** (right / west). This is Paria Canyon's deepest point. The distant rims are 2700 ft (823 m) above the river.

35 mi (56.4 km)
Chocolate-brown Moenkopi sandstone is now evident.

35.9 mi (57.8 km)
Enter Glen Canyon National Recreation Area.

37.2 mi (59.9 km)
Having passed a rusty hulk of a 1920s car and an abandoned cabin, pass a solid **corral** still used today.

37.3 mi (60.1 km)
Pass the **trail register**.

37.7 mi (60.7 km)
Pass **Lonely Dell cemetery**. Straight leads to Lonely Dell. Turn turn left (east) onto a **dirt road**.

38 mi (61.2 km)
At road's end, across from the gauging station, is the **final river ford**. On the far bank, turn right and resume southeast.

38.4 mi (61.9 km)
After ascending a steep, rocky slope above a bend in the river, enter the **Lees Ferry trailhead** parking lot, at 3150 ft (960 m), just above the Colorado River.

TRIP 13

HACKBERRY CANYON & YELLOW ROCK

LOCATION	Grand Staircase-Escalante National Monument between Kanab UT and Page AZ
ROUND TRIP	4.2 mi (6.8 km)
ELEVATION GAIN	800 ft (244 m)
KEY ELEVATIONS	trailhead 4760 ft (1451 m), Yellow Rock 5524 ft (1684 m)
HIKING TIME	2½ to 3½ hours
DIFFICULTY	moderate
MAP	USGS *Calico Peak*

OPINION

A physician devoted to spinal health once told us, "Patterns are what we don't want to see. Patterns are non-adaptation, which is unhealthy." It was sage advice not just for maintaining a strong back, but for living a full life. We took it to mean, "Embrace change and dance with it."

So here's an exercise in adaptation. Instead of dropping into a canyon and dutifully plodding through it to the end, briefly probe the Hackberry Canyon narrows then reverse out. Mix it up. Find the challenging exit route, overlook the narrows from above, then freelance your way across sweeping slickrock to the summit of Yellow Rock and a 360° panorama extending from southern Utah into northern Arizona.

A 1½-hour round-trip stroll in Hackberry Canyon is a relaxing tour of a beautiful, impressive gorge. It's also a warm-up for the shortest but most taxing stage of this three-pronged dayhike: a demanding clamber out of Cottonwood Creek wash to the Hackberry Canyon rim. From there, the final leg is a fun, exhilarating wander up the massive, Navajo sandstone dome.

Yellow Rock assumes a commanding stance atop a wedge-shaped mesa between Cottonwood Canyon, Hackberry Canyon, and the Box of the Paria River. And it's not just yellow. As if created by a soft-serve ice-cream machine extruding all 31 flavors at once, it's a swirling mix of white, orange, red, yellow, rust, and mauve.

Parallel fracture lines perpendicular to the crossbedding of the sandstone divide the surface of Yellow Rock into a thousand rectangles, much like Zion National Park's Checkerboard Mesa. If you're timing is right, you might see fluorescent blooms—perhaps fuchsia monkeyflower or red-orange Indian paintbrush—sprouting from those cracks.

If your time is limited, it's possible to hike either Hackberry or Yellow Rock. We recommend the Rock. And if you have plenty of time, it's possible to free-camp along the trailhead access road through Cottonwood Canyon. Camping, after all, is the ultimate adaptive activity.

FACT

BY VEHICLE

The Cottonwood Canyon Road, which accesses the trailhead, is rough: washboarded in places, sandy in others. If dry, it's usually passable in a 2WD vehicle, though 4WD is always preferable here. If wet, don't even attempt it in a high-clearance Baja beast, because the road's bentonite clay surface transforms into a diabolical combination of gumbo and grease.

From the Grand Staircase-Escalante National Monument visitor center at the east edge of Kanab, drive Hwy 89 east 45.2 mi (72.8 km). This is 3 mi (4.8 km) east of the BLM Paria River contact station on White House Road.

From the Grand Staircase-Escalante National Monument visitor center in Big Water, drive Hwy 89 west 10.5 mi (16.9 km).

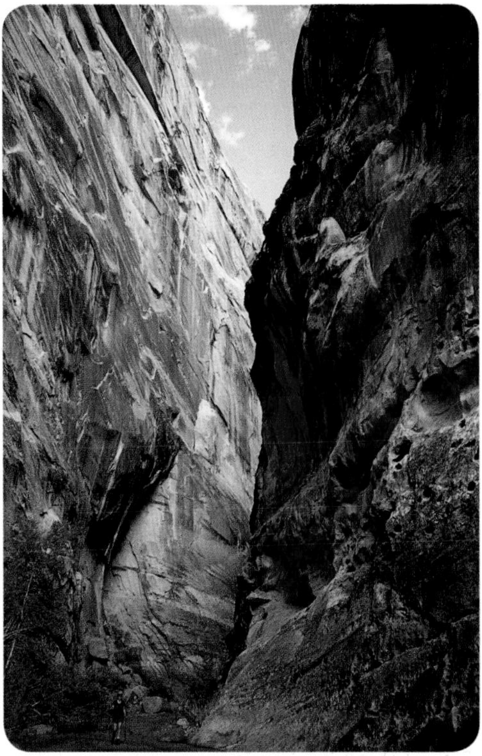

Hackberry Canyon

From either approach, turn north onto unpaved Cottonwood Canyon Road, between mileposts 17 and 18, and reset your trip odometer to 0. A sign states distances to points north: Cottonwood Canyon 8 mi, Grosvenor Arch 30 mi, Cannonville 46 mi.

0 mi (0 km)
Starting north on Cottonwood Canyon Road 400.

1.4 mi (2.2 km)
Bear left on the main road.

6.4 mi (10.4 km)
Curve north.

10.3 mi (16.6 km)
Maintain momentum through a sandy stretch. Don't stop.

10.5 mi (16.9 km)
Pass beneath powerlines.

11.8 mi (19.1 km)
Proceed straight, ignoring the left fork to the Paria River.

12.2 mi (19.6 km)
Proceed straight, ignoring the left fork to the Paria Box trailhead.

13 mi (20.9 km)
The sandstone dome of Yellow Rock is visible ahead. Descend through a pass, then cross a cattleguard.

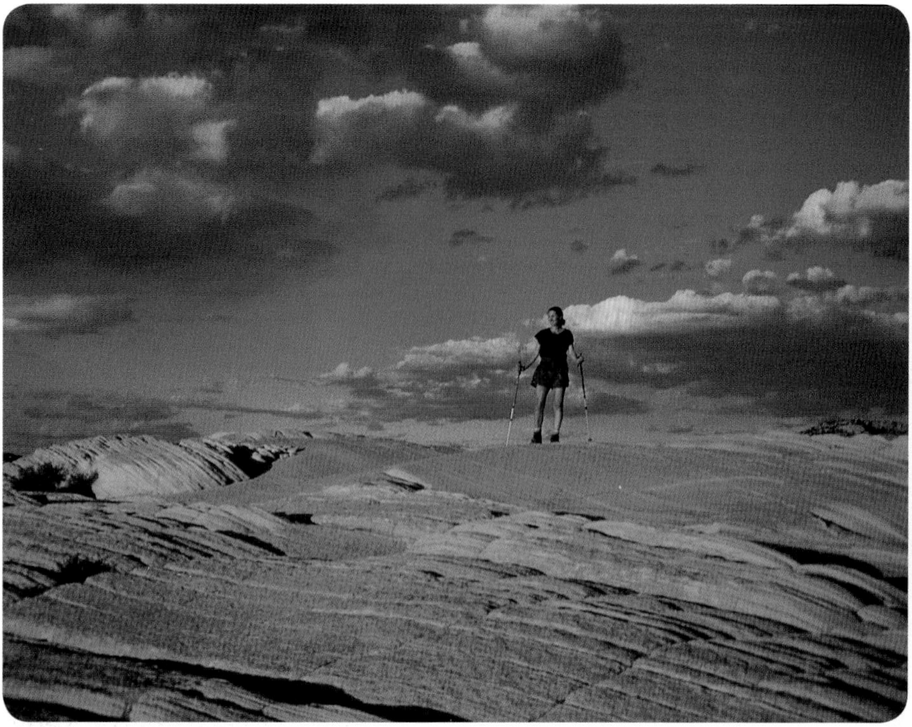

The summit of Yellow Rock

13.2 mi (21.3 km)
Proceed straight. The left spur leads to a primitive campsite beneath cottonwoods.

14.3 mi (23 km)
Cross a cattleguard and proceed straight where Brigham Plain Road 430 forks right.

14.6 mi (23.5 km)
Reach the small, unimproved, trailhead parking area on the left (west), near the confluence of Cottonwood and Hackberry canyons, at 4760 ft (1451 m).

ON FOOT

Yellow Rock is the prominent slickrock dome visible on the western horizon. A BLM signpost indicates the trailhead. Facing Cottonwood Creek (west), Hackberry Canyon is right (upstream), and the route to Yellow Rock is left (downstream).

Hackberry Canyon

Drop into Cottonwood Creek's broad, sandy wash. The water, if flowing, is usually only a couple inches deep. Go right (north), upstream. At 0.2 mi (0.3 km) bear left (northwest) into Hackberry Canyon.

The ensuing 0.4 mi (0.6 km) is a narrow, sheer-walled, 600-ft (183-m) deep rift through The Cockscomb. About 40 minutes upstream the Navajo sandstone walls begin subsiding and the canyon broadens. Most hikers will want to turn around within an hour.

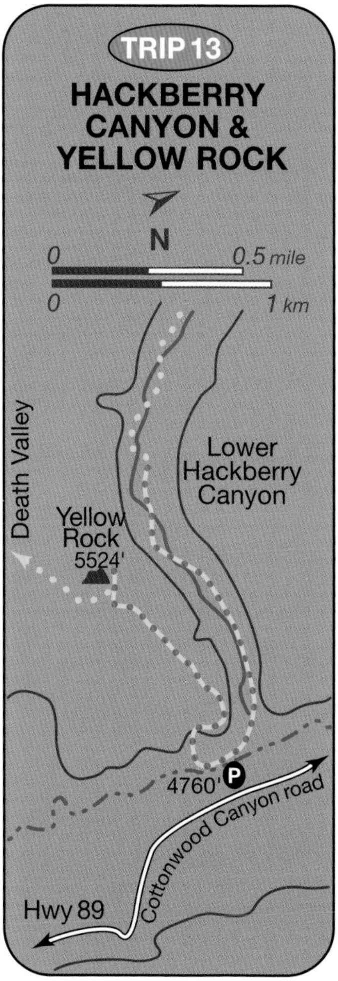

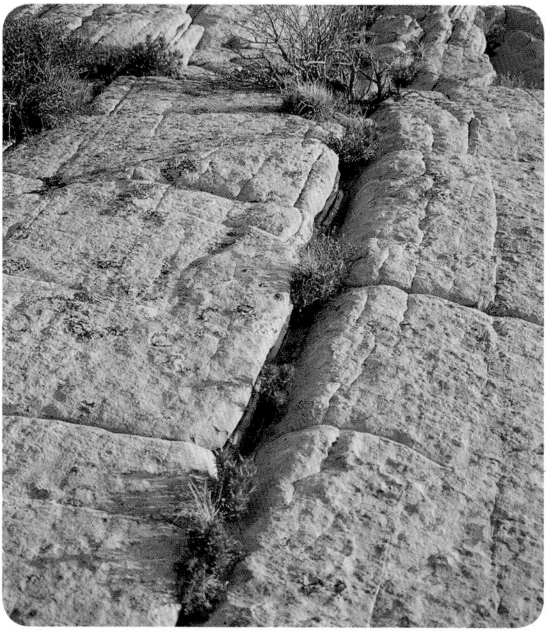

Paintbrush in Navajo sandstone

Yellow Rock

After retracing your steps down Hackberry Canyon, turn right (south) and follow Cottonwood Creek wash downstream. Pass the trailhead parking area (left / east) and within 0.3 mi (0.5 mi) turn right (west) into the **first tributary drainage**.

Short and steep, it appears to be a box canyon. Follow the wash about 50 yd/m to a rugged route ascending loose rock and dirt on the left slope. It quickly drops back to the wash.

About 10 yd/m farther, pick up a very steep route ascending the **rocky chute** on the right. Gain 200 ft (61 m) in the next 220 yd (200 m) by kickstepping footholds and firmly planting your trekking poles on this precarious passage. The grade eases on a rocky rib.

Skirt a gorge and soon arrive at a notch on a **ridge** where Hackberry Canyon is visible 300 ft (92 m) immediately below. Cottonwood Canyon is north, bound on the east by The Cockscomb. To the south are the Paria River, the Paria Plateau, and the Vermilion Cliffs.

From the notch, the sharp, sandstone ridge west affords a moderate ascent route. Reach a **cluster of spires** at 5400 ft (1646 m). The dome of Yellow Rock is visible ahead. Cross the ridge just east of the spires.

Head generally west between slickrock mounds and sandy pockets harboring piñon and ponderosa pine, juniper, manzanita, and scrub oak. Enter a **broad bowl**.

Cross a minor wash and continue west to the south base of your destination. Then work your way up its east slope, cresting the 5524-ft (1684-m) summit of **Yellow Rock** about 1.5 mi (2.4 km) from the trailhead.

TRIP 14

LICK WASH

LOCATION	Grand Staircase-Escalante National Monument northeast of Kanab
ROUND TRIP	8 mi (13 km)
ELEVATION CHANGE	330-ft (100-m) loss and gain
KEY ELEVATIONS	trailhead 6330 ft (1930 m), Park Wash 6000 ft (1830 m)
HIKING TIME	3 to 4 hours
DIFFICULTY	easy
MAPS	BLM brochure *Grand Staircase-Escalante National Monument*, USGS *Deer Spring Point*

OPINION

Driving northeast from Kanab, through gently rolling ranchland cloaked in sagebrush and juniper, you might think the only reason to stop the car is to pee. But all is not as it seems. Throughout southern Utah, surprises crouch just beneath the surface of apparent banality. Dispiriting trailheads are rabbit-hole entrances to worlds of wonder. Many, however, are flagged with alluring names suggesting revelations within. Lick Wash? The landscape is lusterless *and* the name is repellent. Nevertheless, a few minutes down Lick Wash, you'll behold a scene of Zionesque beauty and magnitude.

Lick Wash penetrates the White Cliffs atop Grand Staircase plateau. After a short, impressive narrow section, the wash opens into a voluminous canyon with solid, sheer, 600-ft (183-m) walls. Ponderosa pines—always a dramatic sight—are especially impressive in canyons. Here they grace many of the ledges and benches.

If you're seeking solitude, hike Lick Wash midweek. You'll likely share it with others on weekends. But it's never crowded. Thankfully, not all of Utah's desert-varnished cliffs and cross-bedded domes were lassoed into national parks.

Because Lick Wash is remote, consider also hiking Willis Creek (Trip 19) while you're in the area. Both trailheads are on Skutumpah Road, between Kanab (Hwy 89, southeast of Zion Park) and Cannonville (Hwy 12, southeast of Bryce Park). The optimal plan is to camp nearby, either at Kodachrome Basin State Park or at a quiet, primitive site in the P-J forest (piñon and juniper) along lonely, Skutumpah Road.

Don't let our lengthy *By Vehicle* directions put you off. The drive to Lick Wash is straightforward. We've provided way more detail then you'll likely need. Plus we've described how to reach both trailheads—Lick *and* Willis—from either approach, so you don't have to flip through the book seeking further guidance should you want to complete a one-way tour.

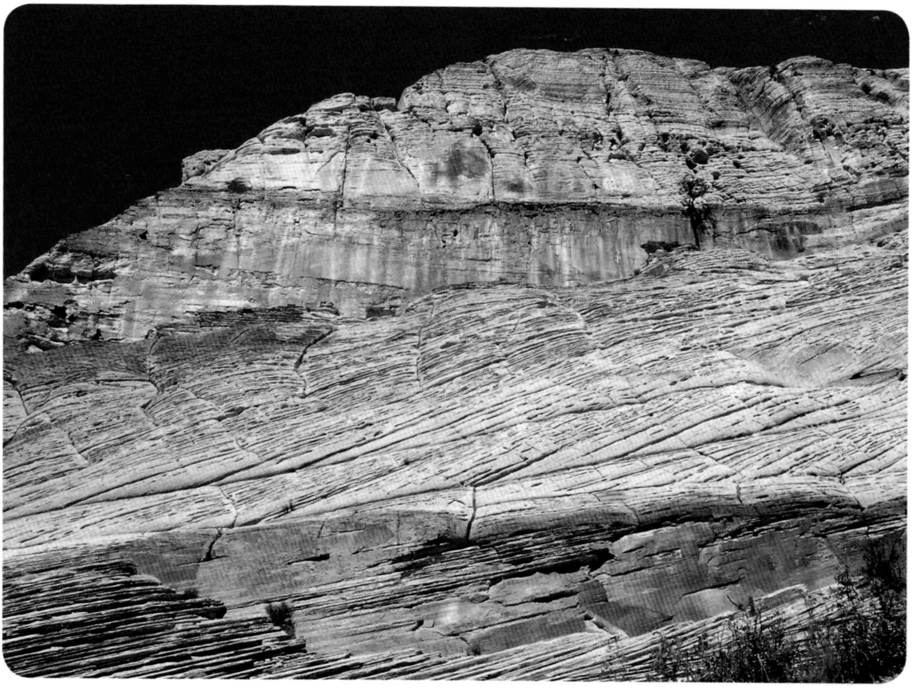

Lick Wash has stupendous, cross-bedded sandstone domes like nearby Zion National Park.

FACT

BEFORE YOUR TRIP

Skutumpah Road, particularly the northeast end near Cannonville, is treacherous when wet because the clay surface makes traction impossible. Do not risk driving it after recent rain or if the forecast calls for rain. The road's northeast end also has steep, narrow sections that, even when dry, might traumatize an inexpert trailer tugger.

BY VEHICLE

From Cannonville

Cannonville is on Hwy 12, southeast of Bryce Park. It's 33 mi (53.1 km) southeast of Panguitch, and 36 mi (58 km) southwest of Escalante. From either approach, turn south onto paved Cottonwood Canyon Road and reset your trip odometer to 0.

0 mi (0 km)
Drive south on paved Cottonwood Canyon Road, which is signed for Kodachrome Basin State Park.

2.8 mi (4.5 km)
Just before (west of) a bridged crossing of the upper Paria River, turn right (southwest) onto unpaved Skutumpah Road, signed for Bull Valley Gorge (9 mi) and Kanab (61 mi). Kodachrome Basin is 6.7 mi (10.8 km) ahead (southeast) on the paved Cottonwood Canyon Road.

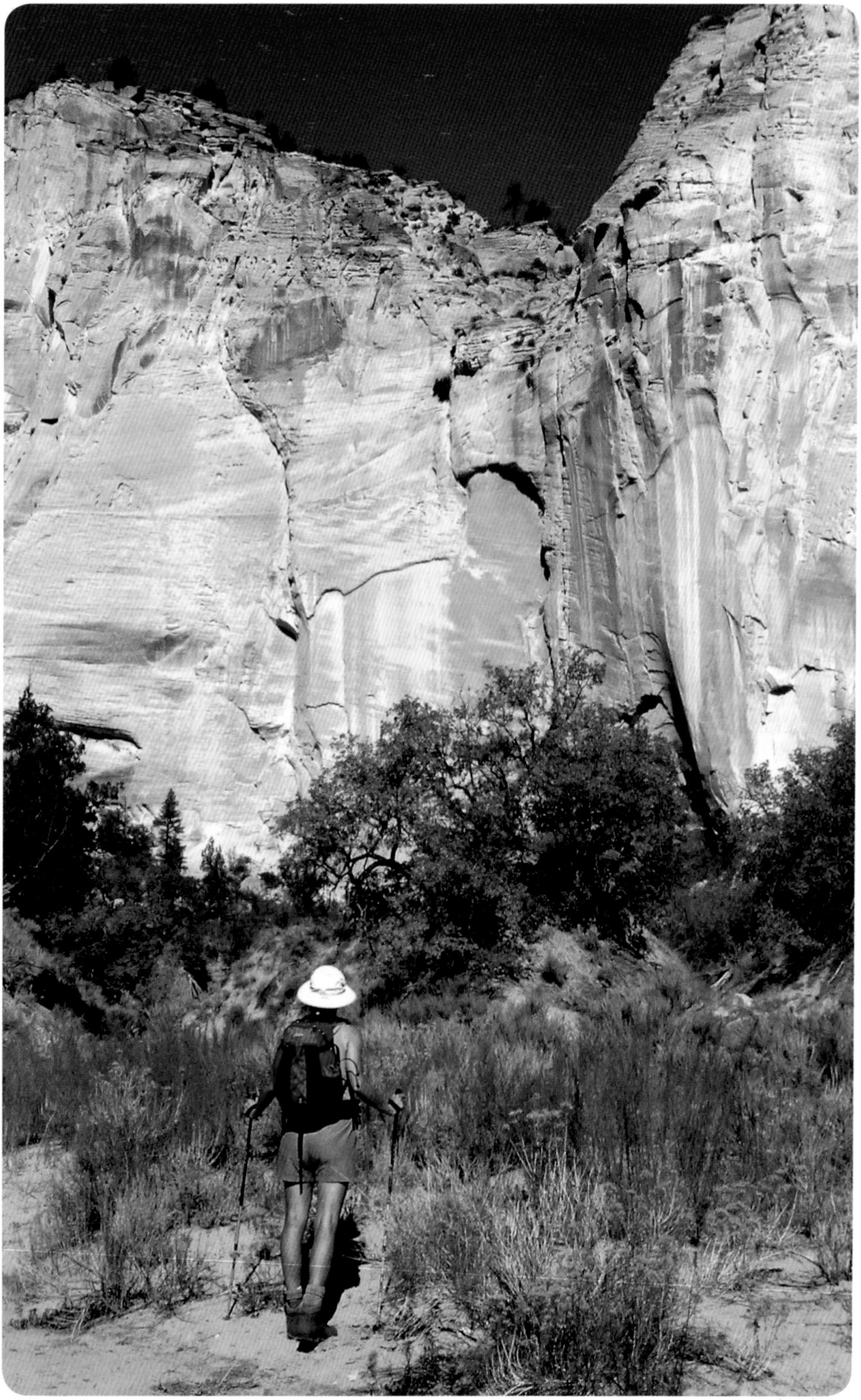

Lick Wash

Proceed on Skutumpah Road (also known as Road 500). Immediately cross Yellow Creek wash—usually dry. If it's wet, the road will be impassable. Stop. Do not continue.

3 mi (4.8 km)
Enter Grand Staircase-Escalante National Monument.

3.4 mi (5.5 km)
Proceed straight. The pink sandstone of Bryce Canyon National Park is visible right (northwest).

4 mi (6.4 km)
Proceed straight.

5.6 mi (9 km)
Bear right to cross runoff below the small concrete spillway of a dam spanning Sheep Creek wash.

6.1 mi (9.8 km)
After ascending a ridge, descend to cross a dry wash.

6.5 mi (10.5 km)
Proceed straight, ignoring the right fork. Avoid the shoulder of the road, which tends to erode and slough off.

7.5 mi (12.1 km)
Descend into a dry wash and climb another ridge.

8.2 mi (13.2 km)
Fork left near the ridgecrest.

9 mi (14.5 km)
Reach **Willis Creek** (Trip 19) trailhead parking area on the right, just north of the creek, at 6000 ft (1829 m).

Continuing southwest to Lick Wash

10.8 mi (17.4 km)
Stop in the pullout, then walk 110 yd (100 m) to see the unique, earthen bridge spanning Bull Valley Gorge. Look for the truck that fell into the gap in the 1940s.

22.1 mi (35.6 km)
Just before a cattleguard, turn left to enter **Lick Wash** trailhead parking area at 6330 ft (1930 m).

Continuing southwest to Hwy 89

36 mi (58 km)
Turn left onto paved Johnson Canyon Road.

52.1 mi (83.9 km)
Reach Hwy 89. Kanab is right (west). Page, Arizona, is left (east).

From Kanab or Big Water

Kanab is on Hwy 89, southeast of Zion Park. Big Water is on Hwy 89, northwest of Page, Arizona.

From the junction of Hwys 89 and 89A in Kanab, drive Hwy 89 east 10 mi (16 km).

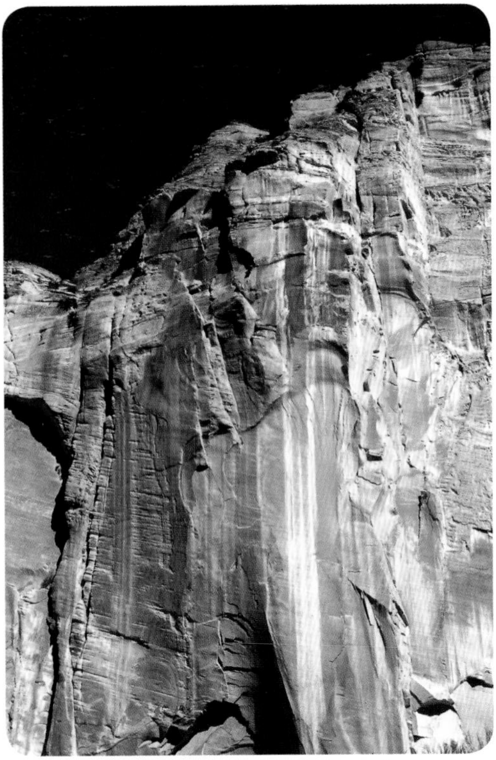

The White Cliffs of the Grand Staircase plateau

From the Big Water exit on Hwy 89, drive west 55 mi (88.6 km).

From either approach, turn north onto paved Johnson Canyon Road (just east of milepost 55) and reset your trip odometer to 0.

0 mi (0 km)
Starting north on paved Johnson Canyon Road.

11.5 mi (18.5 km)
Enter Grand Staircase-Escalante National Monument.

16.1 mi (26 km)
Turn right onto unpaved Skutumpah Road (also known as Road 500), signed for Deer Springs Ranch (13 mi) and Cannonville (38 mi).

17.7 mi (28.5 km)
Bear right, ignoring the left fork. Proceed through a broad, dusty basin rife with sagebrush.

19.4 mi (31.2 km)
Proceed straight, ignoring the left fork.

22.4 mi (36.1 km) / 27 mi (43.5 km) / 27.6 mi (44.5 km) / 28 mi (45 km)
Bear left, ignoring right forks.

28.4 mi (45.8 km)
Bear right.

30 mi (48.4 km)
Proceed straight, ignoring the right fork. Cross a cattle guard and, just before the wash, turn right to enter **Lick Wash** trailhead parking area at 6330 ft (1930 m).

Continuing northeast to Willis Creek (Trip 19)

30.6 mi (49.3 km) / 35.2 mi (56.6 km) / 37.3 mi (60 km)
Proceed on the main road, ignoring minor spurs.

37.4 mi (60.2 km)
Slow down. Just beyond, the road descends steeply then remains narrow for the next 5 mi (8 km).

41.2 mi (66.3 km)
Reach Bull Valley Gorge. Stop in the pullout, then walk 30 yd/m left to see the unique, earthen bridge. Look for the truck that fell into the gap in the 1940s.

43.1 mi (69.4 km)
Reach **Willis Creek** (Trip 19) trailhead parking area on the left, just north of the creek, at 6000 ft (1829 m).

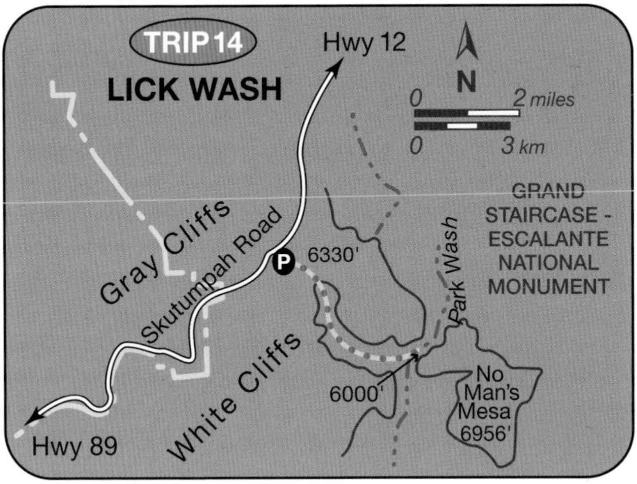

Continuing northeast to Cannonville

43.8 mi (70.5 km)
Proceed on the main road, ignoring a left fork.

48.1 mi (77.5 km)
The road descends. Beware of sand.

49.3 mi (79.3 km)
Intersect paved Cottonwood Canyon Road. Turn left (north) to reach Cannonville and intersect Hwy 12 in 2.8 mi (4.5 km). Turn right (southeast) to reach Kodachrome Basin State Park in 6.7 mi (10.8 km).

ON FOOT

Follow the wash south-southeast into the canyon mouth. Big juniper and tall ponderosa pine are prevalent.

Within five minutes, the canyon narrows to 25 ft (7.6 m). About 20 minutes along, the walls are just 10 ft (3 m) apart. Watch for a couple giant Douglas firs. Within 40 minutes, the canyon widens to 50 ft (15 m).

About an hour from the trailhead, the wash curves east-southeast. On the left, soaring 600 ft (183 m), are great walls of white Navajo sandstone punctuated with ponderosa pines. On the right (south) are crossbedded-slickrock waves and domes; beyond are distant cliffs.

At 3.5 mi (5.6 km), 6000 ft (1830 m), the canyon is considerably broader. The right side is now beyond peripheral eyesight. Lick Wash deepens as it approaches its confluence with **Park Wash**, in an open valley.

Watch left for an alcove-sized scallop in the sandstone cliff. When you're beneath it, look for a cow path ascending left, up the north bank of the wash onto a sage-covered bench.

To better appreciate the area, continue several minutes along the path atop the bench. No Man's Mesa is visible ahead (east-southeast), beyond Park Wash. No Man's is the canyon-country equivalent of a Galapagos Island. It harbors numerous plant and animal species that are rare or endangered elsewhere on the Colorado Plateau.

TRIP 15

RAINBOW BRIDGE & BEYOND

LOCATION	Rainbow Bridge National Monument Lake Powell, east of Dangling Rope Marina
ROUND TRIP	23 mi (27 km)
ELEVATION CHANGE	2640-ft (805-m) gain and loss
KEY ELEVATIONS	boat dock and trailhead 3600 ft (1098 m), confluence of Bridge and Redbud creeks 4100 ft (1250 m) Redbud Pass 4400 ft (1341 m), plateau above Oak Creek Canyon 4880 ft (1487 m)
HIKING TIME	2 to 3 days
DIFFICULTY	challenging
MAPS	Trails Illustrated *Glen Canyon NRA* USGS *Rainbow Bridge, Utah-Ariz*

OPINION

Rainbow Bridge is the touchstone between the Earth and the spirit world according to Navajo legend. Perhaps you'll feel why when you stand beneath it. What you'll see is the world's largest and most famous natural bridge.

Natural bridges were formed by streams. That's what distinguishes them from natural arches, which were created by weathering and/or a combination of erosional forces. Two Utah arches—Kolob (Trip 2) and Landscape (Trip 47)—are longer than Rainbow. And Tushuk Tash, a 1,200-ft (366-m) high arch in China, is much taller.

So Rainbow Bridge—standing 290 ft (88 m) high and spanning 275 ft (84 m) —is neither the longest nor the tallest arcing expanse of stone, but we're convinced it's the most beautiful.

The canyon setting is magnificent. And Rainbow is much more than simply huge. It's an astonishing fusion of elegant symmetry and stalwart resilience. Like the Taj Mahal, you can study photos of it, you can imagine it, yet it's overwhelming when you witness it: an artful sweep of aerial rock soaring between Navajo Mtn and Lake Powell.

Archaeologists believe Natives camped near Rainbow Bridge 2000 years ago. In deference to its spiritual potency, Natives today will not walk beneath it. Paiutes and Navajos now share stewardship of *Nonnezoshe*—the Navajo term for "rainbow turned to stone."

The first white people to see the stone rainbow were guided there by Paiute guides Nasja Begay and Jim Mike in 1909. The group included pre-eminent archaeologist John Wetherill. News of their "discovery" spread rapidly. The following year, President Taft established Rainbow Bridge National Monument.

President Teddy Roosevelt and author Zane Grey were among early travelers who made the arduous, multi-day trek to see the natural colossus. When rafting the Colorado River through Glen Canyon became popular, the 14-mi (22.5-km)

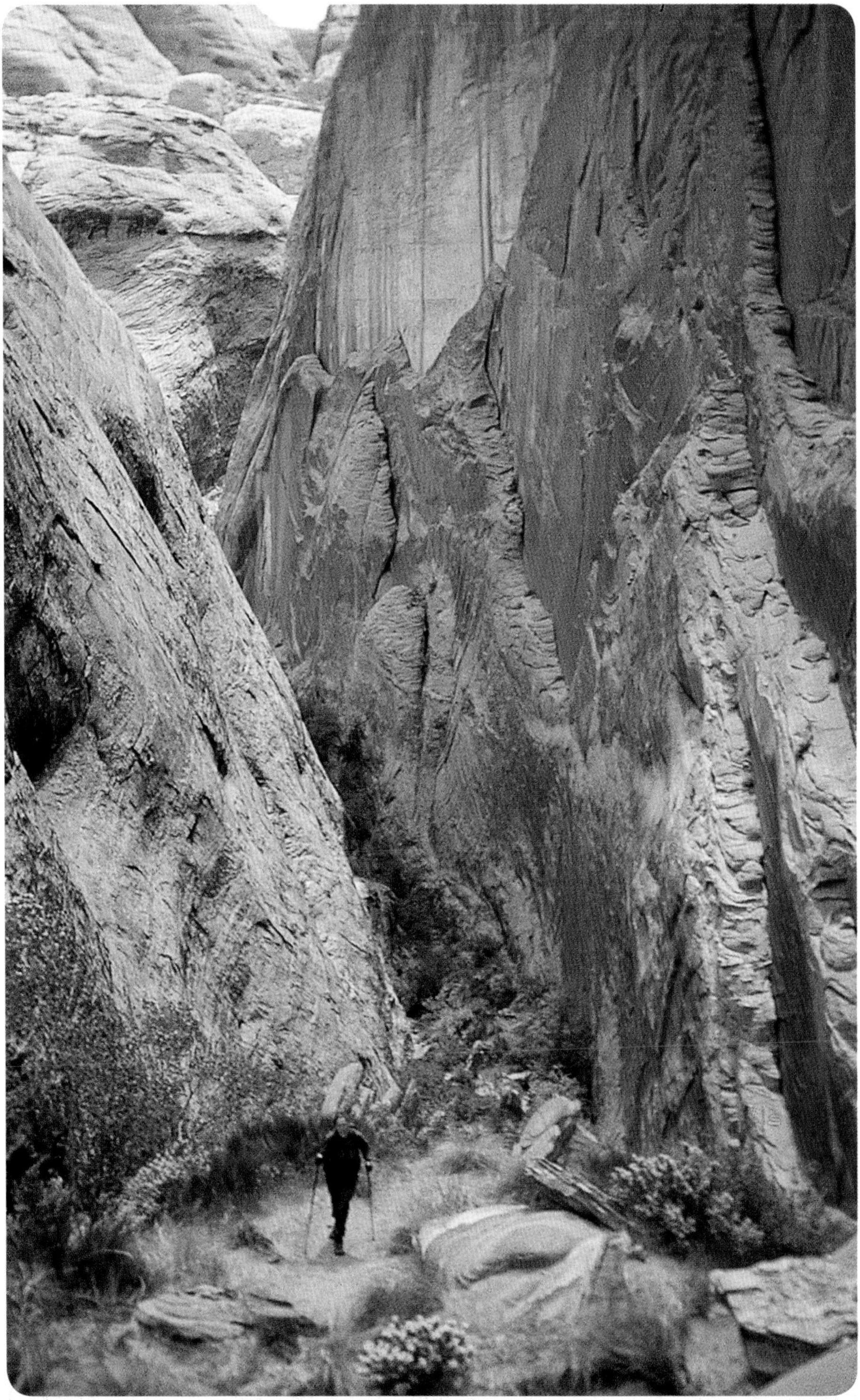

Cliff Canyon

round-trip hike to the Rainbow Bridge was a premier sidetrip. In the 1950s, tourists could jetboat upstream from Lees Ferry, then hike to the bridge. After Glen Canyon Dam was built, halting flow of the Colorado River, the tributary canyons were inundated by 1963. Suddenly tour boats could motor 50 mi (81 km) up-lake from Wahweap Marina nearly to the bridge. Visitors flocked here.

In 1974, the Navajo Nation filed suit to preserve religious sites being flooded by Lake Powell. The U.S. District Court ruled against the Navajos. Water storage was a more pressing need, the court said. In 1980, the Tenth District Court of Appeals ruled that Rainbow Bridge was a public site and said closing it for Navajo religious ceremonies would violate the U.S. Constitution, which protects the religious freedom of all citizens.

Five tribes have historical claims to Rainbow Bridge: the Navajo, Hopi, San Juan Southern Paiute, Kaibab Paiute, and White Mesa Ute. After consulting with them, the National Park Service adopted a management plan in 1993. The tribes' primary request was that Rainbow Bridge, in keeping with its sacred status, be protected and visited respectfully. They also expressed concern about visitors approaching or walking beneath the bridge. Today, the National Park Service simply asks that, while in the presence of Rainbow Bridge, you remain mindful of those who revere it as a supremely spiritual site.

Today, 300,000 people from around the world visit Rainbow Bridge each year. Most consider it the highlight of their trip to Lake Powell, though the lake itself is also a marvel: a vast, sinuous, web of water where, obviously, water should be scarce. It's 150 mi (242 km) long, averages 400 ft (122 m) deep, and has 2,000 mi (610 km) of vibrantly colorful sandstone shoreline punctuated by cliffs, buttes, mesas, domes, and gorges.

Infinite water amid eternal desert is a bizarre and therefore alluring concept. In truth, the water is not infinite, but only seems so. Even the desert surrounding it is impermanent. So while Lake Powell is sublimely scenic and a milestone in the history of human ingenuity, it's also a monument to human conceit.

Our view is that Glen Canyon Dam should never have been built. It replaced a natural wonder with an artificial one. We gained a reservoir of questionable, temporary value (see www.glencanyon.org) at the expense of a canyon of immense, enduring value. Glen Canyon was as resplendent as the Grand Canyon. We flooded a Cistine Chapel so we could float near the ceiling.

But avoiding Lake Powell, turning your back on its seductions, is an ineffective protest. Depriving yourself of the unique experiences it offers will serve nothing. The reservoir exists, at least for now. Might as well enjoy it. Boating to Rainbow Bridge then hiking beyond is a fine way to do that.

The backpack trip described here is a shortcut: the easiest way to see Rainbow Bridge and sample the intriguing wilderness beyond, on the lower slopes of Navajo Mtn. The alternative—more time consuming, physically demanding and logistically complex—is to start at one of two, remote trailheads on Navajo land, then complete a one-way journey on the trail skirting the west half of Navajo Mtn. For information sources, skip below to *Before your trip*.

Despite the throngs who pay homage to Rainbow Bridge via boat, you'll likely be the only one among them shouldering a backpack. Keep hiking past the bridge, and you'll surely find solitude in the depths of Bridge Canyon. You'll also find an oasis where you can camp amid lush foliage. But overall, this is a harsh, intimidating land: topographically tortuous and eerily tranquil. Though beautiful, intrinsic to that beauty is a mysterious atmosphere that lends ineffable credence to the Navajo beliefs about Rainbow Bridge.

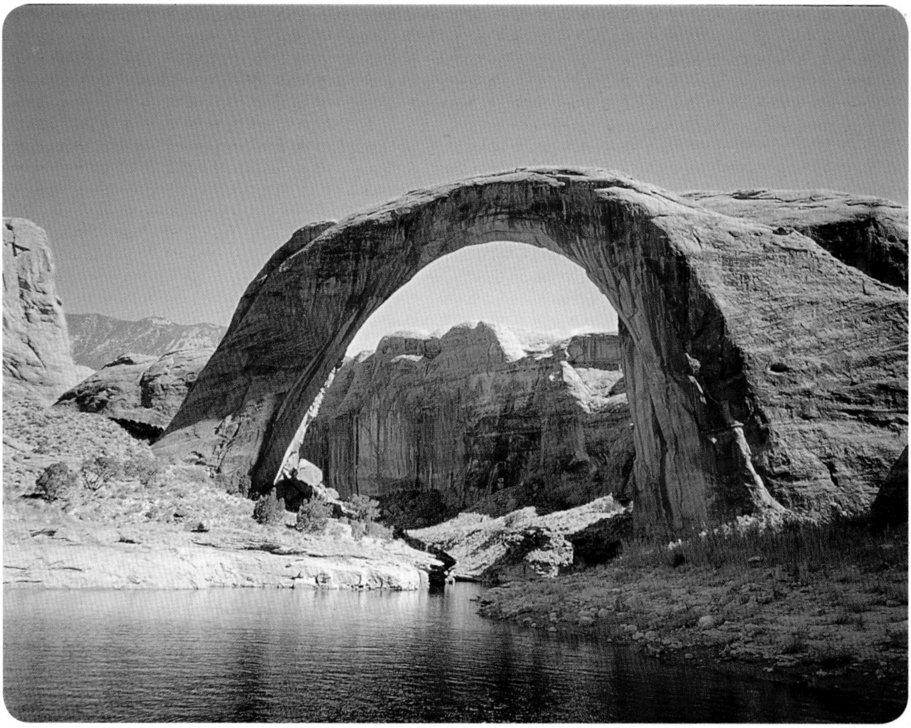

Rainbow Bridge, at the beginning of the hike

The optimal time to hike here is when the weather is neither too hot nor too cold: April, May, September, or October. We recommend pitching your tent near the confluence of Bridge and Redbud creeks at 3 mi (4.8 km), then dayhiking beyond. On day one you should have time to probe either fork. On day two, an early start will allow you to probe the other fork, then return to the boat dock below Rainbow Bridge.

FACT

BEFORE YOUR TRIP

The trail beyond Rainbow Bridge soon enters the Navajo Nation, so you must get a permit to hike on their land. Visit www.navajonationparks.org, email navajoparks@yahoo.com, or phone Antelope Canyon Travel Park at (928) 698-2807.

Make a reservation at least one month in advance for round-trip boat transportation with Lake Powell Resorts & Marinas, an authorized concessioner of the National Park Service. Visit www.visitlakepowell.com, or phone (928) 645-2433 or (888) 896-3829.

All narrow canyons, regardless how easy to enter, are dangerous, because even distant rain can cause an overwhelming volume of water to suddenly rush through them. Hike here only during a period of sunny weather, when there's little risk of a flash flood. Check the forecast at Wahweap Marina.

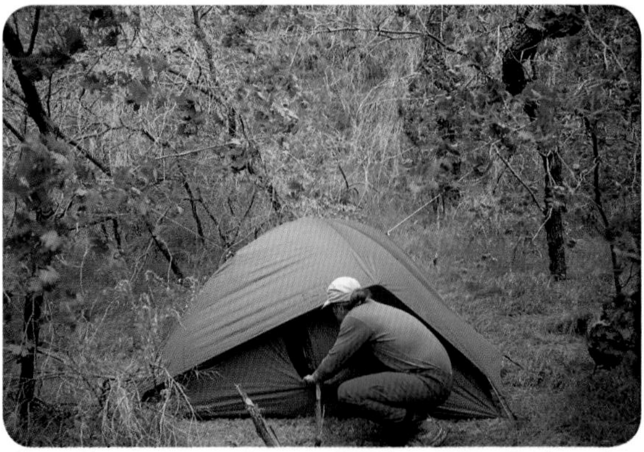
Campsite near the confluence of Bridge and Redbud creeks

Visit www.nps.gov/rabr to learn more about Rainbow Bridge National Monument. Visit www.nps.gov/glca to learn more about Glen Canyon National Recreation Area.

The trip described here is only a portion of the complete, semicircular route skirting the west half of Navajo Mtn—an arduous, 27-mi (43.5-km), one-way journey. To contemplate hiking it, you'll need the USGS topo maps *Chaiyahi Flat* and *Navajo Begay*. You'll also need detailed information regarding the complex access to the two trailheads. Visit www.navajonationparks.org, email navajoparks@yahoo.com, or phone Antelope Canyon Travel Park at (928) 698-2807.

BY VEHICLE

From Page, Arizona, drive Hwy 89 north. Cross Glen Canyon Dam and proceed northwest. Shortly beyond, turn right to enter Wahweap Marina, at the southwest end of Lake Powell.

From Kanab, Arizona, drive Hwy 89 east, past Big Water, then southeast. Shortly before crossing Glen Canyon Dam to Page, Arizona, turn left to enter Wahweap Marina, at the southwest end of Lake Powell.

BY BOAT

April through October, Lake Powell Resorts & Marinas (see contact info above) offers a three-hour trip from Wahweap Marina to Rainbow Bridge. Their schedule is based on Arizona Mountain Standard Time. The final approach is via narrow Forbidding Canyon. Reach the boat dock at approximately 3600 ft (1098 m). This elevation changes, of course, depending on the current lake level.

ON FOOT

Years ago, Lake Powell extended up Forbidding Arm just beyond Rainbow Bridge. But a protracted drought has lowered the lake significantly. Until the Colorado Plateau receives above-average rainfall for several consecutive years, Lake Powell will remain well below full pool.

Recently, the lake level has necessitated at least a 1-mi (1.6-km) hike from the boat dock, southeast to Rainbow Bridge via the left (northeast) side of the drainage.

Pass beneath **Rainbow Bridge** at 3740 ft (1140 m). A plaque near the base of the bridge commemorates the Paiute guides who led the first white men here. The trail continues up the drainage (southeast) along its left (northeast) side, beneath walls 500 ft (152 m) high.

Near 1.5 mi (2.4 km) the trail veers right and meanders southwest. Near 2.1 mi (3.4 km) it curves left and wanders generally southeast. Heading up-canyon, it crosses the usually-dry creekbed several times.

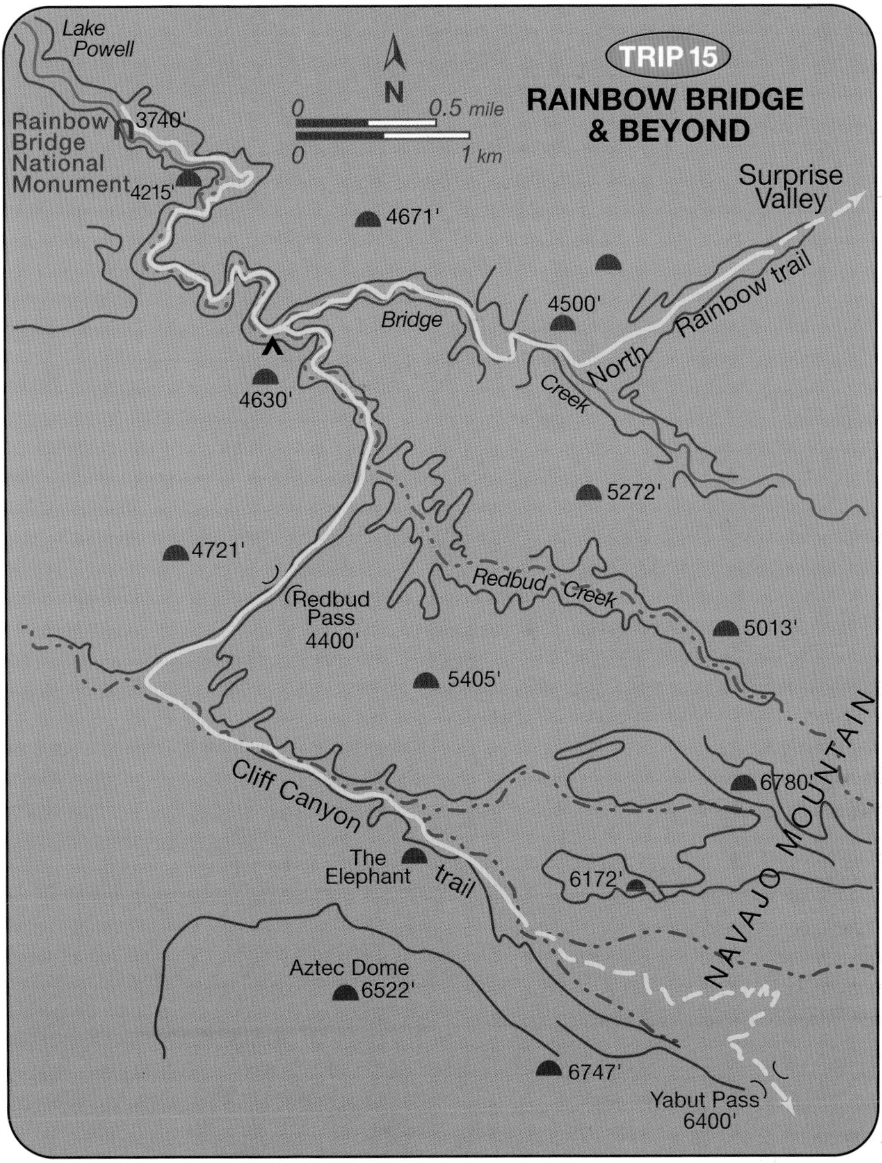

Just after a campsite on a sandy bench in a lush glen, reach the **confluence of Bridge and Redbud creeks** at 3 mi (4.8 km), 4180 ft (1274 m). A dome divides the drainages. Cairns indicate where the trail forks near a tall juniper.

Redbud Pass and Cliff Canyon

Fork right (southeast) into **Redbud Creek Canyon**, where the walls abate. Beware of cacti in the trailside brush.

Follow the winding creekbed up-canyon. After heading generally south, the canyon forks at 1 mi (1.6 km), 4200 ft (1280 m). Left (east-southeast) is the creek drainage. Bear right (south-southwest).

Gradually curving right (southwest), the canyon narrows. About 50 minutes along, ascend a rockslide to crest 4400-ft (1341-m) **Redbud Pass** at 1.5 mi (2.4 km).

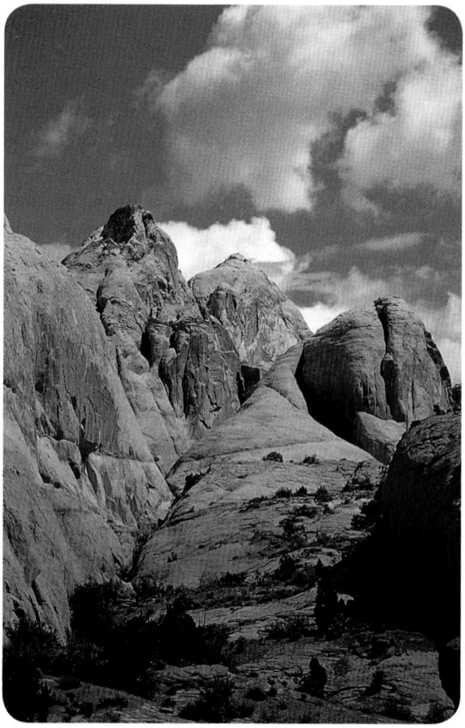
Redbud Creek Canyon

Descend southwest on slickrock. At 2.3 mi (3.7 km), 4180 ft (1274 m), the trail curves sharply left (southeast) into **Cliff Canyon**. White sandstone domes rise above salmon cliffs. Look for pink wild roses near 3 mi (4.8 km). The trail is increasingly rough and brushy.

At 3.5 mi (5.6 km), 4440 ft (1354 m), beneath 6522-ft (1988-m) **Aztec Dome** (right / south), the canyon forks again. Visible ahead (southeast) is 10,388-ft (3167-m) Navajo Mtn. End your foray here, and you'll complete a 7-mi (11.3-km) round trip by the time you return to your campsite near the confluence of Bridge and Redbud creeks.

Should you resume hiking southeast from the canyon fork beneath Aztec Dome, within 0.5 mi (0.8 km) the trail ascends madly. It gains 1600 ft (488 m) in just 1.5 mi (2.4 km) over loose talus to 6400-ft (1951-m) **Yabut Pass** at 6.5 mi (10.5 km). Here, the view extends right (southwest) into Dome Canyon, and ahead (south-southwest) into Arizona.

Oak Canyon

From the cairned junction at the confluence of Bridge and Redbud creeks, fork left (northeast) into **Bridge Creek Canyon**. The trail is initially above the creek's right (southeast) bank but ahead crosses it repeatedly.

The ascent is gentle. Bedrock is often underfoot. Soon visible right (southeast) is 10,388-ft (3167-m) Navajo Mtn. Nearly one hour along, reach a creekside campsite among juniper at 1.5 mi (2.4 km), 4400 ft (1341 m).

After rising onto a bench heading northeast, the trail undulates. Within the next 30 minutes, climb to 4700 ft (1433 m) amid slickrock domes and attain a clear view of Navajo Mtn right (south-southeast).

Ascend briefly. Descend south then east to cross the **first of Oak Creek Canyon's three upper forks** at 3 mi (4.8 km). Resume ascending to a sandy, 4890-ft (1491-m) flat between the first and middle forks. The trail then veers left (northeast) and drops to cross **Oak Creek's second upper fork** at 4680 ft (1427 m).

Another short ascent leads to a sage-covered **plateau**. At 4 mi (6.4 km), 4880 ft (1487 m), about two hours along, the trail nearly levels heading generally east. End your foray here, and you'll complete an 8-mi (12.9-km) round trip by the time you return to your campsite near the confluence of Bridge and Redbud creeks.

Should you resume hiking east across the plateau, the trail soon curves left (northeast), drops to cross **Oak Creek's third upper fork**, then continues rising northeast into more constricted terrain until easing across **Surprise Valley** at 5.4 mi (8.7 km), 4520 ft (1378 m).

TRIP 16

FAIRYLAND

LOCATION	Bryce Canyon National Park
LOOP	8 mi (12.9 km)
ELEVATION GAIN	1670 ft (509 m)
KEY ELEVATIONS	trailhead 7775 ft (2370 m) rim highpoint 8155 ft (2486 m) lowpoint 7150 ft (2180 m)
HIKING TIME	3 to 4½ hours
DIFFICULTY	moderate
MAP	Trails Illustrated *Bryce Canyon National Park*

OPINION

"Do these shoes go with this dress?" "Do my shirt and tie clash?" We're so timid when it comes to fashion. Instead we should learn from Mother Earth. She's beautiful because she's bold. At Bryce Canyon National Park, where she's applauded daily by an endless crowd of international critics, she sashays in a florid, orange-and-pink designer original by Dr. Suess.

Seen from below, Bryce Canyon does resemble the hem of a showy gown. That's because it's not a canyon in the strictest sense, but rather a dozen ravines along the east edge of a plateau. They were formed by rain and melting snow flowing off the Pink Cliffs to the Paria River. Among the ravines are hundreds of ridges, or fins, that have eroded into bizarre, vertical shapes known as *hoodoos*. Soil rich in oxidized manganese and iron creates their vibrant shades of white, yellow, pink, orange and red.

The park's most outlandish scenery is concentrated near the Navajo, Peekaboo, and Queens Garden trails (Trip 17), and that's where you should hike despite the crowd. But if you have a second day here, or you're willing to sacrifice spectacle for serenity, hike the Fairyland loop. You'll still see why Bryce is famous. You just won't be in downtown hoodooville. You'll be in the suburbs.

Strong, ambitious hikers, however, don't have to choose. They can hike both in a single day. Start at Fairyland Point, follow the Fairyland loop directions below, but upon intersecting the canyon rim trail, detour left (south) to Sunrise Point, continue southwest along the rim to Sunset Point, then follow the directions for Trip 17. After returning to Sunrise Point, retrace your steps north, bear left, and resume the Fairyland loop. Your total distance will be 14.4 mi (23.2 km)—about a six-hour task.

Though hiking always beats gawking, allow time before or after your hike to join the gawkers at the 14 viewpoints along the paved park road. All are on the canyon rim, which soars to 9115 ft (2778 m), so they afford dazzling aerial perspectives of the Pink Cliffs immediately below and spectacular panoramas extending south toward the Grand Canyon and east toward Lake Powell.

The optimal time for photographing Bryce? Sunrise, definitely. The rapidly changing light and shifting shadows turn the extraordinary topography into the

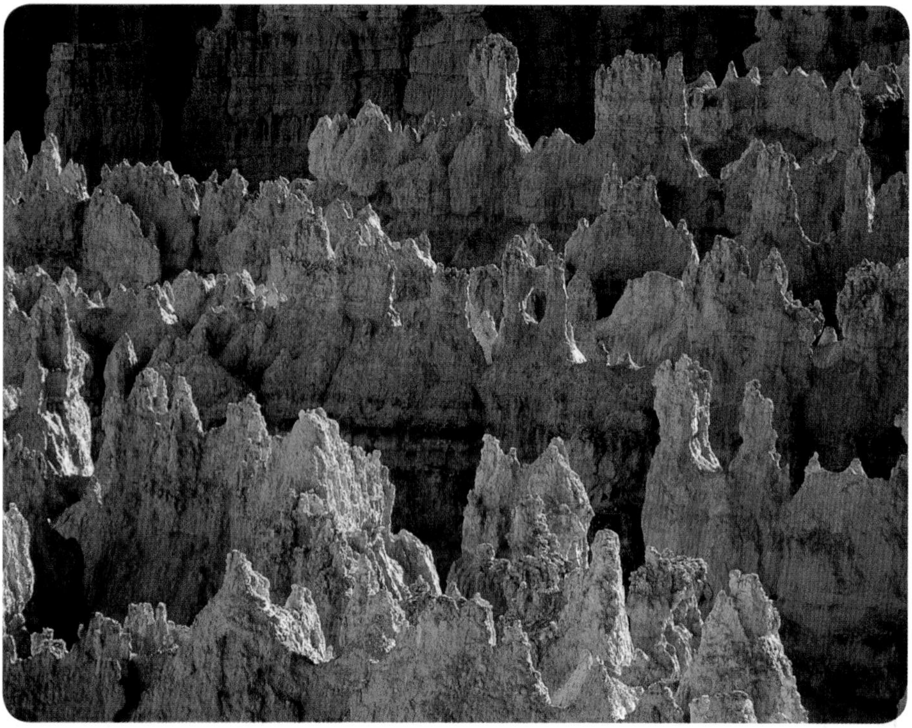

Bryce National Park

visual equivalent of an earsplitting hurrah. Sunsets are disappointing because the Pink Cliffs face generally east and are therefore in shadow when the sun sinks in the west.

Looking at a park map, you'll see numerous trails. This book describes what we believe are the most rewarding two. The Under the Rim trail offers shuttle-assisted dayhiking or overnight backpacking, both of which are rewarding. The one trail we suggest you avoid is the 8.5-mi (13.7-km) Riggs Spring Loop starting at Rainbow Point. It's quiet but heavily forested and scenically dull.

So what does the name *Bryce* have to do with this crazy, colorful land? When the national park was established in 1924, it was named after the region's first white settler, a Mormon farmer—Ebenezer Bryce—who was neither crazy nor colorful.

FACT

BEFORE YOUR TRIP

Hikers can legally enter Bryce Canyon National Park free-of-charge on this trail. It begins near the park's north edge, at the Fairyland Point trailhead, which is accessed outside the park gate. Hiking elsewhere in Bryce will require you to pay the expensive entrance fee. Amortize the cost by purchasing an annual pass valid at all U.S. national parks.

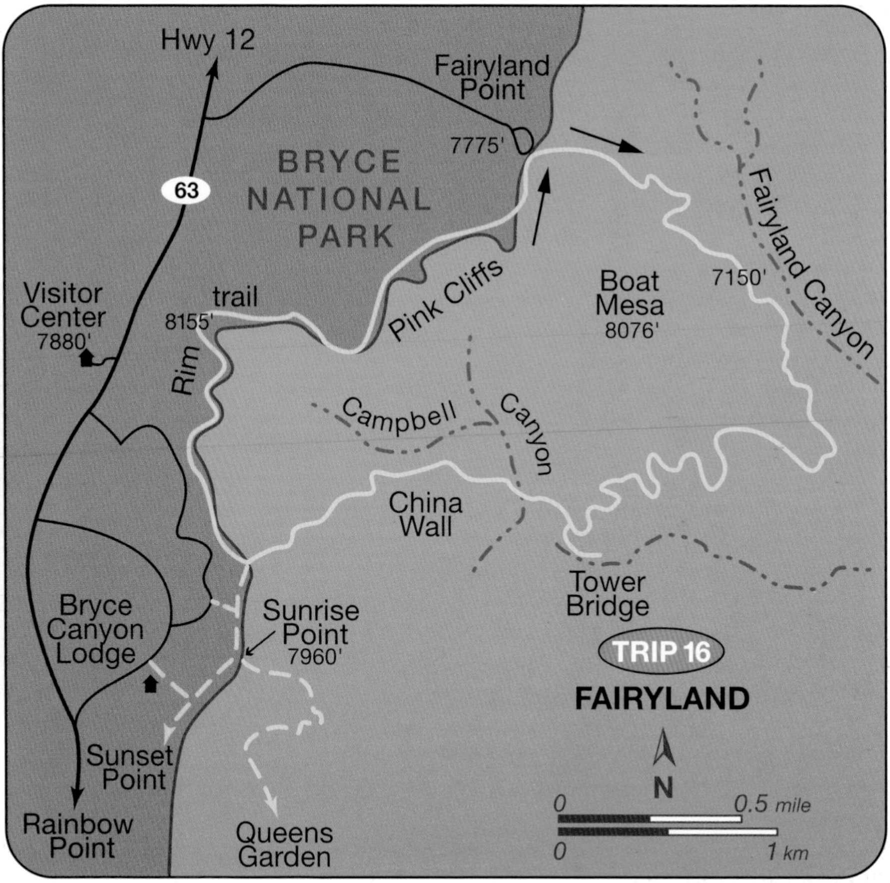

This and Trip 17 are the highest elevation trails in Utah canyon country. The Bryce visitor center, for example, is at 7880 ft (2402 m), while the Zion visitor center is at 4000 ft (1219 m). In spring or fall, expect it to be 15°F (9°C) cooler here than in Zion. Pack accordingly.

Despite cold winter temperatures, Bryce is open year round. During the six months when snow is present, the national park loans snowshoes to visitors free-of-charge. That makes the entrance fee a bargain.

BY VEHICLE

From Hwy 89, southeast of Panquitch, drive Hwy 12 east 14 mi (22.5 km).

From Escalante, drive Hwy 12 southwest to Cannonville, north to Tropic, then continue 7.5 mi (12.1 km) north-northwest.

From either approach, turn south onto Hwy 63 and reset your trip odometer to 0.

At 3 mi (4.8 km), where straight (south) enters the park, turn left (east). Reach road's end and the Fairyland Point trailhead parking lot at 4 mi (6.4 km), 7775 ft (2370 m).

ON FOOT

Descend a narrow ridge left (generally east), among limber, bristlecone, and ponderosa pines, on the edge of a hoodoo studded amphitheater. Curving right (southeast), overlook the upper reaches of **Fairyland Canyon** left (northeast).

After swerving right (southwest) into a dry gully, the trail veers left (southeast) again. Ascend to the left (east) side of a colorful, eroded cliff, then drop to the loop's 7150-ft (2180-m) **lowpoint** near the floor of Fairyland Canyon.

Ascend briefly, contour at 7250 ft (2210 m) for about ten minutes, then ascend to 7375 ft (2248 m) at the loop's **southeast corner**. From here the trail wriggles generally west, contouring beneath 8076-ft (2462-m) Boat Mesa (right / north) and above Campbell Canyon (left / south).

Switchback down to the loop's **midpoint**—4 mi (6.4 km), 7230 ft (2204 m)—where a left spur detours east-southeast 200 yd (183 m) to the foot of **Tower Bridge** (technically an arch or window). Visible south-southwest is 7678-ft (2341-m) Mormon Temple.

From the midpoint spur, the main trail goes right (north), crosses a draw, curves left (west), and crosses another draw. A steep ascent ensues generally west along a ridge just north of **China Wall**.

The ascent continues southwest until intersecting the **canyon rim trail** at 5.5 mi (8.9 km), 7980 ft (2433 m). Left leads south 0.25 mi (0.4 km) to Sunrise Point (Trip 17). Turn right and hike generally north-northwest, then north, along the rim.

After swerving right (east), nip over an 8155-ft (2486-m) knoll— the loop's **highpoint**. Proceed east. Descend southeast to 7850 ft (2393 m), then cruise generally northeast above the pinnacled **Pink Cliffs**. The trail finally curves left (north) to reach **Fairyland Point**, where the loop ends at 8 mi (12.9 km).

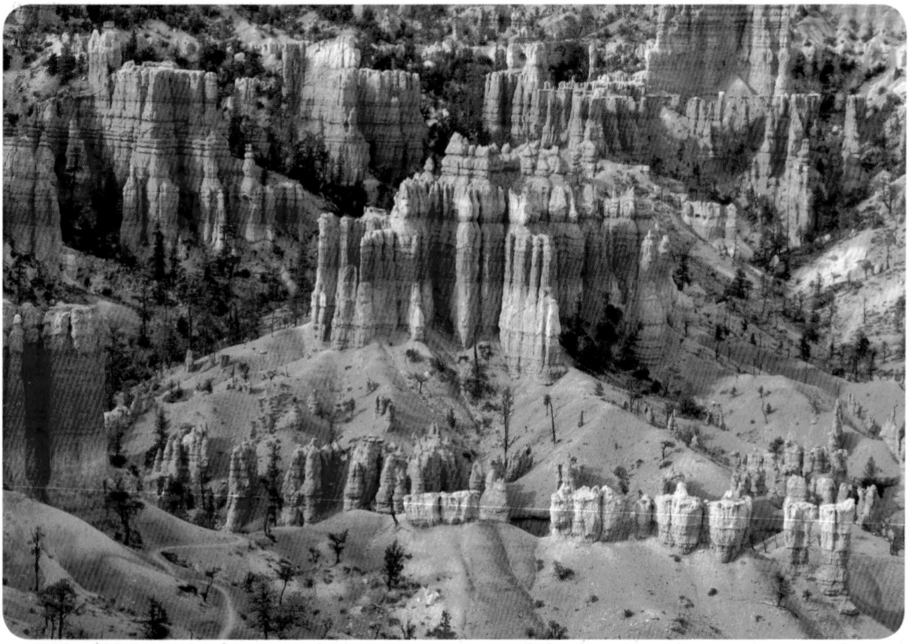

Fairyland

TRIP 17

NAVAJO / PEEKABOO / QUEENS GARDEN

LOCATION	Bryce Canyon National Park
CIRCUIT	1.4 mi (2.3 km) for Navajo 4.8 mi (7.7 km) for Navajo and Peekaboo 6.4 mi (10.3 km) for Navajo, Peekaboo and Queens Garden
ELEVATION CHANGE	505-ft (154-m) loss and gain for Navajo 1020-ft (311-m) loss and 1145-ft (349-m) gain for either of the longer circuits
KEY ELEVATIONS	trailhead 7985 ft (2434 m), lowpoint near Bryce Creek 7420 ft (2262 m), Queens Garden 7600 ft (2317 m)
HIKING TIME	40 minutes for Navajo 2 to 2½ hours for Navajo and Peekaboo 3 to 3½ hours for Navajo, Peekaboo, and Queens Garden
DIFFICULTY	easy to moderate
MAP	Trails Illustrated *Bryce Canyon National Park*

OPINION

Bryce Canyon National Park is surreal. Not in the shallow way the word is commonly used, but in it's true sense: super realistic.

The great surrealist painters—André Masson, René Magritte, Salvador Dali, Max Ernst—saw their art as a weapon against the restrictions of society. They attempted to startle the viewer by showing what they considered the deeper or truer aspects of human nature.

So you're in for a shock, a jolt of hyper realism, because hiking in Bryce Canyon is as close as you'll get to entering one of Max Ernst's mysterious, rocky landscapes. Strange creatures seem to emerge from patterns of paint spread haphazardly over his canvases. And so it is here, where the spires, pinnacles, turrets and towers come alive to the imaginative observer.

Most of Utah canyon country was created from a red-orange color palette. It seems strikingly original until you arrive at Bryce and witness the furthest extreme: orange sherbet, cotton-candy pink, and subtle variations that give the impression of frozen fire.

The Bryce trails plunge off the canyon rim then wiggle through a riot of spasmodic shapes. Gazing down from the park's scenic overlooks, it's difficult to believe you can penetrate such convoluted topography. But each twisting passage leads to another. It's constantly engaging and often surprising.

Starting at Sunset Point, you have several options. The Navajo loop is excellent but too short. Combine it with the Peekaboo loop for the minimum hike necessary to adequately sample the park. If you hike the longest of the

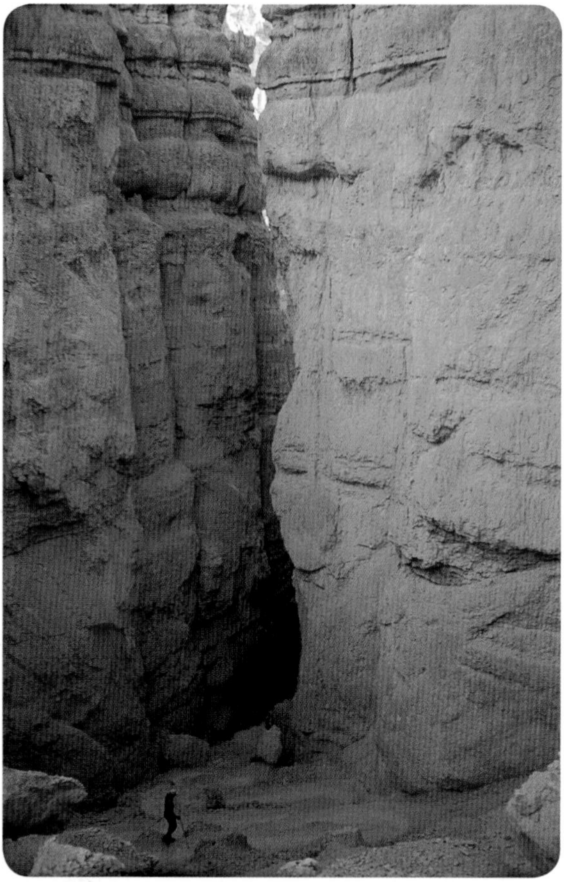

Wall Street, on the Navajo loop

three circuits described here, you'll have a much more complete experience. Afterward, drive south to 9015-ft (2748-m) Rainbow Point and hike the 1-mi (1.6-km) Bristlecone loop, where you'll commune with 1,600-year-old bristlecone pines—the world's oldest trees.

When hiking the Peekaboo loop, be prepared to encounter one of the twice-daily horseback tours. Serious hikers wince at how it heightens the Disney-esque atmosphere, but most agree it's worth tolerating.

FACT

BEFORE YOUR TRIP

The entrance fee for Bryce Canyon National Park is expensive. Amortize the cost by purchasing an annual pass valid at all U.S. national parks. Trip 16 describes how to legally enter Bryce free-of-charge by starting your hike near the park's north edge, at the Fairyland Point trailhead, which is accessed outside the park gate. It will add a 5.5-mi (8.9-km) round trip to your total circuit distance, however, so you'll have to be fit and keen in addition to frugal.

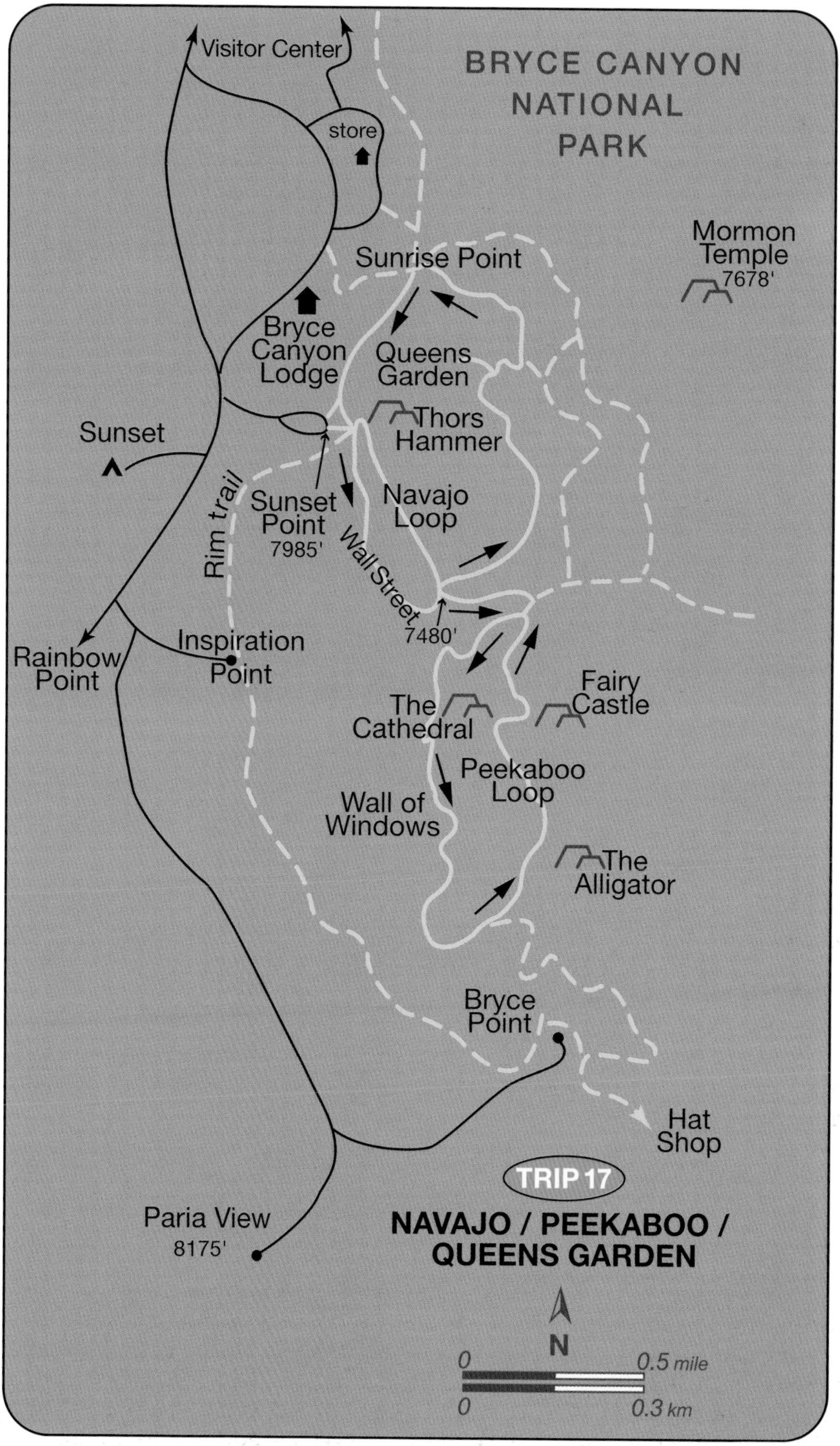
BRYCE CANYON NATIONAL PARK
Visitor Center
store
Sunrise Point
Mormon Temple 7678'
Bryce Canyon Lodge
Queens Garden
Thors Hammer
Sunset
Rim trail
Sunset Point 7985'
Navajo Loop
Wall Street
7480'
Inspiration Point
Rainbow Point
Fairy Castle
The Cathedral
Peekaboo Loop
Wall of Windows
The Alligator
Bryce Point
Hat Shop
TRIP 17
NAVAJO / PEEKABOO / QUEENS GARDEN
Paria View 8175'
N
0 0.5 mile
0 0.3 km

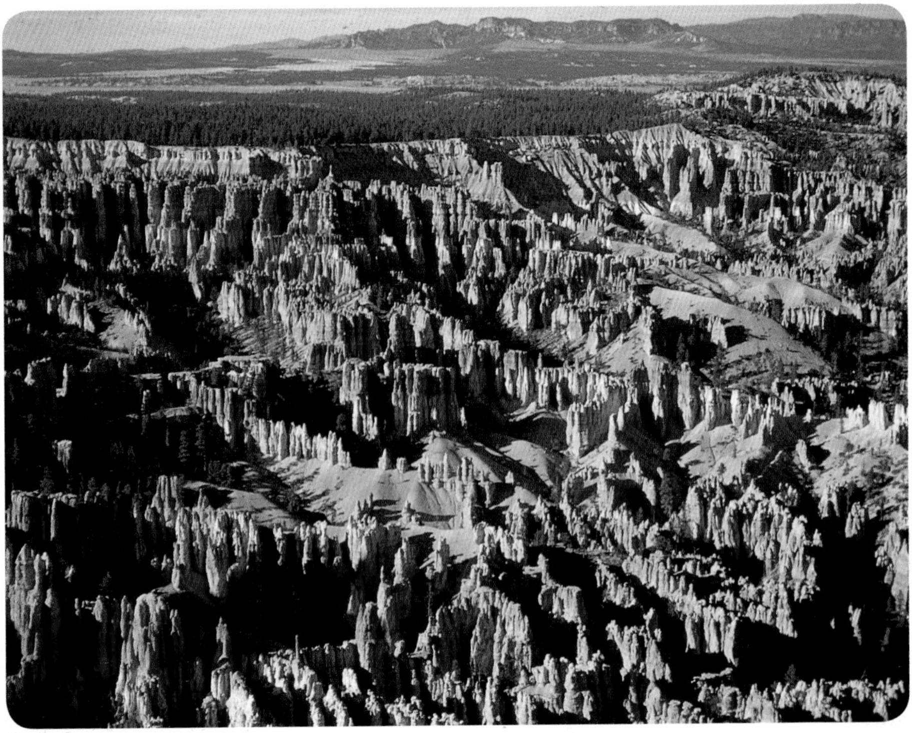

Overlooking the Peekaboo area, from Bryce Point

This and Trip 16 are the highest elevation trails in Utah canyon country. The Bryce visitor center, for example, is at 7880 ft (2402 m), while the Zion visitor center is at 4000 ft (1219 m). In spring or fall, expect it to be 15°F (9°C) cooler here than in Zion. Pack accordingly.

Despite cold winter temperatures, Bryce is open year round. During the six months when snow is present, the national park loans snowshoes to visitors free-of-charge. That makes the entrance fee a bargain.

BY VEHICLE

From Hwy 89, southeast of Panquitch, drive Hwy 12 east 14 mi (22.5 km).

From Escalante, drive Hwy 12 southwest to Cannonville, north to Tropic, then continue 7.5 mi (12.1 km) north-northwest.

From either approach, turn south onto Hwy 63 and reset your trip odometer to 0.

At 2.8 mi (4.5 km) proceed straight (south). Left leads 3.7 mi (6 km) east to the Fairyland Point trailhead, where Trip 15 begins.

At 3.5 mi (5.6 km), reach the park gate and fee station. Immediately beyond is the visitor center. Proceed straight (south). Turn left (east) at 4.8 mi (7.7 km). Reach the Sunset Point trailhead parking lot at 5 mi (8 km), 7985 ft (2434 m).

ON FOOT

Begin on the far right (south) trail departing the trailhead. Hike southeast 110 yd (100 m) to the **canyon rim**.

Follow signs for **Wall Street**. A switchbacking descent leads generally south among the towering formations comically reminiscent of Manhattan skyscrapers.

In 20 minutes reach a **junction** at 0.75 mi (1.2 km), 7480 ft (2280 m). Turn right, initially descending south. Left immediately splits again, affording two options: ascending left (northwest) via the Navajo loop back to Sunset Point where your total distance will be 1.4 mi (2.3 km), or descending right and winding generally north to Sunrise Point via Queens Garden.

After turning right (south) at the 0.75-mi (1.2-km) junction, follow the **Peekaboo connector** trail curving left (east). At 0.9 mi (1.5 km), 7420 ft (2262 m), about 25 minutes along, reach another **junction**. A horse trail descends left (northeast). Turn right and ascend south-southwest to reach the **Peekaboo trail** in 100 yd (110 m). Then turn right (west) and continue a moderate ascent.

At 1.3 mi (2.1 km) Wall Street is visible north-northwest. The colorful hoodoos of Silent City are northwest. Inspiration Point is west, on the canyon rim. Soon pass **The Cathedral** (left / east). Crest the Peekaboo loop's 7875-ft (2401-m) highpoint.

About 45 minutes from the trailhead, a **tunnel** grants passage through orange cliffs at 1.75 mi (2.8 km). Shortly beyond is the **Wall of Windows**. After a series of short ups and downs, the trail contours at 7750 ft (2363 m) before descending left (northeast). Bryce Point is visible right (southeast) on the canyon rim.

Five minutes farther, a right (southeast) spur leads to a spring-fed drinking fountain, picnic tables, and toilets. Follow the main trail left (north), past the **horse corral**, to continue the Peekaboo loop. Ascend briefly through forest to a **junction** at 2.7 mi (4.4 km), 7685 ft (2343 m). Strong hikers arrive here about one hour after departing the trailhead.

Right, initially ascending east, climbs 600 ft (183 m) in 1 mi (1.6 km) to the paved road on the canyon rim, near Bryce Point. To resume the Peekaboo loop, turn left and begin a switchbacking descent northwest. Bryce Point is again visible behind you (south).

At 3 mi (4.8 km) cross a wash. Ascend to a ridge just west of **Fairy Castle**. Switchback down to a **junction**. You're on familiar ground. Left (west) is the way you began the Peekaboo loop, which you've now completed. Bear right and descend north-northeast 110 yd (100 m) to another **junction**, at 4 mi (6.5 km), 7420 ft (2262 m). A horse trail descends right (northeast). Go left and follow the **Peekaboo connector** trail west.

Still on familiar ground, reach the **Navajo loop junction** at 4.2 mi (6.8 km), 7480 ft (2280 m). Left is the trail you initially descended from the trailhead through Wall Street. Go right. The trail immediately splits again, affording two options: ascending left (northwest) via the Navajo loop to Sunset Point where your total circuit distance will be 4.8 mi (7.7 km), or descending right and continuing to Sunrise Point via Queens Garden. Time and energy permitting, go right.

After turning right at the 4.2-mi (6.8-km) junction, follow the trail east. It gradually curves left (north). Reach **Queens Garden** at 5 mi (8 km), 7600 ft (2317 m). A left spur detours to Queen Victoria—a white-topped pinnacle. The main trail winds generally east to a **junction**. Right is a horse trail. Go left. Heading north, then ascending northwest, reach **Sunrise Point** at 5.9 mi (9.5 km), 7960 ft (2426 m).

Turn left at Sunrise Point. Follow the trail contouring southwest, then south along the **canyon rim**. Reach **Sunset Point** at 6.4 mi (10.3 km).

TRIP 18

RED CANYON

LOCATION	Hwy 12, just east of Hwy 89, between Panguitch and Bryce
DISTANCE	6-mi (9.7-km) round trip, 13.7-mi (22.1-km) circuit
ELEVATION GAIN	480 ft (146 m) for round trip, 1000 ft (305 m) for circuit
KEY ELEVATIONS	trailhead 7120 ft (2170 m), Losee/Cassidy junction 7600 ft (2316 m), Brayton Point 7880 ft (2402 m)
HIKING TIME	2½ to 7 hours
DIFFICULTY	easy to moderate
MAPS	Red Canyon brochure (free, available at visitor center), Trails Illustrated *Paunsaugunt Plateau/Mount Dutton/Bryce Canyon*

OPINION

Anything touting itself as a "miniature this" or a "gateway to that" is essentially trumpeting its inferiority. It's desperate, parasitic advertising that surely by now most of us ignore because we see through it. Yet those are the phrases that most often precede descriptions of Red Canyon.

Is it really a miniature Bryce Canyon? No. It's near the celebrated national park, has comparable geologic formations and the same pink-and-orange color scheme, but the similarities end there. Bryce isn't merely bigger. It's much more spectacular.

Calling Red Canyon "the gateway to Bryce," however, suggests it's just a doormat. And it shouldn't be; not if you're a hiker. Most tourists, rushing to see Bryce, roar through Red Canyon on Hwy 12 and merely glimpse it. And that makes Red Canyon distinctly different and, in one respect, superior: few people stop to explore it, whereas Bryce is constantly inundated.

A carnival atmosphere is pervasive in Bryce. Not only are the trails crowded, but you can often look up and see non-hikers peering down at you from the scenic overlooks, as if hiking were a spectator sport. Or worse, as if hikers were lab rats in a maze.

Red Canyon lacks the magnificently freakish appearance that earns Bryce Canyon its world-wonder status. But the tranquility you'll almost certainly enjoy while hiking in Red Canyon goes a long way toward compensating for less dramatic scenery.

Besides, "less dramatic" does not mean "undramatic." Red Canyon's brilliantly hued, almost neon walls—sculpted with alcoves, punctuated with strange, sand-castle-like hoodoos, decorated with stately ponderosa pines—are beautiful.

Red Canyon even has a colorful history, having served as a hideout for Butch Cassidy, the infamous outlaw who was born in nearby Circleville.

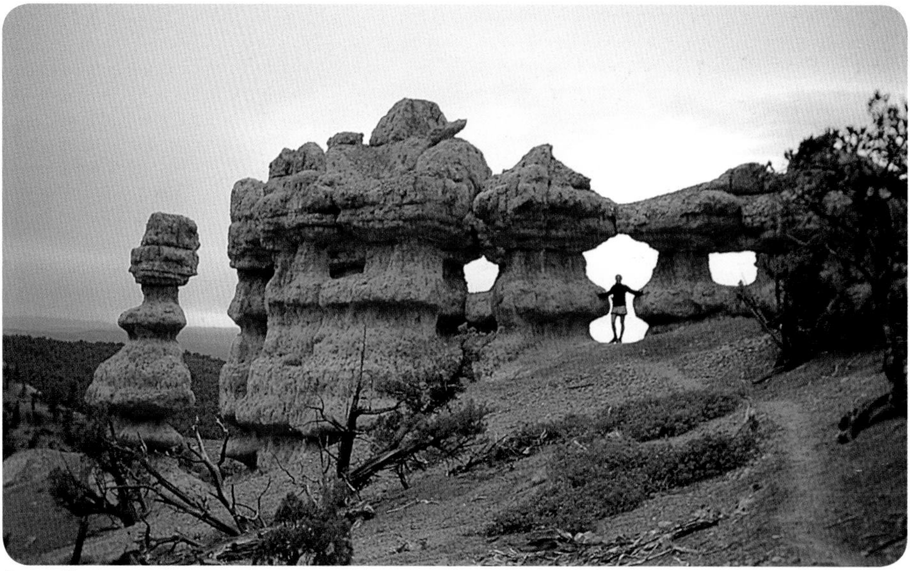

Losee Canyon

As the story goes, Butch was at a dance in Panguitch, got into a brawl over a girl, threw a punch and knocked his rival to the floor. Thinking he'd killed him, Butch fled. A posse immediately gave chase, but Butch eluded his pursuers in Red Canyon. Meanwhile the victim turned out to be merely unconscious.

The Cassidy trail—part of our recommended hiking route—is named after Butch. As for the name *Red Canyon*, it refers to the area in general and specifically to the corridor through which Hwy 12 passes. Following our directions, you won't be hiking in Red Canyon itself, but instead accessing the area via Losee Canyon.

Your other option would be to enter the area via Casto Canyon, farther north. But ATVs are allowed there, so hikers should stay away. Mountain bikers and equestrians are permitted on the Losee Canyon trail, but you're unlikely to see many.

BEFORE YOUR TRIP

You'll be hiking between 7000 and 8000 ft (2134 and 2438 m), so expect cool temperatures and pack accordingly. In late April, for example, when the daytime high might be 78°F in Escalante, the mercury might rise no higher than 63°F at Red Canyon.

Before completing the drive to the trailhead, pick up a free brochure/map at the Red Canyon visitor center. It's on the north side of Hwy 12, 3.2 mi (5.2 km) east of Hwy 89 (1.3 mi / 2.1 km beyond Casto Canyon Road), or 1 mi (1.6 km) west of Red Canyon trailhead.

Before or after hiking the Losee Canyon trail, hike the Arches trail—a 0.7-mi (1.1-km) loop accessing 15 small arches. It starts at the Losee trailhead.

The Red Canyon campground is a convenient, inviting place to stay before or after your hike. It's on the south side of Hwy 12, just east of the visitor center. Yes, it has showers.

FACT

BY VEHICLE

From Hwy 89, southeast of Panquitch, drive Hwy 12 east 1.9 mi (3.1 km). Or, from Hwy 63, north of Bryce Park, drive Hwy 12 northwest 12 mi (19.3 km). From either approach, turn north onto unpaved Casto Canyon Road and drive 2 mi (3.2 km) to the Losee Canyon trailhead parking area, on the right (east), at 7120 ft (2170 m).

ON FOOT

After departing the east side of the parking area, the trail meanders generally east through an arid, open forest of manzanita, juniper, and ponderosa and limber pine.

Following the usually-dry wash draining **Losee Canyon**, begin a gently ascending tour of the orange-and-pink limestone hoodoos and alcoves along the canyon's north wall.

The trail then curves northeast, intersecting the **Cassidy trail** at 3 mi (4.8 km), 7600 ft (2316 m). There's an outhouse and corral here. Turn around now to complete a 2½-hour round trip.

Want to continue a short distance? Left leads generally north through the Little Desert (a miniature badlands) then east to Casto Canyon. About 30 minutes in that direction entails a 330 ft (100 m) ascent and will earn you a view west toward low mountains.

Want to complete a longer circuit? Turn right and follow the Cassidy trail south-southeast. Its soon veers west. Shortly after curving south again, reach a **fork** at 4.5 mi (7.2 km). Right is the Rich trail—a short detour you might opt for on the return. For now, continue left (south) on the Cassidy trail.

At 4.8 mi (7.7 km), reach a **four-way junction**. The Rich trail crosses the Cassidy trail here. Right (north) is the detour you declined at the last fork. Straight ahead, the Cassidy trail leads northwest to Brayton Point—another short detour you might opt for on the return. For now, turn left onto the **Rich trail** and hike south. Traverse a hillside, then descend generally west.

Intersect the **Cassidy trail** at 5.3 mi (8.5 km). Right (north) is the Brayton Point detour you declined at the last junction. Turn left onto the Cassidy trail, then immediately reach a **junction**. Left is the Cassidy trail on which you'll return via the circuit. For now, turn right and follow the **Rich trail** south.

Cross a saddle, descend past **The Gap** (a wash between buttes), ascend along a wash, then angle toward another saddle. Reach a **fork**. The Rich trail continues left (east). Go right for a short detour south to **Ledge Point** (a scenic overlook), then loop north.

Soon rejoin the **Rich trail**. Turn right and hike generally east. Drop beneath sandstone cliffs, above a drainage. The rocky path soon begins a switchbacking descent. Pass more hoodoos and alcoves.

At the end of the draw, again intersect the **Cassidy trail**. Right leads south 0.8 mi (1.3 km) to Red Canyon trailhead on Hwy 12. Go left. Soon reach a confluence of washes, surmount a hill, and briefly follow a ridge among Douglas firs.

Reach a **junction** at 7.7 mi (12.4 mi). You're now on familiar ground. Left is the Rich trail, which you previously followed south to Ledge Point. Turn right, resume on the **Cassidy trail,** and immediately reach a fork.

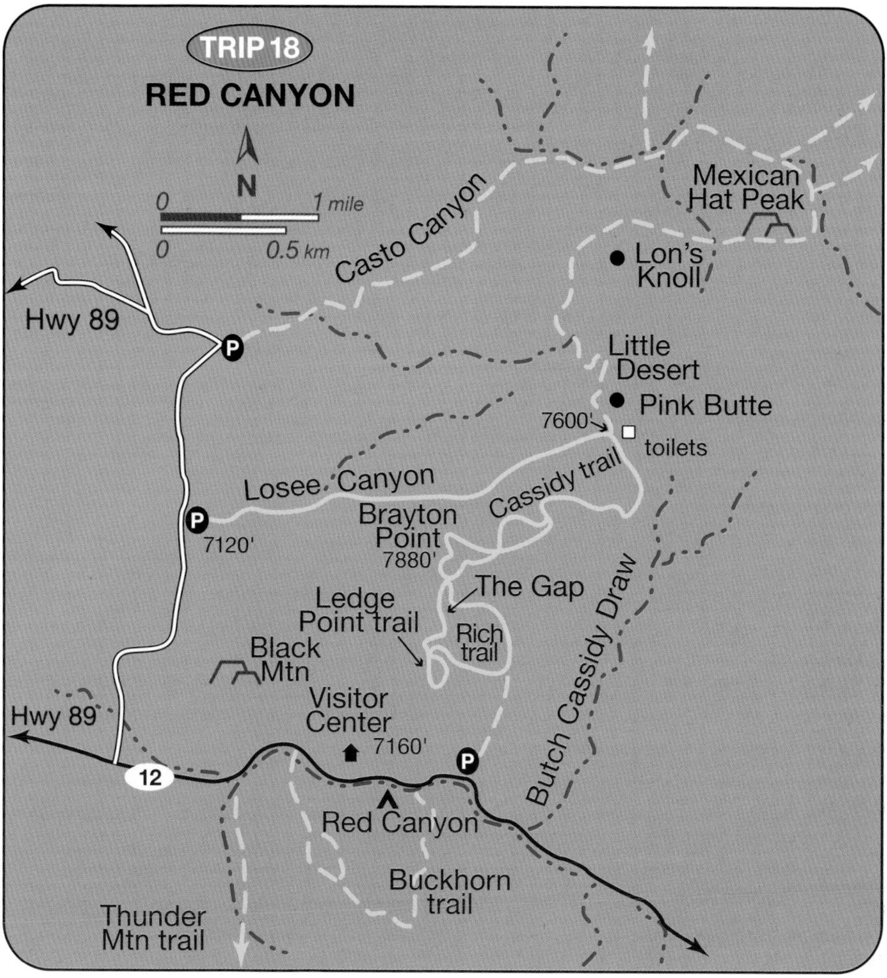

Turn right again to retrace your steps along the Rich trail. Or proceed straight (north) on the Cassidy trail and detour to **Brayton Point**—a panoramic vantage at 7880 ft (2402 m).

Digressing to Brayton will add only 0.5 mi (0.8 km) to your total distance and is scenically worthwhile. From the point, continue right (southeast) to the **four-way junction** where the Rich trail crosses the Cassidy trail.

Right (south) is the Rich trail, which you followed previously. Left (north) is also the Rich trail—a detour that allows you to vary your return route yet adds only 0.2 mi (0.3 km) to your total distance. Straight ahead is the Cassidy trail—the most direct way to retrace your steps to the trailhead.

If you opt for the short Rich-trail detour (left / north), you'll quickly intersect the **Cassidy trail** again. Once more, you're on familiar ground. Turn left. Follow the Cassidy trail north, east, then north to a junction with the **Losee Canyon trail**.

You've now hiked 10.7 mi (17.2 km) if you opted for both detours on the return, or 10 mi (16.1 km) if you declined them both. Turn left to follow the Losee Canyon trail southwest, then generally west to the trailhead.

TRIP 19

WILLIS CREEK CANYON

LOCATION	Grand Staircase-Escalante National Monument south-southwest of Cannonville
ROUND TRIP	4.8 mi (7.7 km)
ELEVATION CHANGE	300-ft (91-m) loss and gain
KEY ELEVATIONS	trailhead 6000 ft (1829 m), lowpoint at Willis/Sheep confluence 5700 ft (1737 m)
HIKING TIME	2 to 3 hours
DIFFICULTY	easy
MAPS	BLM brochure *Grand Staircase-Escalante National Monument* for general orientation, USGS *Bull Valley Gorge*

OPINION

Canyons are terrestrial lacerations. They range from gaping wounds—Mexico's Copper Canyon, for example—to mere paper cuts like Willis Creek Canyon.

Willis is what's known as a *slot*—a surgical incision in the earth's skin. Deep and exceedingly narrow, slot canyons are seductive, but exploring them tends to require technical climbing proficiency most hikers lack.

Willis, however, is a rarity among slots. You don't have to climb into or out of it. You can simply stroll through it. The virtually level canyon floor—mostly gravel and smooth stone—poses no obstacles.

Water draining off the pink cliffs of Bryce Canyon National Park feeds Willis Creek. Initially a broad wash, it traipses across wooded terraces until arriving at the Navajo sandstone of the White Cliffs, where it becomes a canyon-cutting scalpel.

The result is a 1.3-mi (2.1-km) stretch where the canyon floor is 200 to 300 ft (61 to 91 m) below the surface of the adjacent land, and the slickrock walls narrow to a claustrophobic 6 ft (2 m) apart. These mysterious, serpentine hallways, echoing with exquisitely delicate water music, are as captivating as any comparable length of trail anywhere.

Because Willis Creek is remote, consider also hiking Lick Wash (Trip 14) while you're in the area. Both trailheads are on Skutumpah Road, between Kanab (Hwy 89, southeast of Zion Park) and Cannonville (Hwy 12, southeast of Bryce Park). The optimal plan is to camp nearby, either at Kodachrome Basin State Park or at a quiet, primitive site in the P-J forest (piñon and juniper) along lonely, Skutumpah Road.

Don't let our lengthy *By Vehicle* directions put you off. The drive to Willis Creek Canyon is straightforward. We've provided way more detail then you'll likely need. Plus we've described how to reach both trailheads—Willis *and* Lick—from either approach, so you don't have to flip through the book seeking further guidance should you want to complete a one-way tour.

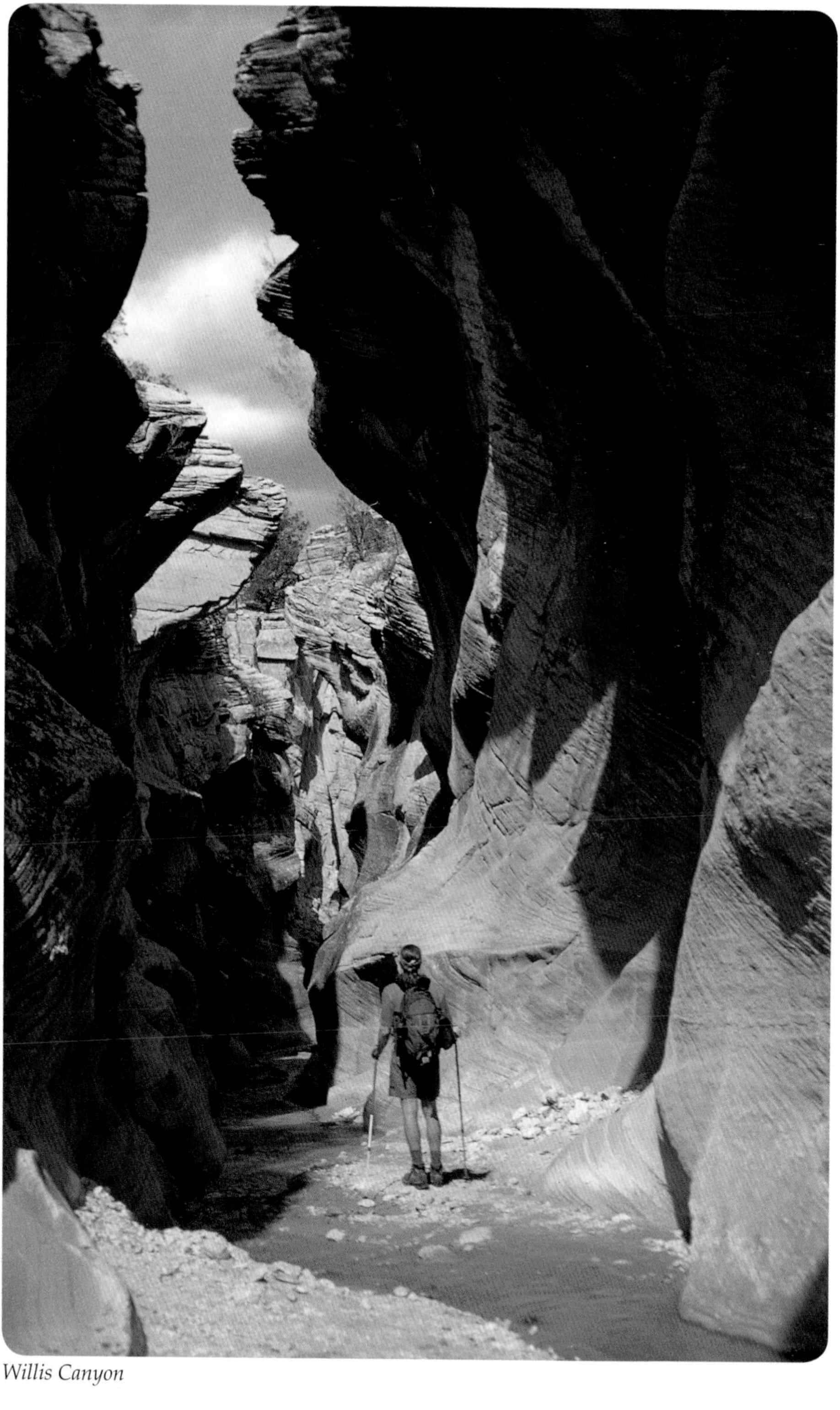

Willis Canyon

FACT

BEFORE YOUR TRIP

Skutumpah Road, particularly the northeast end near Cannonville, is treacherous when wet because the clay surface makes traction impossible. Do not risk driving it after recent rain or if the forecast calls for rain. The road's northeast end also has steep, narrow sections that, even when dry, might traumatize an inexpert trailer tugger.

All slot canyons, regardless how easy to enter, are dangerous, because even distant rain can cause an overwhelming volume of water to suddenly rush through them. Hike here only during a period of sunny weather, when there's little risk of a flash flood. Check the forecast at the BLM offices in Cannonville or Kanab.

Willis Creek is often a trickle: shallow enough to walk in without soaking your footwear, narrow enough to easily hop across. But in case it's not, amphibious footwear is preferable. Technical sandals designed for hiking are ideal. Fabric hiking boots you don't mind dunking are fine, too. Insulating neoprene socks will ensure wet feet ≠ frigid feet. Or, if it's a hot day, go barefoot.

BY VEHICLE

From Cannonville

Cannonville is on Hwy 12, southeast of Bryce Park. It's 33 mi (53.1 km) southeast of Panguitch, and 36 mi (58 km) southwest of Escalante. To reach Willis Creek trailhead, you'll drive four minutes on pavement, then 20 minutes on the steep end of unpaved Skutumpah Road.

0 mi (0 km)
Drive south on paved Cottonwood Canyon Road, which is signed for Kodachrome Basin State Park.

2.8 mi (4.5 km)
Just before (west of) a bridged crossing of the upper Paria River, turn right (southwest) onto unpaved Skutumpah Road, signed for Bull Valley Gorge (9 mi) and Kanab (61 mi). Kodachrome Basin is 6.7 mi (10.8 km) ahead (southeast) on the paved Cottonwood Canyon Road.

Proceed on Skutumpah Road (also known as Road 500). Immediately cross Yellow Creek wash—usually dry. If it's wet, the road will be impassable. Stop. Do not continue.

3 mi (4.8 km)
Enter Grand Staircase-Escalante National Monument.

3.4 mi (5.5 km)
Proceed straight. The pink sandstone of Bryce Canyon National Park is visible right (northwest).

4 mi (6.4 km)
Proceed straight.

5.6 mi (9 km)
Bear right to cross runoff below the small concrete spillway of a dam spanning Sheep Creek wash.

6.1 mi (9.8 km)
After ascending a ridge, descend to cross a dry wash.

6.5 mi (10.5 km)
Proceed straight, ignoring the right fork. Avoid the shoulder of the road, which tends to erode and slough off.

7.5 mi (12.1 km)
Descend into a dry wash and climb another ridge.

8.2 mi (13.2 km)
Fork left near the ridgecrest.

9 mi (14.5 km)
Reach **Willis Creek** trailhead parking area on the right, just north of the creek, at 6000 ft (1829 m).

Continuing southwest to Lick Wash (Trip 14)

10.8 mi (17.4 km)
Stop in the pullout, then walk 110 yd (100 ft) to see the unique, earthen bridge spanning Bull Valley Gorge. Look for the truck that fell into the gap in the 1940s.

22.1 mi (35.6 km)
Just before a cattleguard, turn left to enter **Lick Wash** (Trip 14) trailhead parking area at 6330 ft (1930 m).

Continuing southwest to Hwy 89

36 mi (58 km)
Turn left onto paved Johnson Canyon Road.

52.1 mi (83.9 km)
Reach Hwy 89. Kanab is right (west). Page, Arizona, is left (east).

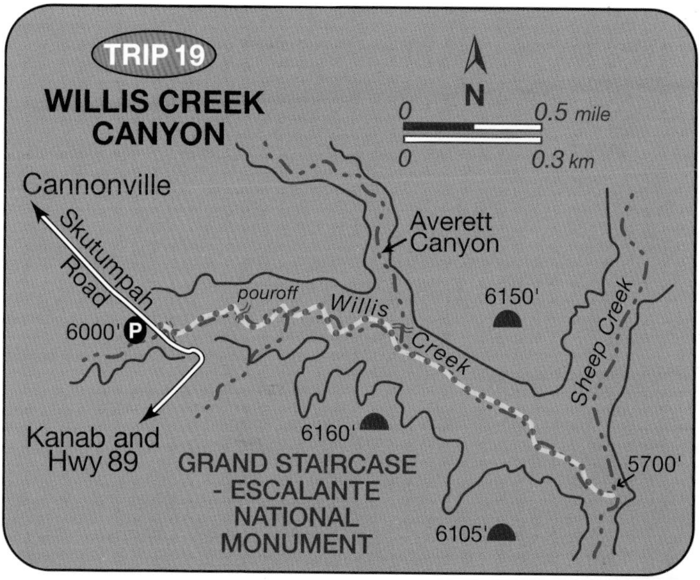

From Kanab or Big Water

Kanab is on Hwy 89, southeast of Zion Park. Big Water is on Hwy 89, northwest of Page, Arizona. From the junction of Hwys 89 and 89A in Kanab, drive Hwy 89 east 10 mi (16 km). From the Big Water exit on Hwy 89, drive west 55 mi (88.6 km). From either approach, turn north onto paved Johnson Canyon Road (just east of milepost 55) and reset your trip odometer to 0.

0 mi (0 km)
Starting north on paved Johnson Canyon Road.

11.5 mi (18.5 km)
Enter Grand Staircase-Escalante National Monument.

16.1 mi (26 km)
Turn right onto unpaved Skutumpah Road (also known as Road 500), signed for Deer Springs Ranch (13 mi) and Cannonville (38 mi).

17.7 mi (28.5 km)
Bear right, ignoring the left fork. Proceed through a broad, dusty basin rife with sagebrush.

19.4 mi (31.2 km)
Proceed straight, ignoring the left fork.

22.4 mi (36.1 km) / 27 mi (43.5 km) / 27.6 mi (44.5 km) / 28 mi (45 km)
Bear left, ignoring right forks.

28.4 mi (45.8 km)
Bear right.

30 mi (48.4 km)
Proceed straight, ignoring the right fork. Cross a cattle guard and, just before the wash, turn right to enter **Lick Wash** (Trip 14) trailhead parking area at 6330 ft (1930 m).

Continuing northeast to Willis Creek

30.6 mi (49.3 km) / 35.2 mi (56.6 km) / 37.3 mi (60 km)
Proceed on the main road, ignoring minor spurs.

37.4 mi (60.2 km)
Slow down. Just beyond, the road descends steeply then remains narrow for the next 5 mi (8 km).

41.2 mi (66.3 km)
Reach Bull Valley Gorge. Stop in the pullout, then walk 30 yd/m left to see the unique, earthen bridge. Look for the truck that fell into the gap in the 1940s.

43.1 mi (69.4 km)
Reach **Willis Creek** trailhead parking area on the left, just north of the creek, at 6000 ft (1829 m).

Continuing northeast to Cannonville

43.8 mi (70.5 km)
Proceed on the main road, ignoring a left fork.

48.1 mi (77.5 km)
The road descends. Beware of sand.

49.3 mi (79.3 km)
Intersect paved Cottonwood Canyon Road. Turn left (north) to reach Cannonville and intersect Hwy 12 in 2.8 mi (4.5 km). Turn right (southeast) to reach Kodachrome Basin State Park in 6.7 mi (10.8 km).

ON FOOT

Cross the road and walk south to the creek. Go left (downstream) about 30 yd/m, pass a low pouroff, then drop off the left (north) side of the wash into the **streambed**. Within five minutes, sculpted Navajo sandstone walls rise on both sides. Proceed down-canyon, generally east.

The incipient chasm snakes along then suddenly deepens and constricts dramatically into a classic slot. Past the first **narrows**, the height of the walls and their distance apart varies. Where the canyon briefly opens, the slickrock walls relax into benches harboring piñon and ponderosa pine, juniper, and gambel oak.

At 0.6 mi (1 km) ascend left onto a slickrock ledge to bypass an 11-ft (3.3-m) **pouroff**, then drop back into the streambed. The canyon's journey-to-the-center-of-the-earth atmosphere continues until **Averett Canyon** (left / north) intersects it at 1.3 mi (2.1 km), 5800 ft (1768 m). Though the narrows end here, Willis remains an engaging canyon and affords easy walking.

Just after a 200-ft (61-m) cliff appears to block passage ahead, the clear water of Willis Creek flows into muddy **Sheep Creek** at 2.4 mi (3.9 km), 5700 ft (1737 m). The Sheep also ends soon, flowing into the Paria River.

Turn around at the Willis/Sheep confluence and appreciate the Willis narrows again while retracing your steps to the trailhead. If you didn't notice them previously, look for a pair of rough arches above the north wall just upstream from Averett Canyon.

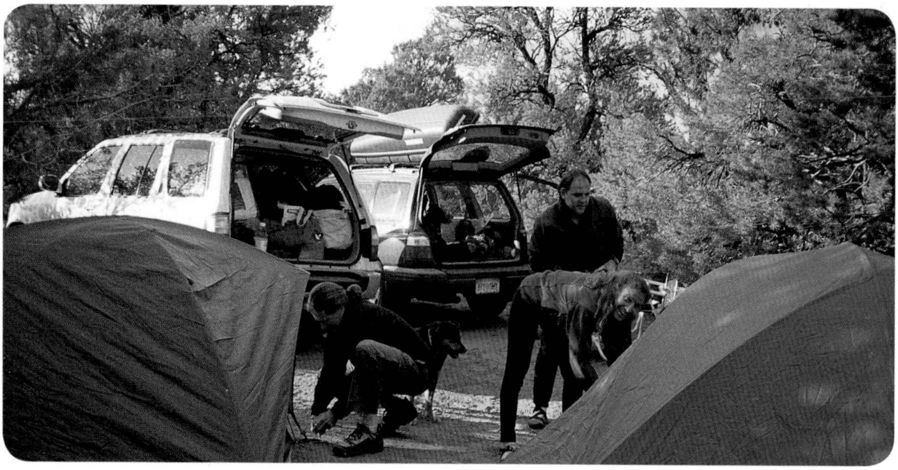

Primitive camping in Grand Staircase - Escalante National Monument

TRIP 20

PINE CREEK

LOCATION	Box-Death Hollow Wilderness north of Escalante, west of Boulder
DISTANCE	8.5 mi (13.7 km) one way
ELEVATION LOSS	1300 ft (396 m)
KEY ELEVATIONS	Upper Box trailhead 7720 ft (2354 m) Deep Creek 7020 ft (2140 m) Lower Box trailhead 6420 ft (1957 m)
HIKING TIME	3 to 4 hours
DIFFICULTY	easy
MAP	Trails Illustrated *Canyons of the Escalante*

OPINION

Peaceful canyon. Sandstone cliffs. Cream. Mustard. Salmon pink. Graceful spruce. Towering ponderosas. Half mountain, half desert. Clear water. Gentle path. Beside the creek, never in it. Only an occasional hop across. One way hike, all downhill. No cows. No roads. No crowds. Not too long. Not too short. Not too far from town. Just enough to empty your mind. Maybe just what you need.

On a summer day, when it's too hot for the Hole-in-the-Rock Road trails, a cooler, shadier world awaits on the lower slopes of the Aquarius Plateau and Boulder Mtn. Here, a short drive north of Escalante, you can spend a relaxing day following Pine Creek downstream.

Pine Creek Canyon is also known as *The Box*—an odd name given that it's not a box canyon, but a steep-walled, open-ended drainage carved by a perennial stream. Along with the upper reaches of neighboring Death Hollow, Pine Creek is protected in Box-Death Hollow Wilderness.

If you have amigos with a second vehicle, a shuttle is easy to arrange and will allow you the luxury of a one-way hike. The alternative, which has worked for us, is to park at the lower trailhead and hitchhike to the upper trailhead. Enough explorers travel the Hells Backbone Road between Escalante and Boulder that it's worth trying.

Lacking a shuttle and failing to catch a ride, a round trip starting at the lower trailhead is still rewarding. Within 30 minutes you'll see dramatic, colorful cliffs. After hiking upstream, generally north, occasionally crossing to which ever bank appears easiest, turn around in 1¾ hours. At that point you'll have seen the canyon's narrowest and most scenic stretch.

FACT

BEFORE YOUR TRIP

It's possible to complete the hike without soaking your feet. We have. But you must cross the creek numerous times, and trekking poles will help you vault over. The creek is narrow and shallow—perhaps ankle to calf deep—so even if fording is necessary, it should be easy, especially if you pack a pair of sandals for that purpose.

BY VEHICLE

From Hwy 12, at the east edge of Escalante, 0.5 mi (0.8 km) northwest of the high school, turn north onto Posy Road and reset your trip odometer to 0. Posy Road is also called *Pine Creek Road* and is signed for Hells Backbone Road.

0 mi (0 km)
Starting north on paved Posy Road.

0.5 mi (0.8 km)
Cross a bridge over the Escalante River.

0.6 mi (1 km)
Bear right at the Y-junction.

3.4 mi (5.5 km)
Pavement ends. Proceed northwest.

7.1 mi (11.4 km)
Enter Dixie National Forest.

7.3 mi (11.8 km)
The right spur leads 0.3 mi (0.5 km) to the **Lower Box trailhead** parking area at 6420 ft (1957 m). Leave your shuttle vehicle here, where the one-way hike ends. Resume north on Pine Creek Road.

13.8 mi (22.2 km)
Intersect Hells Backbone Road. Left (initially northeast) leads to Posy Lake. Go right (east). Pine Creek Canyon is soon visible right (east)

18.3 mi (29.5 km)
Reach the **Upper Box trailhead**, on the right, at 7720 ft (2354 m). Begin hiking here. Just 0.2 mi (0.3 km) ahead, immediately before the road crosses Pine Creek, a left spur leads 0.5 mi (0.8 km) north to Blue Spruce campground. Hells Backbone Road intersects Hwy 12, near Boulder, at 40 mi (64.4 km).

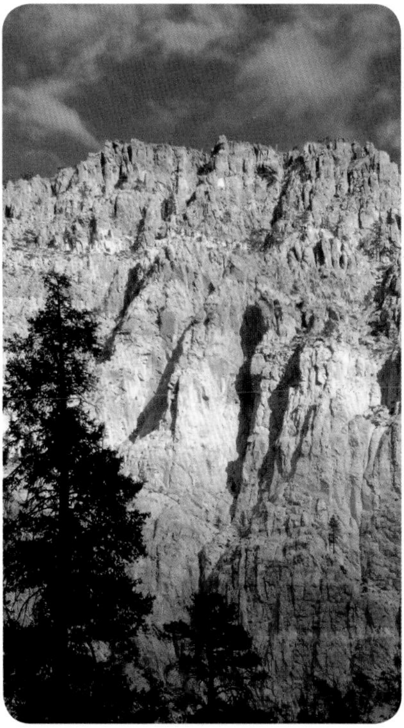
The Box

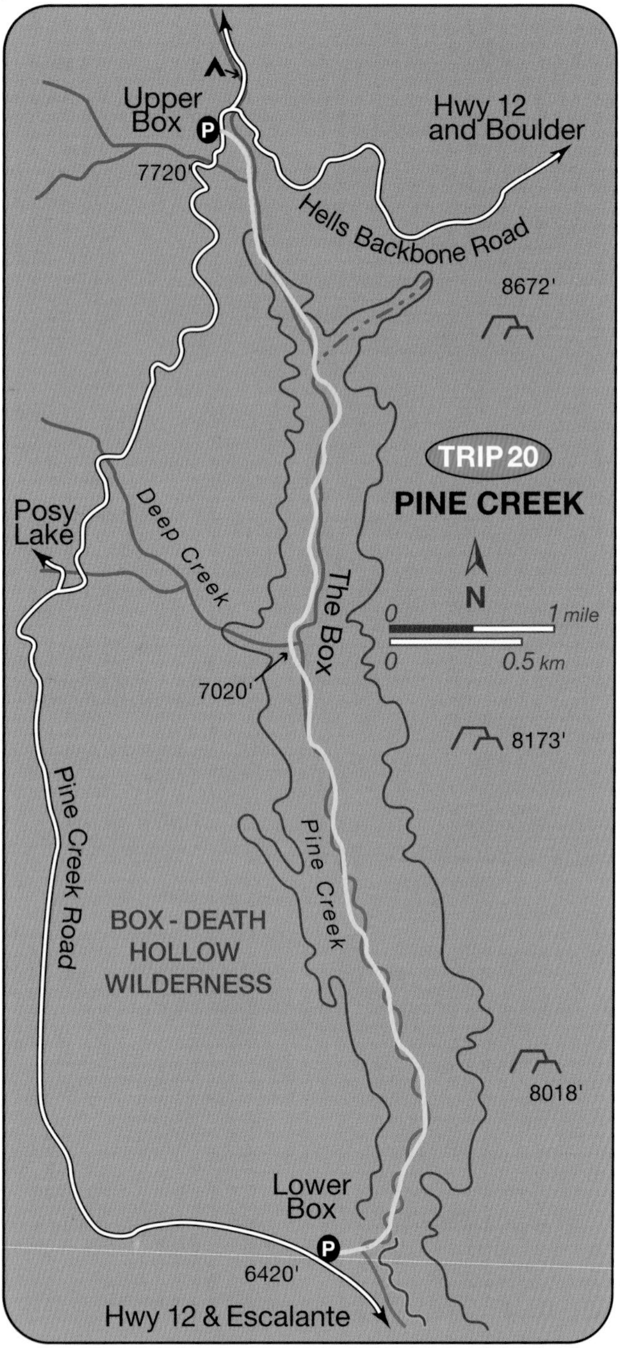

Upper Box
7720'
Hwy 12 and Boulder
Hells Backbone Road
8672'
TRIP 20
PINE CREEK
N
0
1 mile
0
0.5 km
Posy Lake
Deep Creek
The Box
7020'
8173'
Pine Creek
Pine Creek Road
BOX - DEATH HOLLOW WILDERNESS
8018'
Lower Box
6420'
Hwy 12 & Escalante

ON FOOT

From the road, descend the pine-needle covered slope one minute to Pine Creek. Turn right and follow the trail downstream (initially southeast) among spruce and Douglas fir above the creek's right (southwest) bank.

Within two minutes pass a trail register and map/sign. Cross the creek. Proceed through a hiker's maze, which allows people but not cows to pass through the fence.

About 15 minutes along, enter Box-Death Hollow Wilderness at 7555 ft (2303 m). Where the path is vague, just continue downstream on whichever bank is most accommodating. Your general direction of travel will remain south.

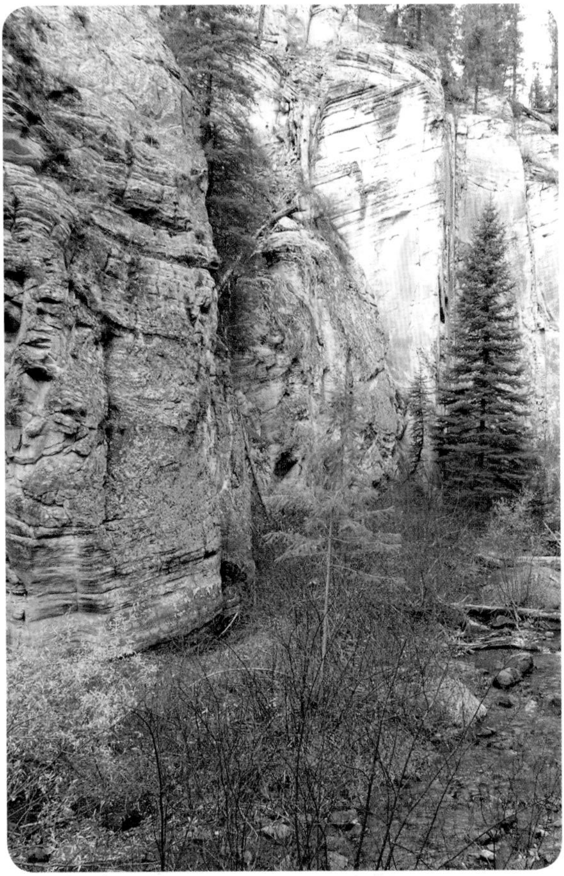
Pine Creek

The canyon gradually constricts. Nearly 30 minutes from the trailhead, the walls are occasionally just 20 yd/m apart. Pass an inviting campsite near a deep pool at 7320 ft (2232 m). After the trail makes an overzealous ascent right, it returns to the canyon floor.

At 7180 ft (2189 m), about 1½ hours along, the canyon widens but remains deep. The east wall rises 1000 ft (305 m) to a long, narrow plateau separating Pine Creek Canyon (also known as *The Box*) from Death Hollow. The trail is increasingly sandy due to the eroding sandstone slopes.

Reach the **Deep Creek** confluence at 4 mi (6.4 km), 7020 ft (2140 m), about two hours from the trailhead. This tributary drainage, entering from the right (west-northwest), is fenced just upstream. Continue following Pine Creek downstream (south) among ponderosa pine.

Necessary creek crossings become more frequent about 2¾ hours along. After 3¼ hours the sandstone walls are particularly colorful. Five crossings within 15 minutes signal you've nearly reached your destination. The trail and the creek suddenly exit the canyon. Just ahead is the **Lower Box trailhead** at 8.5 mi (13.7 km), 6420 ft (1957 m).

HISTORY

THE HOLE-IN-THE-ROCK ROAD

The Escalante River flows generally southeast from the town of Escalante to Lake Powell. Above and southwest of it, the Straight Cliffs parallel the river. Between the cliffs and the river are numerous drainages—tributaries of the Escalante—where you'll find seven of Utah's premier canyon-country hikes: Trips 21 through 27. All are accessed via the Hole-in-the-Rock Road.

The road too angles southeast, between and parallel to the cliffs and the river. It appears to be just another of the countless unpaved tracks that make the map of southeast Utah look like a shattered windshield. But this road is unique—in the state, in the nation, in the world—because it wasn't built with machinery but instead forged by the faith and desperation of 70 families on an epic journey.

Mormon emigrants led by Brigham Young reached the Great Salt Lake Basin in 1847. "This is the place," he said, and so it became. The theocratic colony numbered 40,000 within a decade. Increasingly confident, the Latter-day Saints asserted their independence from the U.S. by openly practicing polygamy. Increasingly furious, President Buchanan dispatched an army of 2500 to restore federal law in the defiant kingdom of Zion.

Hostilities persisted through the 1870s. Determined to expand Mormon dominion, Young sent missions to establish settlements in Idaho, Colorado, Wyoming, Arizona, even Mexico. Young anticipated decamping all the Saints south of the border if their polygamous doctrine provoked civil war.

After Young's death in 1877, the church continued colonizing aggressively. When his successors heard miners and ranchers were sifting into the wilderness of southeast Utah from Colorado, they scrambled to settle the area before the Gentiles (the Saints' term for non-Mormon whites) were ensconced. The Hole-in-the-Rock expedition was underway.

But only in retrospect was it called that, because the expedition could have, perhaps should have, chosen a different route. Their starting point was Cedar City. Their goal was the confluence of Montezuma Creek and the San Juan River. A reconnaissance mission reached it by detouring south into Arizona, then looping back north roughly along the path of today's Hwy 191 and Interstates 70 and 15. They were forced to hand-drill for water. They were constantly menaced by Navajos whose homeland they'd invaded. They barely survived.

So the colonizing expedition—70 families in 83 wagons, plus 1200 horses and cattle—declined both the south and north routes. Instead they would cut directly across the Escalante Desert, which no white person had seen much less traversed. They departed Cedar City in October, 1879. A month later, they passed through the town of Escalante—the final Mormon hamlet en route—where they reprovisioned.

With supplies for six weeks they entered terra incognita on a pilgrimage that would ultimately take six months.

Wagon travel is slow at best. Having to first build a road through raw desert slowed the expedition to a crawl. By late November they were camped only 40 mi (64.4 km) southeast of Escalante. But winter was upon them. Snow was accumulating. Retreat was impossible. And "no way forward" was their scouts' report. They were trapped.

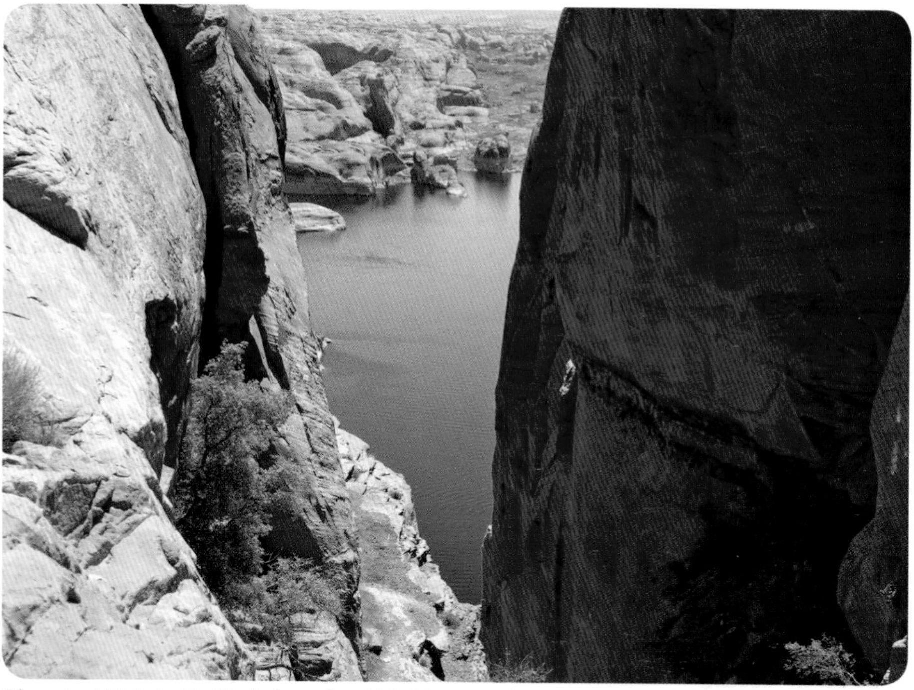

The actual Hole in the Rock through which Mormon pioneers built a wagon road to the Escalante River

Hope, however, was not diminishing as fast as their provisions. They sent the scouts out again.

Meanwhile the entire camp ranged across the desert gathering what meager forage they could find for their stock. They also dragged in sagebrush and black shadscale (a bushy weed), which they burned for warmth and cooking. It took a bale of it to boil an egg.

They slaughtered the cattle they were herding to their new home. They ground and ate the seed they'd intended to plant in the spring. They cheered themselves with singing and dancing. They gathered on a huge, south-facing, natural amphitheater, where the caravan's three fiddlers filled the desert night with music, and couples twirled across the level sandstone. They called it *Dance Hall Rock.*

Mostly they leaned on their faith. It was the yoke that kept them all pulling together as one. Food was scarce, meals spare, but church services nourished their will to endure. They were God's people, chosen to spread the truth. Speaking through his Mormon prophets, God said "go." So the expedition dutifully persisted through the Valley of the Shadow of Death.

The second scouting party returned. "Maybe," they said this time, "if we had dynamite." So the wagon train inched ahead while the leader, Silas Smith, slogged all the way back to Salt Lake City where he implored the church legislature to grant another $2,500 for explosives.

In mid-December, having lumbered 57 mi (92 km) from Escalante, they arrived at "maybe"—a cavernous fault in the rim of Glen Canyon, 1800 ft (550 m) above the Colorado River. For 70 families on the brink of starvation, it must have looked like suicide. This was the hole in the rock. And if it didn't soon

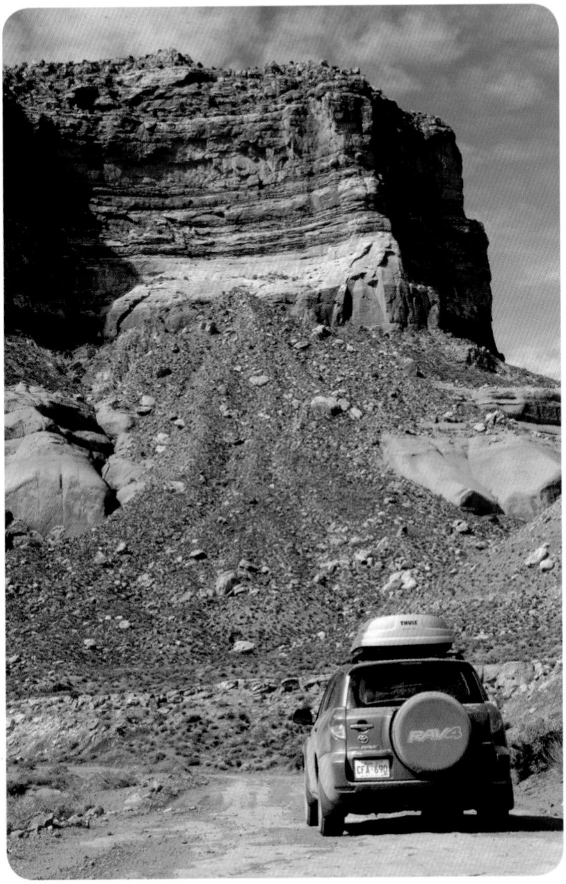

The Hole in the Rock Road at Fiftymile Point

resemble a road, it would be a mass grave instead. Construction on the Hole-in-the-Rock Road began immediately.

They dangled in barrels over the precipice, drilled holes in the stone, filled them with dynamite, and blasted. When the powder ran out, they made do with muscle. They hacked, pounded, scraped, chiseled and shoveled. When they tried to lead the horses down to feed at the river, nine animals fell and died. So they kept hacking, pounding, scraping, chiseling and shoveling.

While the men labored, the women and children shivered. Wood was too precious to waste for mere warmth. Yet the daytime highs were only 10° to 20° F (-12° to -7° C). Six inches (2.4 cm) of snow blanketed their dismal camp on Christmas Eve. They had no presents to exchange, yet all the pioneers were grateful. Having survived thus far was a miraculous gift.

Still their continued survival remained in doubt. They couldn't build a continuous rock road wide enough for the wagons. So they settled for a ledge supporting only the inside wheels. They drilled holes beneath it, pounded in long stakes made from scavenged scrub-oak, then piled driftwood, brush and rocks on this oak-stake platform until it approximated a road: partially on the canyon wall, largely a makeshift extension suspended above the abyss.

Construction continued eleven hours a day for six weeks. On January 25, 1880, the Hole-in-the-Rock Road was as wagon-worthy as time and energy allowed.* Initially it dropped one yd/m for every yd/m forward. The average angle of descent was 50 degrees. They rolled the first wagon into place, chained two wheels to prevent a runaway disaster, then began lowering the rig with ropes held by a dozen men, a few horses, and several posts wedged into cracks.

By February 1, every wagon, man, woman, child, and most of the livestock had safely completed the descent into Glen Canyon. They'd reached the Colorado River. Yet the gauntlet of struggle and deprivation resumed.

They floated the wagons across, but the stock spooked midstream and scattered. The pioneers rounded them up and drove them across the torrent again. Ascending the far canyon wall took a full week, with each wagon pulled by eight to fourteen horses or oxen. What had appeared to be a plateau above was wildly unlevel.

Their scouts nearly died of hunger and thirst. Once, a lucky glimpse of galloping bighorn sheep revealed a hidden passage. They skidded the wagons down slickrock cascades. They pushed them through deep sand. They built causeways across arroyos and carved dugways into stone. They skirted canyon after canyon, including a lengthy, gaping rift they named *Grand Gulch.* They hewed through dense piñon and juniper forests. They whipped their exhausted animals, who stumbled repeatedly, leaving a trail of dried blood and matted hair gouged from their forelegs. The expedition averaged 2 mi (3.2 km) a day.

High on Cedar Mesa, the scouts feared they were lost. Trudging in thigh-deep snow, one of them finally glimpsed the Abajo Mtns, which he recognized from the previous reconnaissance mission. They were on course. They named the viewpoint *Salvation Knoll.* It's beside Hwy 95, near Mule Canyon roadside ruin.

On April 6, 1880, after six months of fighting their way across 260 mi (420 km) of the baddest badlands on Earth, they collapsed at Cottonwood Wash, beside the San Juan River. Just 18 mi (29 km) shy of their goal, Montezuma Creek, they could stagger no farther. They'd lost not one human life. But there was little life left in any of them. It was flat here. That, plus a scrap of pasture and few cottonwoods, was enough. They pitched camp and stayed.

What they'd seized from the Gentiles eventually became the town of Bluff. But the Gentiles, it turns out, didn't covet the place. The location was resource poor. The settlement never succeeded. Natives were a constant threat. The flood-happy San Juan destroyed dams, irrigation ditches, crops, years of toil. Twice the colonists begged the church to relinquish them from their woebegone outpost. Within 30 years, most quit farming, took up ranching, moved north to Blanding or Monticello, which remain Mormon strongholds. Today, Bluff's 300 residents consider their town the least Mormon in Utah.

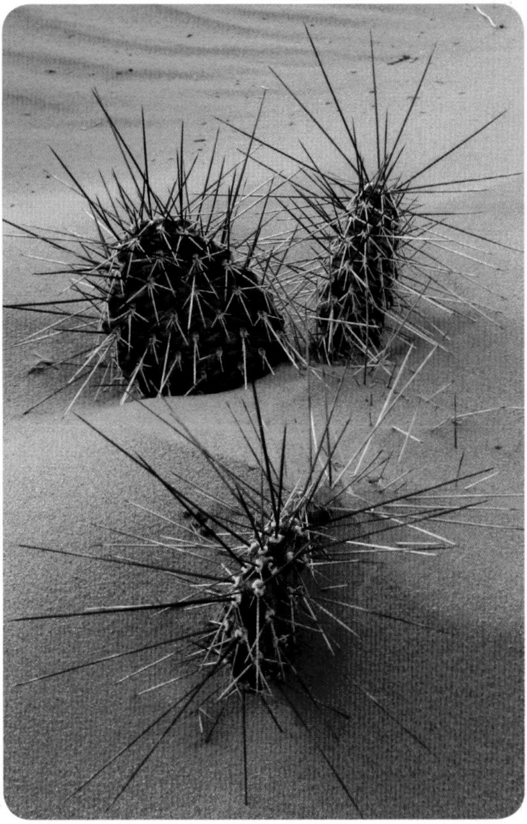

*Entirely by chance, it was January 25, 2008 when we finished writing this account of the Hole-in-the-Rock expedition. That was the 128th anniversary of the day the Mormon pioneers finished constructing the road.

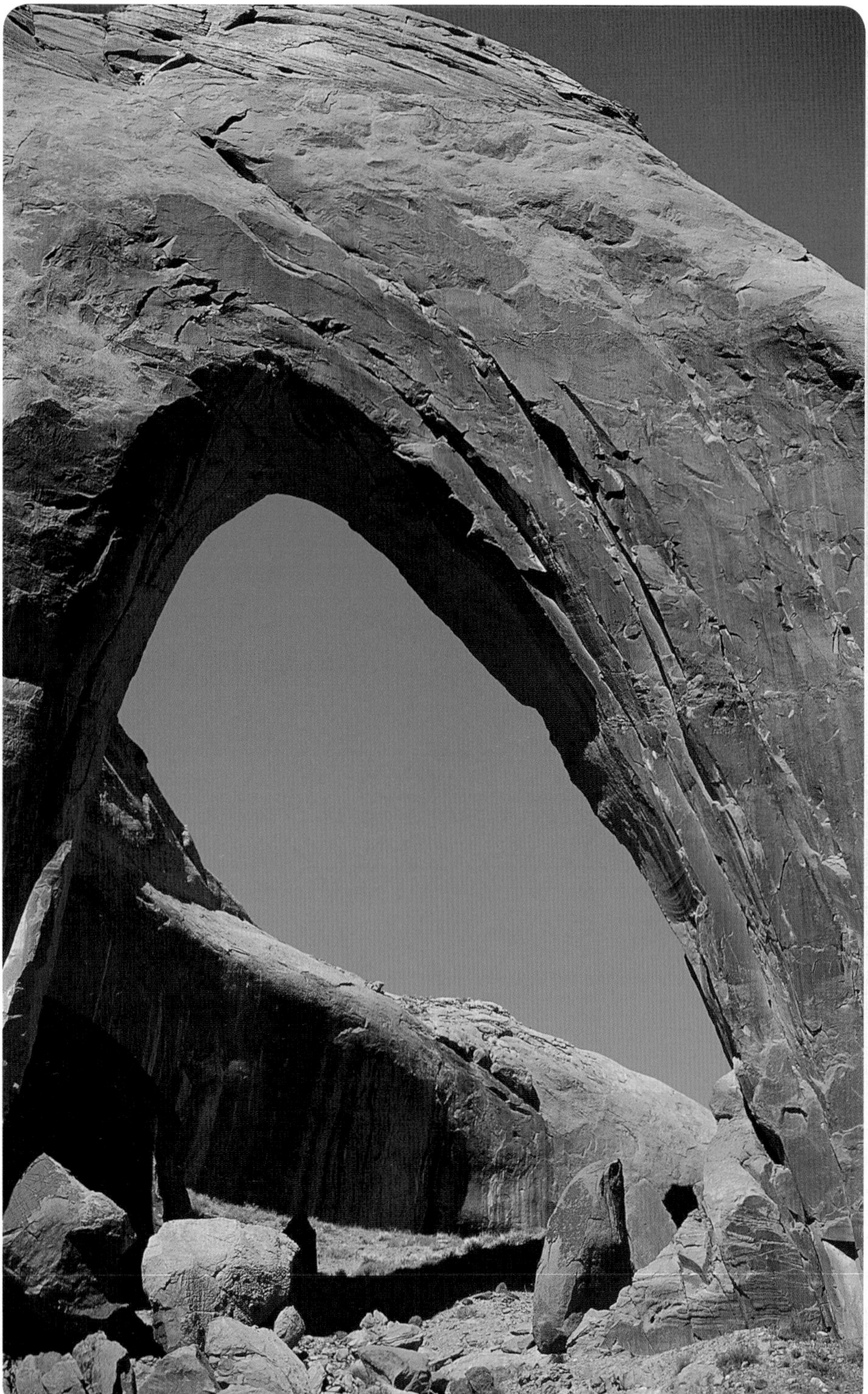

Broken Bow Arch, Willow Gulch (Trip 26)

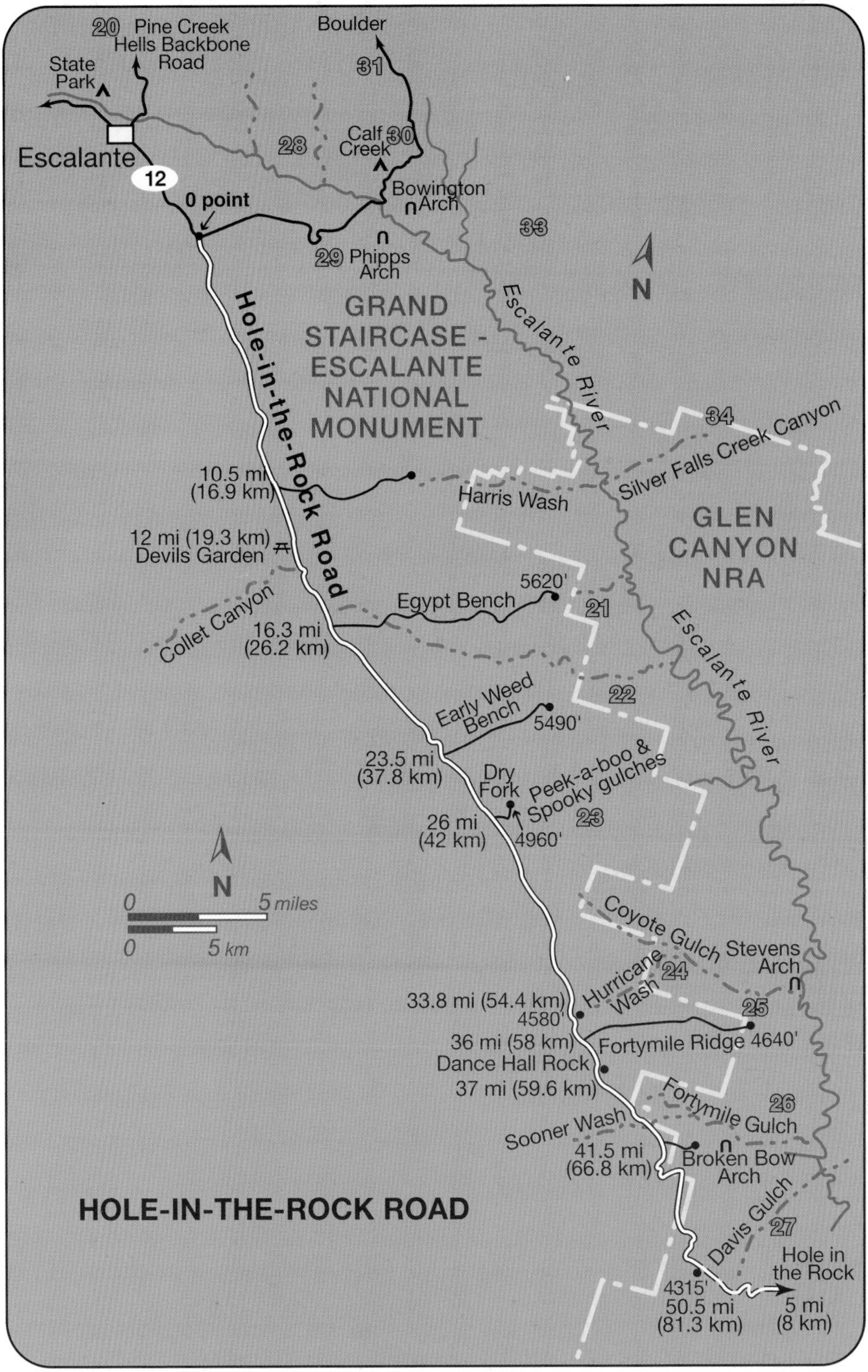
20 Pine Creek
Hells Backbone
Road
Boulder
31
State
Park
Escalante
12
28
Calf
Creek
30
Bowington
Arch
0 point
33
29 Phipps
Arch
N
Hole-in-the-Rock Road
GRAND
STAIRCASE -
ESCALANTE
NATIONAL
MONUMENT
Escalante River
34
Silver Falls Creek Canyon
10.5 mi
(16.9 km)
Harris Wash
GLEN
CANYON
NRA
12 mi (19.3 km)
Devils Garden
5620'
Egypt Bench
21
Collet Canyon
16.3 mi
(26.2 km)
Escalante River
22
Early Weed
Bench
5490'
23.5 mi
(37.8 km)
Dry
Fork
Peek-a-boo &
Spooky gulches
26 mi
(42 km)
4960'
23
N
0
5 miles
0
5 km
Coyote Gulch
Stevens
Arch
Hurricane
Wash
24
33.8 mi (54.4 km)
4580'
25
36 mi (58 km)
Fortymile Ridge 4640'
Dance Hall Rock
37 mi (59.6 km)
26
Fortymile Gulch
Sooner Wash
41.5 mi
(66.8 km)
Broken Bow
Arch
Davis Gulch
27
HOLE-IN-THE-ROCK ROAD
Hole in
the Rock
4315'
50.5 mi
(81.3 km)
5 mi
(8 km)

TRIP 21

NEON CANYON & GOLDEN CATHEDRAL

LOCATION	Hole-in-the-Rock Road Glen Canyon National Recreation Area
ROUND TRIP	9.2 mi (14.8 km)
ELEVATION CHANGE	1260-ft (384-m) loss and gain
KEY ELEVATIONS	trailhead 5620 ft (1713 m) Escalante River at Fence Canyon 4540 ft (1384 m) Neon Canyon at Golden Cathedral 4720 ft (1439 m)
HIKING TIME	3½ to 4½ hours
DIFFICULTY	moderate
MAPS	Trails Illustrated *Canyons of the Escalante*, USGS *Egypt*

OPINION

National Geographic Adventure magazine published a cover photo of the Golden Cathedral in the late 90s. This relatively obscure canyon-country destination was suddenly as famous and popular as it deserved to be.

It's a stupendous Wingate sandstone grotto in Neon Canyon. Long ago, whenever water rushed through Neon, it would cascade over the grotto lip, pool up on the canyon floor far below, then sedately flow into the Escalante River. Gradually the grit-laden water scoured potholes above the grotto. Eventually those potholes collapsed, leaving two, gaping, Pantheon-like apertures in the grotto ceiling.

Climbers like to absail through the holes, down to the green pool in the lower canyon. Hikers like to approach this awesome, natural temple from below, wade into the pool, and stare up at the blue yonder through the stone skylights.

While the Cathedral is a premier destination, the hike to and from is only moderately appealing until Neon Canyon, which is impressively deep and narrow. Bear in mind you must ford the Escalante River en route, which adds spice or hassle, depending on your perspective.

FACT

BEFORE YOUR TRIP

Stop at the Escalante Interagency Visitor Center before driving the Hole-in-the-Rock Road. Get a current weather report, ask about the condition of the road, and find out how deep the Escalante River is likely to be.

Start hiking in boots. Most of the trip is on dry terrain. But you'll ford the Escalante River at least twice, and if you prefer not to do it barefoot then pack a pair of sandals. Trekking poles are also useful for probing water depth, staying upright while fording, and negotiating steep, sandy riverbanks.

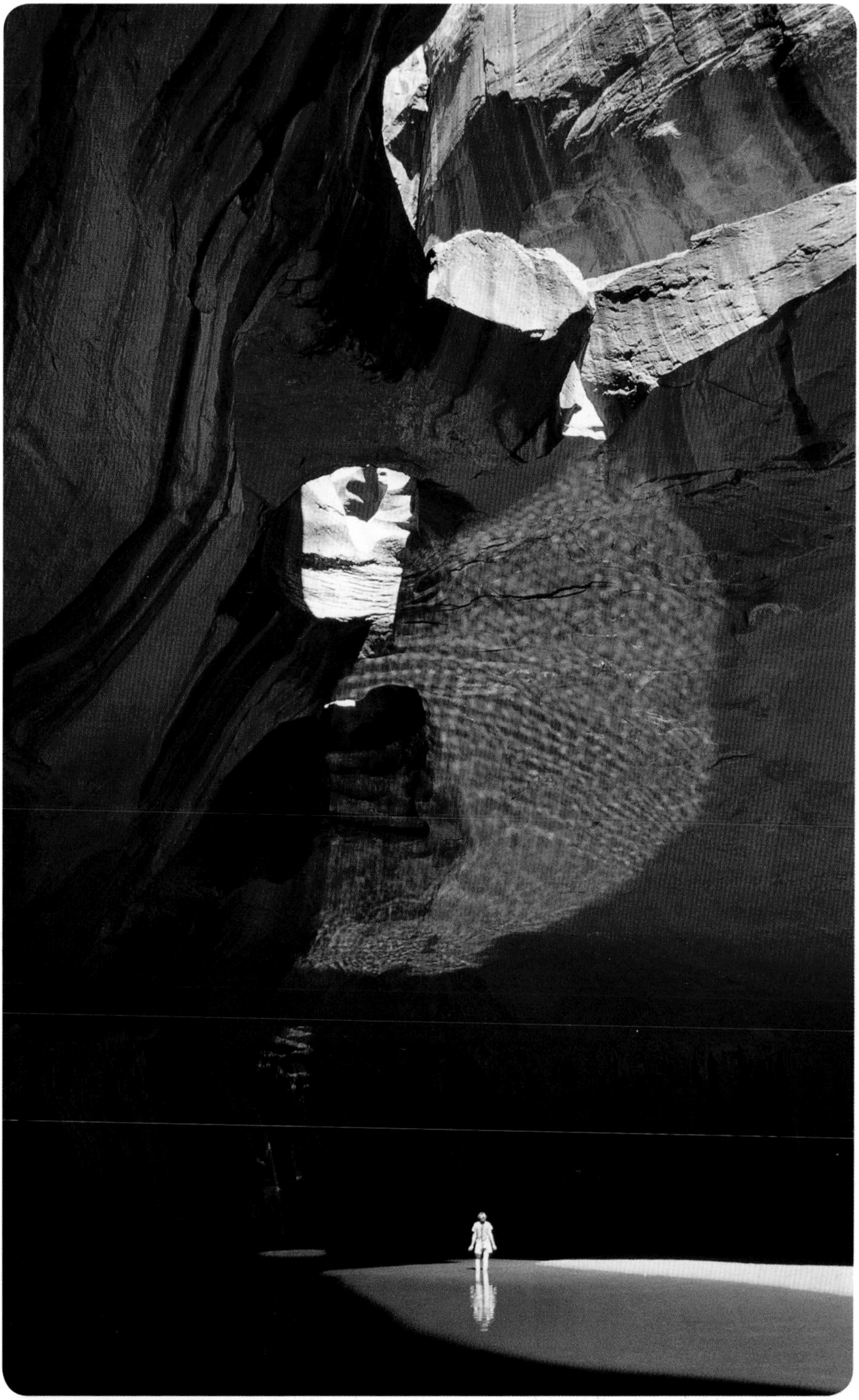

Golden Cathedral, Neon Canyon

BY VEHICLE

From Boulder, at the junction of Hwy 12 and Burr Trail Road, drive Hwy 12 west, then generally south. At 12.7 mi (20.4 km), just past Calf Creek Rec Area, reset your trip odometer to 0 on the Escalante River bridge. Proceed south. At 4.5 mi (7.2 km) stop at the scenic overlook, then proceed west. At 9.5 mi (15.3 km) turn left (south) onto the signed, unpaved Hole-in-the-Rock Road.

From the southeast edge of Escalante, near the high school, drive Hwy 12 generally southeast. At 4.5 mi (7.3 km) turn right (south) onto the signed, unpaved Hole-in-the-Rock Road.

From either approach, depart Hwy 12, reset your trip odometer to 0, and follow the Hole-in-the-Rock Road southeast. At 16.3 mi (26.2 km) turn left (east-northeast) onto Egypt Bench Road.

Reset your trip odometer to 0 again and follow Egypt Bench Road generally northeast. At 2.9 mi (4.6 km) pass the trailhead parking area for Twentyfive Mile Wash. (See Trip 22 for our recommended alternative access to the lower, deeper reaches of Twentyfive Mile Wash.) The road deteriorates beyond, crossing several washes. At 6.4 mi (10.3 km) slow down for a sharp right turn then drop into a wash. At 7.4 mi (11.9 km) confront a short, rough, steep incline. Fork right at 9.3 mi (15 km). Reach Egypt trailhead parking area at 9.9 mi (15.9 km), 5620 ft (1713 m).

ON FOOT

The trail descends northeast. Follow cairns down the slickrock bowl. Sandstone steps, chiseled by ranchers, drop to sand at 0.4 mi (0.6 km), 5150 ft (1570 m). Proceed northeast.

Cross a shallow **wash**—the tail of Fence Canyon—at 0.8 mi (1.3 km). Do not follow the wash. Continue northeast above the northwest rim of the incipient canyon.

Cairns, and probably bootprints, indicate the way. Pause occasionally and look back, so you can confidently retrace your steps to the trailhead.

The route undulates over sandstone ledges, through patches of sand, past juniper trees. The canyon's lower reaches are visible below. Proceed among huge cottonwoods about 45 minutes along.

Bear right at 2 mi (3.2 km), 4950 ft (1494 m). Begin a steep descent generally east. Reach a sandy bench at 4580 ft (1396 m). Then follow a stock trail right (southeast) into the mouth of **Fence Canyon**.

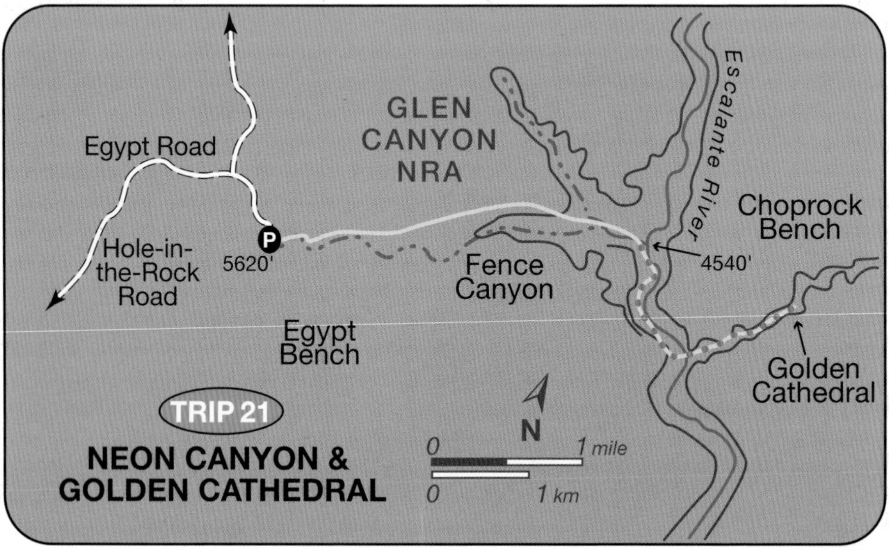

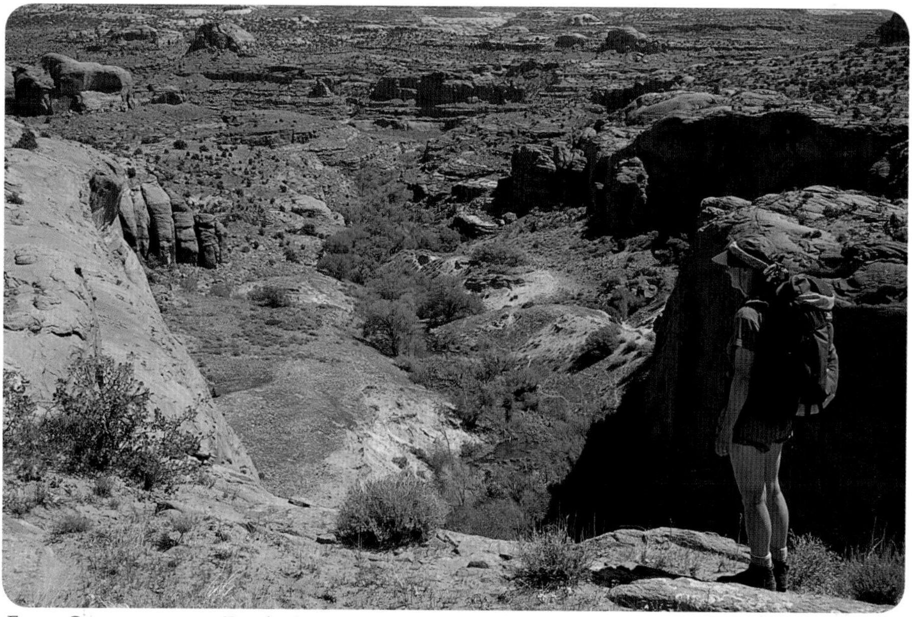

Fence Canyon route to Escalante River

Pause again. Study the area so you'll know where to tag onto the stock trail when you exit the canyon. Then continue down-canyon (east). Reach the **Escalante River** at 2.8 mi (4.5 km), 4540 ft (1384 m), about 1¼ hours from the trailhead. Turn right and follow the river downstream, looking for the easiest place to **ford** to the far bank.

The riverbed and its riparian vegetation can change dramatically with each flood. So it's impossible to predict where the optimal ford will be when you arrive. Bootprints indicate where others have crossed but are no assurance of safety or ease. Use your own judgment and be cautious.

Remember: rivers tend to be shallowest where they're widest. The Escalante is typically knee to thigh deep, but can be much deeper. The current, usually languid, can be strong. And the turbid water makes it difficult to judge depth. If fording appears dangerous, turn back.

In the ensuing 0.9 mi (1.4 mi), seek the path of least resistance while proceeding downstream, generally southeast. You might have to ford the river again. You'll almost certainly have to tunnel through tamarisk, willow, Russian olive, and cottonwoods.

After approximately 20 minutes of downstream progress, you should be hiking east, on the left (north) bank. Study the south-facing canyon wall for two petroglyph panels. Just ten minutes farther, at 3.7 mi (6 km), reach the mouth of **Neon Canyon**—the first tributary drainage below Fence Canyon—near a massive, ancient cottonwood.

Turn left, enter Neon Canyon, and follow it generally north-northeast. Within 20 minutes, enter the **Golden Cathedral** at 4.6 mi (7.4 km), 4720 ft (1439 m) —a soaring, dome-like cavern with two pouroff holes in the roof. Hikers are forced to turn around here.

After exiting Neon Canyon, either retrace your route upstream to Fence Canyon, or lengthen your dayhike by turning left (south) and resuming downstream another 0.9 mi (1.4 km)—about 30 minutes—to explore **Ringtail Canyon** (left / east).

TRIP 22

FOX CANYON & TWENTYFIVE MILE WASH

LOCATION	Hole-in-the-Rock Road Glen Canyon National Recreation Area
ROUND TRIP	15.2 mi (24.5 km)
ELEVATION CHANGE	1030-ft (314-m) loss and gain
KEY ELEVATIONS	trailhead 5490 ft (1673 m), confluence of Fox Canyon and Twentyfive Mile Wash 4580 ft (1396 m) Escalante River 4460 ft (1360 m)
HIKING TIME	2 to 3 days
DIFFICULTY	challenging
MAPS	Trails Illustrated *Canyons of the Escalante*, USGS *Egypt*

OPINION

It's a long trudge to the Escalante River via Twentyfive Mile Wash, and it's a rather mundane boulevard most of the way. But you can shorten the round trip by 14 mi (22.5 km) and significantly increase the reward-to-effort ratio by dropping into Twentyfive's impressive lower reaches via Fox Canyon.

To do so you must navigate cross-country to Fox Canyon, then enter it by way of a short but steep friction-walk. If you have any routefinding experience, the 1 mi (1.6 km) across trail-less terrain will pose no difficulty as long as you carry a compass in one hand and the 1:24 000 topo map in the other. As for dropping into Fox, the slickrock-ramp entry appears more committing than it actually is. A nervous novice might manage it on the seat of his hopefully double-bottomed shorts if not on the soles of his boots.

The entire trip is scenic. From the trailhead, you'll hike on rolling sandstone across the outer edge of Early Weed Bench, with sweeping views of canyon country. Fox Canyon is short but intriguingly narrow. And while "wash" aptly describes most of Twentyfive Mile, the stretch you'll be hiking is a full-blown canyon. The bulbous sandstone walls tower above and occasionally overhang the meandering trickle you'll follow to the Mother Escalante.

Beyond the confluence of Fox Canyon and Twentyfive Mile Wash, navigation is simple: just head downstream, without being diverted up the four primary tributary drainages. The hiking, however, might not be a total cakewalk. In the past, the riparian vegetation has been thick and ornery á la Southeast Asia.

FACT

BEFORE YOUR TRIP

Stop at the Escalante Interagency Visitor Center before driving the Hole-in-the-Rock Road. Get a current weather report, ask about the condition of the road, and find out how deep the Escalante River is likely to be.

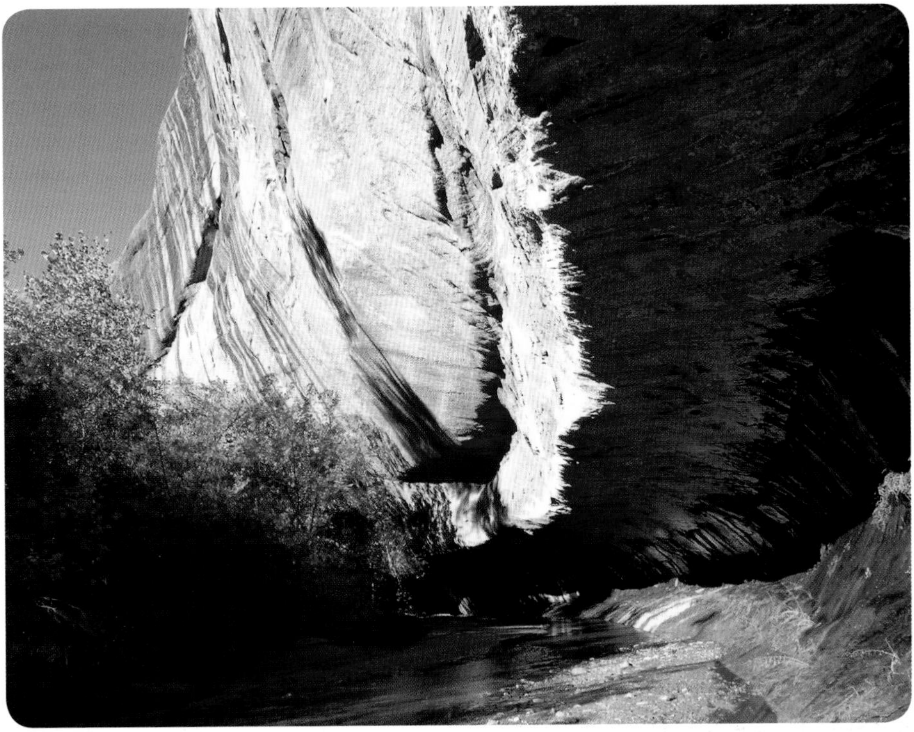

Twentyfive mile Wash

The stream in lower Twentyfive Mile is often a trickle: shallow enough to walk in without soaking your footwear, narrow enough to easily hop across. But in case it's not, amphibious footwear is preferable. Wear technical sandals designed for hiking, or fabric hiking boots you don't mind dunking. If you intend to continue in the Escalante River, dunkable boots are essential.

BY VEHICLE

From Boulder, at the junction of Hwy 12 and Burr Trail Road, drive Hwy 12 west, then generally south. At 12.7 mi (20.4 km), just past Calf Creek Rec Area, reset your trip odometer to 0 on the Escalante River bridge. Proceed south. At 4.5 mi (7.2 km) stop at the scenic overlook, then proceed west. At 9.5 mi (15.3 km) turn left (south) onto the signed, unpaved Hole-in-the-Rock Road.

From the southeast edge of Escalante, near the high school, drive Hwy 12 generally southeast. At 4.5 mi (7.3 km) turn right (south) onto the signed, unpaved Hole-in-the-Rock Road.

From either approach, depart Hwy 12, reset your trip odometer to 0, and follow the Hole-in-the-Rock Road southeast. At 23.5 mi (37.8 km) turn left onto Early Weed Bench Road, reset your trip odometer to 0, and follow it northeast. At 4.7 mi (7.6 km), bear right (east) ignoring the 4WD road forking left. Reach the trailhead at 5.2 mi (8.4 km), 5490 ft (1673 m). Park here. A sandstone knoll is visible on the rim directly east. The road continues east-southeast to the Early Weed Bench trailhead at 5.6 mi (9 km).

ON FOOT

Study the 1:24 000 topo map before departing. Your immediate goal, Fox Canyon, is easy to identify though it's unlabeled. It's about 1 mi (1.6 km) north-northeast of the trailhead. It runs generally north / south, along the left (west) boundary of Glen Canyon National Rec Area.

Begin hiking north, over the rim. Follow the path of least resistance across undulating sandstone, gradually bearing right (north-northeast). The steep canyon walls near the confluence of Fox Canyon and Twentyfive Mile Wash are visible north.

Aim for the prominent, brown-topped butte. At 1 mi (1.6 km), 4880 ft (1488 m), proceed generally north, above the left (west) **rim of Fox Canyon**. Cross the shallow tail of a minor tributary.

Shortly beyond, curve right (northeast) and begin a steep friction-walk on a **slickrock ramp** dropping to a sandy bench. Follow a path right (south) down to the **floor of Fox Canyon**. Then turn left (north) and hike down-canyon.

At 1.8 mi (2.9 km), 4580 ft (1396 m), intersect **Twentyfive Mile Wash**. Follow it downstream (right / east), soon curving left (north). It meanders constantly, but your generally direction of travel will remain northeast all the way to the Escalante River.

Water within Twentyfive Mile Wash should be less turbid and contaminated than the Escalante, so refill water bottles en route.

At 3.6 mi (5.8 km) continue east, ignoring a tributary drainage (left / north). At 4.1 mi (6.6 km), continue northeast, ignoring a sheer-walled tributary drainage (right / south). Ignore two more tributary drainages (left / north, and right / south) within the ensuing 2 mi (3.2 km).

Reach the **Escalante River** at 7.6 mi (12.2 km), 4460 ft (1360 m). Look for possible campsites above the river's far (east) bank, or 0.4 mi (0.6 km) downstream above the right (west) bank.

After exploring the Escalante either upstream or down as far as time, energy and curiosity permit, retrace your steps to the trailhead through Twentyfive Mile Wash and Fox Canyon.

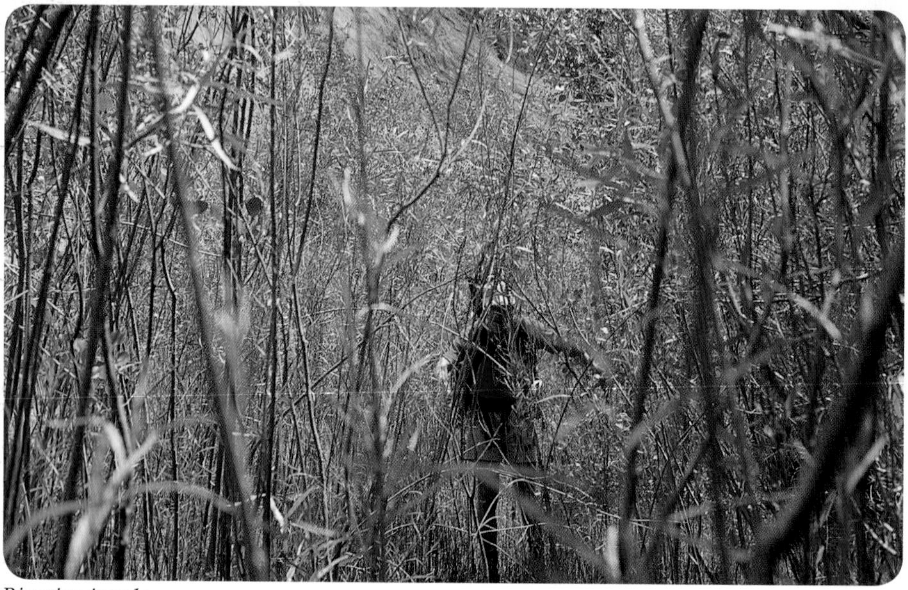

Riparian jungle

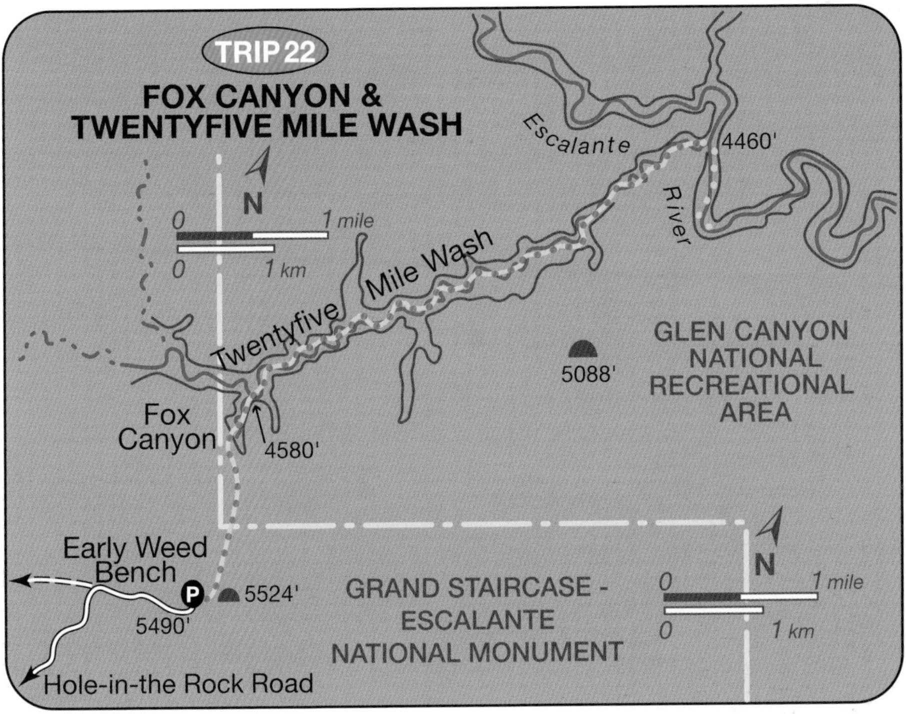

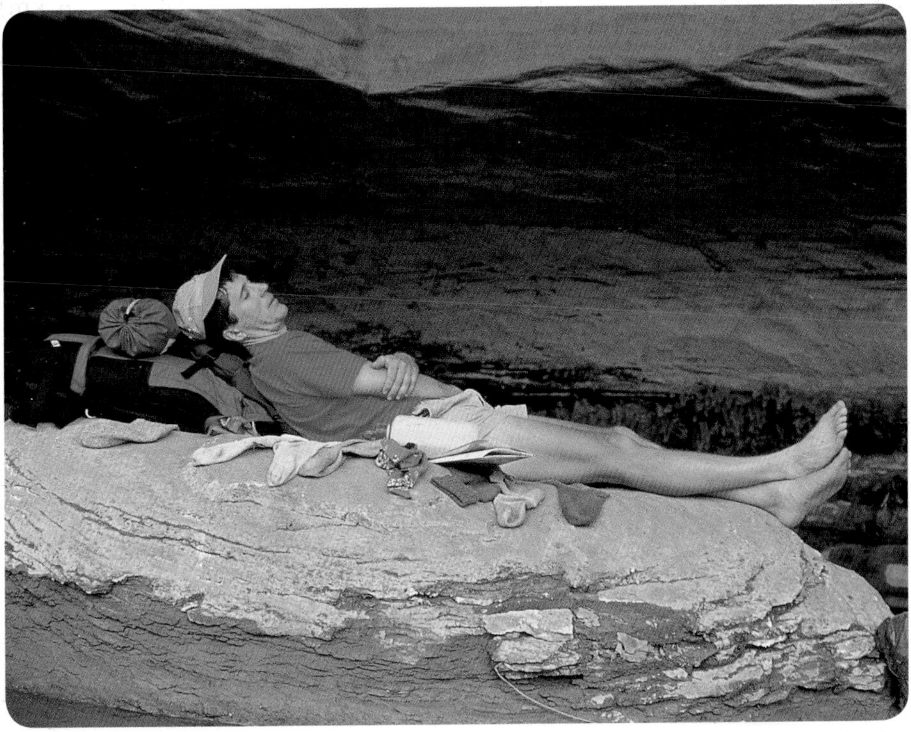

Preventing heat exhaustion

TRIP 23

PEEK-A-BOO, SPOOKY & BRIMSTONE GULCHES

LOCATION	Hole-in-the-Rock Road Grand Staircase-Escalante National Monument
DISTANCE	4.8 mi (7.7 km)
ELEVATION GAIN	565 ft (172 m)
KEY ELEVATIONS	trailhead 4960 ft (1512 m), bottom of Peek-a-boo 4720 ft (1439 m), highpoint / traverse to Spooky 4880 ft (1487 m), bottom of Spooky 4640 ft (1414 m), lowpoint / bottom of Brimstone 4580 ft (1396 m)
HIKING TIME	2½ to 3 hours
DIFFICULTY	moderate
MAPS	Trails Illustrated *Canyons of the Escalante* USGS *Big Hollow Wash, Egypt*

OPINION

Man loses 283 lbs simply by walking.

As the tabloids occasionally remind us, the simple act of walking is more effective than any miracle diet. Healthier, too. But this is one hike you should avoid if you're overweight. Peek-a-boo, Spooky, and Brimstone gulches are so narrow, it's actually possible for a girthy guy or gal to get stuck.

These are among the most popular slot canyons in Utah. Access is easy, you can probe all three in a day, and hikers without technical canyoneering equipment or skills can enjoy a significant portion of each.

All are sensuously sculpted. Their fluid shapes and liquid appearance mirror the rushing water that created them. To the imaginative eye, their serpentine sandstone walls seem to shudder and waft upwards like the throaty, echoing laugh of a ghoul.

Bear in mind, the distance and time figures stated above are rough estimates only. There are many ways to vary this trip. And hiking speed is difficult to predict in terrain where you might spend several minutes slithering just a few feet.

Peek-a-boo

The shortest and shallowest of the three, this is the slot most hikers will feel comfortable probing. It's possible to hike up Peek-a-boo, then down Spooky.

Spooky

Longer and slimmer than Peek-a-boo, Spooky forces even anorexic hikers to carry their daypacks, turn sideways, and wiggle through. A few short drops and a chokestone jungle add intrigue.

Brimstone

You'd have to be a shapeshifter to slip all the way through Brimstone. It's the darkest and narrowest of the trio and poses serious obstacles even before it becomes impassable. Still, it's well worth inserting yourself into, if only to check your immunity to claustrophobia.

If it's rained recently, you might encounter pools in Peek-a-boo or Spooky, but their floors are usually dry and sandy. Brimstone tends to retain water, so expect to wade if you probe it very far. The regional weather forecast suggests it *might* rain? Stay away. Slot canyons can instantly become flashflood death zones.

Slot-canyon photography is tricky. Peek-a-boo is brighter than the others, so it's possible to handhold your camera and still obtain a sharp image if you set your digital to ISO 400. Spooky is darker, and Brimstone darker yet. Both will probably require a tripod. All three are brightest around midday.

FACT

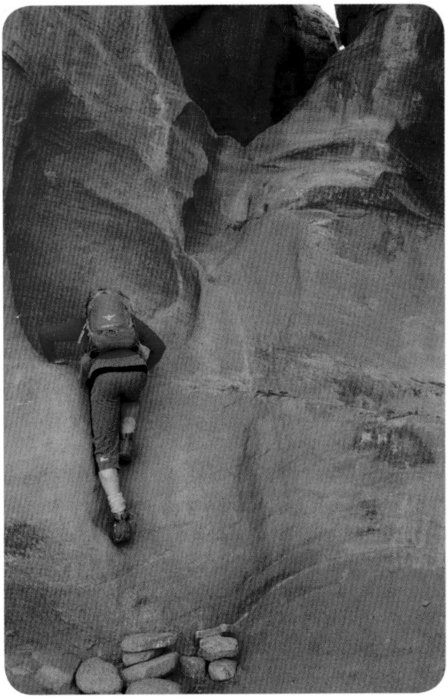

Mouth of Peekaboo Gulch

BEFORE YOUR TRIP

Stop at the Escalante Interagency Visitor Center before driving the Hole-in-the-Rock Road. Check the current weather report, ask about the condition of the road, and confirm that the trailhead access has remain unchanged.

All three gulches are in the Scorpion Wilderness Study Area, which is within Grand Staircase-Escalante National Monument. For years, authorities have considered moving the spur road and establishing a new trailhead outside the WSA. Access to the spur would continue to be via Hole-in-the-Rock Road. But the trail would lead to Spooky first, rather than to Peek-a-boo as it does now. At the time of publication, we were assured this still might not happen and certainly wouldn't happen soon. Just in case it does, however, a quick visit to the Escalante Interagency Visitor Center could spare you some minor inconvenience.

BY VEHICLE

From Boulder, at the junction of Hwy 12 and Burr Trail Road, drive Hwy 12 west, then generally south. At 12.7 mi (20.4 km), just past Calf Creek Rec Area, reset your trip odometer to 0 on the Escalante River bridge. Proceed south. At 4.5 mi (7.2 km) stop at the scenic overlook, then proceed west. At 9.5 mi (15.3 km) turn left (south) onto the signed, unpaved Hole-in-the-Rock Road.

From the southeast edge of Escalante, near the high school, drive Hwy 12 generally southeast. At 4.5 mi (7.3 km) turn right (south) onto the signed, unpaved Hole-in-the-Rock Road.

From either approach, depart Hwy 12, reset your trip odometer to 0, and follow the Hole-in-the-Rock Road southeast. At 26 mi (42 km) turn left onto the unsigned spur leading to Dry Fork Coyote Gulch, reset your trip odometer to 0, and follow it east. Soon fork left and curve north. Reach the road's end trailhead at 1.7 mi (2.7 km), 4960 ft (1512 m).

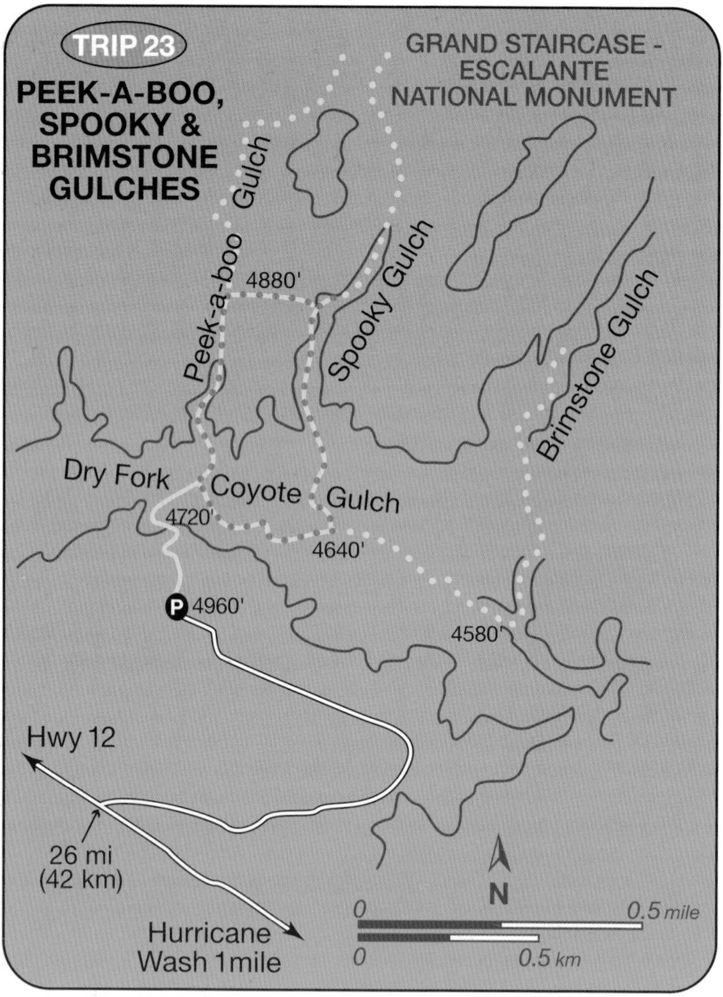

ON FOOT

A brief orientation is all you should need to find and enjoy these three slot canyons, so here goes.

Dry Fork Coyote Gulch runs generally left (west-northwest) to right (east-southeast). The trailhead is above Dry Fork's south side. From left to right (west to east), Peek-a-boo, Spooky, and Brimstone are parallel tributary slots draining into the dry fork's north side. All three slots run generally north/south.

The mouth of Peek-a-boo is basically across Dry Fork from the trailhead. The mouths of Spooky and Brimstone are a short distance right (east-southeast) down Dry Fork.

After dropping into Dry Fork, simply probe each of the slots as far as curiosity, energy, time, and ability allow. Or, part way up Peek-a-boo, you can traverse to Spooky, creating a loop: up one, down the other.

Never proceed where it appears you'll be unable to reverse out. Stay within your comfort zone. If you're deeply hesitant, trust your instinct: find another way forward (perhaps by ascending, then following the rim of the slot) or turn back.

Want more detailed directions? Keep reading.

From the trailhead, follow the cairned trail switchbacking generally north, over ledges, down into **Dry Fork Coyote Gulch**. In about 15 minutes, bottom out in the **wash**.

The tail of Dry Fork is left. Heading generally west-northwest, it quickly slots up and is worth a short detour. For Peek-a-boo, Spooky, and Brimstone, turn right and hike down-canyon.

In about 100 yd (91 m) turn left to follow **Peek-a-boo** generally north. Steps carved into the sandstone offer assistance on the initial 20-ft (6-m) ascent.

Though only about 50 ft (15 m) deep, Peek-a-boo narrows dramatically. Soon pass a double bridge. A bit farther are two more small, natural bridges. Where the slot constricts so much you cannot continue, ascend out, proceed along the rim for a couple minutes, then drop back in.

The slot ends in a **broad, sandy wash**, about 35 to 40 minutes from Dry Fork. You have two choices:

(a) Turn around and **descend** south **through Peek-a-boo**. When you reach Dry Fork, go left. Proceed down-canyon (east-southeast) about 15 minutes to the mouth of Spooky. Turn left (north), ascend Spooky as far as you please, then turn around and return to Dry Fork.

(b) **Traverse** right (east) across a low ridge for about ten minutes **to Spooky**—the first broad, sandy wash you intersect—drop into it, turn right, and follow it south to Dry Fork. You can also hike south atop Spooky's right (west) rim, then drop into Dry Fork on a sandslide.

So you've explored Peek-a-boo and Spooky, and you're now in **Dry Fork** at Spooky's mouth. Go left (east-southeast) to check out Brimstone, or right (west-northwest) to return to the trailhead.

Brimstone is about 25 minutes down-canyon from Spooky. En route, Dry Fork narrows and a chokestone blocks passage. Scramble around it on the right. Shortly past a prominent, white guano stain on the right wall, turn left (north) into the broad, sandy mouth of **Brimstone**.

The walls of Brimstone soon constrict into a deep, dark, technically challenging slot. It's impossible to continue all the way through, but squeezing yourself into it for 15 minutes or so is fun. It's also possible to ascend a sandslide from the mouth to the rim, then follow along the top, peering into and leaping across the slender rift.

After exiting Brimstone to Dry Fork, either retrace your steps up-canyon to the trailhead, or continue down-canyon a couple minutes to a slickrock slab (right / southwest). Ascend it to the **rim of Dry Fork**, then bear right and hike generally west-northwest, along the rim, back to the trailhead.

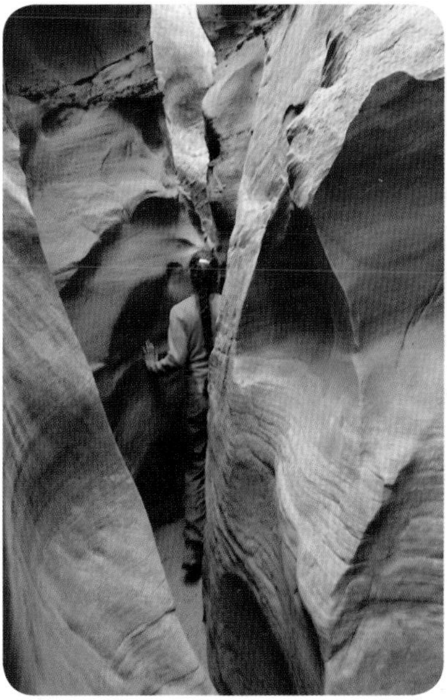

Spooky Gulch

TRIP 24

HURRICANE WASH & COYOTE GULCH

LOCATION	Hole-in-the-Rock Road Glen Canyon National Recreation Area
ROUND TRIP	18 mi (29 km) to Coyote Natural Bridge 26.8 mi (43.1 km) to the Escalante River
ELEVATION CHANGE	680-ft (207-m) loss and gain for Coyote Natural Bridge 880-ft (268-m) loss and gain for the Escalante River
KEY ELEVATIONS	trailhead 4580 ft (1396 m) Jacob Hamblin Arch 4050 ft (1235 m) Coyote Natural Bridge 3900 ft (1189 m) Escalante River 3700 ft (1128 m)
HIKING TIME	9 hours to 2 days
DIFFICULTY	easy
MAPS	Trails Illustrated *Canyons of the Escalante* USGS *Big Hollow Wash, King Mesa*

OPINION

What evening light does to canyon-country stone is alchemy.

Of the countless places to witness that wondrous, twilight transformation, one of the most memorable will be reclining at your campsite on a sandy bench within a soaring alcove deep in Coyote Gulch.

The distinction between *gulch* and *canyon* being arbitrary, Coyote is as beautiful and intriguing as any canyon on the Colorado Plateau. The Navajo sandstone walls are massive, vaulting high overhead, and sensuously sculpted with frequent amphitheaters. It harbors a perennial stream, two arches, a natural bridge, numerous cascades, several waterfalls, and plentiful springs. Plus it's replete with appealing campsites.

That's why it's the most popular backpack trip off the Hole-in-the-Rock Road, and why you shouldn't hike here during April, May, or October. The solitude necessary to appreciate wilderness will be impossible to find. Instead, come in early March or early November. The nights will be chilly, but the days will be pleasant, and you won't hear other hikers' idiotic chit chat and annoying laughter constantly pinging off the canyon walls.

Entering Coyote Gulch via Hurricane Wash, as described here, is gradual but easy and simple: just follow the broad streambed into the ever deepening canyon. Crack in the Wall (Trip 25) offers a short, very sharp descent directly to the mouth of Coyote Gulch near its confluence with the Escalante River. The two routes are distinctly different. We recommend Hurricane Wash for backpacking, Crack in the Wall for dayhiking.

It is possible, however, for athletic keeners to complete the 18-mi (29-km) round trip from Hurricane Wash trailhead to Coyote Natural Bridge in eight or nine hours' hiking time. The elevation loss and gain is imperceptible. The terrain underfoot is smooth. It's sandy, but without the burden of a full pack, you'll stride rather than plod through the initial stretch of dry sand.

Still, it's better to backpack—if you can do it when the canyon is not flooded with raucous students on spring break. While determined dayhikers might tag the natural bridge before turning around, Coyote Gulch extends far below and is highly scenic the entire way. Plus it's difficult to appreciate the evening alchemy while racing the setting sun back to the trailhead. Better to slow down and live within the canyon's embrace for at least 24 hours.

FACT

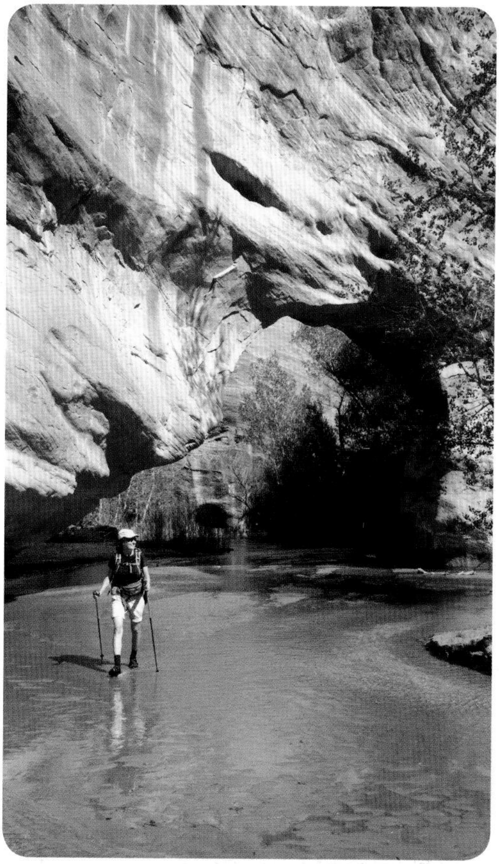

Coyote Natural Bridge

BEFORE YOUR TRIP

Stop at the Escalante Interagency Visitor Center before driving the Hole-in-the-Rock Road. Check the current weather report, ask about the condition of the road, and, if you intend to backpack, get a no-fee permit. Permits are also available at the trail register.

A perennial stream flows in lower Hurricane Wash and Coyote Gulch. Though it tends to be only ankle deep, you'll cross it repeatedly. And the easiest, least impactful route is usually the streambed itself, rather than the multiple, sandy, often steep "shortcut" paths across benches. So amphibious footwear is preferable. Wear technical sandals designed for hiking, or fabric hiking boots you don't mind dunking. If you intend to continue in the Escalante River, dunkable boots are essential.

BY VEHICLE

From Boulder, at the junction of Hwy 12 and Burr Trail Road, drive Hwy 12 west, then generally south. At 12.7 mi (20.4 km), just past Calf Creek Rec Area, reset your trip odometer to 0 on the Escalante River bridge. Proceed south. At 4.5 mi (7.2 km) stop at the scenic overlook, then proceed west. At 9.5 mi (15.3 km) turn left (south) onto the signed, unpaved Hole-in-the-Rock Road.

From the southeast edge of Escalante, near the high school, drive Hwy 12 generally southeast. At 4.5 mi (7.3 km) turn right (south) onto the signed, unpaved Hole-in-the-Rock Road.

From either approach, depart Hwy 12, reset your trip odometer to 0, and follow the Hole-in-the-Rock Road southeast. Reach the Hurricane Wash trailhead parking area at 33.8 mi (54.4 km), 4580 ft (1396 m), on the right (west) side of the road.

ON FOOT

Experienced hikers will find a detailed route description unnecessary and tedious. Simply follow Hurricane Wash generally northeast until intersecting Coyote Gulch at 5.5 mi (8.9 km). Then turn right and follow Coyote Gulch down-canyon. Here the stream meanders constantly, but your general direction of travel will be east to Cliff Arch, then northeast to the Escalante River at 13.4 mi (21.6 km). But if you prefer the unabridged version, here you go…

Cross to the east side of the road and follow a sandy, **4WD spur** east along the north side of the shallow tail of Hurricane Wash. At 0.3 mi (0.5 km), reach the 4WD parking area and the **trail register**. Beyond, follow the former road into the **wash**. Within 12 minutes, proceed through a hiker's maze, which allows people but not cows to pass through the fence.

At 1.8 mi (2.9 km), about 30 minutes along, bear right (east-northeast) at a fork in the road. Continue following the wash. After another hiker's maze, the route alternates between the wash and the low benches.

About 50 minutes along, where the former road ascends right, bear left and descend into the sandy wash near a scrim of piñon pine. Within an hour, slickrock domes border the wash. It's evident you're in a canyon. The walls are 80 to 150 ft (24 to 46 m) high.

Enter **Glen Canyon Recreation Area** at 3 mi (4.8 km), 4280 ft (1305 m). Eight minutes farther, the canyon briefly constricts to just 18 ft (5.5 m), then broadens again. About 1½ hours along, pass a tributary drainage (right /southwest). Expect to encounter water approximately 2 in (5 cm) deep in the wash ahead. Slip through yet another hiker's maze.

After hiking 1¾ hours, reach an inviting campsite on a sandy bench, within earshot of the gentle water music, beneath an overhanging, desert-varnished, 250-ft (76-m) high wall. The canyon is now 50 to 60 ft (15 to 18.3 m) wide. Cottonwoods and willows are profuse here.

Intersect **Coyote Gulch** at 5.4 mi (8.7 km), 4067 ft (1240 m), about two hours from the trailhead. Proceed down-canyon by bearing right (south) and immediately curving left (east). The stream, which you'll follow all the way to the Escalante River, has more volume below this confluence. A sandy bench here is the first of Coyote's many superb campsites.

Amphitheaters rise 500 ft (152 m) at nearly every bend. Hanging gardens flourish where water seeps from the shaded walls. About 2 hours and 20 minutes along, pass a tributary drainage (left / north). And 2½ hours along, just beyond a sandy point affording several campsites, pass a signed toilet (left / north) at 6.8 mi (10.9 km).

After curving through Coyote's grandest amphitheater, **Jacob Hamblin Arch** is visible at 7 mi (11.3 km), 4050 ft (1235 m). The sandy bench opposite the arch provides a campsite for a lucky few. The man for whom the arch is named served as a scout and Indian missionary for Brigham Young.

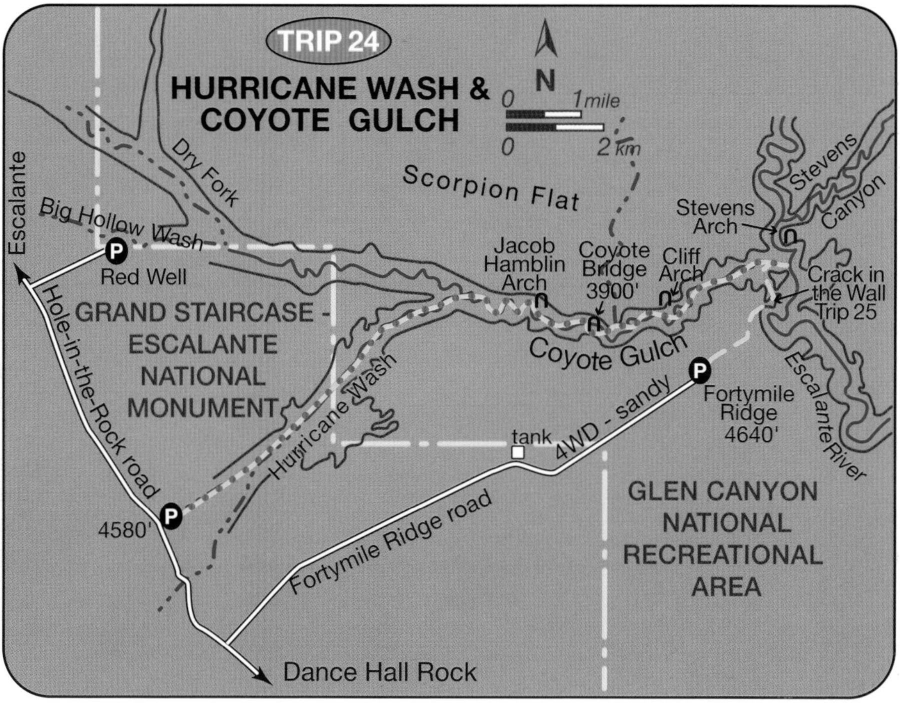

Immediately past the arch, watch left (north) for a series of reliable springs. Pass another signed toilet 110 yd (100 m) beyond the arch. The canyon walls soar to 600 ft (183 m) here.

At 8.5 mi (13.7 km) the canyon constricts and the stream cascades over slickrock. Pass **Coyote Natural Bridge** at 9 mi (14.5 km), 3900 ft (1189 m). Just beyond, a reliable spring dribbles down the left (north) wall.

About 20 minutes farther, enter a broad park beneath a long, shallow alcove (left / north). A **pictograph panel** is visible near the alcove's right edge, about 125 ft (38 m) up. One of the huge figures resembles a centipede.

Continuing downstream, favor the left north bank. Within 20 minutes, where the stream veers right (south), opt for a scenic shortcut. Bear left and ascend to a slickrock saddle at 11 mi (17.7 km). **Cliff Arch** is visible immediately ahead, just above head height. Below, the stream cascades among boulders between massive fins. Descend via the obvious slickrock draw and resume down-canyon.

Soon encounter two 15-ft (4.6-m) **waterfalls**. Bypass both on the right. Skirting the second one, switchback left (toward the falls) while descending the slickrock ledges.

Pass a showering spring (left / north)—refreshing, but unhelpful for topping up your supply. After a small alcove affording the canyon's final campsite, reach another **waterfall**. Bypass it on the right. A couple minutes farther, a small draw (left / north) hides a reliable, convenient spring.

Reach a **junction** at 13 mi (21 km), 3760 ft (1146 m). Right ascends south via Crack in the Wall (Trip 25) to Fortymile Ridge trailhead, granting a view of Stevens Arch en route. Proceed straight (east) to reach the **Escalante River** at 13.4 mi (21.6 km), 3700 ft (1128 m).

TRIP 25

CRACK IN THE WALL

LOCATION	Hole-in-the-Rock Road Glen Canyon National Recreation Area
ROUND TRIP	5.2 mi (8.4 km) to Coyote Gulch 13.2 mi (21.3 km) to Coyote Natural Bridge
ELEVATION CHANGE	880-ft (268-m) loss and gain
KEY ELEVATIONS	trailhead 4640 ft (1415 m), Coyote Gulch 3760 ft (1146 m)
HIKING TIME	3 to 4 hours
DIFFICULTY	moderate
MAPS	Trails Illustrated *Canyons of the Escalante* USGS *King Mesa, Stevens Canyon South*

OPINION

The human imagination doesn't constantly burn at full flame. Sometimes we need a squirt of lighter fluid.

Canyon country serves that purpose. Hiking here is often a search for secretive, elusive passageways. Finding and slipping through them can be exultant, stimulating us to think creatively and seek surprising solutions to all kinds of problems.

Crack in the Wall is a classic example. After hiking nearly an hour across rolling slickrock, you approach the rim of Escalante River Canyon. You think you'll need wings or a suicide note to continue, until a portal appears. The cliff is sheer, but there's a safe descent route afterall.

Invisible until your boots are upon it, the Crack is a shoulder-width stone corridor. Stepping into it is like a trip to Diagon Alley. Suddenly everything changes.

One minute you're atop sunblasted slickrock where the view is panoramic. The next you're squeezing through the dark, cool Crack. Then you're glissading down a massive sand dune into the mouth of Coyote Gulch near its confluence with the Escalante River. From there you can quickly access the river or follow Coyote Gulch up-canyon.

Coyote is as beautiful and intriguing as any chasm on the Colorado Plateau. The Navajo sandstone walls are massive, vaulting high overhead, and sensuously sculpted with frequent amphitheaters. It harbors a perennial stream, two arches, a natural bridge, numerous cascades, several waterfalls, and plentiful springs.

If dayhiking, you might go as far as Coyote Natural Bridge before turning back and retracing your steps to the rim via the Crack. Backpacking into Coyote Gulch via the Crack is also an option, but we recommend dayhiking here. Wrangling big packs through the Crack is awkward, and trudging *up* that sand dune is toilsome enough without bearing a full load. Backpackers should opt for the gradual approach via Hurricane Wash (Trip 24) rather than this abrupt entrance.

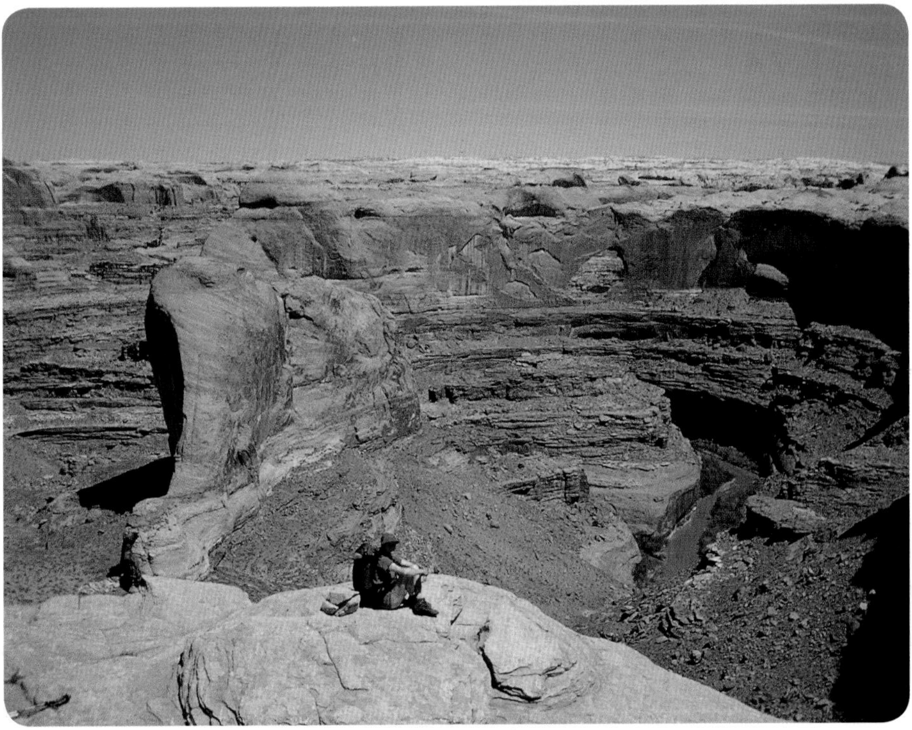

Overlooking the Escalante River, from Crack in the Wall

FACT

BEFORE YOUR TRIP

Stop at the Escalante Interagency Visitor Center before driving the Hole-in-the-Rock Road. Get a current weather report, ask about the condition of the road, and find out how deep the Escalante River is likely to be.

Read the *By Vehicle* section below, so you're aware of the sand and the exposed cattleguard on the final approach to the trailhead.

The steep, rough descent from the trailhead demands sturdy, supportive hiking boots. But a perennial stream flows in Coyote Gulch, and you'll cross it repeatedly en route to Coyote Natural Bridge. So wear fabric boots you don't mind dunking, or pack a pair of amphibious sandals you can change into. If you intend to continue in the Escalante River, dunkable boots are essential.

Bring enough lightweight nylon cord to lower packs down a 20-ft (6-m) cliff.

BY VEHICLE

From Boulder, at the junction of Hwy 12 and Burr Trail Road, drive Hwy 12 west, then generally south. At 12.7 mi (20.4 km), just past Calf Creek Rec Area, reset your trip odometer to 0 on the Escalante River bridge. Proceed south. At 4.5 mi (7.2 km) stop at the scenic overlook, then proceed west. At 9.5 mi (15.3 km) turn left (south) onto the signed, unpaved Hole-in-the-Rock Road.

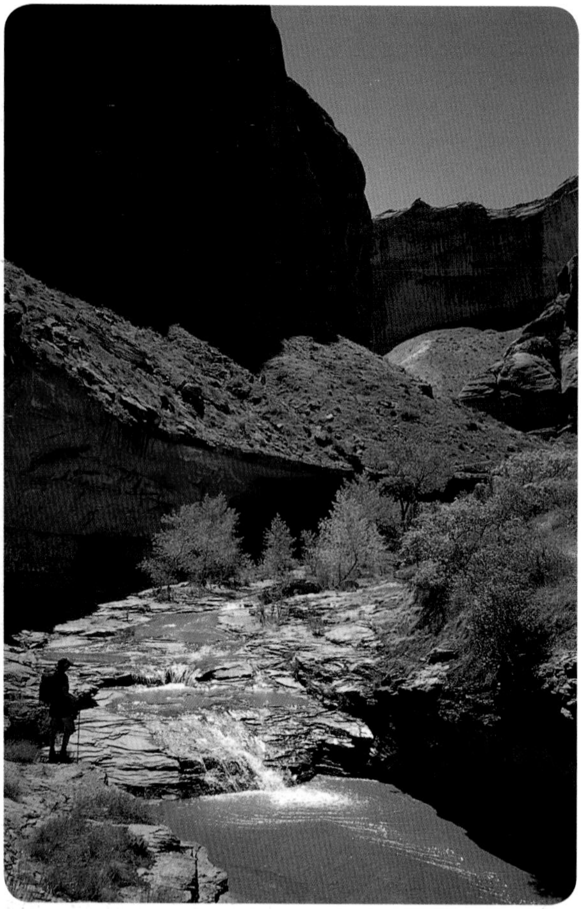

Lower Coyote Gulch

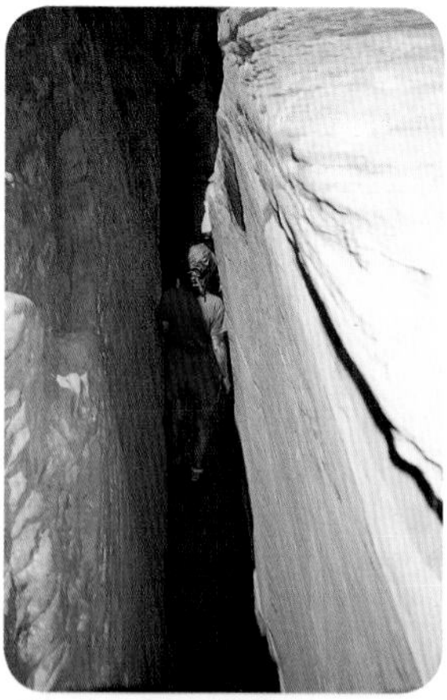

Crack in the Wall

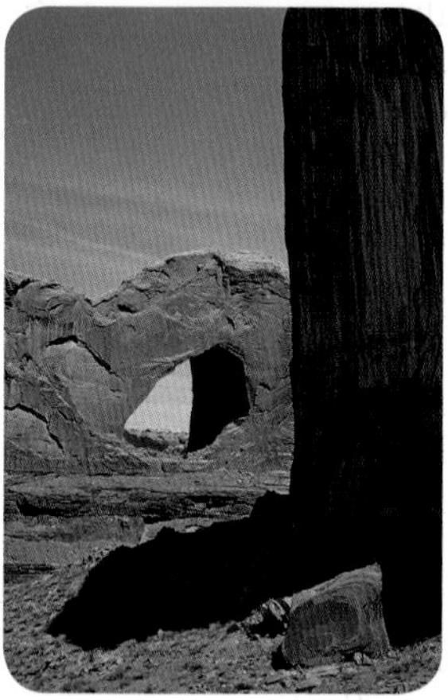

Stevens Arch

From the southeast edge of Escalante, near the high school, drive Hwy 12 generally southeast. At 4.5 mi (7.3 km) turn right (south) onto the signed, unpaved Hole-in-the-Rock Road.

From either approach, depart Hwy 12, reset your trip odometer to 0, and follow the Hole-in-the-Rock Road southeast. At 36 mi (58 km) turn left onto Fortymile Ridge Road, reset your trip odometer to 0, and follow it northeast.

Bear right at 4.2 mi (6.8 km) where a left spur ascends to a knoll-top parking area near water tanks. At 5 mi (8.1 km) proceed through deep sand that requires you to maintain momentum. Skilled drivers manage this final stretch in low-clearance 2WD cars, but high-clearance 4WD is preferable. Beware of the protruding cattleguard at 5.3 mi (8.6 km). Reach the trailhead parking area at 6.8 mi (10.9 km), 4640 ft (1415 m).

Shortly after leaving the trailhead to drive back to the Hole-in-the-Rock Road, stay alert when approaching the cattle guard. In the past, the sand at its base has been deeply eroded, leaving the metal bars high above ground: a serious obstacle for low-clearance vehicles. If the gate to the left is open, drive through it and bypass the cattleguard.

ON FOOT

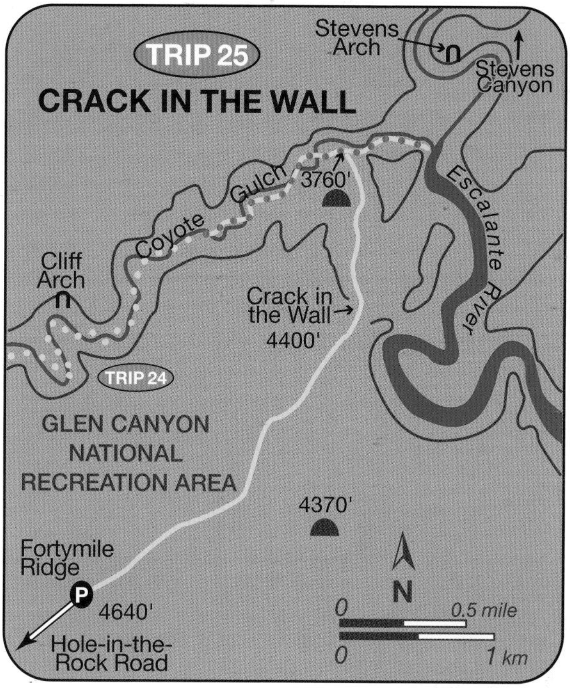

Your general direction of travel will be northeast all the way to the rim of Escalante River Canyon. En route, a sweeping expanse of Navajo sandstone is visible from left (north) to right (southeast).

From the trail register, descend the wide sandy path to a shrubby flat amid slickrock slopes. The path soon narrows. Follow cairns over a patch of slickrock, then resume on sand. Within 30 minutes, keep following cairns across **slickrock**.

Reach the **rim of Escalante River Canyon** at 1.8 mi (2.9 km), 4400 ft (1341 m), about 50 minutes from the trailhead. The meandering river is visible below. Stevens Arch is north-northeast, high above a broken wall. North, at the foot of the rim, is a trail descending a sand dune, which you'll eventually follow to the mouth of Coyote Gulch. The Straight Cliffs are west, rising 3000 ft (915 m) to the Kaiparowits Plateau. A two-minute detour east will reveal another perspective of the river below (southeast).

To reach the sand dune below, proceed over the rim, turn left, and descend through the **Crack in the Wall**—a very slim, 150-ft (46-m) long passage between the cliff and a series of three, vertical, sandstone slabs.

The initial drop is easy, with comfortable footholds. The third section of the crack is the narrowest. Before slithering through, you'll probably have to take off your pack and use a rope to lower it down outside the crack.

About 20 minutes after entering the crack, reach the base of the cliff and the **top of the sand dun**e at 4040 ft (1232 m). Then follow the trail generally north down the dune. About 20 minutes farther, or about 1½ hours from the trailhead, intersect the **Coyote Gulch** trail at 2.6 mi (4.2 km), 3760 ft (1146 m).

Right (east) leads to the river. Stay on the lower and safer of several paths descending the steep, ledgy slope. After the final drop—made possible by a tree trunk placed vertically against an overhang—follow the stream to its confluence with the **Escalante River** at 3 mi (4.8 km), 3700 ft (1128 m).

Turn left (west) at the 2.6-mi (4.2-km) junction to hike up-canyon into Coyote Gulch. Follow the path of least resistance, wading and crossing the stream as necessary. Bypass four waterfalls en route. Reach **Coyote Natural Bridge** at 6.6 mi (10.6 km), 3900 ft (1189 m).

TRIP 26

WILLOW & FORTYMILE GULCHES

LOCATION	Hole-in-the-Rock Road Glen Canyon National Recreation Area
LOOP	7.7 mi (12.4 km)
ELEVATION CHANGE	430-ft (131-m) loss and gain
KEY ELEVATIONS	trailhead 4190 ft (1277 m) Broken Bow Arch 3820 ft (1165 m) confluence of Willow and Fortymile 3760 ft (1146 m)
HIKING TIME	4½ to 6 hours
DIFFICULTY	easy hiking, entry-level routefinding
MAPS	Trails Illustrated *Canyons of the Escalante* USGS *Sooner Bench, Davis Gulch*

OPINION

The connection was terminated due to lack of activity.

That's why most of humankind has so little understanding of and appreciation for nature. We have no relationship with it, because we've ignored it. Turned our attention elsewhere: toward the shallow and fleeting, away from the deep, the enduring, the earthly.

Hiking, particularly when routefinding rather than heedlessly following a trail, reboots our connection with nature. It requires us to engage it directly. And canyon country is the ideal place to venture into trail-less terrain, because the canyons themselves tend to prevent you from straying far off course.

The loop linking Willow and Fortymile gulches involves only a little routefinding—not so much that intermediate hikers will be overwhelmed, but enough to keep anyone's connection with terra firma from terminating.

Both gulches are impressive, beautiful, and narrow. Neither is choked with a riparian jungle. Willow harbors Broken Bow Arch, which, if it were less remote, might garner as much applause as Rainbow Bridge (Trip 15) or at least Corona Arch (Trip 50). But Fortymile is the more constricted of the two passages. Negotiating its slot-like narrows is the journey's climax.

At the confluence of Willow and Fortymile you have the option of detouring downstream toward the Escalante River arm of Lake Powell. The canyon quickly widens and becomes less scenic, but we enjoyed splashing along the wash bottom, which resembles a tidal flat.

Once you drop into Willow, it'll be at least three hours before you emerge from Fortymile. Identifying Fortymile Gulch, so you'll know where to exit Willow, is not difficult. The confluence is obvious. Even the short cross-country route, from upper Fortymile back to the Willow trailhead, should be straightforward.

Bring a compass, of course. And if you have the USGS 1:24 000 topo maps in hand, navigation should be extremely easy. Of the two, *Sooner Bench* is the most useful because it shows the bulk of the route, including the overland finale.

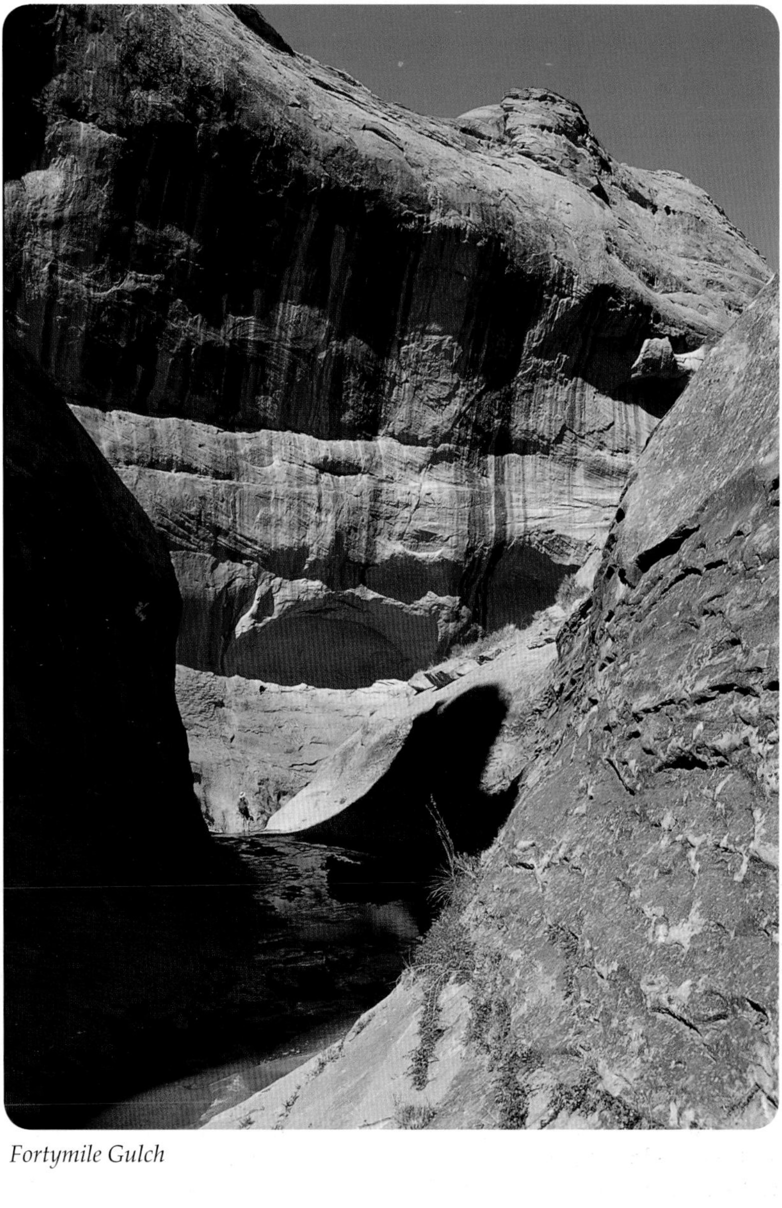

Fortymile Gulch

You'll almost certainly encounter water in the lower reaches of both Willow and Fortymile. It will likely be shallow, perhaps ankle deep, most of the way. But be prepared to wade or even swim through a couple deep holes. At one point in Fortymile, we held our packs overhead while the clear water rose nearly to our armpits. It was fun and refreshing.

You can always turn back if what you see unnerves you. The loop's relatively short length should allow time to retrace your steps to the trailhead. That's another reason why this trip is a good choice for hikers who want to begin developing navigation skills.

FACT

BEFORE YOUR TRIP

Stop at the Escalante Interagency Visitor Center before driving the Hole-in-the-Rock Road. Get a current weather report, ask about the condition of the road, and find out how high Lake Powell might extend up the Escalante River into Willow Gulch.

Most of the hike is on dry terrain, so wear sturdy, supportive hiking boots. But you might be wading, possibly swimming. So wear fabric boots you don't mind dunking, or pack a pair of amphibious sandals you can change into.

BY VEHICLE

From Boulder, at the junction of Hwy 12 and Burr Trail Road, drive Hwy 12 west, then generally south. At 12.7 mi (20.4 km), just past Calf Creek Rec Area, reset your trip odometer to 0 on the Escalante River bridge. Proceed south. At 4.5 mi (7.2 km) stop at the scenic overlook, then proceed west. At 9.5 mi (15.3 km) turn left (south) onto the signed, unpaved Hole-in-the-Rock Road.

From the southeast edge of Escalante, near the high school, drive Hwy 12 generally southeast. At 4.5 mi (7.3 km) turn right (south) onto the signed, unpaved Hole-in-the-Rock Road.

From either approach, depart Hwy 12, reset your trip odometer to 0, and follow the Hole-in-the-Rock Road southeast.

At 40.5 mi (65.2 km), about 1½ hours from Hwy 12, descend into deep Sooner Wash. The Entrada sandstone domes here invite freelance slickwalking. Just beyond the wash, spurs lead to inviting campsites.

At 41.5 mi (66.8 km), atop Sooner Bench, turn left (east) onto a spur and proceed 1.4 mi (2.3 km) to Willow Gulch trailhead parking area at 4190 ft (1277 m).

ON FOOT

From the trail register, follow the faint path northeast down a sand slide and over a brushy sand dune.

Pass a hoodoo shaped like a graduation cap. Go right (east) to descend slickrock. In five minutes, reach a **wash bottom** at 0.2 mi (0.3 km), 4020 ft (1226 m). Bear right and follow this tributary drainage southeast.

Within 15 minutes, at 0.6 mi (1 km), ignore the minor tributary drainage (right / south) and the small draw (left /northeast). Proceed straight (east-southeast) in the main wash.

About 25 minutes along, at 1 mi (1.6 km), 3960 ft (1207 m), intersect **Willow Gulch** beneath its 200-ft (61-m) west-facing wall. Expect to find water trickling down-canyon. Cottonwoods and the namesake willows thrive here. Right (south) is the tail of the gulch. Go left (northeast) and hike downstream.

Brushy benches line the wash. As the gulch broadens, the right (southeast) walls remain sheer, while the left (northwest) side is open and broken. Hike in the streambed or on segments of bootbeaten path.

Watch the left (north) wall for **Broken Bow Arch** at 2 mi (3.2 km), 3820 ft (1165 m). A path leads beneath it. It was named in 1930 by Escalante teacher Edison Alvey, who found a broken Native bow nearby.

Continuing down-canyon, within ten minutes encounter a knee- to hip-deep pool. Either wade in or skirt it by bashing through willows. The canyon narrows beyond, but you can probably hike beside the stream or hop across it.

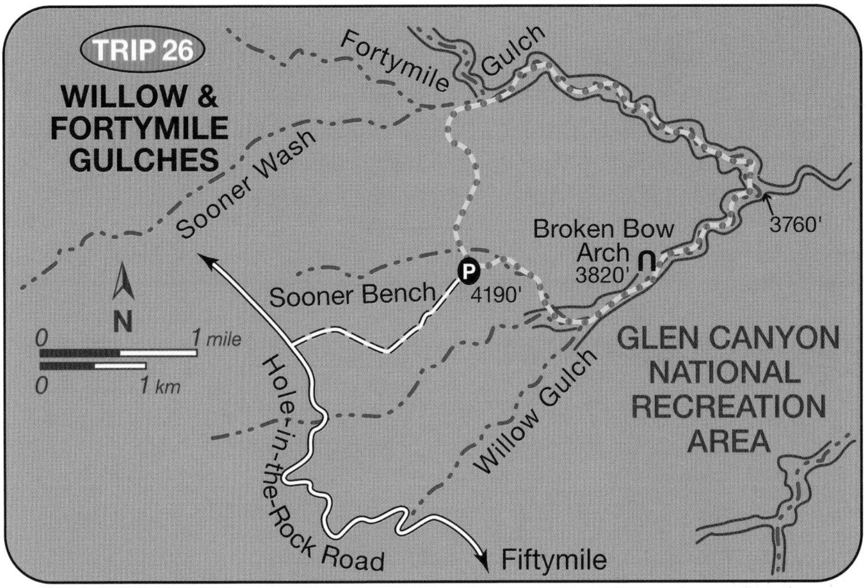

Reach the **Fortymile Gulch confluence** at 3 mi (4.8 km), 3760 ft (1146 m), about 1¼ hours from the trailhead. Downstream (right / initially north) continues through lower Willow Gulch generally east-northeast to the Escalante River. Go left (northwest) to loop back to the trailhead via Fortymile Gulch.

It's about 5 mi (8 km) to the **Escalante River**, though the actual distance varies depending on the level of Lake Powell. Just five minutes in that direction is a campsite, among cottonwoods and juniper, on a bench. Five minutes farther, the sandy wash bottom is smooth. The canyon widens beyond.

Heading generally northwest up-canyon through **Fortymile Gulch**, about 50 minutes from the confluence reach the first obstacle: a 3.5- to 5-ft (1- to 1.5-m) **pool**. It could be dry, but expect to wade or perhaps swim. Fifteen minutes farther, pass a slender **cascade** flowing over convoluted slickrock. Soon after, at 5.4 mi (8.7 km), 3960 ft (1207 m), bear left (southwest) past a **major tributary drainage** (right / northwest).

Once you've hiked about 1¼ hours from the confluence, the rest of Fortymile Gulch will likely be dry. Go left (south) onto a bushy slope. Pass an attractive campsite among cottonwoods on a bench, then another on a higher, grassy bench about eight minutes farther.

In another ten minutes, near 6.2 mi (10 km), 3970 ft (1210 m), pass the mouth of a **tributary drainage** (right / northwest) and a **park-like expanse of grass** beneath cottonwoods on a bench. The trailhead is still an hour distant. Continue hiking in the wash.

The walls of Fortymile Gulch subside near 6.5 mi (10.5 km). Proceed from sand onto slickrock. Watch for a cairn guiding you up and out. Look for more cairns above. Curve left (south) where the terrain allows. Aim for where the drainage pinches out into a U-shape. Then angle left up a slickrock ramp. You've now hiked about 1¾ hours from the confluence, or 30 minutes beyond the grassy park.

Heading cross-country, generally south-southeast, watch for your vehicle at the trailhead. Set a course directly toward it. Cross the shallow tail of an arroyo and rise onto a plateau. Proceed southeast. Beyond two more shallow dips, reach the **trailhead** at 7.7 mi (12.4 km).

TRIP 27

DAVIS GULCH

LOCATION	Hole-in-the-Rock Road Glen Canyon National Recreation Area
ROUND TRIP	4.6 mi (7.4 km) to Bement Arch view 8 mi (12.9 km) to Davis Gulch below stock trail
ELEVATION CHANGE	755-ft (230-m) loss and gain to Davis Gulch below stock trail
KEY ELEVATIONS	trailhead 4315 ft (1316 m), Bement Arch view 4100 ft (1250 m), Davis Gulch below stock trail 3760 ft (1146 m)
HIKING TIME	4 hours for Bement Arch view 7 to 8 hours for Davis Gulch below stock trail
DIFFICULTY	easy hiking, moderate routefinding
MAPS	Trails Illustrated *Canyons of the Escalante* USGS *Davis Gulch*

OPINION

In a sandstone wall near Bement Arch in Davis Gulch is a mysterious inscription: *NEMO 1934*

The author was Everett Ruess, a 20-year-old artist, writer and wanderer devoted to beauty, silence, isolation, and wilderness. He roamed the high desert for months at a time, with two burros his only companions. He explored much of northern Arizona and southern Utah. Where Natives and old-timers said he shouldn't go, he went anyway. In 1934 he departed Escalante on yet another couple-month sojourn. He vanished without a trace.

His last known campsite was in Davis Gulch. The inscription he left behind might be the Greek word for "no one." It might refer to Captain Nemo, who shunned mankind by disappearing under the sea in Jules Verne's *Twenty Thousand Leagues Under the Sea*. It might be a terse statement of desire to become one with the austere beauty of canyon country and hence no one.

Ruess had previously written this seemingly prophetic statement in a letter to a friend: *When I go I leave no trace.*

And in one of his journals he'd written: *I have been thinking more and more that I shall always be a lone wanderer in the wilderness.*

Perhaps he achieved that goal. Some believe he was murdered. Others think he got lost or fatally injured himself. But his remains have never turned up. Ranchers, miners, even a Navajo tracker searched for Ruess over several months. They found his starving burros but no clue suggesting what happened to the young, high-desert drifter.

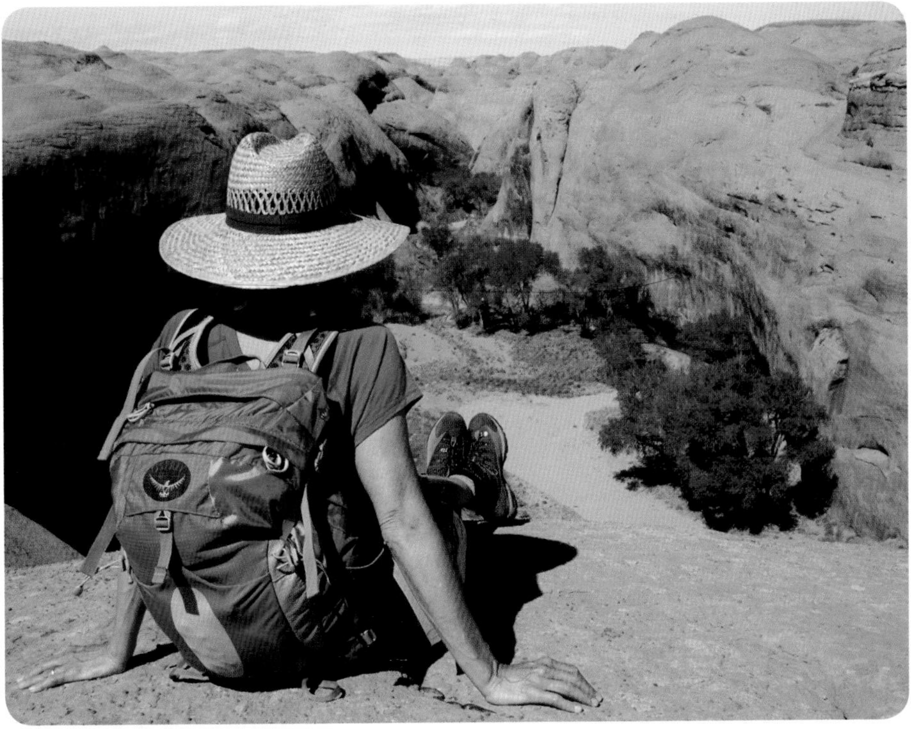

Overlooking Davis Gulch

Now, with the story of Everett Ruess fresh in mind, you can imagine the Davis Gulch environs. Had he known his end was near, this is precisely the kind of place he would have chosen for his pilgrimage into the unknown. It's vast, lonely, mysterious, spectacular, tranquil. He was a contemplative soul, and this is an ideal place for soulful contemplation of canyon-country wilderness.

We don't, however, recommend dropping directly into Davis Gulch. The upper reaches pose a severe canyoneering challenge. Attempt it only if you have climbing skills and equipment, and confidence born of substantial slot-canyon experience.

Instead, hike along the rim of Davis Gulch. It's one of the great slickwalks in this book. The scenery is panoramic. You can also frequently gaze *into* the gulch, admire the austere beauty of its secret recesses, and wonder… just what the heck *did* happen to Everett Ruess?

You'll be freelancing—devising your own route, meandering across rolling, trail-less terrain, probably covering no more than about one linear mile (1.6 linear kilometers) per hour. There's enough relief to the topography that someone in your group should carry a compass and be a competent cross-country navigator. But simply keeping the gulch in view should prevent you from getting lost.

About two-thirds of the way along, an old stock trail offers a reasonable descent route to the floor of Davis Gulch. If you have time and energy, accept the invitation, then hike back up the gulch, perhaps to the base of Bement Arch where you can commune with the beatific ghost of Everett Ruess.

FACT

BEFORE YOUR TRIP

Stop at the Escalante Interagency Visitor Center before driving the Hole-in-the-Rock Road. Check the current weather report, and ask about the condition of the road.

BY VEHICLE

From Boulder, at the junction of Hwy 12 and Burr Trail Road, drive Hwy 12 west, then generally south. At 12.7 mi (20.4 km), just past Calf Creek Rec Area, reset your trip odometer to 0 on the Escalante River bridge. Proceed south. At 4.5 mi (7.2 km) stop at the scenic overlook, then proceed west. At 9.5 mi (15.3 km) turn left (south) onto the signed, unpaved Hole-in-the-Rock Road.

From the southeast edge of Escalante, near the high school, drive Hwy 12 generally southeast. At 4.5 mi (7.3 km) turn right (south) onto the signed, unpaved Hole-in-the-Rock Road.

From either approach, depart Hwy 12, reset your trip odometer to 0, and follow the Hole-in-the-Rock Road southeast. In about two hours, park near the shallow tail of Davis Gulch (a minor slickrock draw bisecting the road) at 50.5 mi (81.3 km), 4315 ft (1316 m). The steep escarpment right (southwest) is Fiftymile Point.

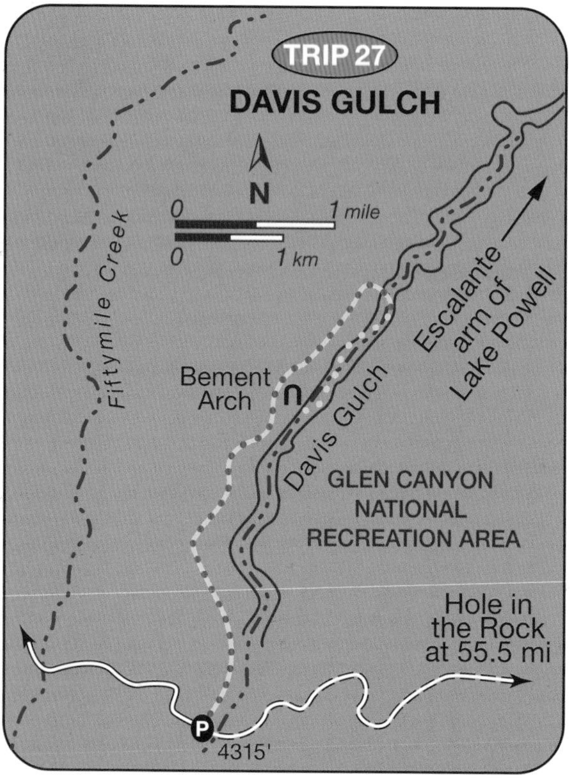

The Hole-in-the-Rock Road continues generally east. It soon deteriorates, requiring high-clearance 4WD. It ends at 55.5 mi (89.4 km), on the rim of Glen Canyon, above a short, steep arm of Lake Powell.

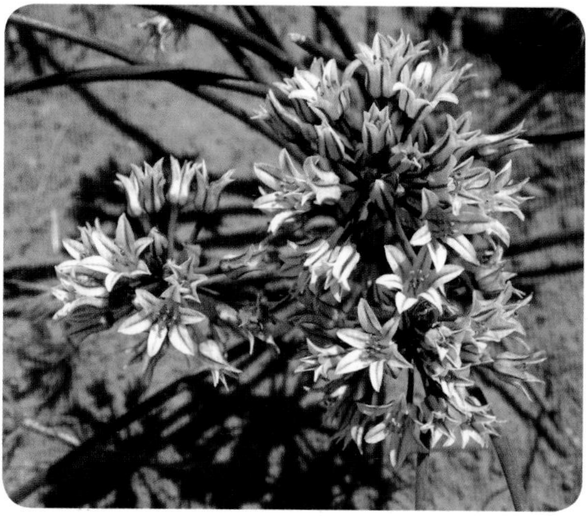

Wild onion, April

ON FOOT

The tail of Davis Gulch is a 4-ft (1.2-m) deep slickrock draw where the road crosses it. Depart the road on the northwest side off the gulch, which soon constricts into a slot. Hike north-northeast above its left (west) rim.

Paralleling the gulch, proceed across the vast, **undulating slickrock**. Gradually angle north. Traverse sandy pockets dotted with scrubby vegetation (blackbrush, sagebrush, mormon tea, yucca). Boulder Mtn is visible north. The Escalante River basin is north to northeast. The Henry Mtns are northeast. Navajo Mtn is southeast. Behind you is Fiftymile Point—the steep escarpment just beyond the road. It will serve as a landmark when returning to the trailhead.

Despite ups and downs, you'll generally maintain an elevation of about 4100 ft (1250 m). Near 1 mi (1.6 km) reach a **tributary drainage** extending west-southwest. Detour about 0.25 mi (0.4 km) left to contour around its tail.

Resuming north, a **broad tributary drainage** at 1.5 mi (2.4 km) requires another brief detour. Descend left (northwest) into its upper end. Beyond, continue generally north-northeast on gentle slickrock ridges, closely paralleling Davis Gulch. It's about 150 to 200 ft (45.7 to 61 m) deep here. Cottonwoods and alcoves are visible below.

About two hours along, at 2.3 mi (3.7 km), 4100 ft (1250 m), **Bement Arch** is visible beneath the northwest wall of the gulch. It's evident from here that the floor of the gulch is rough hiking terrain: benches to work around or over, thick vegetation to bash through, beaver dams to mince across.

About two hours along, at 3.7 mi (6 km), glance ahead (north-northeast) for an old **stock trail** accessing the floor of the gulch. It descends through the first significant break in the northwest wall, past two black stones standing on end. A butte, visible east across the gulch, is a helpful landmark. Beneath that butte, a Navajo sandstone chute drops to a thick grove of gambel oak and cottonwoods in a draw.

Cairns offer guidance along the stock trail. Gouged steps provide assistance on the final descent. Intersect a bootbeaten path on the **floor of Davis Gulch** at 4 mi (6.4 km), 3760 ft (1146 m). Left leads down-canyon, generally northeast, to Lake Powell. The distance depends on the ever-changing lake level. Right leads up-canyon, generally southwest. Bement Arch is 1.8 mi (2.9 km) in that direction.

TRIP 28

ESCALANTE RIVER

LOCATION	Grand Staircase-Escalante National Monument between Calf Creek and Escalante
DISTANCE	15.5 mi (25 km)
ELEVATION GAIN	760 ft (232 m)
KEY ELEVATIONS	Calf Creek trailhead 5200 ft (1585 m) Death Hollow confluence 5380 ft (1640 m) Escalante trailhead 5960 ft (1817m)
HIKING TIME	6 to 9 hours
DIFFICULTY	moderate
MAPS	Trails Illustrated *Canyons of the Escalante* USGS *Calf Creek, Escalante*

OPINION

"Where you from?" he asked.

"Near Banff National Park," we said.

He screwed up his face, shook head. "Never heard of it."

"In the Canadian Rockies," we explained, "a few hours north of US Glacier Park."

"I don't know where that is. How's the fishing?"

"We don't fish."

"Do you hunt?" he asked enthusiastically.

"No. We hike."

"No horses?" he asked in dismay.

"Nope."

After eyeing us with curiosity, he finally said, "My grandaddy told me never go anywhere without a purpose."

"Well," we said, "we like to explore new areas."

He nodded thoughtfully, smiled, and turned away. He was a native of Escalante. And his attitude toward the surrounding land, we gradually learned, was common among locals. They agree it's beautiful, but they prize how useful it is. We, on the other hand, like most hikers, appreciate canyon country solely for its beauty.

That's why you'll rarely meet a longtime local hiking in Grand Staircase-Escalante National Monument. They see no purpose in it. But if you're here strictly in search of beauty, hiking the Escalante River Canyon—from the Calf Creek confluence to the town of Escalante—affords as beautiful an experience as it's possible to have, not just in canyon country but anywhere on Earth.

Though the canyon is deeper downstream (paralleling the Hole-in-the-Rock Road), this section is comparably impressive. It's also much to easier to hike, because the river is shallower and the banks are less choked with riparian vegetation (willow, tamarisk, thorny Russian olive).

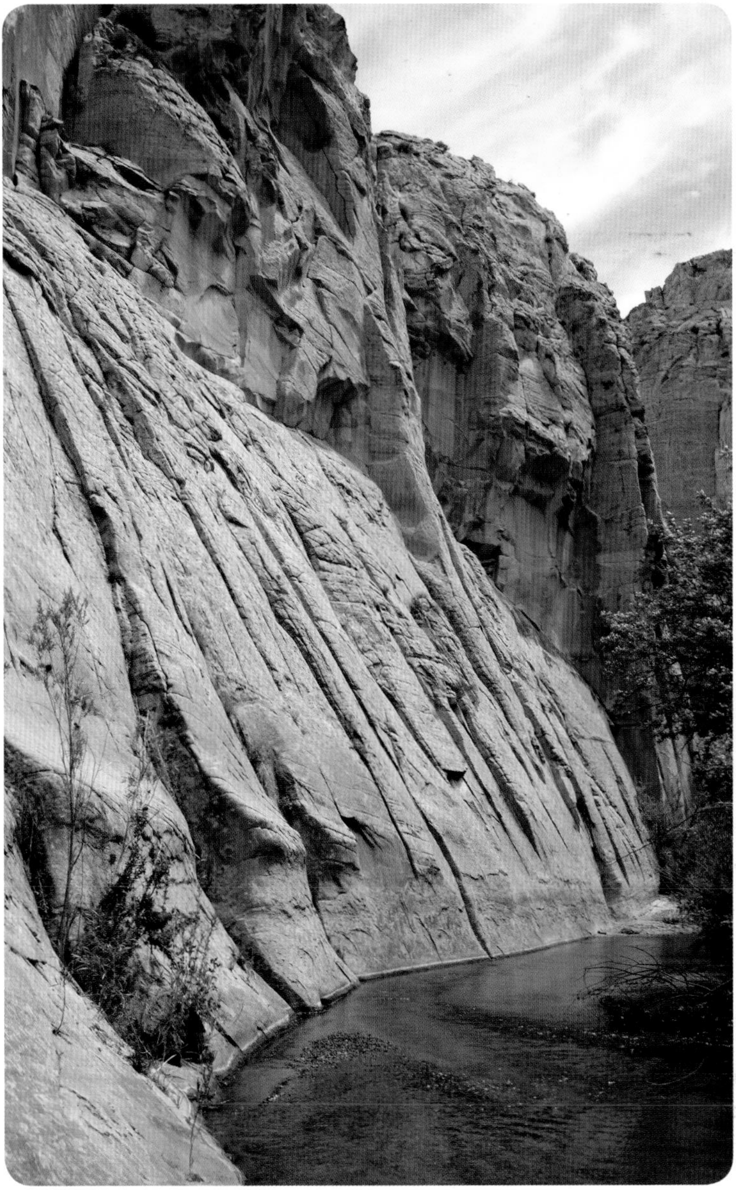

Escalante River Canyon

Much of the way, your path will be the river itself. On a warm, sunny day in spring or fall, splashing along in the ankle- to knee-deep water while gazing up at the sculpted, Navajo sandstone walls is a joy. And traveling end to end—constantly witnessing new scenery—heightens the sense of exploration.

We recommend hiking east to west. That's upstream and uphill. But at normal flow, the current is negligible. And the elevation gain is imperceptibly gradual. The advantages are that the canyon builds to a climax in this direction and, if you're unable to arrange a two-car shuttle and must therefore hitchhike, you'll end up at the edge of town.

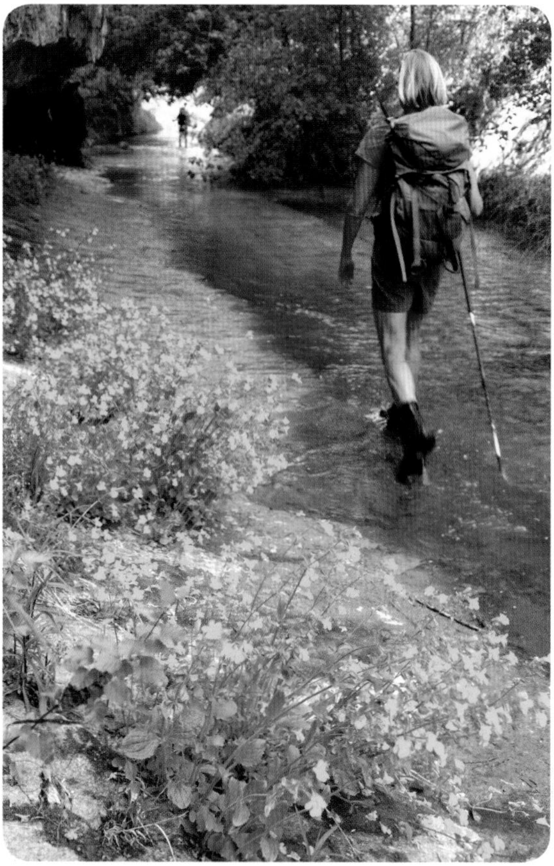

Probing Death Hollow, a tributary of the Escalante River

FACT

BEFORE YOUR TRIP

Stop at the Escalante Interagency Visitor Center. Check the current weather report and find out how deep the Escalante River is likely to be.

You'll be in the river frequently, so wear amphibious boots. Those designed specifically for hiking in water are ideal, but a sturdy pair of fabric hiking boots you don't mind dunking are fine too. Wear insulating neoprene socks to keep your feet warm. Leave your sandals behind; they lack sufficient ankle support and allow pebbles to lodge beneath your feet.

The Escalante River is silty and contaminated. Drink it only as a last resort, and then only after you've filtered or purified it. Ideally, carry all the drinking water you'll need for the entire trip: at least three quarts (liters) per person. If it appears you'll need more, fill up about midway, from the creek flowing out of Death Hollow, although it too must be filtered or purified.

BY VEHICLE

Escalante trailhead

From Hwy 12, on the east edge of Escalante, turn north onto the cemetery road. It's 0.25 mi (0.4 km) southeast of the high school, and 3.8 mi (6.1 km) northwest of the Hole-in-the-Rock Road. Pass the cemetery and bear right (east). Curve left (north) at 0.4 mi (0.6 km). Reach the trailhead parking area at 0.6 mi (1 km), 5960 ft (1817 m). Leave your shuttle vehicle here, where the one-way hike ends.

Calf Creek trailhead

From the southeast edge of Escalante, near the high school, drive Hwy 12 generally east then north. At 14.1 mi (22.7 km) cross the Escalante River bridge. Immediately after, turn left (south) into the trailhead parking area at 5200 ft (1585 m). Begin hiking here.

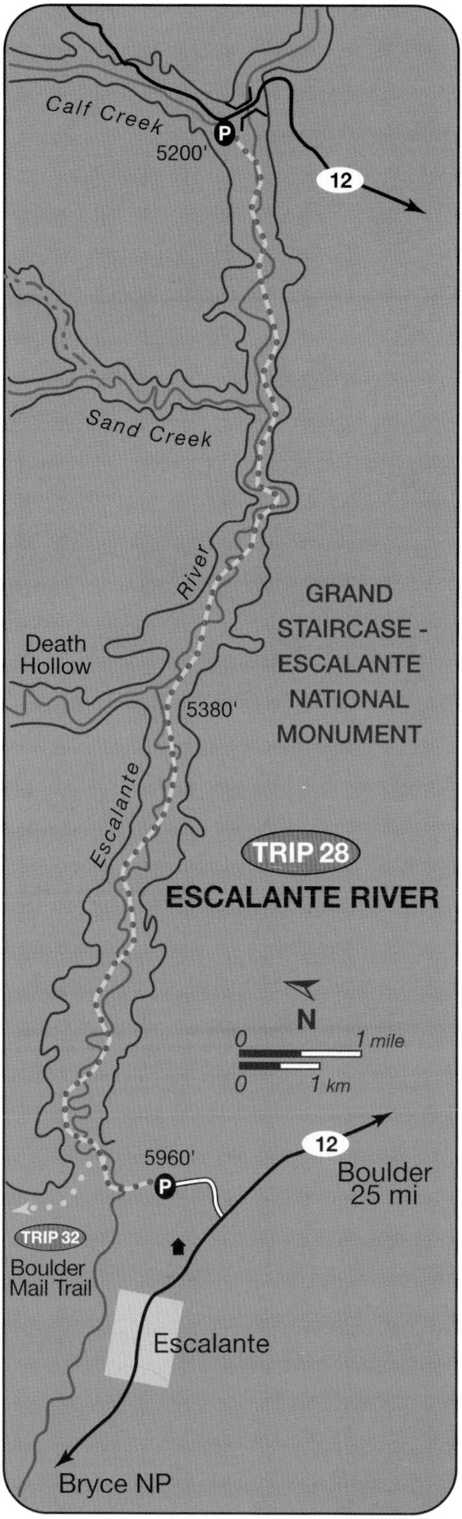

ON FOOT

Ford the river to the south bank, turn right (east), and follow the path upstream among sagebrush and cottonwoods through the broad canyon. Your general direction of travel will be west until you exit the canyon near Escalante.

About 20 minutes along, it's necessary to ford the river three times in quick succession. Upstream—several bends ahead (west)—an arch is visible on the skyline. Before passing beneath it, however, look left (southwest) for **Escalante Natural Bridge**. It's on the canyon's left (south) wall at 1.8 mi (2.9 km), about 35 minutes from the trailhead, just past a tributary drainage (right / north). It's 130 ft (40 m) high and spans 100 ft (30.5 m).

Ford the river again about four minutes farther, then look left (southwest) for a ruin in a small, rough alcove about a third of the way up the canyon wall. Ford the river again and attain a better view.

At 2.2 mi (3.5 km), about 50 minutes along, pass beneath the **skyline arch** (left / south) you saw earlier. After fording the river for perhaps the seventh time, follow a path across a sandy bench among sagebrush and thorny Russian olive trees. After fording the river for perhaps the tenth time, about 1¼ hours along, reach a grassy flat opposite a cottonwood grove.

Pass the **Sand Creek** confluence (right / north) at 2.7 mi (4.3 km). About two hours along, at 4.5 mi (7.2 km), the canyon constricts, and the Navajo sandstone walls are 400 ft (1220 m) high. About three hours along, riparian vegetation—including Russian olive—is more profuse. You'll probably find it easier to hike in the river.

Reach the **Death Hollow** confluence (right / north-northwest) at 7.5 mi (12.1 km), 5380 ft (1640 m).

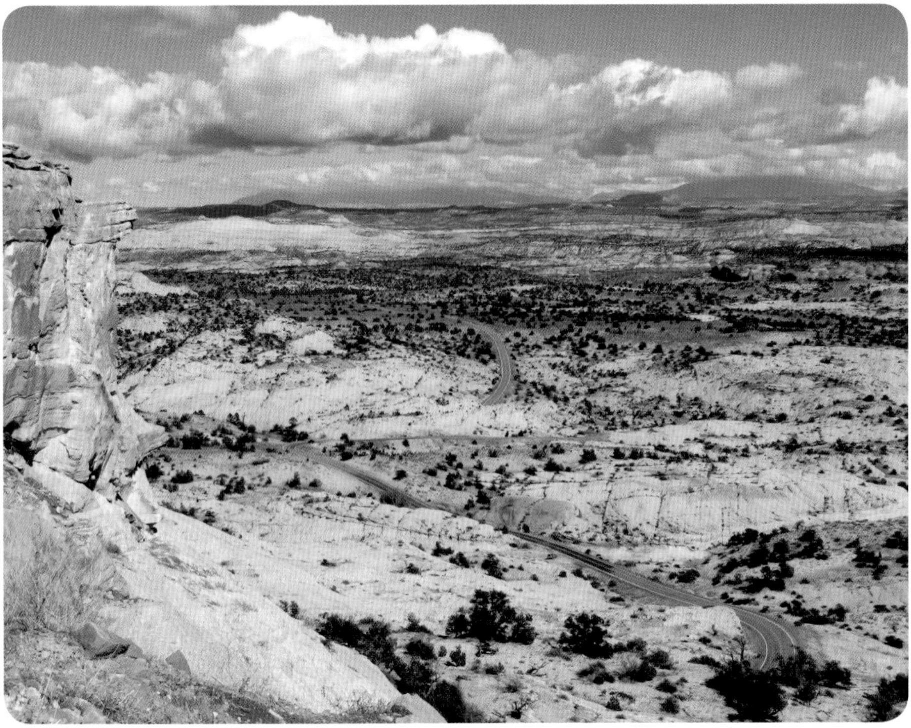

Grand Staircase – Escalante National Monument, between Escalante and Boulder

The mouth is choked with willow and Russian olive. Bear left (south-southwest) to continue upstream along the Escalante River. Ahead, the canyon is more sinuous, and the walls are 700 ft (213 m) high.

Look for a **snake pictograph panel** on the right (north) wall at 8.8 mi (14.2 km). About four hours along, the canyon is particularly scenic, with smooth, sheer, pink, cream and mauve walls. Ponderosa pines are now present. Near 12 mi (19.3 km), at the apex of a north-trending bend, look for more pictographs in an alcove.

At 13 mi (21 km), 5640 ft (1720 m), about 5½ hours along, the canyon walls diminish from cliffs to broken ledges. Pass the **Pine Creek** confluence (right / northwest) and a water gauge at 14.5 mi (23.3 km), 5680 ft (1732 m). Exiting the canyon, follow a trail southwest across an open bench.

Proceed through a **hiker's maze**, which allows people but not cows to pass through the fence. Ford the Escalante River for the last time. Bear left (south). Soon pass through the fence again. Attain a view of the town. Still heading south, ascend an old road. Aim for the knoll near the trailhead.

Reach the **Escalante trailhead** at 15.5 mi (25 km), 5960 ft (1817 m). Fast hikers will arrive about six hours after departing the Calf Creek trailhead. If you did not park here and intend to hitchhike back to your vehicle, continue walking the road south then west to **Hwy 12**, which is only 0.6 mi (1 km) away. Then go right (northwest) 0.25 mi (0.4 km) to the gas station.

TRIP 29

PHIPPS ARCH

LOCATION	Grand Staircase-Escalante National Monument between Hole-in-the-Rock Road and Escalante River southeast of Hwy 12
ROUND TRIP	8 mi (12.9 km)
ELEVATION CHANGE	840-ft (256-m) loss and gain
KEY ELEVATIONS	trailhead 5720 ft (1743 m), lowpoint in Phipps Wash 5220 ft (1591 m), Phipps Arch 5560 ft (1725 m)
HIKING TIME	4 to 5 hours
DIFFICULTY	easy
MAPS	Trails Illustrated *Canyons of the Escalante* USGS *Tenmile Flat, Calf Creek*

OPINION

Driving Highway 12 is torture. Between Escalante and Boulder, it swoops through the northern reaches of Grand Staircase-Escalante National Monument, affording constant views of a strikingly bizarre and beautiful land. Yet sheer cliffs, hairpin turns, blind corners and narrow passages demand drivers remain vigilantly attentive to the road while their passengers ooh and ahh in rapturous wonder.

So DO NOT DRIVE STRAIGHT THROUGH. Plan to stop. Not just at the scenic overlooks for a brief gander, but long enough to stride well off the highway and appreciate this unique wilderness with your sinew as well as your eyes. An exciting place to do it is Phipps Wash.

A gentle but impressive tributary of the Escalante River, Phipps Wash has two enticing features. The first is a long, trail-less approach mostly on slickrock. The second is Phipps Arch—a secretive stunner that keeps hikers eagerly searching for it until they almost bump into it. En route, the wash constricts beneath soaring walls and is itself well worth the walk.

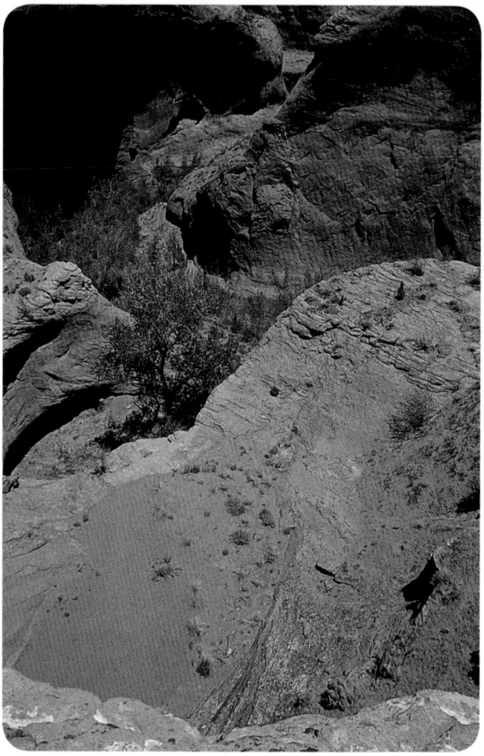

Descending into Phipps Wash

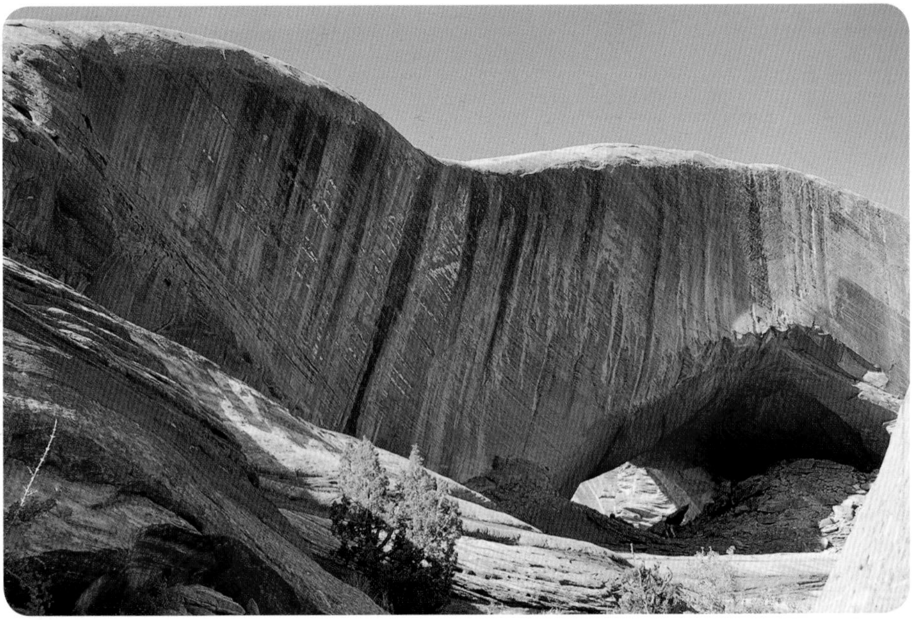

Phipps Arch

The trail-less approach also means Phipps isn't so popular as other hiking destinations off Hwy 12 and will likely grant you more solitude. Even the Hole-in-the-Rock hikes (Trips 21 through 27), though less convenient, are much better known. The trail-less approach to Phipps, however, does require you to be confident in your ability to routefind. Lacking experience in cross-country navigation, you should instead hike the nearby trail to Lower Calf Creek Falls (Trip 30).

There are actually two ways to reach Phipps Arch. The other begins at the confluence of Calf Creek and the Escalante River. It's shorter than our recommended route but far less enjoyable. It requires you to ford the river and thrash through riparian vegetation. It denies you the joy of slickwalking, the intrigue of finding your way into the canyon, and the pleasure of seeing its narrower, upper reaches.

After paying homage to Phipps Arch, you have the option of also visiting Maverick Bridge. It will add only 1.6 mi (2.6 km) to your round-trip mileage, but won't significantly boost the day's wow factor. Maverick is a small, virtually subterranean natural bridge: a curiosity, not a marvel.

FACT

BY VEHICLE

From Boulder, at the junction of Hwy 12 and Burr Trail Road, drive Hwy 12 west, then generally south. Pass Calf Creek Rec Area, cross the Escalante River Bridge, and pass Boynton Overlook. Proceed southwest. Near 15.5 mi (25 km)—before ascending through a west-pointing hairpin turn—park on the left (south), in an unsigned, unpaved pullout, where slickrock extends above and below. This is immediately east of milepost 71. Elevation: 5720 ft (1743 m).

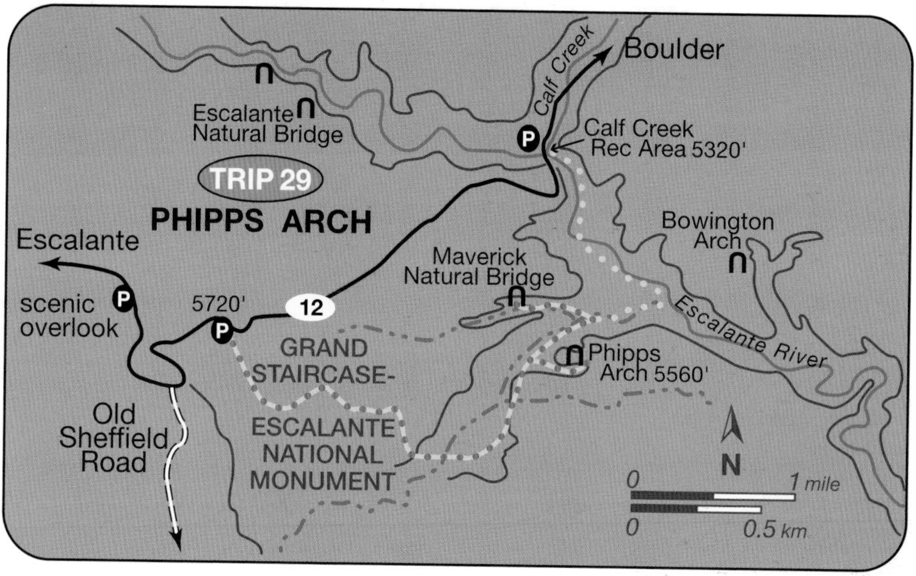

From the southeast edge of Escalante, near the high school, drive Hwy 12 southeast. Pass Hole-in-the-Rock Road, Head of Rocks Overlook, and Sheffield Road. Continue descending, curving left (north). Proceed through a left (west) pointing hairpin turn. The road then levels, heading northeast. Near 11.1 mi (17.9 km), park on the right (south), in an unsigned, unpaved pullout, where slickrock extends above and below. Elevation: 5720 ft (1743 m).

ON FOOT

Descend generally south. Hiking on slickrock or sand, avoiding cryptogamic soil, skirting pouroffs, and passing a series of tenajas (depressions sometimes holding water), gradually curve left (southeast) into a shallow, upper, **tributary drainage** of Phipps Wash.

Quickly reach a large, semicircular dryfall. Bypass it on the right. Resume in the wash, bearing right (south-southeast). About 30 minutes along, reach a second dryfall. Bypass it on the left, then descend slickrock back into the sandy wash among cottonwoods. Immediately after, descend left of a third dryfall. A couple minutes farther, the wash veers abruptly right (south-southwest) to a fourth dryfall, about 150-ft (46-m) high. Bypass it on the right (west) by ascending slickrock, continuing about 0.25 mi (0.4 km) along the rim, then descending a sandslide left (southeast) into **Phipps Wash**, about 1¼ hours from the highway.

Turn left (east) and follow broad, sandy, Phipps Wash down-canyon. About 1½ hours along, the canyon curves left (north) and begins constricting. Cottonwoods are more profuse. Negotiate brush, willows, and stagnant water. Watch for sections of bootbeaten path. Pass a broad, shallow, 300-ft (91-m) high **alcove** (right / east). It has just enough overhang to offer shelter from rain.

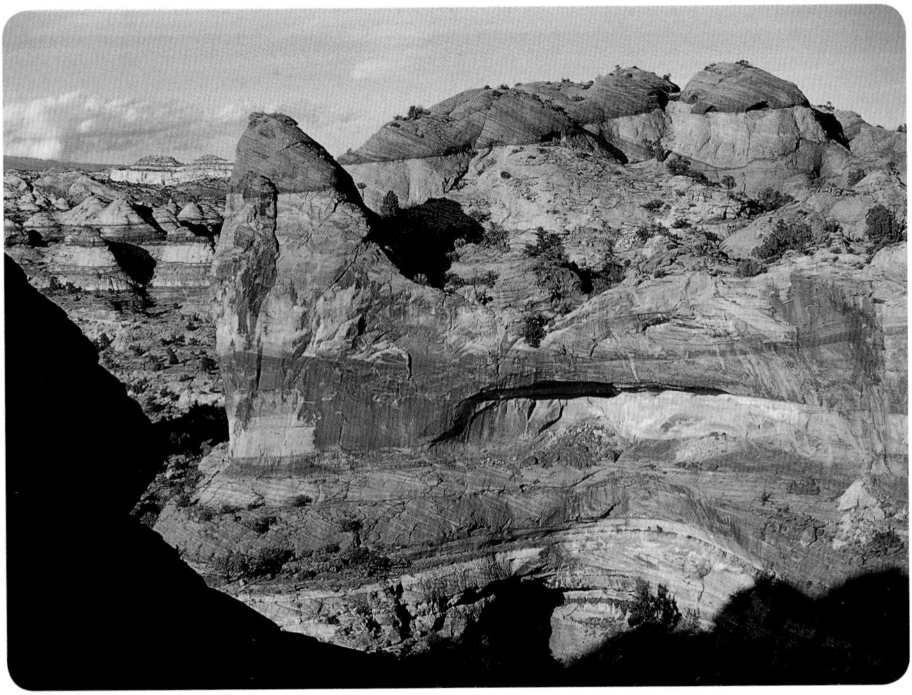

Phipps Wash

The canyon soon opens somewhat and a path allows easier, faster progress. After passing two bays (right / east), turn right (southeast) into the **first substantial draw**. Phipps Arch is just ahead, though it will remain hidden from view until you're upon it.

Watch for cairns on the left. Follow them, ascending northeast over slickrock ledges. Negotiate a steep, friction pitch. Above, follow a prominent ledge right for several yd/m. Then curve left into a shallow draw. It leads directly to **Phipps Arch**, at 4 mi (6.4 km), 5560 ft (1725 m).

The chunky arch is on the skyline, surrounded by Kayenta sandstone domes. It's 100 ft (30 m) long and 30 ft (9 m) high. Enjoy a cool refuge in the shade of its underbelly while you admire the view.

After returning to Phipps Wash, retrace your steps left (south) up-canyon to the highway. Or extend your hike by detouring right (north, gradually curving northeast) down-canyon.

Continuing down Phipps Wash, the first draw on the left (west), before the prominent tower, harbors **Maverick Bridge**. (The USGS topo erroneously indicates the bridge is in the second draw, which trends north.) The bridge is about 0.8 mi (1.3 km) from the mouth of Phipps Arch draw. Phipps Wash intersects the **Escalante River** about 1.2 mi (1.9 km) from the mouth of Phipps Arch draw.

TRIP 30

LOWER CALF CREEK FALLS

LOCATION	Grand Staircase-Escalante National Monument south of Boulder
ROUND TRIP	6 mi (9.7 km)
ELEVATION GAIN	260 ft (79 m)
KEY ELEVATIONS	trailhead 5320 ft (1622 m), base of falls 5500 ft (1677 m)
HIKING TIME	2 to 3 hours
DIFFICULTY	easy
MAP	Trails Illustrated *Canyons of the Escalante*

OPINION

On a 1-to-10 scale, the hike to Lower Calf Creek Falls earns widely varying scores depending on which aspect of it you're judging.

The 126-ft (38-m) waterfall is a unique spectacle and deserves a 10 for beauty. You want to go swimming in the desert? The plunge pool beneath the falls is irresistible on a hot day and also earns a 10. The canyon itself is relatively short yet quite impressive, so we'll give it a 6. The ancient ones built only two, small granaries here, but the one rock-art panel they created earns a 3 for archaeology. However, this is among the best-known, most popular hikes between Bryce and Capitol Reef national parks. Plus it begins at a campground and is initially within sight and sound of the nearby highway. So it scores a zero for wilderness atmosphere. Finally, there's a nominal but galling day-use fee for which we ding it a minus 2.

Conclusion? You should hike here. Seniors, fledgling striders, and parents with young hikers-in-training appreciate the convenient, paved trailhead, the easy-to-walk trail, and the security of knowing others are nearby. Experienced canyon-country hikers wince at all that yet are wowed by the refreshing oasis at trail's end. They also have time to visit Upper Calf Creek Falls the same day. (Read a comparison of these bookend trails in Trip 31.)

True high-desert aficionados think of Lower Calf Creek Falls as simply an obligatory sight, a stunning anomaly, a one-view wonder. Most would agree any of the nearby hikes—including the Escalante River (Trip 28), Phipps Arch (Trip 29), Pine Creek (Trip 20), the Boulder Mail Trail (Trip 32), Little Death Hollow (Trip 33), or Upper Muley Twist (Trip 35)—afford a richer overall experience.

All those options are *not* options, however, during rainy weather, when narrow canyons are vulnerable to flashfloods and unpaved access roads are impassable. If it's simply a drizzle, not a downpour, Lower Calf Creek is *the* place to hike, because the trailhead is paved, the canyon is broad, and the path to the falls remains a safe distance above the creek for most of its length.

So, how did the creek earn its name? Pioneer stockmen used this box canyon as a natural corral. Many a calf was weaned here.

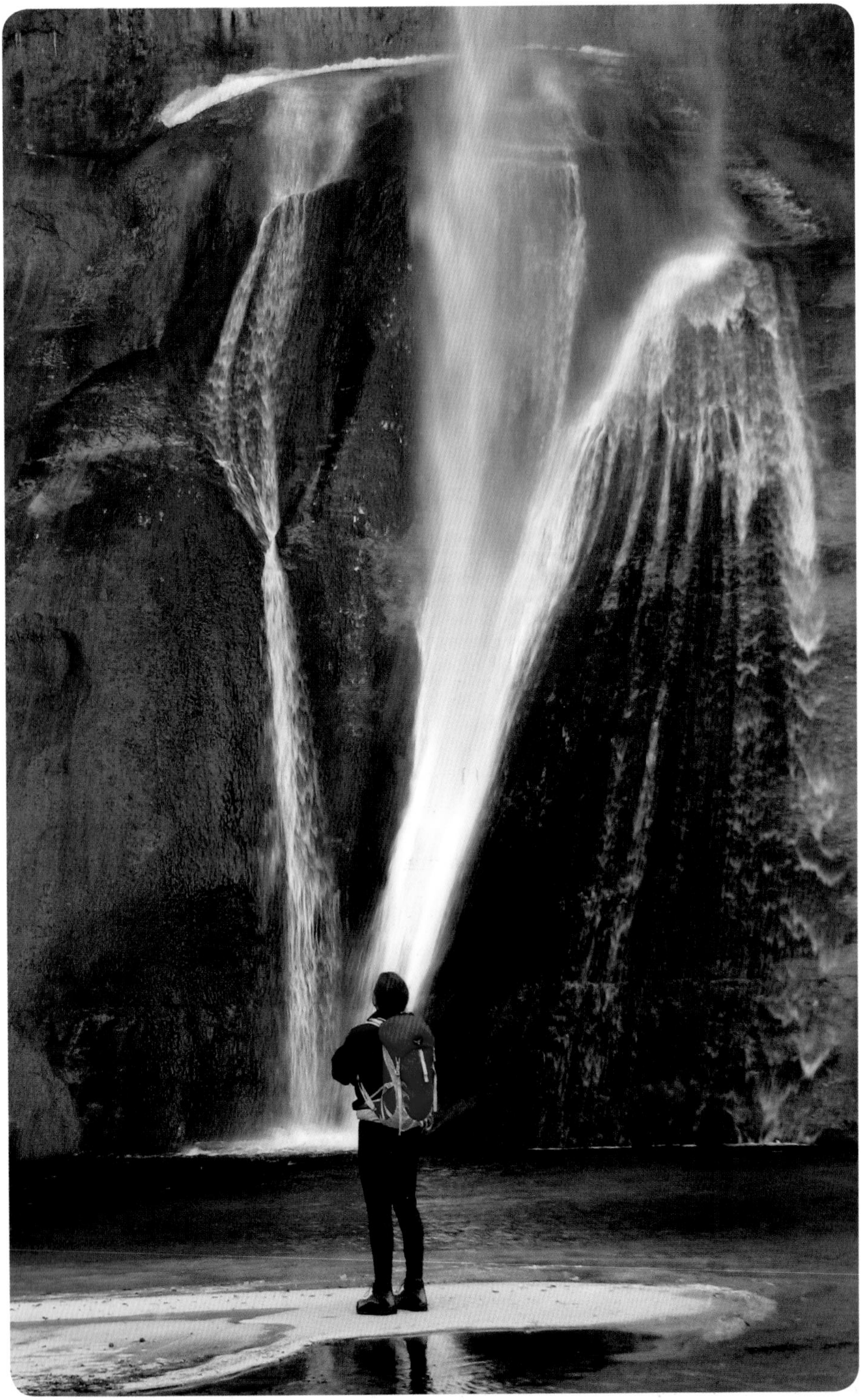

Lower Calf Creek Falls

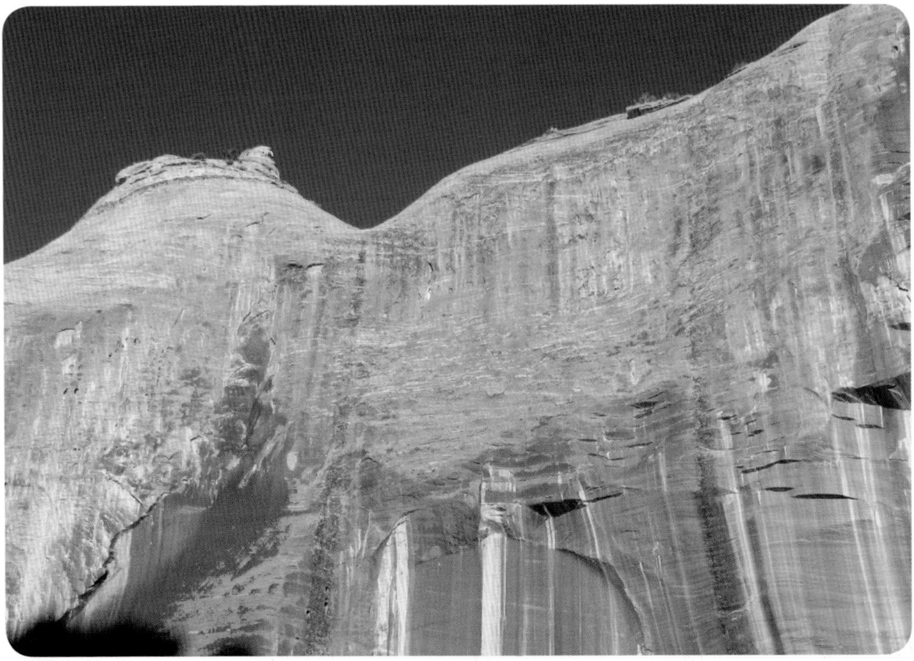

Calf Creek Canyon

FACT

BY VEHICLE

From Boulder, at the junction of Hwy 12 and Burr Trail Road, drive Hwy 12 west, then generally south. At 11 mi (17.7 km) turn right (northwest) into Calf Creek Rec Area.

From the southeast edge of Escalante, near the high school, drive Hwy 12 generally east then north. At 14.1 mi (22.7 km) cross the Escalante River bridge. At 15.2 mi (24.5 km) turn left (northwest) into Calf Creek Rec Area.

From either approach, descend the paved access road. In 0.2 mi (0.3 km) arrive at the day-use parking lot. Elevation: 5320 ft (1622 m). Pay the day-use fee and get an interpretive brochure. It illuminates the area's geology, biology, and 1,000-year human history by describing numerous posted sites along the trail.

ON FOOT

Follow the paved road north through the campground. Just before the road drops to the creek, go left onto the **signed trail** rising along the left (west) wall of the Navajo sandstone canyon.

The wide, frequently sandy trail leads up-canyon, generally north, above the left (west) bank of Calf Creek. Beaver felled the cottonwood trees that once thrived here. What remains are P-J (piñon pine and juniper), gambel oak, water birch, box elders, and rabbitbrush.

Within ten minutes bear right at the mouth of a **gully**, then ascend onto a ledge. Don't follow the gully left.

About 16 minutes along, reach **signpost 6**. Stop here and look directly east. A granary (a short, circular, stone wall with a dark opening) is visible near the top of the far canyon wall.

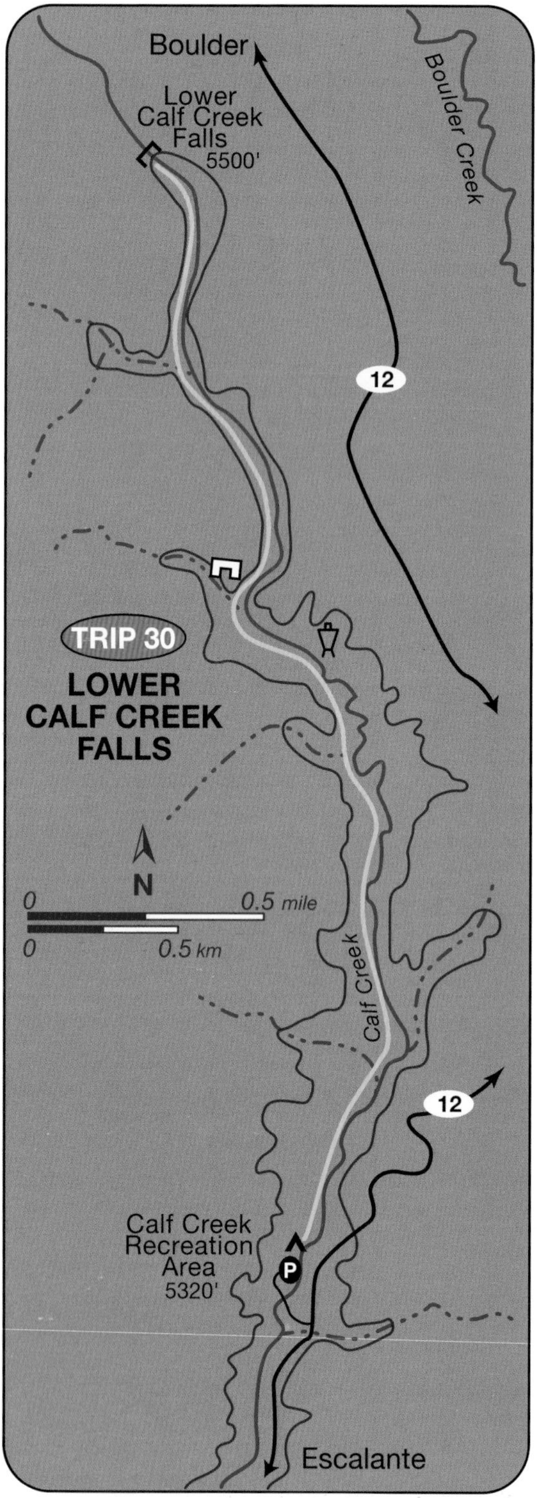

Reach **signpost 9** about 25 minutes from the trailhead. Stop here and again scan the far canyon wall. You'll see two bays divided by a fin jutting toward you. In the left (upstream) of the two bays, are two broad, vertical streaks of desert varnish. Look north-northeast, midway between those streaks, at the base of the cliff, just above the broken rock. You'll see a pictograph panel comprising a trio of large, red, human figures holding hands.

Ahead, occasionally glance up at the top of the canyon's right (east) wall. You'll see where Hwy 12 slices through the slickrock. Highway signs are even visible. It's a reminder that we humans are still exercising our ingenuity in precarious settings.

About 35 minutes along, reach **signpost 10**. Stop here and look straight ahead (north-northwest), in the direction the trail continues. On the right side of that tributary drainage is a southwest-facing wall. About halfway up the wall, in a shallow alcove, is granary whose door is facing you.

About 40 minutes along, the canyon begins to narrow and the trail nears the creek. After hiking 3 mi (4.8 km) from the actual trailhead at the end of pavement, reach the plunge pool beneath **Lower Calf Creek Falls**. Elevation: 5500 ft (1677 m). Seeps ringing the amphitheater nurture hanging gardens of maidenhair fern and alcove columbine. Fast hikers will arrive here in about 50 minutes.

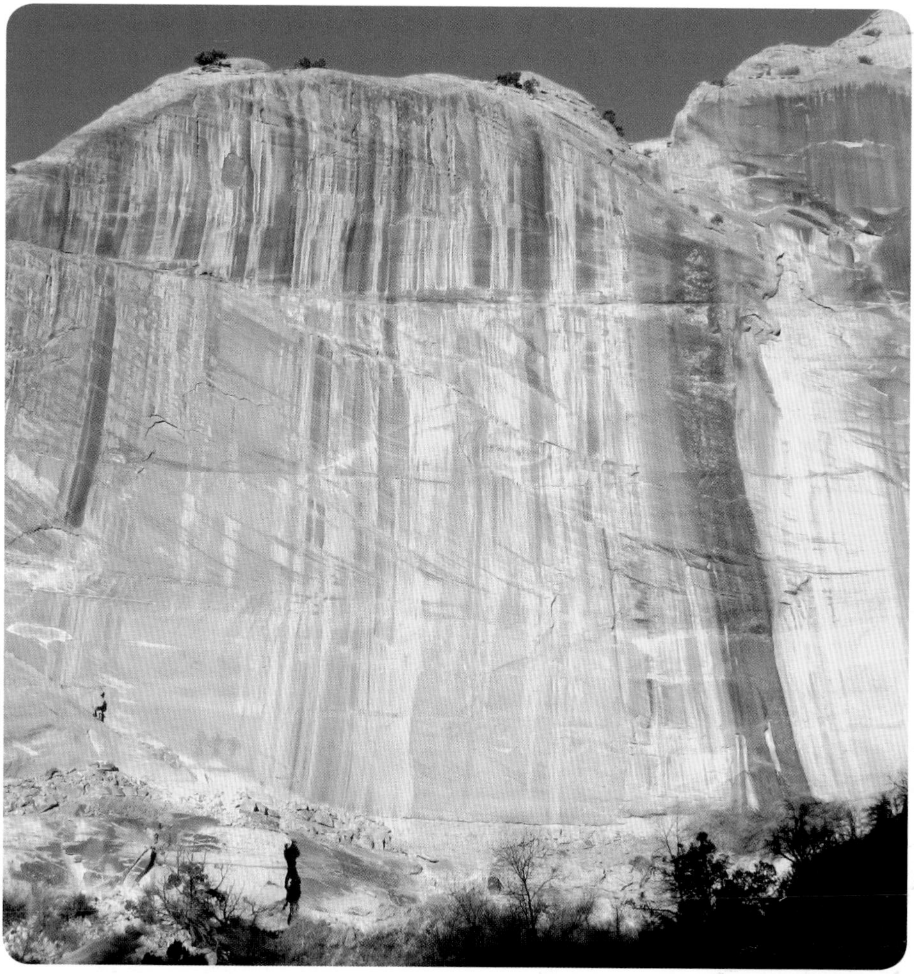

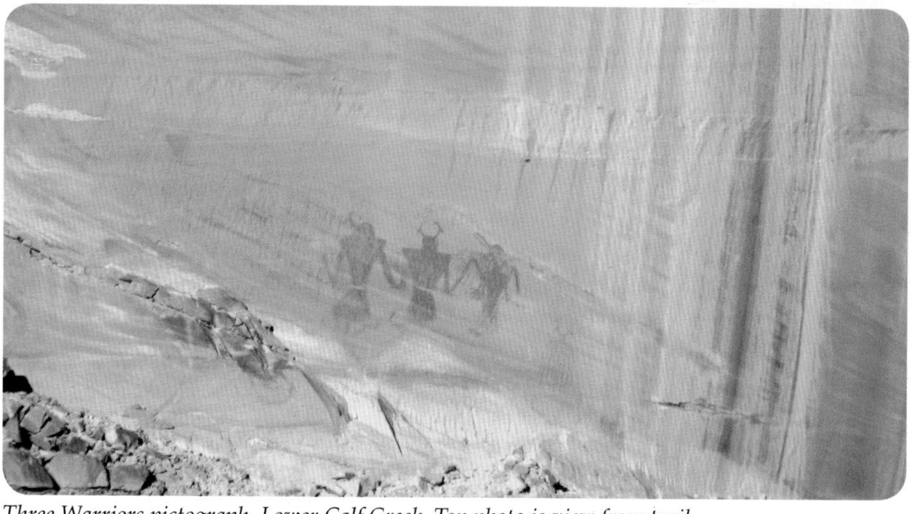

Three Warriors pictograph, Lower Calf Creek. Top photo is view from trail.

TRIP 31

UPPER CALF CREEK FALLS

LOCATION	Grand Staircase-Escalante National Monument south-southwest of Boulder
ROUND TRIP	2.2 mi (3.5 km)
ELEVATION CHANGE	657-ft (200-m) loss and gain
KEY ELEVATIONS	trailhead 6527 ft (1990 m), base of falls 5870 ft (1790 m)
HIKING TIME	1 to 1½ hours
DIFFICULTY	moderate
MAP	Trails Illustrated *Canyons of the Escalante*

OPINION

Highway 12—linking the towns of Escalante, Boulder, and Torrey—is as scenic as any stretch of pavement anywhere. It's also a marvel of engineering, particularly the stretch between Calf Creek and Hell's Backbone Road, where it snakes along the slender Hogback.

Motorists—pupils dilated, eyebrows arched, heads swiveling—snatch only fleeting views for fear of ending up airborne á la Thelma and Louise. To see anything, you have to stop at one of the pullouts. To appreciate what see, you need to hike here. Fortunately, there's a trailhead atop the narrow isthmus. It leads to Upper Calf Creek Falls.

The 50-ft (15-m) plume spills over a sandstone balcony to a pool within a small, sheer-walled amphitheater. It's a soothing sight, yet startling too. Water bursting forth and creating a moist, green sanctuary seems a miracle in this arid land.

But even without the falls as a destination, this would be a premier hike. Beautiful Navajo sandstone—ranging from creamy white to burnt gold—is visible in every direction. It's also underfoot, where you'll appreciate it with each step on the initial descent: a steep, fun, friction walk. And the sandstone is littered with exclamation points: 20-million-year-old, black, volcanic boulders. Glacial meltwater transported them here about 10,000 years ago from high on 10,000-ft (3048-m) Boulder Mountain.

Because it's possible to visit Upper Calf Creek Falls in a couple hours, consider also hiking to Lower Calf Creek Falls (Trip 30) the same day. This bookend trail starts near the bottom of the Hogback.

If you must choose between them, here's how they compare. The upper-falls trail affords a grand vista and a palpable sense of wilderness. It's less known, starts at an obscure trailhead, and begins with a sharp descent that might alarm wimps, neophytes, and parents with small children.

The lower-falls trail is entirely on the canyon floor; you'll see imposing walls but nothing beyond. It's virtually level, therefore easy, and starts at an inviting campground, so it's too popular to grant solitude.

As for the falls themselves, the lower one is more impressive: the amphitheater is broader, the precipice over which the water spills is higher, the pool it splashes into is bigger.

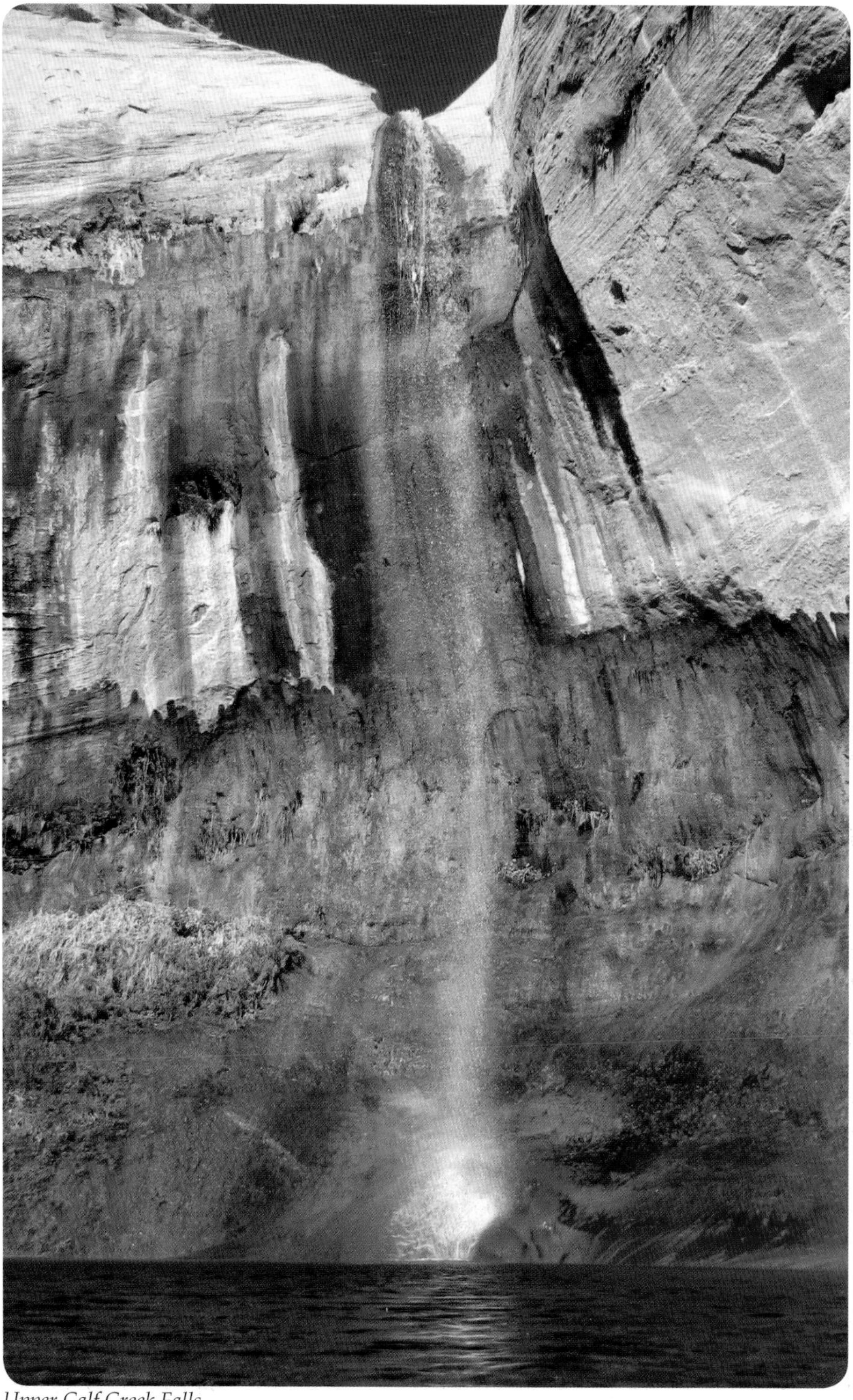

Upper Calf Creek Falls

FACT

BY VEHICLE

From Boulder, at the junction of Hwy 12 and Burr Trail Road, drive west on Hwy 12. At 3 mi (5 km) pass Hells Backbone Road (right). At 5.2 mi (8.4 km) pass milepost 81. Immediately south of it, at 5.4 mi (8.7 km), turn right (west) onto an unsigned, unpaved spur.

From the southeast edge of Escalante, near the high school, drive Hwy 12 generally east then north about 22 mi (35.4 km). Just before milepost 81, turn left (west) onto an unsigned, unpaved spur.

From either approach, reach the circular, trailhead parking area within two minutes. The signed trail departs the far (west) side of the loop, at 6527 ft (1990 m).

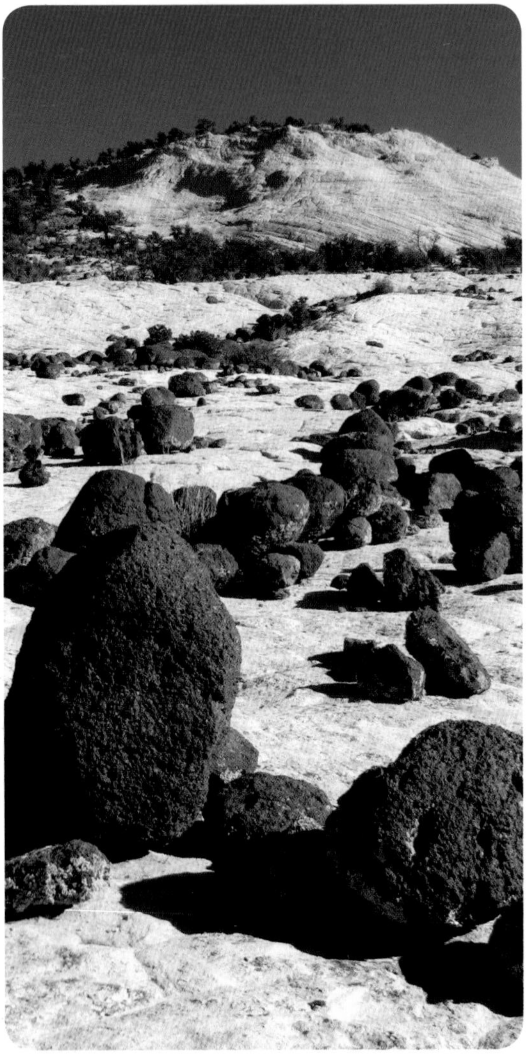

Ancient, volcanic boulders on Navajo sandstone

ON FOOT

Instantly attain an aerial view of upper Calf Creek canyon and the ridges beyond it. The Straight Cliffs, at the edge of the Kaiparowits Plateau south of Escalante, are visible on the southwest horizon.

A steep descent ensues on slickrock (Navajo sandstone) scattered with black, volcanic boulders. The way forward is evident, alternating between cairned route and rock-lined path, heading generally southwest.

In about three minutes, the descent eases on a sandy trail. Within six minutes, you'll be about 300 ft (91 m) below the rim. In season, evening primrose, goldenweed and spiderwort bloom here. Within 20 minutes, having descended 560 ft (171 m), the desert-varnished walls of the inner canyon are visible and Calf Creek is audible.

The route veers right (northwest), contours up-canyon, then forks. Right (northwest) ascends to the top of the falls. For now, go left (west) and complete the descent to the bottom of the falls.

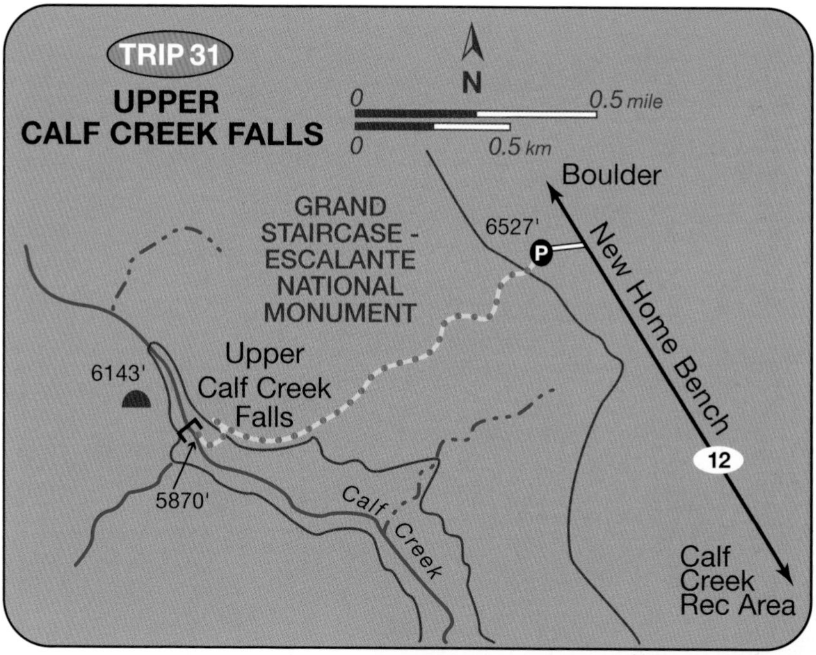

About 30 minutes from the trailhead, reach the **pool at the base of Upper Calf Creek Falls**. Elevation: 5870 ft (1790 m). Hanging gardens soften the sheer walls embracing it. Thick, thorny vegetation crowds the water's edge.

From the fork above, it's only two minutes to the **pool at the top of Upper Calf Creek Falls**. Elevation: 5965 ft (1819 m). Step carefully here. The mossy stream bed is slippery, and the falls below is not visible; don't risk your life trying to peer over.

Experienced cross-country navigators can cross the creek near the upper pool, ascend west on slickrock, and roam for hours.

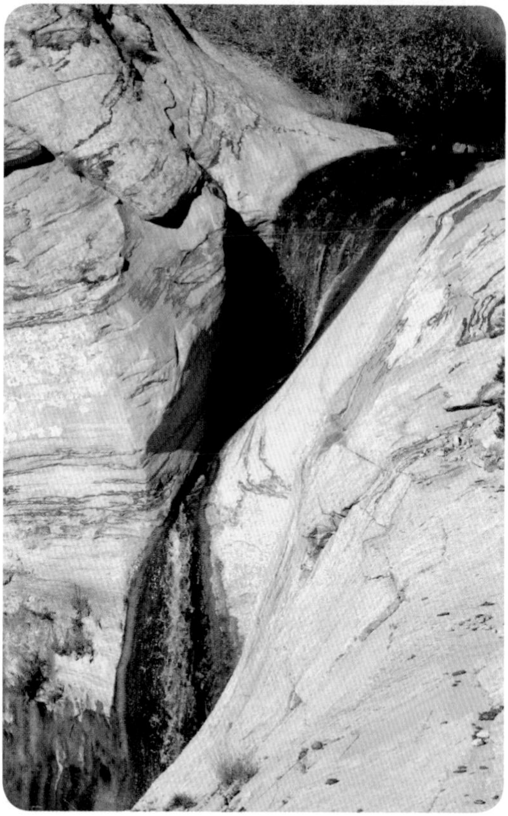

Lip of Upper Calf Creek Falls

TRIP 32

BOULDER MAIL TRAIL

LOCATION	Grand Staircase-Escalante National Monument between Boulder and Escalante
DISTANCE	15 mi (24.2 km) one way
ELEVATION CHANGE	3320-ft (1012-m) loss, 2500-ft (762-m) gain
KEY ELEVATIONS	Boulder trailhead 6780 ft (2066 m) Sand Creek 6100 ft (1859 m) Death Hollow 5740 ft (1750 m) Mamie Creek 6020 ft (1835 m) confluence of Pine Creek & Escalante River 5680 ft (1732 m) Escalante trailhead 5960 ft (1817m)
HIKING TIME	7- to 9-hour dayhike, or two-day backpack trip
DIFFICULTY	challenging dayhike, moderate backpack trip
MAPS	Trails Illustrated *Canyons of the Escalante* USGS *Calf Creek, Escalante*

OPINION

In 1908, the first Model T rolled out of the Ford Motor Company in Detroit. They ceased producing the revolutionary automobile in 1927 after selling 15 million of them. By then, people were driving all kinds of cars on paved roads throughout the world. Traffic and smog were growing problems.

But not in Boulder, Utah. The community was so tiny and isolated that in 1924, residents' mail still arrived on the backs of mules. To reach the lonely outpost, the mule train traversed a vast, turbulent expanse of slickrock via the route you're now contemplating hiking: the Boulder Mail Trail.

Boulder is still small and remote. But if you were standing there, chatting with a local about how Hwy 12 wasn't completed until 1940, how this was the last place in the U.S. to gain automobile access, how the highway wasn't entirely paved until 1971, and how this remains the farthest hamlet from a U.S. interstate, your conversation might be momentarily interrupted by a UPS or Fedex delivery truck zooming past.

Today you can send a package from Boulder to Hong Kong and expect it to arrive in a couple days. And while you can now transport yourself through Boulder in all of about 10 seconds from behind the wheel of your zippy hybrid, you can also stop at the Hell's Backbone Grill (www.hellsbackbonegrill.com) and savor a dining experience touted in *The New York Times*. And you can spend the night at the Boulder Mountain Lodge (www.boulder-utah.com), which *Outside Magazine* raved about in an article titled "The Perfect 10: Adventure Lodges We Love."

Both the restaurant and the lodge were built by a local who's obviously a master craftsman but who's also a blackbelt climber. And he'll tell you, if he thinks you need reminding, that no matter how much Boulder has changed, *the* reason to come here is still the surrounding canyon-country wilderness, which has changed very little since the Desert Archaic Indians arrived in AD 1.

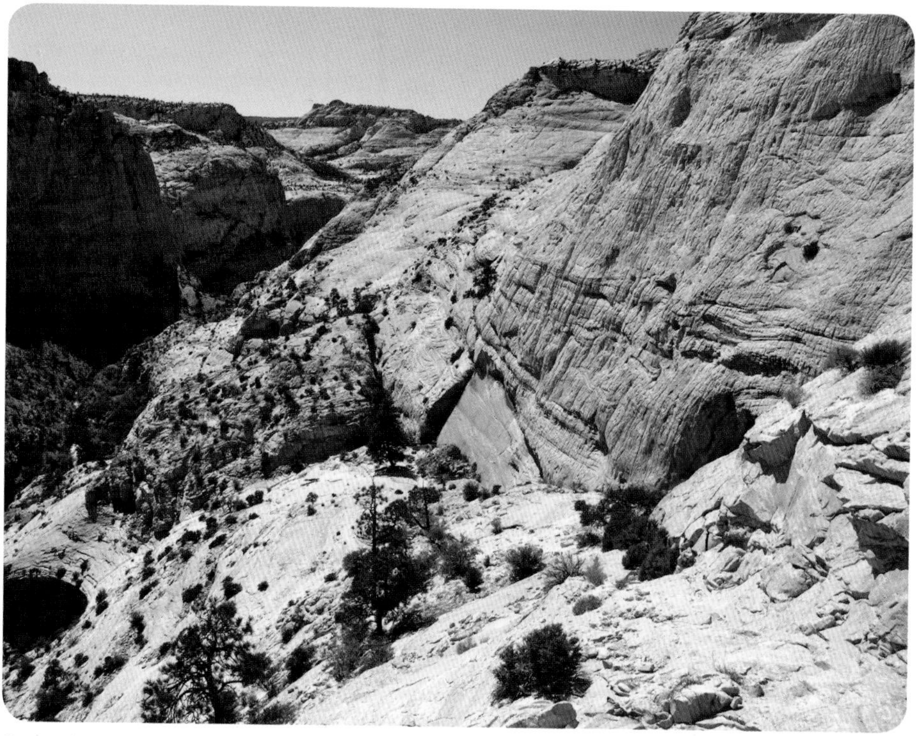

Route descending into Death Hollow

To experience as much of that wilderness as possible in a single day, we recommend a hearty dinner at the grill, a sound sleep at the lodge, then an early start for a one-way through-hike of the Boulder Mail Trail, crossing the profound chasm of Death Hollow en route, and ending in the town of Escalante.

Though frequently traveled at one time, the Boulder Mail Trail bears little evidence that others have preceded you. Were it not for the cairns indicating the route, it would pose an orienteering challenge. That's because much of the way is on solid rock: beautiful Navajo sandstone ranging from creamy white to burnt gold. It also plies sandy benches, pierces piñon and juniper forest, and dips (or nose-dives) into canyons bisecting the route, then muscles its way skyward again.

Keen, swift striders who are also experienced, confident cross-country navigators can flash the Boulder Mail Trail in seven hours' hiking time. Others will probably need nine hours' hiking time. But everyone should allow themselves more daylight than they anticipate will be necessary. If you're not at least a strong, intermediate hiker with a little routefinding under your boots, it would be wise to leave this one on your "someday" list. Or plan only an in-and-out journey as far as Death Hollow.

A two-day backpack trip is also an option, of course. Camping in Death Hollow—perhaps in an alcove, or beneath ponderosa pines within earshot of the creek—holds great appeal. Allow three days, and you could spend day two probing Death Hollow either up- or down-canyon. Still, we prefer the freedom of minimal weight and the exhilaration of trekking far and fast in a single day.

About those cairns you'll be relying on: Don't rely on them entirely. Buy the topos, get familiar with them, and bring them on the hike, along with your compass. Fools, thoughtlessly assuming cairns are simply cute and decorative, often build them for their own amusement. They think they've left behind a backcountry garden gnome. What they've actually done is mislead others. On the Boulder Mail Trail, however, you occasionally have another guide: segments of the telegraph line that in 1910 linked Boulder and Escalante.

FACT

BEFORE YOUR TRIP

Stop at the Escalante Interagency Visitor Center. Check the current weather report, and ask how much water might be flowing in Sand Creek, Death Hollow, Mamie Creek, Pine Creek, and the Escalante River, all of which you'll cross.

Though called a "trail," this is actually a route: long, challenging, across rough terrain, marked only by cairns. Carry a compass and the three USGS 1:24 000 topo maps.

If you intend to hike the entire one-way trip in a single day, start earlier than you think necessary. Even a minor navigational error could prevent you from accomplishing your goal, so be prepared to spend the night out.

BY VEHICLE

Escalante trailhead

From Hwy 12, on the east edge of Escalante, turn north onto the cemetery road. It's 0.25 mi (0.4 km) southeast of the high school, and 3.8 mi (6.1 km) northwest of the Hole-in-the-Rock Road. Pass the cemetery and bear right (east). Curve left (north) at 0.4 mi (0.6 km). Reach the trailhead parking area at 0.6 mi (1 km), 5960 ft (1817m). Leave your shuttle vehicle here, where the one-way hike ends.

Boulder trailhead

From the southeast edge of Escalante, near the high school, drive Hwy 12 generally east then north. At 24.2 mi (39 km)—3 mi (5 km) shy of the Hwy 12 / Burr Trail Road junction—turn left (northwest) onto Hells Backbone Road, also signed for Salt Gulch. Reset your trip odometer to 0, proceed only 110 yd (100 m), then turn left onto unsigned, unpaved, McGath Point Road leading southwest. At 0.4 mi (0.7 km) cross the Boulder airstrip. Just beyond, the road is briefly studded with boulders. (Too rough for your vehicle? Park before the airstrip.) Reach the trailhead parking area (left) at 0.6 mi (1 km), 6780 ft (2066 m).

ON FOOT

Immediately before the trailhead parking area is a **sign and trail register** (right). The trail departs here. Initially hike west, into P-J forest. (Do not follow the road south.)

In twelve minutes, enter a sandy wash. A minute farther, cairns lead left onto trail. Just beyond, resume in a wash for several minutes. Cairns again lead left onto trail passing above a low escarpment (right). Cross sage flats, then head generally south through forest.

About 30 minutes along, the trail bends right (south-southwest). Five minutes farther, at 6600 ft (2012 m), arrive at the **rim of Sand Creek Canyon**.

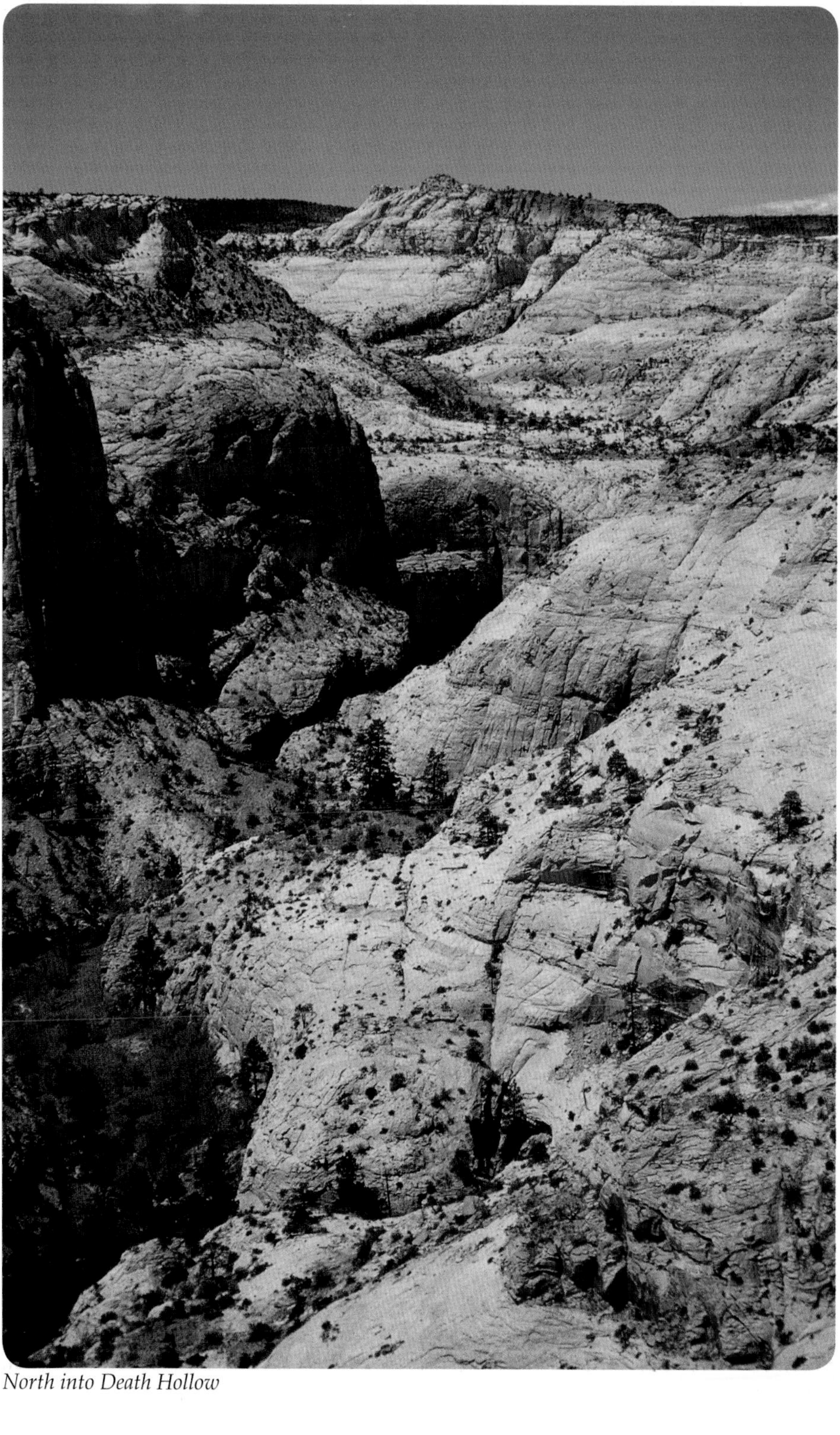

North into Death Hollow

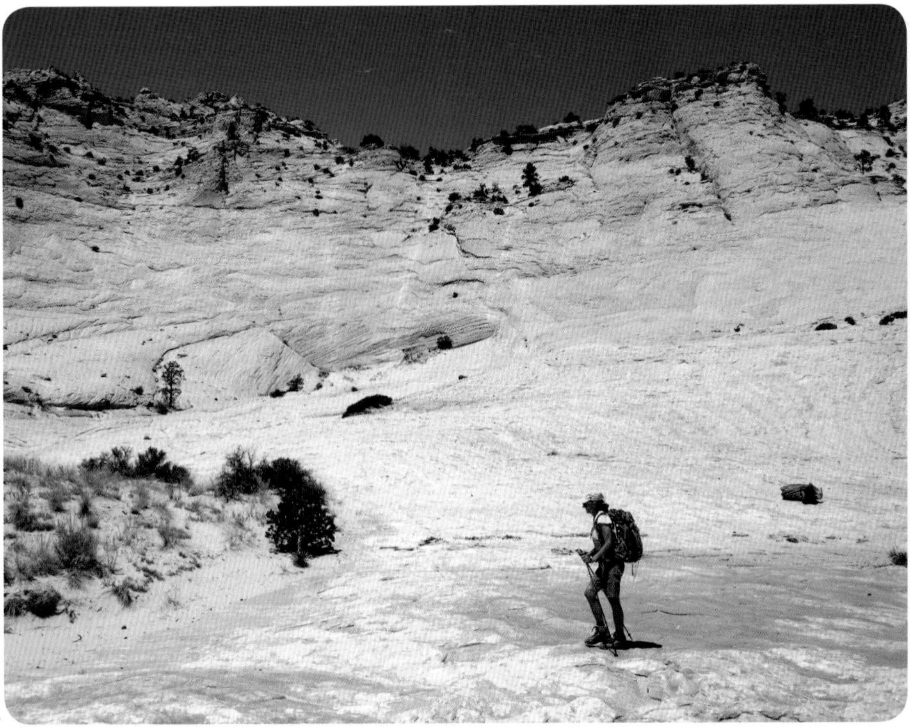

Descending to Sand Creek

Descend southwest into a sandstone bowl. The trail is again in sand. Just over an hour from the trailhead, drop onto slickrock at 6430 ft (1960 m). Cairns lead down the drainage. After hiking about 1⅓ hours, cross **Sand Creek** among cottonwoods, willows, and cliffrose bushes (tiny, fragrant, yellow-white flowers), at 2.8 mi (4.5 km), 6110 ft (1863 m).

Briefly hike downstream. A minute after jumping to the **west bank**, follow the trail right (northwest), switchbacking up and out of the drainage. Pass a campsite (right). Above, continue ascending. The route remains evident: bootbeaten into sand, cairned on slickrock.

At about 2½ hours, just west of and below a multi-spired **dome**, the route follows a wire strung between trees. This is the historic, **telegraph line** that once linked Boulder and Escalante. Ahead, you'll occasionally see it again. Between two, prominent ponderosa pines, ascend steeply left (southwest) onto cairned slickrock. Rounding the dome, bear left to pick up the sandy path above.

Long stretches of meandering, sandy path lead generally southwest. Top out at 6560 ft (2000 m) on **Slickrock Saddle Bench** at about 2¾ hours. Boulder Mountain dominates the view north-northeast. McGath Point fills the near horizon (east-northeast to southeast). The sandy path bends south-southeast.

Crest the **east rim of Death Hollow** at about 3 hours. Ahead, a very deep section of the chasm is visible below (left / south-southwest). Follow the sandy path west, then drop right, onto slickrock. Following cairns, traverse north-northwest, then descend sharply. Sections of the route were obviously leveled to grant pack animals better footing. Though the Boulder Mail Trail was established more than a century ago, in 1902, scrape marks from shod hooves are still evident.

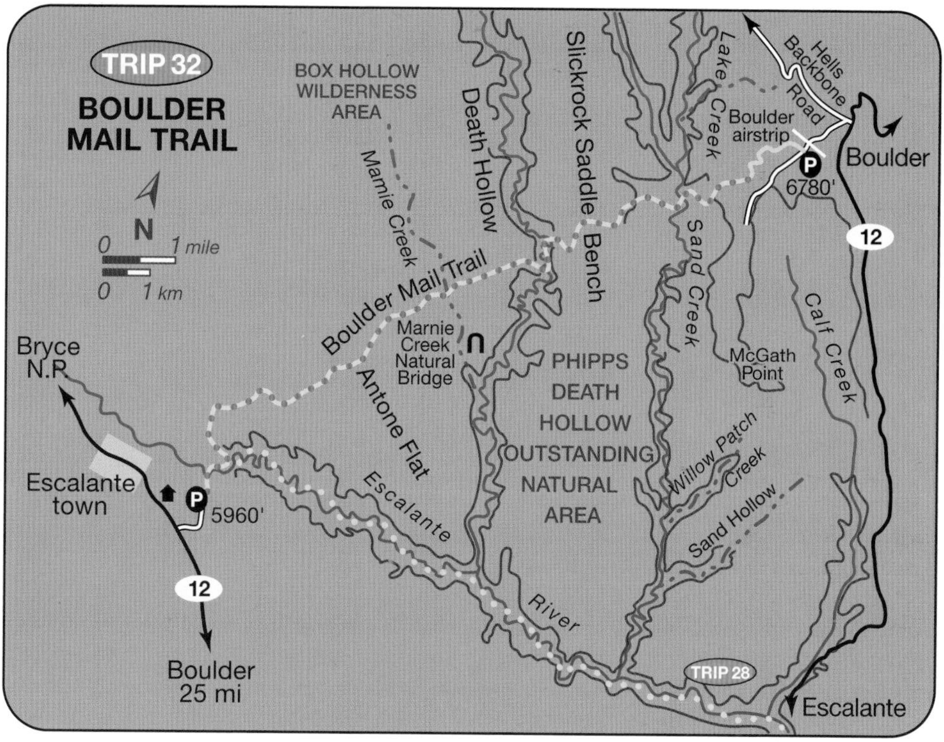

On the final switchbacking descent south, pass an inviting, sheltered campsite in a huge alcove, on the right, just above the canyon floor. About 30 minutes after departing the rim, bottom-out in **Death Hollow** at 5.7 mi (9.2 km), 5780 ft (1762 m), near the foot of a prominent, east-jutting sandstone fin.

Follow the path downstream, rockhopping or fording the creek as necessary. Pass an excellent campsite on a sandy bench, beneath ponderosa pines, across from a weeping-wall spring. Watch for and avoid poison ivy (bright-green shrubby plant, 2 to 3 ft / 0.6 to 0.9 m high, three leaves at the end of each stem, yellowish-white pea-sized berries).

After hiking downstream 0.6 mi (1 km) in about 15 minutes, look right (west) for an eye-level cairn indicating the exit route. It's at 5740 ft (1750 m), near where the creek flows right (west) after the sixth bend in the canyon (counting the east-jutting one where you arrived). If you've been watching closely, you'll see this is the first place where hiking up and out is conceivable.

Departing the downstream Death Hollow trail, turn right here and follow subsequent cairns northwest. The broken slope is moderately steep. After a 30-minute ascent, crest the canyon's sandy, **west rim** at 6540 ft (1993 m). The route then curves left to resume progress southwest.

Enjoy a level respite while crossing a sandy plateau among P-J forest. Blazes on trees indicate the route until cairns resume. About 30 minutes beyond Death Hollow's west rim, overlook the **Mamie Creek** drainage, then descend into it. Though shallower than the previous canyons, Mamie is more awkward to enter. The telegraph line crosses overhead.

Bottom-out beside the creek at 8 mi (12.9 km), 6020 ft (1835 m). Backpackers with time for a detour should hike down the wash generally southeast about 1 mi (1.6 km) to a 30-ft (9-m) natural bridge towering above a pouroff and pool. To continue following the main route, hike down the wash only about 90 yd (82 m), then ascend right on a slickrock ramp above a pouroff and pool. The Escalante trailhead is about 7 mi (11.3 km) farther. Strong hikers will cover that distance in about three hours.

Beyond the southwest rim of Mamie Creek drainage, drop across sand into a shallow draw, then ascend beneath the telegraph line. Curve left (south), staying close to the line. After the line ends, proceed south-southwest on slickrock. Pass several natural water-tanks on 6400-ft (1951-ft) **Antone Flat**. Keep following the cairns.

At 10 mi (16.1 km) ascend right (northwest) around the head of a minor drainage. Soon curve left (south), and at 10.5 mi (16.9 km) curve right (southwest) again. Just ahead, about 1½ hours from Mamie, top out at 6760 ft (2060 m). Hike southwest on a sandy trail affording a panorama of the terrain you've traversed. The view extends northeast to the Henry Mtns and north-northwest to the Aquarius Plateau. Soon attain an aerial view southwest over Escalante and the agricultural land surrounding it.

Curving right (west) at 11.4 mi (18.4 km), 6640 ft (2024 m), begin the final, long, steep descent. Near 11.8 mi (19 km), 6200 ft (1890 m), curve left (southwest) again. Briefly rise over the bluff bearing the giant, whitewashed, block letter E, which is visible from the town. Resume descending.

The final 0.6-mi (1-km) plunge north is particularly rugged. Reach **Pine Creek** at 12.7 mi (20.4 km), 5740 ft (1750 m). Bear left (south) and follow it downstream. Stay on the east bank, avoiding the private property on the west bank. At 13.2 mi (21.3 km) follow the creek left (east).

Reach the confluence of Pine Creek and the **Escalante River**, near a water gauge, at 13.9 mi (22.4 km), 5680 ft (1732 m). Turn right (south) and follow the river upstream, soon curving right (west). Exiting the canyon, follow a trail left (southwest) across an open bench.

Proceed through a hiker's maze, which allows people but not cows to pass through the fence. Ford the river. Bear left (south). Soon pass through the fence again. Still heading south, ascend an old road. Aim for the knoll near the trailhead.

Reach the **Escalante trailhead** at 15 mi (24.2 km), 5960 ft (1817 m). If you did not park here and intend to hitchhike back to your vehicle, continue walking the road south then west to **Hwy 12**, which is only 0.6 mi (1 km) away. Then go right (northwest) 0.25 mi (0.4 km) to the gas station.

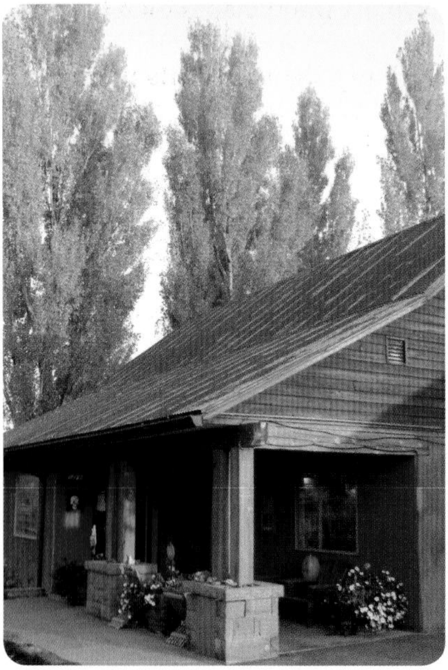

Boulder Mountain Lodge

TRIP 33

LITTLE DEATH HOLLOW

LOCATION	Grand Staircase-Escalante National Monument south of Burr Trail Road
LOOP	15.2 mi (24.5 km)
ELEVATION GAIN	665-ft (203-m) loss and gain
KEY ELEVATIONS	trailhead 5560 ft (1695 m), confluence of Little Death Hollow and Horse Canyon 5000 ft (1524 m)
HIKING TIME	7 to 9 hours
DIFFICULTY	moderate
MAPS	Trails Illustrated *Canyons of the Escalante* USGS *Pioneer Mesa, Silver Falls Bench* *Red Breaks, King Bench*

OPINION

Little Death seems a rather unnerving name. Until you're there. Then it's easy to read a deeper meaning into it. Or rather feel a deeper feeling.* Because while walking in this fantastic, otherworldly slot canyon, you might experience a little death: a dissolution of your conscious self as your spirit reaches out, groping to fathom the strange, cosmic artistry of what you see.

Loop dayhikes are rare in canyon country. Typically, it's down and in, then retrace your steps up and out. But after hiking into Little Death Hollow, you can return via Horse and Wolverine canyons. This loop option makes for a long day but significantly sharpens Little Death's appeal.

Both Wolverine and Little Death are enticingly slender. At its narrowest, Little Death is more groove than canyon. Slots like this usually pose serious, technical hurdles, but a boulder jam is the only difficulty in Little Death. Precisely what you'll encounter there will depend on the volume of recent rain and the strength of subsequent floods. If you're unable to either negotiate or bypass this obstacle… checkmate. Game over. Thanks for coming out to play. Time to the return to the trailhead.

Assuming you slip through (last time, we did it by crawling beneath one of the boulders), then it's clear striding ahead. But don't expect to dispatch the first half of the loop quickly. Little Death is so engaging it will probably slow your pace. If so, you might arrive at the boulder jam in about two hours, the chokestone (easy to stem around) in four hours, and the confluence with Horse Canyon within five hours. If you then quicken your pace, you can expect to reach the Horse / Wolverine confluence in 5½ hours, the south fork of Wolverine in 6¾ hours, and the Wolverine Loop Road (near the trailhead) in 8 hours.

*The French call sexual orgasm *la petite mort* or *the little death*. It refers to the fleeting, climactic release from physicality, the momentary coalescing of two spirits as one. So perhaps melding with creation can also be an orgasmic experience, oui?

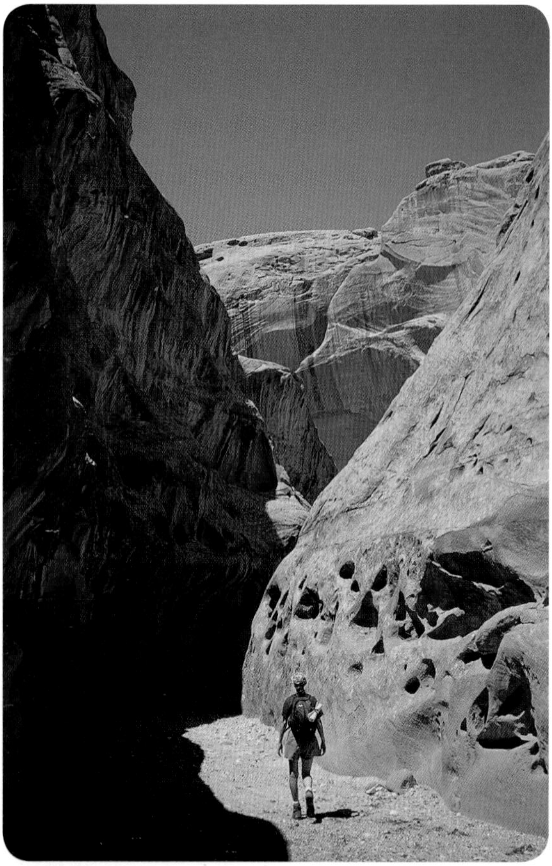

Little Death Hollow

FACT

BEFORE YOUR TRIP

Stop at the Escalante Interagency Visitor Center. Check the current weather report, and ask about the condition of the Wolverine Loop Road.

If you find water en route (and you might not), it will require purifying or filtering. Carry more than you'll need for the entire hike: at least three quarts (liters) per person.

BY VEHICLE

From Boulder, at the junction of Hwy 12 and Burr Trail Road, drive Burr Trail Road east. At 18.5 mi (29.8 km) turn right (south) onto the west Wolverine Loop Road, reset your trip odometer to 0, and follow it generally south.

Bear left at 5.5 mi (8.9 km). Reach a T-junction at 10.7 mi (17.2 km). Right (southwest) leads to the north fork Wolverine trailhead. Go left (east) on the main road. Bear left again at 11.8 mi (19 km) where right accesses Wolverine Petrified Wood Natural Area and the south fork of Wolverine Canyon. You'll intersect the road near here after exiting Wolverine Canyon's south fork on our recommended loop hike. At 12.5 mi (20.1 km) turn right (south) to enter the Little Death Hollow trailhead. Park near the corral, at 5560 ft (1695 m).

Upon leaving, if you continue following the Wolverine Loop Road east, reach a junction at 19.5 mi (31.4 km). Right (south) leads to Silver Falls Creek Canyon (Trip 34). Left (northeast) intersects Burr Trail Road at 27.5 mi (44.3 km).

ON FOOT

Heading southwest, begin a gradual descent through the broad redrock canyon. About 25 minutes along, look for pictographs on a huge boulder (right), about 12 yd/m off trail.

At 1.5 mi (2.4 km), 5470 ft (1668 m), ignore the tributary drainage (left / east). Bear right (southwest). About 15 minutes farther, at 2.2 mi (3.5 km), 5400 ft (1646 m), the canyon constricts. It opens again about ten minutes ahead.

Reach the crux—a **boulder jam**—at 2.7 mi (4.3 km), 5360 ft (1634 m). In the past, it's been easy to work through and under the boulders. If floods have rearranged the boulders or if water is present, it might be necessary to scramble

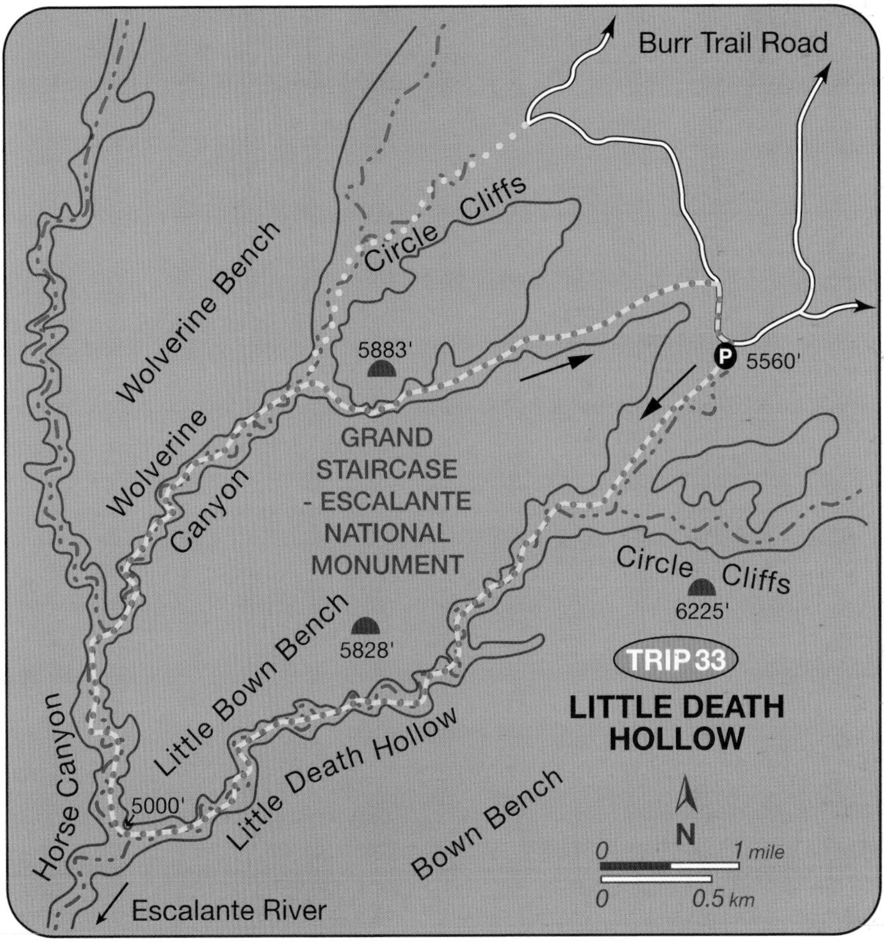

over the boulders. If that appears too challenging, backtrack upcanyon 110 yd (100 m), turn left into a slot, and begin a scrambling ascent west-southwest. Above, follow the bench downcanyon to the top of an east-west peninsula. Then go left (east) and descend a steep chute into the canyon below the boulder jam.

Beyond this crux, Little Death Hollow poses no serious obstacles. Soon enter the **narrows**, where the distance between the walls diminishes to just 6 ft (1.8 m). Ahead, the canyon meanders generally southwest. At one point, where a chokestone creates a slender passage, stem your way through: back against one side, feet against the other. Any reasonably athletic person can manage it.

Petrified wood is scattered through the canyon's lower reaches. Hike in the 30-ft (9-m) inner gorge, beneath a slickrock bench. Bypass a series of pools by ascending right (north).

Intersect **Horse Canyon**—the loop lowpoint—at 6.5 mi (10.5 km), 5000 ft (1524 m). Pass a wire and a pipe spanning the wash. A cottonwood grove on a bench here is an inviting campsite. There's a seasonal spring nearby.

Horse Canyon—initially left (west), then generally south—leads to the Escalante River. To resume the loop, turn right (northwest) and follow it up-canyon. Look for scraps of trail on the sandy bench (left), pass a metal shack,

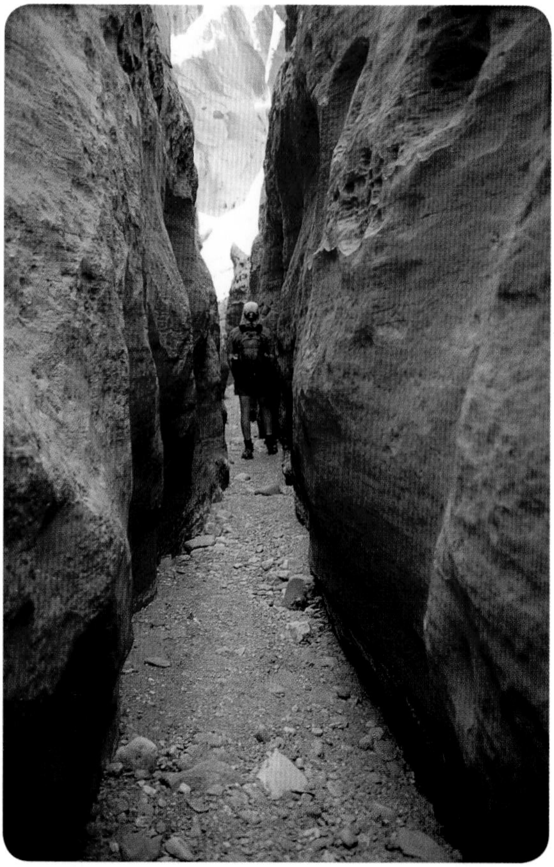
Little Death Hollow slot

and continue on a sandy road. Cross the benches to shortcut the meandering wash. The canyon's salmon and orange-sherbert colored walls are about 110 yd (100 m) apart here.

At 8.5 mi (13.7 km), 5050 ft (1540 m), reach a confluence. Horse Canyon continues left, generally north. Go right (east-northeast) into **Wolverine Canyon**. It soon constricts, averaging 8 to 15 ft (2.5 to 4.5 m) wide. A few sections are even narrower. The Wingate sandstone walls are 400 ft (122 m) high. After several sharp curves, the canyon leads generally northeast. Pass several impressive alcoves.

Wolverine Canyon splits at 11.4 mi (18.4 km), 5440 ft (1660 m). Left (northeast) is the main fork. Go right (east) into the canyon's deeper, narrower **south fork**. It briefly veers southeast before bending east, then finally leading northeast. The canyon walls are Chinle sandstone. Bear right past two, short, tributary drainages (left / north).

At 13.2 mi (21.3 km), 5500 ft (1677 m) approach an escarpment where the canyon forks again. Left (north) leads beneath a talus slope and cliffs. Proceed right (east) in the **wash**. Gradually curve northeast.

Soon reach a triple gully amid large, petrified logs. Bear right. Go over the bank. Continue through a 220-yd (200-m) gap, onto a bootbeaten path across flat, open terrain. Intersect the **Wolverine Loop Road** at 14.5 mi (23.3 km), 5665 ft (1727 m).

Turn right (southeast) and follow the road about 0.7 mi (1.1 km) to the **Death Hollow trailhead**, where the 15.2-mi (24.5-km) loop ends.

TRIP 34

SILVER FALLS CREEK CANYON

LOCATION	Grand Staircase-Escalante National Monument Glen Canyon National Recreation Area, south of Burr Trail
ROUND TRIP	12 mi (19.3 km) to Hobbs inscription 16.6 mi (26.7 km) to Escalante River
ELEVATION CHANGE	660-ft (201-m) loss and gain to Hobbs inscription 750-ft (229-m) loss and gain to Escalante River
KEY ELEVATIONS	trailhead 5440 ft (1659 m), Hobbs inscription 4780 ft (1457 m) Escalante River 4690 ft (1430 m)
HIKING TIME	6 hours or overnight
DIFFICULTY	easy
MAPS	Trails Illustrated *Canyons of the Escalante* USGS *Silver Falls Bench, Horse Pasture Mesa*

OPINION

Silence. It's rarely cited as a reason to go hiking, but it's an increasingly valid one as our world grows louder.

Intrusive, irritating sound can damage more than your hearing. It contributes to rising blood pressure, declining productivity, and higher serum-cholesterol levels.

Studies show that incessant noise makes people less caring, less communicative, less reflective; more apt to feel helpless and powerless. Even routine hospital noise impedes healing.

Ahhh, canyon country. It poses physical challenges that deter human visitation, so it's among the loneliest landscapes on earth. And once you're deep in, you're walled off. Canyons are sanctuaries of silence. Temples of tranquility. Cathedrals of quietude.

Contrary to its name, Silver Falls Creek Canyon harbors no shimmering cascades. It's actually unremarkable compared to many Utah canyons. And therein lies its appeal: it's far less popular than most of the Escalante River tributary drainages. It's beautiful, with soaring red walls streaked with metallic, blue-black desert varnish. And long ago it was a wagon route, so it's easier to walk than most of the neighboring canyons. Yet you'll likely be here alone. In blessed silence.

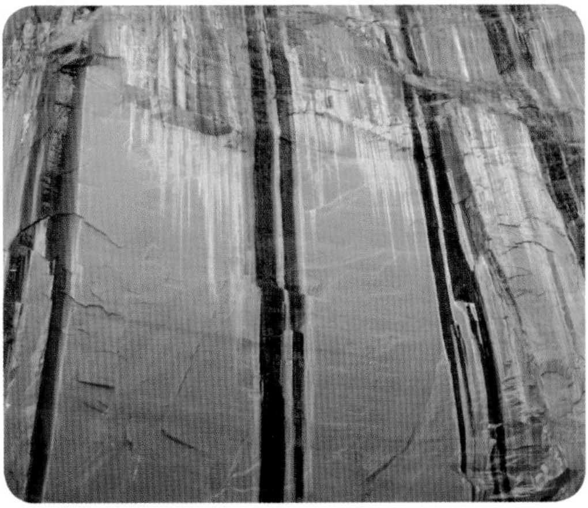

Desert varnish

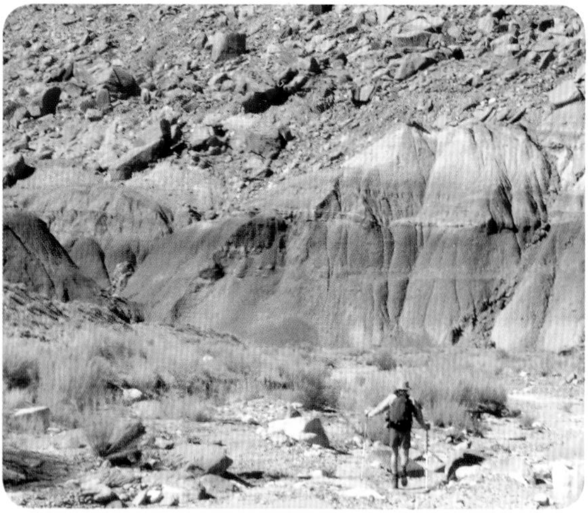

Chinle sandstone, Silver Falls Creek Canyon

The stillness that's always prevailed in Silver Falls Creek Canyon was briefly broken only twice. In 1881, Charles Hall pioneered an easier, safer alternative to the arduous Hole-in-the-Rock Road (see page 140) linking Escalante and the new Mormon outpost of Bluff. His new route eased through the Circle Cliffs via Silver Falls Creek Canyon, crossed the Escalante River, then proceeded up Harris Wash. Later, motorheads in 4WD vehicles followed the old wagon road, but they were banned when Glen Canyon National Recreation Area was established.

If you examine the walls, you'll see evidence of the canyon's shortlived popularity. For example, George Brigham Hobbs passed this way in 1883 and left a billboard of an inscription to remind us of that. He'd previously served as one of four scouts on the frightfully desperate Hole-in-the-Rock expedition. Later, on his 24th birthday, while hauling supplies through Silver Falls Creek Canyon, a blizzard struck and his survival was again in doubt. He spent what he feared would be his final days pecking his name into the canyon wall. So forgive him if his petroglyph strikes you as egotistic. The poor kid thought it was his epitaph.

Not only did young George escape, he eventually had a son who in 1956 at the age of 66 hiked into the canyon to visit the site of his father's frigid ordeal.

Charles Hall inscription

FACT

BEFORE YOUR TRIP

Stop at the Escalante Interagency Visitor Center. Check the current weather report, and ask about the condition of the Wolverine Loop Road.

Silver Falls Creek Canyon is usually dry except for the last couple miles before the Escalante River. If dayhiking, carry all the water you'll need. Though it's tempting for

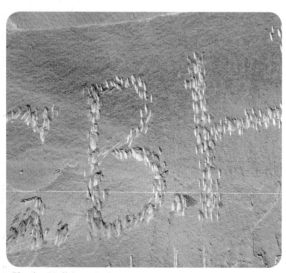

backpackers to assume they'll find water in the lower canyon, they might not. And the Escalante River is often too silty to filter. So backpackers too should carry all the water they'll need.

BY VEHICLE

From Boulder, at the junction of Hwy 12 and Burr Trail Road, drive Burr Trail Road east. At 18.5 mi (29.8 km) pass the west Wolverine Loop Road (right / south). At 29 mi (46.7 km) turn right onto the east Wolverine Loop Road, reset your trip odometer to 0, and follow it generally south.

At 8 mi (12.9 km), bear left (south-southeast). Right (southwest) leads to Little Death Hollow (Trip 33). At 10.7 mi (17.2 km) turn right (west). At 11.4 mi (18.4 km) bear left. At 11.7 mi (18.8 km) the road follows the wash, soon crossing it repeatedly. Depending on the current condition of the road, high clearance and/ or 4WD might be necessary beyond. Reach the trailhead, beside a corral, at 13 mi (21 km), 5440 ft (1659 m).

ON FOOT

From the corral, follow the old road west into the wash. Soon traverse a bench. Your general direction of travel will remain southwest all the way to the Escalante River. En route you'll cross the wash (usually dry) several times.

The variegated Chinle formation (mauve, charcoal, purple, olive) is readily apparent. Rich in uranium, it attracted prospectors in the 1950s. The red walls above it are Wingate sandstone.

At 1.6 mi (2.6 km), 5200 ft (1585 m), about 30 minutes along, enter Glen Canyon National Recreation Area. The Chinle sandstone here is a striking green.

Pass **North Fork Silver Falls Canyon** (right / northwest) at 3 mi (4.8 km), 5060 ft (1543 m), about one hour from the trailhead. Proceed west, down the main canyon, alternating between open benches and the rocky wash.

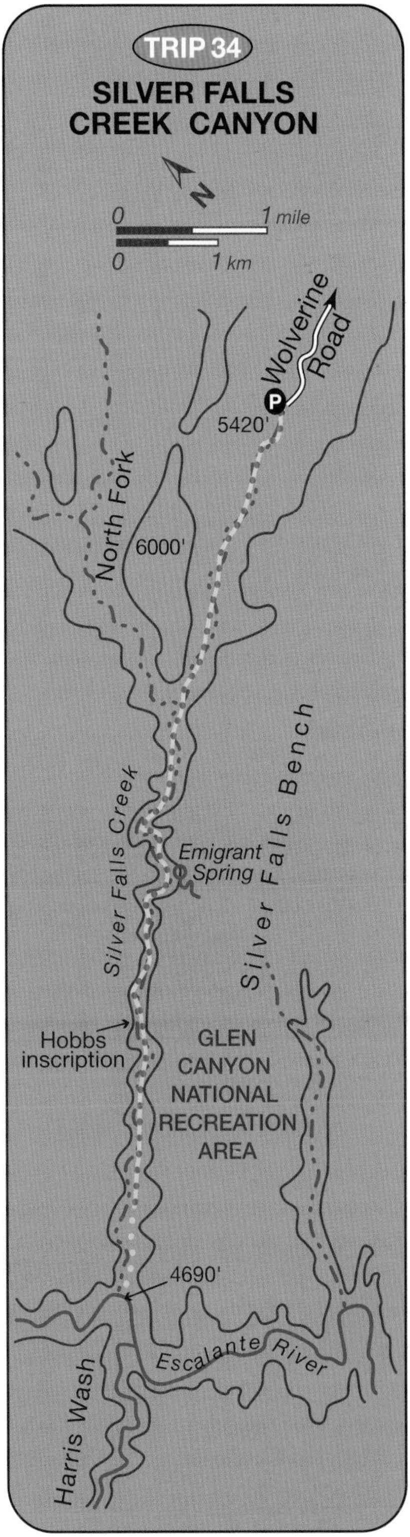

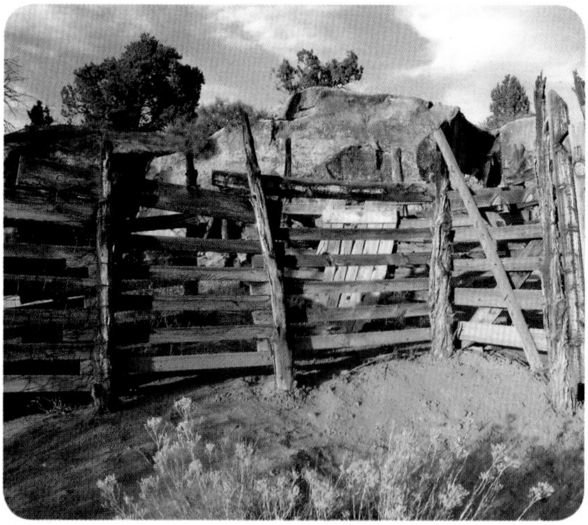

Silver Falls Creek Canyon trailhead

A 5204-ft (1587-m) **sandstone tower** (right / north) punctuates a rincon (an abandoned meander) at 3.6 mi (5.8 km). Beyond, the canyon constricts and the walls become sheer, rising 400 ft (122 m). Hiking is easy on the broad, hard-packed wash.

At 4.7 mi (7.6 km), 4950 ft (1509 m), about two hours from the trailhead, a 200-ft (61-m) **sandstone tower** (left / south) separates two amphitheaters. At the base of the tower are several historic inscriptions, one dated 1921. The second (westernmost) amphitheater harbors **Emigrant Spring**, an unreliable, seasonal seep.

Ahead, massive boulders litter the wash. You'll likely find water beginning to trickle down-canyon. A few pools might be present. Trees are more profuse.

About 2¾ hours along, at 6 mi (9.7 km), 4780 ft (1457 m), look for the **G.B. Hobbs inscription** and a commemorative plaque in a low alcove (right / north).

Soon after, the canyon widens. The walls are now Navajo sandstone. Benches afford comfortable campsites. Reach the **Escalante River** at 8.3 mi (13.4 km), 4690 ft (1430 m).

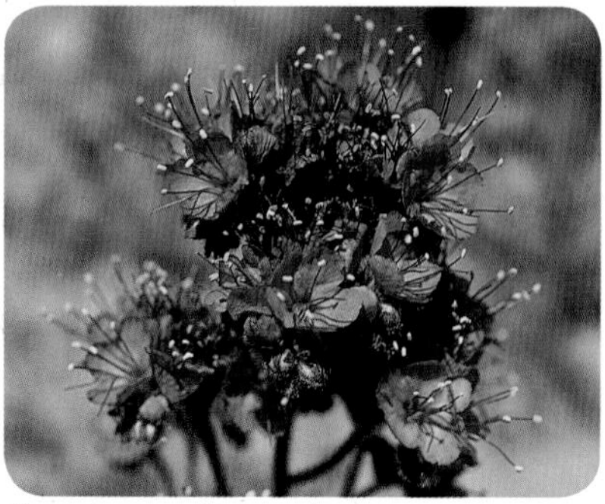

Scorpion weed

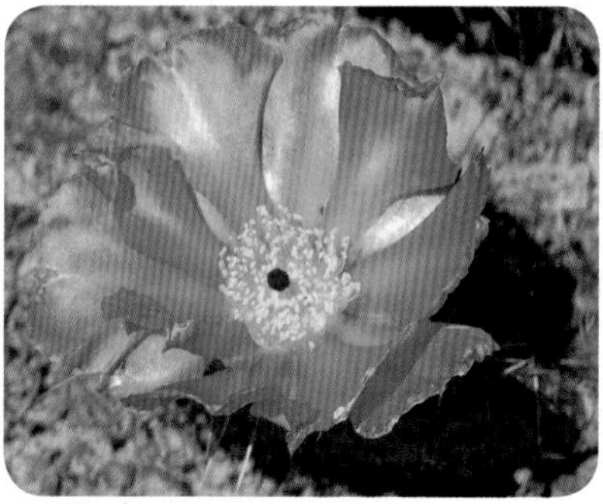

Prickly pear

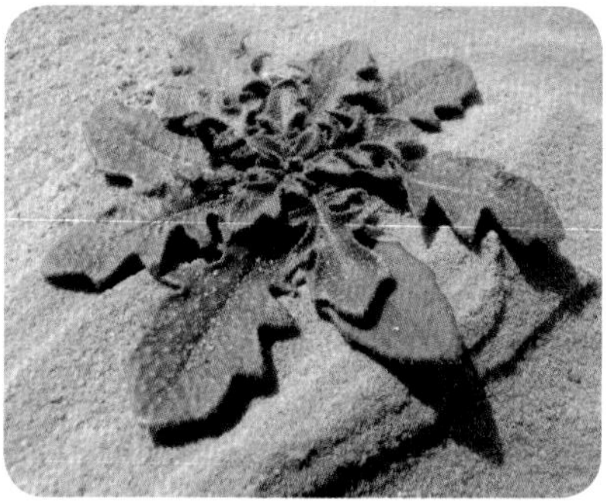

TRIP 35

UPPER MULEY TWIST

LOCATION	Capitol Reef National Park, east end of Burr Trail Road
CIRCUIT	14.2 mi (22.9 km) from 2WD trailhead 9.4 mi (15.1 km) from 4WD trailhead
ELEVATION GAIN	1060 ft (323 m) from 2WD trailhead 920 ft (280 m) from 4WD trailhead
KEY ELEVATIONS	2WD trailhead 5730 ft (1747 m), 4WD trailhead 5870 ft (1790 m) north end of Upper Muley Twist Canyon 6400 ft (1951 m) Rim Route highpoint 6640 ft (2024 m)
HIKING TIME	5 to 8 hours
DIFFICULTY	moderate
MAPS	Trails Illustrated *Capitol Reef National Park* USGS *Bitter Creek Divide, Wagon Box Mesa*

OPINION

In canyon country, wherever flashfloods *and* lightning strikes are potential threats, the hiking will probably be spectacular. That's certainly true here, because the Upper Muley Twist circuit covers extremely varied terrain—from deep and narrow, to high and exposed—within a surprisingly short distance.

It begins in a canyon paralleling the spine of the extraordinary Waterpocket Fold (see Trip 38 for a detailed description). The canyon itself, which harbors numerous arches, is sufficiently beautiful and intriguing to warrant hiking here even if the route didn't continue. But it does, ascending to the crest of the Fold, which you'll follow for a full hour, enjoying constant, sweeping views.

The initial leg of the journey is easy. There's no trail, but none is needed: simply follow the wash up-canyon. Looping back atop the Fold, however, is not for neophytes or acrophobes. Cairns indicate the way up, then you must hike the writhing, squirming route along the crest without guidance. Navigation shouldn't be a problem, because the Fold drops away steeply on both sides, but some might find that alarming in itself. If you're an intermediate hiker with at least a little experience navigating cross-country and scrambling, you'll probably find the Upper Muley Twist circuit mildly challenging yet within your ability.

As for lightning, there's of course little or no danger as long as the regional weather is fair. It's interesting to note, however, that lightning is rarely cited as a concern for canyon-country hikers. Yet all those flashfloods we're constantly, and rightly, warned about are the result of thunderstorms. Utah's relatively high elevations and sudden, radical temperature fluctuations contribute to volatile storms and frequent lightning. And Utah's mineral-rich soil and countless isolated promontories (many with up to 45% iron content) ensure frequent lightning strikes. Add to that scenario vast tracts of bare land, and it becomes obvious why lightning fatalities are more common here than elsewhere in the U.S.

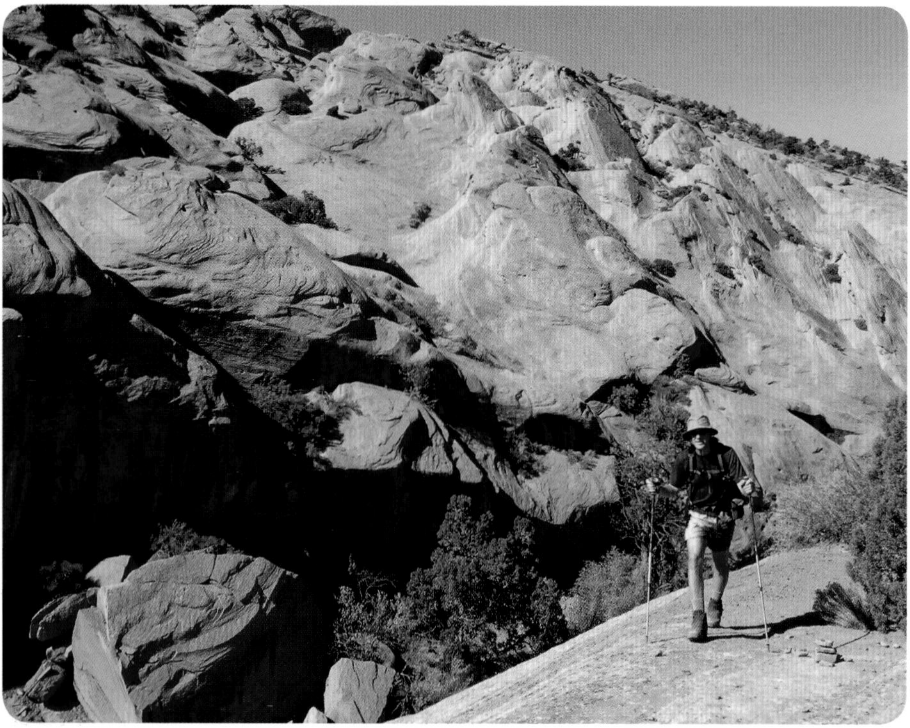
Upper Muley Twist Canyon

FACT

BEFORE YOUR TRIP

Stop at the Capitol Reef National Park Visitor Center. Check the current weather report, and ask about the condition of the Notom and Burr Trail roads.

Expect to find no water en route. Carry more than you'll need for the entire hike: at least three quarts (liters) per person.

BY VEHICLE

From the junction of Hwy 24 and the Notom Road, at the signed east entry to Capitol Reef National Park just west of milepost 89, turn south onto the Notom Road and reset your trip odometer to 0. Pavement ends at 5 mi (8.1 km). The road forks at 33 mi (53 km). Left leads to Bullfrog Marina on Lake Powell and continues to Hwy 276. Turn right onto Burr Trail Road and follow it generally southwest. Soon begin a steep, switchbacking ascent. Immediately after cresting the switchbacks, pass the Lower Muley Twist trailhead (left / south). At 36.2 mi (58.4 km) turn right (northeast) onto Strike Valley Overlook road and reset your trip odometer to 0.

From Boulder, at the junction of Hwy 12 and Burr Trail Road, drive Burr Trail Road east. Enter Capitol Reef National Park at 30.5 mi (49.1 km). Pavement ends. At 33 mi (53.1 km) turn left (northeast) onto Strike Valley Overlook road and reset your trip odometer to 0.

From either approach, reach the 2WD trailhead parking area at 0.4 mi (0.6 km), 5730 ft (1747 m). Or continue to the 4WD trailhead at 2.8 mi (4.5 km), 5870 ft (1790 m).

If the road is dry, the 4WD trailhead might be accessible in a high-clearance 2WD vehicle. Most of the way it follows a broad, level wash. If the road is wet, however, just reaching the 2WD trailhead might be difficult, in which case it's safest to park alongside Burr Trail Road.

ON FOOT

From the **2WD trailhead**, the road drops into the wash. Follow it generally north-northwest.

Look left (west) for **Double Arch** about 35 minutes along. At 2.4 mi (3.9 km), 5870 ft (1790 m), reach the **4WD trailhead**. Our subsequent hiking distances begin here.

Right (east) is a trail ascending generally northeast 0.5 mi (0.8 km) to 5980-ft (1823-m) Strike Valley Overlook atop the Waterpocket Fold. "Strike" is a geological term for the axis of the fold. For now, ignore this detour. You'll attain superior views on the Upper Muley Twist circuit.

So, from the 4WD trailhead, continue following the wash. Your general direction of travel will remain north-northwest all the way to the north end of Upper Muley Twist Canyon. Whenever the wash appears to split, bear right to stay in the main channel.

After hiking 1.5 mi (2.6 km) in about 30 minutes, look for an **arch** 200 ft (61 m) up the left (west) wall. About five minutes farther is **Saddle Arch**, also on the left (west) wall. Reach a signed **junction** here, at 1.8 mi (2.9 km).

Right (east) ascends to the Rim Route. You'll return that way on our recommended clockwise circuit. For now, proceed north through the rocky wash.

At 3.1 mi (5 km), about 1¼ hours from the 4WD trailhead, **two arches** are visible above (left / west) flanking a break in the red Wingate sandstone wall. Yet another **arch** is visible at 3.9 mi (6.3 km), near the bottom of a slot, again on the left (west) wall.

Shortly beyond, the canyon constricts dramatically. Arrive at a **pouroff**. Bypass it via the cairned route on the canyon's right (east) wall. Ascend to a shelf about 100 ft (30.5 m) above the wash. Contour above the **narrows** until the bypass route descends back to the wash at 4.6 mi (7.4 km).

Approaching the **north end of Upper Muley Twist Canyon** at 4.9 mi (7.9 km), 6400 ft (1951 m), be alert for a sign directing you to the **Rim Route**.

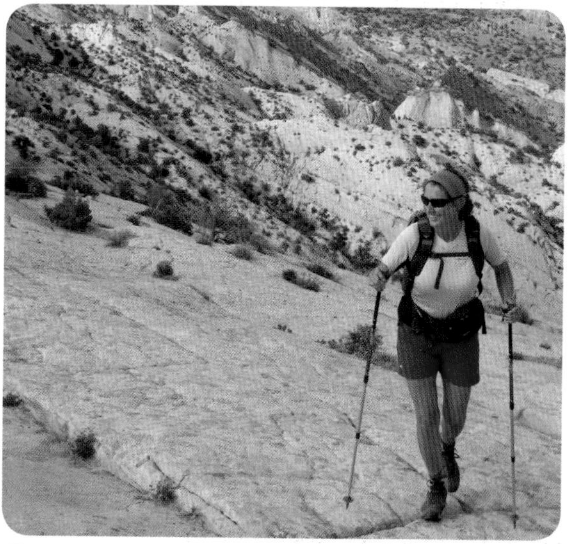

Returning along the top, upper Muley Twist

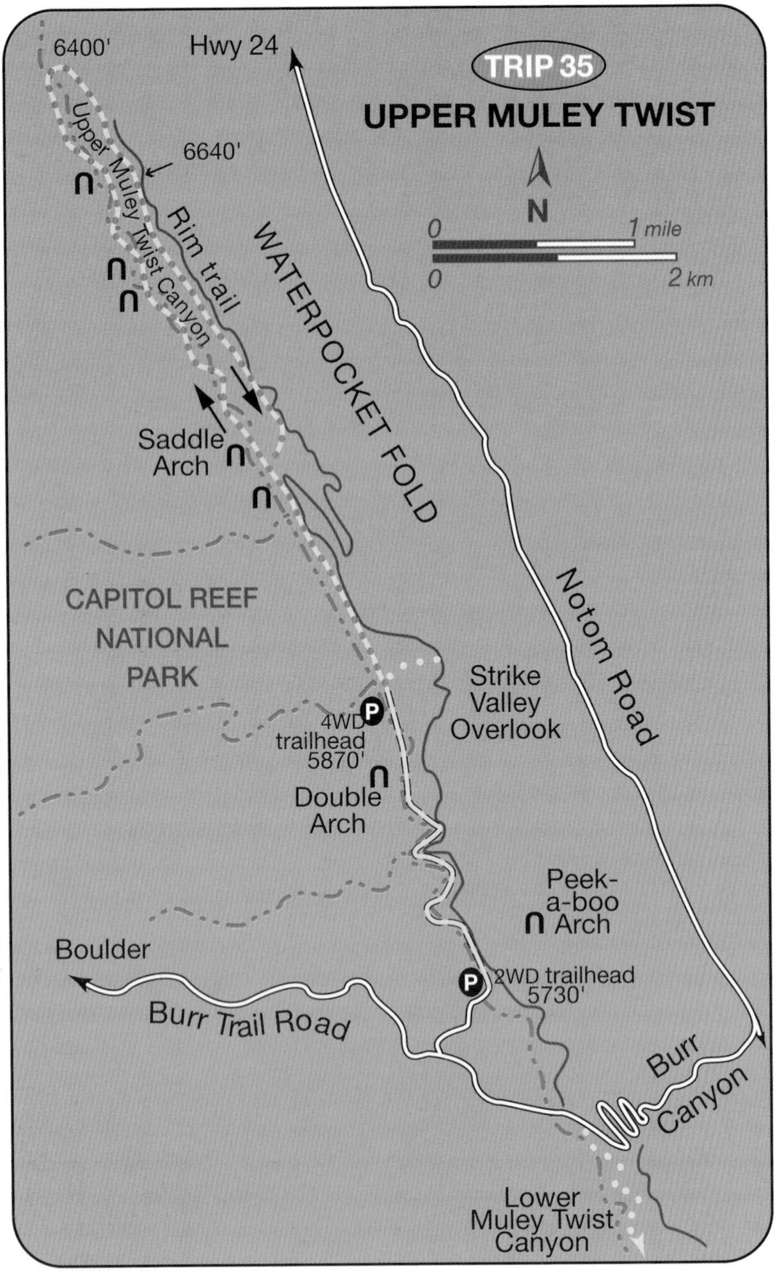
TRIP 35
UPPER MULEY TWIST
N
0
1 mile
0
2 km
6400'
Hwy 24
6640'
Upper Muley Twist Canyon
Rim trail
WATERPOCKET FOLD
Saddle Arch
CAPITOL REEF NATIONAL PARK
Strike Valley Overlook
4WD trailhead 5870'
Double Arch
Notom Road
Peek-a-boo Arch
Boulder
2WD trailhead 5730'
Burr Trail Road
Burr Canyon
Lower Muley Twist Canyon

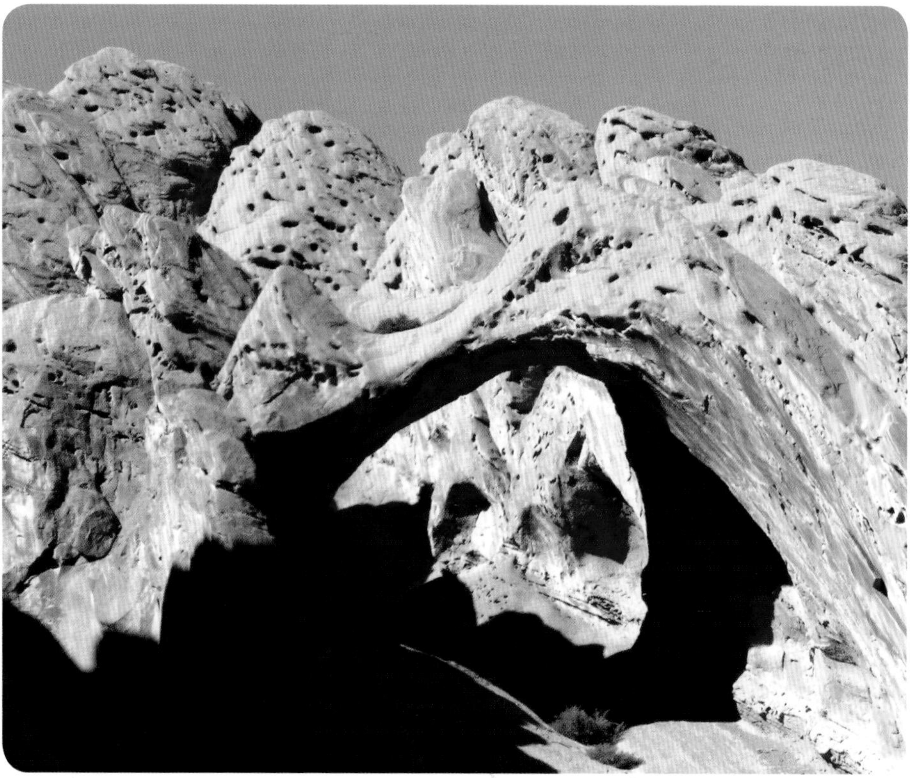

Saddle Arch

Following cairns, ascend the canyon's right (east) wall to the **crest of the Waterpocket Fold**. Then bear right along the crest and follow it generally south-southeast. Proceed over the Rim Route **highpoint**: 6640 ft (2024 m).

The view is panoramic. North are white Navajo sandstone domes in the heart of Capitol Reef National Park. East, paralleling the Fold, is the broad valley known as *Grand Gulch*. (This is not the Grand Gulch on Cedar Mesa, described in Trip 75). West, beyond Upper Muley Twist Canyon, is a massive expanse of Wingate sandstone eroded into myriad shapes.

Near 7.3 mi (11.7 km) be alert for a sign directing you to the **Canyon Route**. Following cairns, descend right (west)—over ledges, across slickrock—into Upper Muley Twist Canyon. Reach the **wash** beneath **Saddle Arch** at 7.6 mi (12.2 km). You're now on familiar ground. Follow the wash generally south-southeast 1.8 mi (2.9 km) to the **4WD trailhead** or, if you didn't park there, another 2.4 mi (3.9 km) to the **2WD trailhead**.

TRIP 36

SPRING CANYON

LOCATION	Capitol Reef National Park
DISTANCE	9.7 mi (15.6 km) one way
ELEVATION CHANGE	250-ft (76-m) gain, 1070-ft (326-m) loss
KEY ELEVATIONS	Chimney Rock trailhead 6050 ft (1845 m) highpoint near Chimney Rock 6300 ft (1920 m) Chimney / Spring canyons confluence 5880 ft (1793 m) Fremont River 5230 ft (1595 m)
HIKING TIME	4 to 6 hours
DIFFICULTY	moderate
MAP	Trails Illustrated *Fish Lake North / Capitol Reef*

OPINION

Walking, observing, simply being. That's enough. It's wealth and fulfillment. But our obsession with trivia and our mania for progress conspire to deny us this refreshing, meditative state. Only in a new setting—someplace extraordinarily strange or beautiful—might we spontaneously step out of the conga line to disillusionment and become human beings rather than human doings.

Spring Canyon is such a place: an exotic, soothing enclave where walking, observing, simply being, is rapturous. Its length, depth and grace rank it among the most magnificent chasms on the Colorado Plateau, along with Paria (Trip 12), Escalante (Trip 28), and Grand Gulch (Trip 75). Yet Spring Canyon is much easier to hike than most. In less than a full day, you can pierce the heart of it.

If you must choose only one hike in Capitol Reef National Park, make it this one or Navajo Knobs (Trip 37). The two are opposites. In Spring Canyon you'll go deep, following a narrow, sandy wash strewn with volcanic boulders between sheer, sandstone walls. En route to Navajo Knobs you'll get high, traversing slickrock ledges while overlooking much of the park. Intimate vs. vast. Mysterious vs. grand. The yin and yang of canyon country.

Spring Canyon runs 23 mi (37 km) from the east shoulder of Thousand Lakes Mtn, through the Waterpocket Fold, to the Fremont River. It's usually dry for most of its length. You'll face only two obstacles—both minor compared to the serious challenges most canyons heave at you.

The first obstacle is about a third of the way along, where you must bypass a pouroff via a narrow trail on a steep, loose slope (acrophobes beware). The second obstacle is a ford of the knee- to thigh-deep Fremont River at the conclusion of the hike. Neither will faze experienced hikers. Yet these obstacles do suggest that north to south is the optimal direction for this one-way shuttle trip.

You'll be leaving a car near the canyon mouth, where the trip ends, so it's convenient to check the ford and make sure it's safe before driving to the trailhead and hiking all the way down-canyon to the river. As for the pouroff bypass, if anyone in your party finds it daunting, it's close enough to the trailhead that turning back is a reasonable option.

So the hike begins with short-but-engaging descent of Chimney Rock Canyon. Where it intersects Spring Canyon, you can choose to explore its upper or lower sections. Following our directions, you'll descend Lower Spring Canyon—impressively narrow, and short enough to dayhike. Upper Spring Canyon soon broadens, so it's less engaging. It's also about twice as long—ideal for a one-night backpack trip.

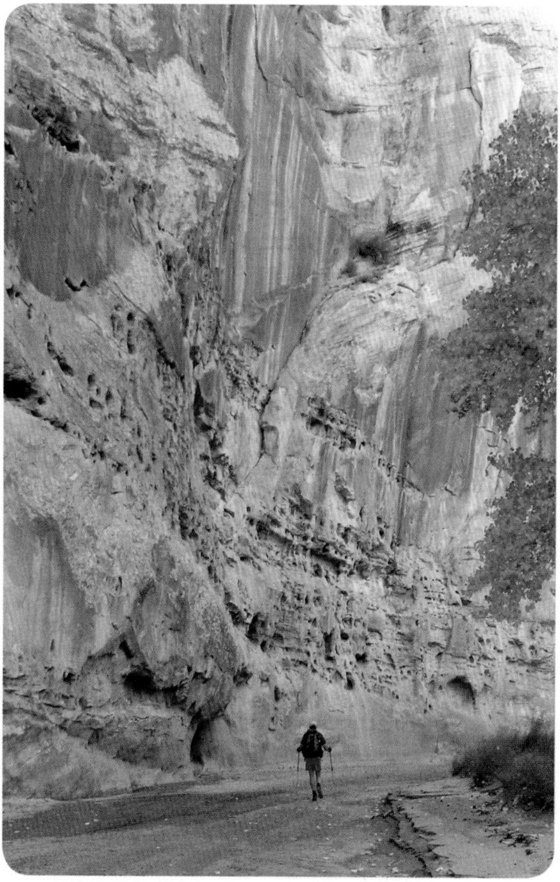

Lower Spring Canyon (also see inside front cover)

FACT

BEFORE YOUR TRIP

Expect to find no water en route. Carry more than you'll need for the entire trip: at least three quarts (liters) per person.

All deep, narrow canyons, regardless how easy to enter, are dangerous. Even distant rain can cause an overwhelming volume of water to suddenly rush through them. Hike here only during a period of sunny weather, when there's little risk of a flashflood. Check the forecast at the nearby visitor center.

If backpacking the upper *and* lower sections of the canyon, go to the park visitor center. Get a backcountry camping permit and a printed description of the route (starting on Holt Draw road just west of the park boundary).

BY VEHICLE

Fremont River trailhead

From the Capitol Reef National Park visitor center, turn right onto Hwy 24 and drive generally east-southeast 3.7 mi (6 km) to the roadside pullouts (both sides) east of milepost 83, at 5230 ft (1595 m). The Fremont River parallels the left

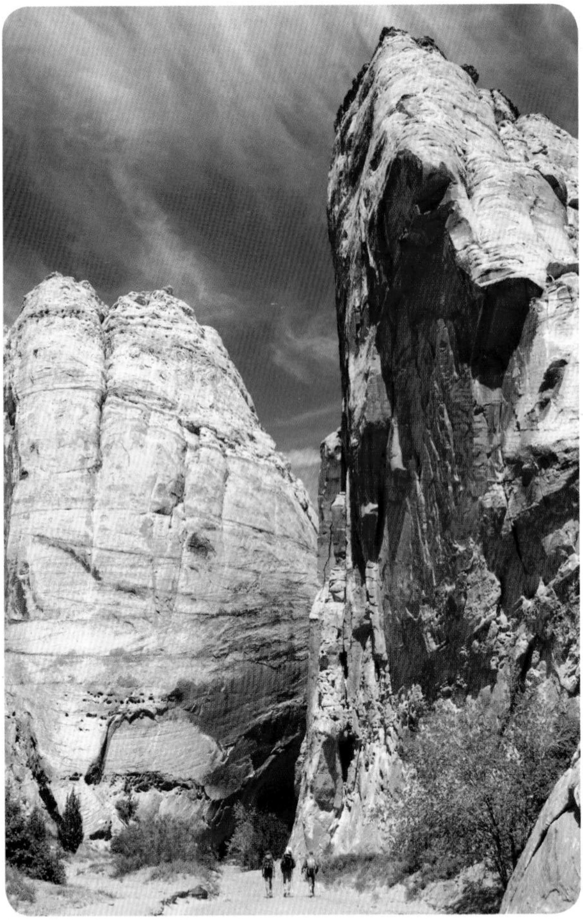
Spring Canyon

(north) side of the highway. After checking the flow to make sure fording will be safe, leave your shuttle vehicle here, where the one-way trip ends.

Chimney Rock trailhead

From the Capitol Reef National Park visitor center, turn left onto Hwy 24 and drive generally northwest 2.9 mi (4.7 km) to the paved Chimney Rock trailhead parking lot on the right (northeast) at 6050 ft (1845 m). Begin hiking here.

ON FOOT

The trail departs the far (north-northeast) end of the trailhead. It gradually curves east around the north side of Chimney Rock.

Soon begin a switchbacking ascent. Reach a junction at 0.5 mi (0.8 km), 6300 ft (1920 m). Right is the Chimney Rock loop, a detour which later rejoins the main trail. Go left and continue generally east.

Aspiring geologists, take note. On this relatively short hike, you'll witness six rock strata: Moenkopi (Chimney Rock itself), Shinarump, Chinle, Wingate and Kayenta walls in the canyon depths, then Navajo sandstone near the Fremont River.

About 20 minutes from the trailhead, at 1.2 mi (1.9 km), 6140 ft (1872 m), reach the next junction. The Chimney Rock loop ascends right (east-southeast) and curves 1 mi (1.6 km) back to the previous junction. For Spring Canyon, go left (northeast) and drop into the wash.

Follow cairns and fragments of bootbeaten path generally northeast along the gently descending wash-bottom. About 45 minutes from the trailhead, bear right (east), passing two tributary drainages (left / northwest). You're in **Chimney Rock Canyon**—a 50-yd/m wide corridor of sheer, 400-ft (122-m) Wingate sandstone cliffs streaked with charcoal, brown, and metallic-purple desert varnish.

At 2.8 mi (4.5 km), 5880 ft (1793 m), about an hour from the trailhead, arrive at the **confluence of Chimney Rock and Spring canyons**. Go right (east) to descend Lower Spring Canyon to the Fremont River and Hwy 24. Left is Upper Spring Canyon. One mile (1.6 km) in that direction (generally north, then northwest) is the canyon's namesake spring, in a cottonwood-camouflaged alcove on the right.

In **Lower Spring Canyon**, your general direction of travel is southeast. At 4 mi (6.4 km) the canyon walls are broken and the floor is scattered with boulders. At 4.6 mi (7.4 km), 5720 ft (1744 m), about 30 minutes from the confluence, easy passage is interrupted by a **pouroff in the narrows**, where the inner canyon constricts dramatically.

For fun, follow the wash bottom into the constriction and peer over the lip of the pouroff. Then walk back to where you can clamber onto the slickrock above and follow the **bypass route**. It contours five minutes along the left (northeast) wall. Beyond the pouroff, the route is a narrow-but-adequate path bootbeaten into steep sand. It then broadens on more solid ground and gradually drops to the canyon floor. Resume hiking generally southeast.

Near its mouth, the canyon widens, and the walls are white-and-mustard Navajo sandstone. Reach the north bank of the **Fremont River** at 9.7 mi (15.6 km). Hwy 24 is immediately beyond. Strong, determined hikers arrive here within four hours of departing Chimney Rock trailhead.

At normal flow, the river is only about 18 inches deep here, so fording should be easy. But be cautious anyway. On the far bank, thrash through the vegetation to the highway, where your shuttle vehicle awaits.

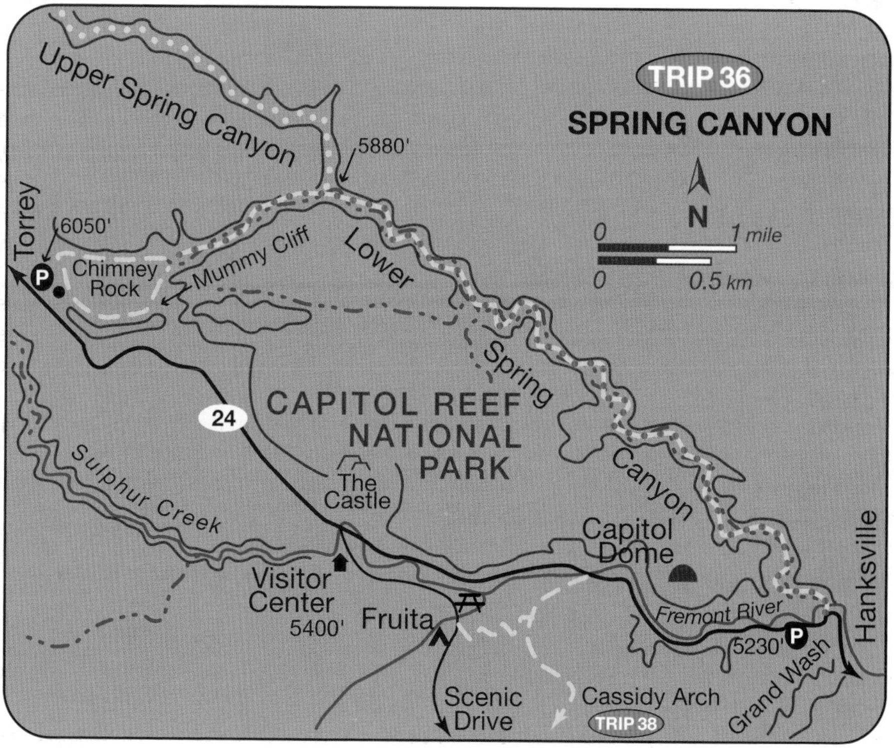

TRIP 37

NAVAJO KNOBS

LOCATION	Capitol Reef National Park
ROUND TRIP	4.5 mi (7.2 km) to Rim Overlook 9 mi (14.5 km) to Navajo Knobs
ELEVATION GAIN	1100 ft (335 m) to Rim Overlook 2500 ft (762 m) to Navajo Knobs
KEY ELEVATIONS	trailhead 5350 ft (1631 m) Rim Overlook 6400 ft (1951 m) Navajo Knobs 6980 ft (2128 m)
HIKING TIME	3 to 5 hours
DIFFICULTY	moderate
MAP	Trails Illustrated *Fish Lake North / Capitol Reef*

OPINION

Down and in. That's generally the way forward when exploring canyon country. But not this time. The hike to Navajo Knobs is up and out.

Starting on trail, continuing on a cairned route, you'll ascend from the Fremont River to the canyon rim high above the Capitol Reef visitor center.

Because you'll mostly be on broad, gently-ramping slickrock ledges where precise foot placement is unnecessary, your eyes will be free to roam across an ever-widening panorama.

By the time you surmount the Navajo sandstone knobs at route's end, this wonderful national park will seem even bigger than the Utah state map suggests. And you'll have witnessed far more of its startling variety than do most of the park's relatively small number of visitors, many of whom drive straight through or stop only for a picnic beneath the cottonwoods.

Of all the nearby trails, this one's the best for appreciating the Waterpocket Fold—the 100-mi (161-km) long wrinkle in the Earth's crust that the park enshrines.

The fold is where massive layers of sediment were deposited in seas, tidal flats, deserts, and other environments that evolved here hundreds of millions of years ago. They were folded during an episode of regional mountain building, then began eroding away. What remains is only a hint of the ancient fold's enormity.

Yet the fold is still a marvel, as you'll see from Navajo Knobs. The elevation change from the fold's upper reaches near Torrey (west) and its lower edge near Hanksville (east) is 2,500 ft (762 m).

Hiking to the knobs is, in our opinion, one of the two most desirable options for serious striders visiting Capitol Reef. The other is Spring Canyon (Trip 36). If you must choose between them, because you have only one day in the park, ask yourself: Do I want depth, or altitude?

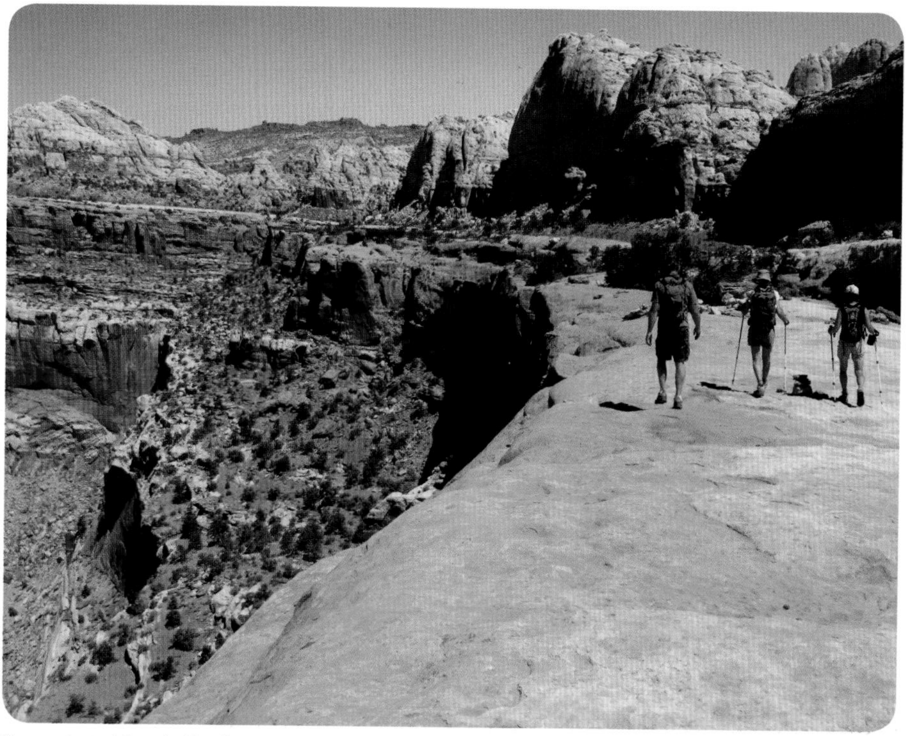
En route to Navajo Knobs

FACT

BEFORE YOUR TRIP

Expect to find no water en route. Carry more than you'll need for the entire hike: at least three quarts (liters) per person.

BY VEHICLE

From the junction of Hwys 24 and 12, on the east edge of Torrey, drive Hwy 24 east. Pass the Capitol Reef National Park visitor center at 10 mi (16.2 km). At 12 mi (19.3 km) turn left (north) into the paved Hickman Natural Bridge trailhead parking lot beside the Fremont River, at 5350 ft (1631 m).

From the junction of Hwy 24 and the Notom Road, at the signed east entry to Capitol Reef National Park just west of milepost 89, drive Hwy 24 west 7.1 mi (11.5 km). Turn right (north) into the paved Hickman Natural Bridge trailhead parking lot beside the Fremont River, at 5350 ft (1631 m).

ON FOOT

Follow the trail downstream (east) along the Fremont River.

In seven minutes, at 0.25 mi (0.4 km), 5490 ft (1675 m), reach a junction. Left (west-northwest) detours to **Hickman Bridge** (skip below for details). Go right (north-northeast) for Rim Overlook and Navajo Knobs. Capitol Dome is nearby east.

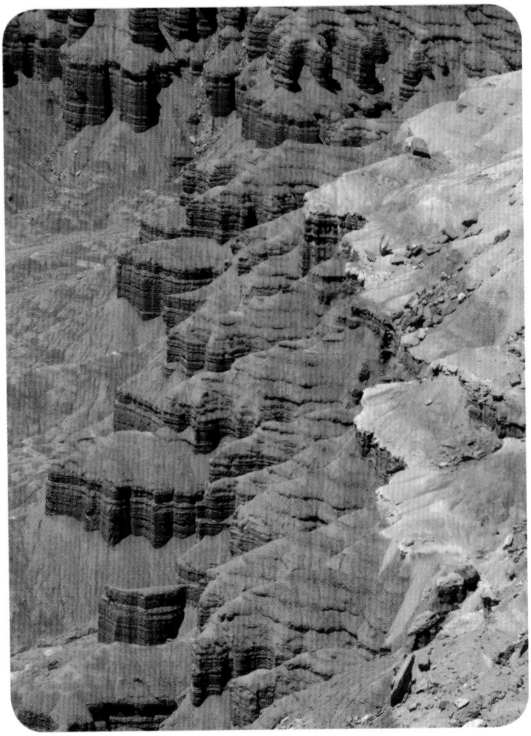
Below Navajo Knobs

Proceed among volcanic boulders. Cross a wash. Curve northwest. At 0.6 mi (1 km), 5680 ft (1732 m), about 25 minutes from the trailhead, reach **Hickman Bridge overlook**. Go left about 30 yd/m off trail to see the bridge spanning a wash below (southwest). From here, you can also see where you'll be hiking: around the sheer point farther west.

Swerve in and out of two box canyons, the second of which drains beneath Hickman Bridge. After ascending out of the second wash, hike through sand among scattered shrubs and trees. The sand is from the Navajo sandstone cliffs above—former sand dunes that were pressed into stone ages ago and are slowly decomposing into sand once again.

Heading generally west, bend in and out of two more drainages. Attain a view of the Golden Throne (southeast) and the Henry Mountains beyond. Follow cairns across slickrock, ramping higher. About an hour from the trailhead, reach **Rim Overlook** at 2.25 mi (3.6 km), 6400 ft (1951 m).

Directly below the cliffs you're standing atop are the visitor center, the Fruita orchards, and the Fremont River, which cuts through the Waterpocket Fold, ventures east into the San Rafael Desert, joins the Dirty Devil River, and ultimately feeds Lake Powell. Dominating the southwest horizon is rounded, forested, 10,908-ft (3326-m) Boulder Mtn. Thousand Lakes Plateau is northwest.

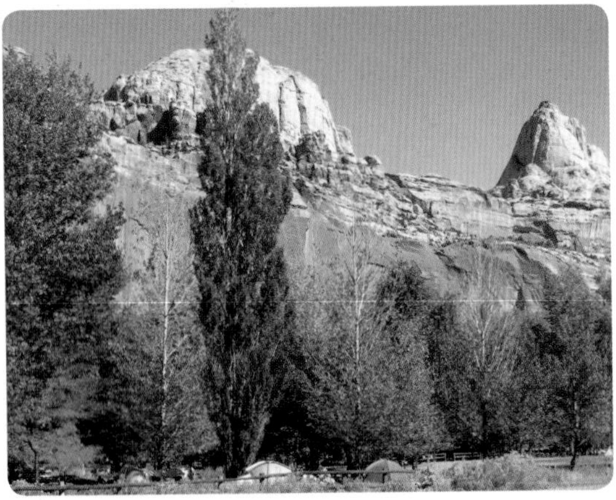
Fruita campground, Capitol Reef

Descending past the overlook, within a minute follow cairns left toward the edge, then hike north. Quickly lose and regain 100 ft (30.5 m). About 15 minutes beyond the overlook, reach the base of a slickrock peninsula topped with a communications gizmo at 6530 ft (1991 m). Drop into the next bay and proceed generally north.

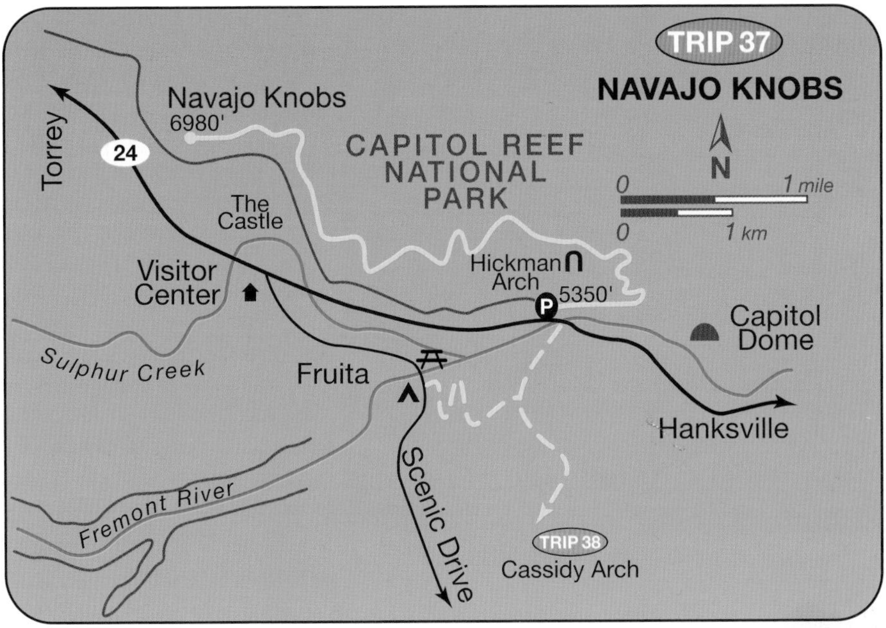

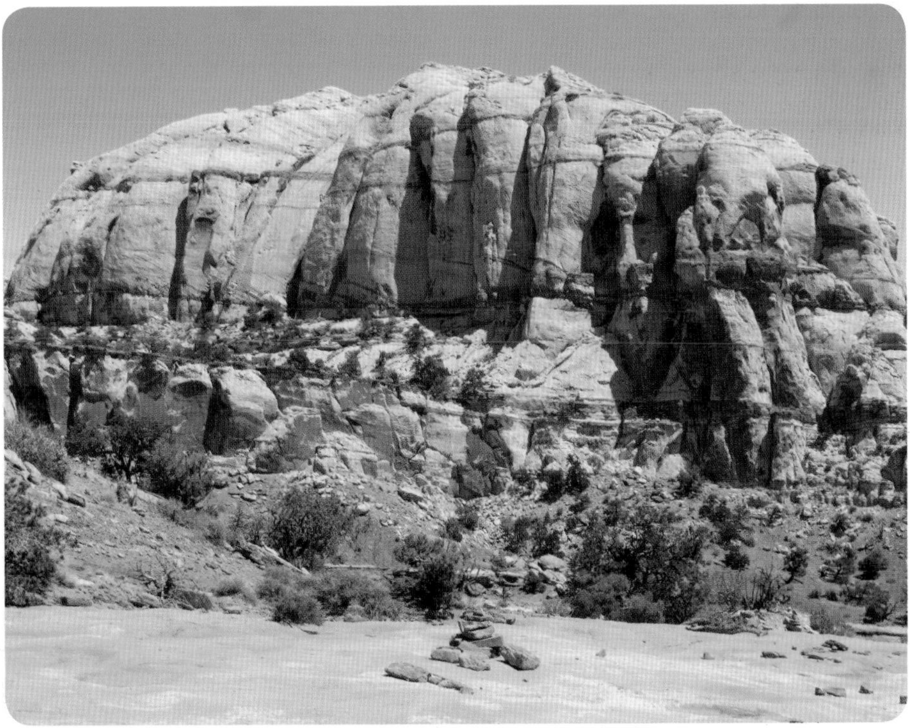

En route to Navajo Knobs

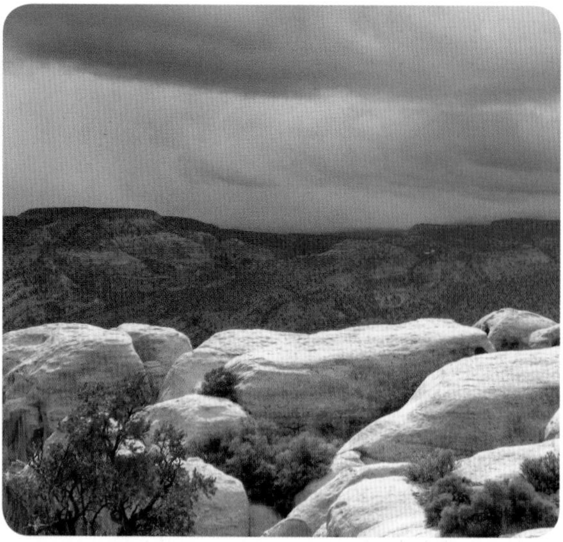

Storm over Boulder Mountain, from Navajo Knobs

About 25 minutes from the overlook, reach the head of the bay at 6315 ft (1925 m). Now ascend left (west). The route twice loses and regains 40 ft (12 m). Finally, about 40 minutes from the overlook, approach **Navajo Knobs**. Your goal, the top of the promontory, is visible ahead.

Just five minutes farther, you're facing the final knob. Go right, cross the peninsula, then follow the cairned route corkscrewing upward. It's steep, but easy and safe. Crest the **summit** at 4.5 mi (7.2 km), 6980 ft (2128 m).

Detour to Hickman Bridge

From the junction on the main trail, 0.25 mi (0.4 km) from the trailhead, go left (west-northwest). Ascend open slopes scattered with volcanic boulders. Cross a minor wash. Proceed generally west. Where the trail splits at 0.5 mi (0.8 km), 5600 ft (1707 m), bear right. Cross slickrock above the wash to arrive at the Navajo sandstone bridge. Elevation: 5650 ft (1723 m). It stands 125 ft (38 m) high, and the span between abutments is 133 ft (41 m). Resuming the circuit, soon reach familiar ground and retrace your steps. Upon intersecting the main trail, you've completed a 0.75-mi (1.2-km) circuit.

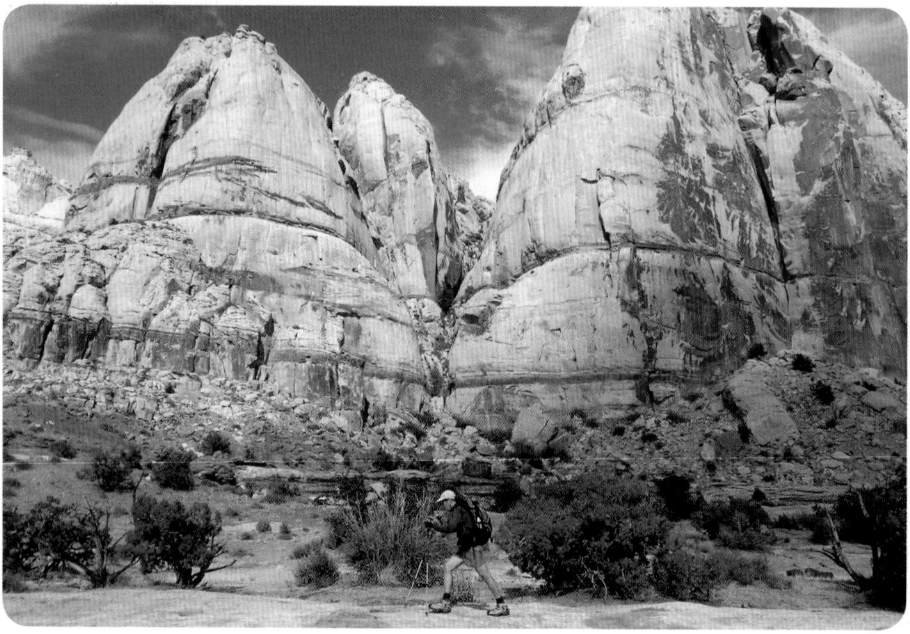

En route to Navajo Knobs

TRIP 38

COHAB CANYON / CASSIDY ARCH / GRAND WASH

LOCATION	Capitol Reef National Park
DISTANCE	6.3 mi (10.1 km) one way to Grand Wash 8.1 mi (13 km) one way through Grand Wash 9.2-mi (14.8-km) round trip to Cassidy Arch
ELEVATION CHANGE	1545-ft (471-m) gain, 1565-ft (477-m) loss to Grand Wash 1545-ft (471-m) gain, 1765-ft (538-m) loss through Grand Wash 2530-ft (771-m) gain and loss to/from Cassidy Arch
KEY ELEVATIONS	Fruita trailhead 5440 ft (1659 m) Frying Pan trail highpoint 6450 ft (1966 m) Cassidy Arch 6000 ft (1829 m), Grand Wash / Scenic Drive trailhead 5400 ft (1646 m) Grand Wash / Hwy 24 trailhead 5200 ft (1585 m)
HIKING TIME	3 to 5 hours
DIFFICULTY	moderate
MAP	Trails Illustrated *Fish Lake North / Capitol Reef*

OPINION

Science and history do not make the Earth interesting any more than a beard and robe make God powerful.

Cohab Canyon to Grand Wash via Cassidy Arch is an enthralling trek, regardless how little you know about the land underfoot and its former residents.

But science and history are piquant spices. So here are two facts—one scientific, the other historic—that might spark your desire to hike here and fire your mind en route:

(1) This is the heart of the Waterpocket Fold—a 100-mi (161-km) long monoclinal flexure in the planet's upper crust. A monocline is a kink in otherwise uniformly horizontal rock. Monoclines are characteristic of the Colorado Plateau. The Fold was kinked by the collision of tectonic plates deep in the Pacific Ocean, off the west coast of North America. The impact, though distant, was sufficiently powerful to send violent tremors rippling far into the continent and uplift the Fold. It's among the longest, continuously exposed monoclines in the world. And it comprises an astonishing array of bizarre landforms made of brilliantly colored sedimentary strata, including arches, natural bridges, slot canyons, monoliths, cathedrals, hogbacks, fins, and domes. You'll see most of them on this hike.

(2) Cassidy Arch is named after Butch, the famous outlaw, who eluded his would-be captors in this incomprehensibly tortuous terrain. Before him, Mormon polygamists, known as *cohabs*, took refuge here in the 1880s, when polygamy was a felony and they were pursued by U.S. marshals. The specific notch in which they secreted themselves, Cohab Canyon, is barely recognizable even when in view from the river plain below. As for the Frying Pan trail—which you'll follow between Cohab Canyon and Grand Wash—perhaps it refers

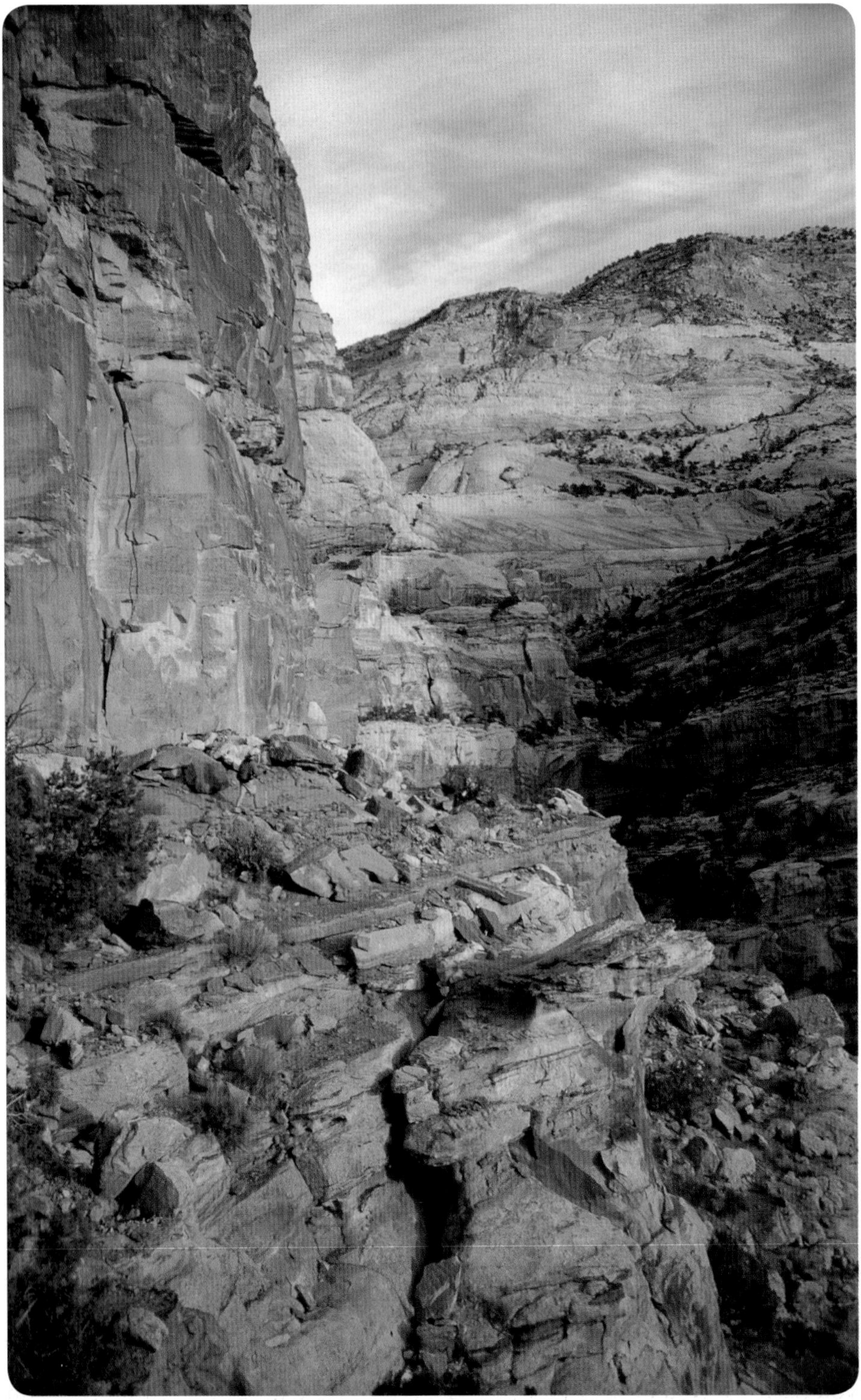

The Frying Pan trail descends into Grand Wash.

to the intense sun, soaring temperatures and endless heat-radiating rock that can make hiking here in summer not just uncomfortable but dangerous.

Starting at the Fruita trailhead, fast hikers can probe Cohab Canyon, follow the Frying Pan trail to Cassidy Arch, and return to Fruita within four hours but should allow more time to admire the constantly engaging scenery and frequent panoramas.

Ideally, hike one way from Fruita, past Cassidy Arch, through Grand Wash, to Hwy 24. If you prefer not to hitchhike, you'll need to arrange a two-vehicle shuttle. If you lack a shuttle slave or buddies with a second vehicle, look for some capable, willing hikers at the Fruita campground, introduce yourself, and propose they join you.

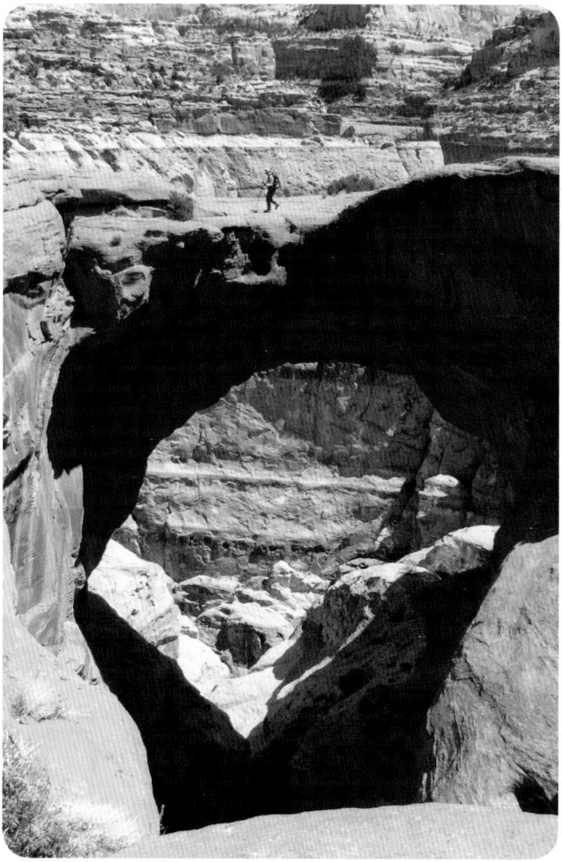

Cassidy Arch

Starting at the Grand Wash / Scenic Drive trailhead, Cassidy Arch is a mere 3.4-mi (5.5-km) round trip gaining 680 ft (207 m), but we don't recommend it. The vantage points just above Cohab Canyon are a more rewarding destination for a short, easy hike. We also prefer entering Cohab Canyon from Fruita, rather than from the Hickman Bridge trailhead on Hwy 24, because the ascent from Fruita affords instantly vast views.

FACT

BEFORE YOUR TRIP

Expect to find no water en route. Carry more than you'll need for the entire trip: at least three quarts (liters) per person.

BY VEHICLE

From Torrey, drive Hwy 24 east into the national park. At 11 mi (17.7 km) turn right (southeast) onto Scenic Drive.

From Hanksville, drive Hwy 24 west. Reset your trip odometer to 0 when you pass the Notom road (left / south) and enter the national park. At 8.7 mi

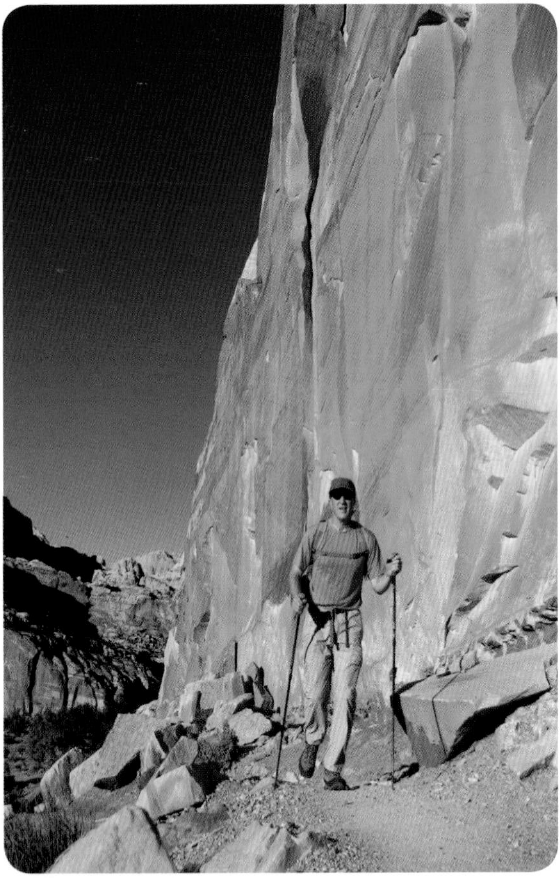
Cohab Canyon trail

(14 km) turn left (southeast) onto Scenic Drive.

From either approach, drive 1 mi (1.7 km) past the visitor center and turn right into the Fruita trailhead parking lot immediately before the historic Gifford farmhouse and beside the Fremont River. Whether hiking a round trip or one way, begin here, at 5440 ft (1659 m).

Grand Wash trailhead on Scenic Drive

Hiking one way *to* Grand Wash? Continue following Scenic Drive another 2.3 mi (3.7 km) south. Turn left (northeast) onto the unpaved spur. Proceed 1.2 mi (1.9 km) to the Grand Wash trailhead parking area at road's end. Elevation: 5400 ft (1646 m). Leave your shuttle vehicle here, where the one-way trip ends.

Grand Wash trailhead on Hwy 24

Hiking one way *through* Grand Wash? Return past the visitor center to Hwy 24. Reset your trip odometer to 0, turn right, and drive east. At 4.4 mi (7.1 km) reach a pullout on the right (west), near the mouth of Grand Wash. Elevation: 5200 ft (1585 m). Leave your shuttle vehicle here, where the one-way trip ends.

ON FOOT

From the Fruita trailhead parking lot, walk south beside Scenic Drive. Pass the farmhouse and barn. The signed trail departs the left (east) side of the road, shortly before the campground entrance on the right (west).

Initially head southeast then immediately switchback left (northeast). The trail ascends Chinle slopes dramatically punctuated with basalt boulders. About eight minutes along, at 5770 ft (1759 m), briefly contour south beneath 200-ft (61-m) Wingate cliffs. Soon reach the hanging rift known as **Cohab Canyon**.

The trail turns left (east) and gently drops into the canyon. The bulbous, tan and orange walls are intricately sculpted. Follow the sandy wash about 0.25 mi (0.4 km) among piñon pine and juniper. The canyon broadens. Follow cairns across slickrock on the left (north-northwest) side.

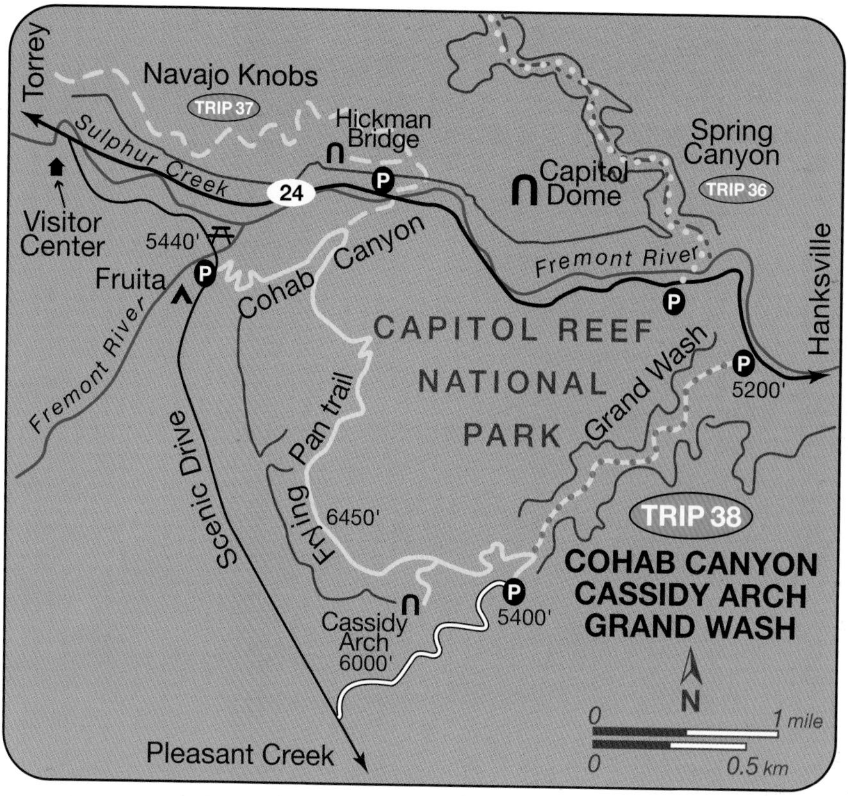

Reach a signed junction at 1 mi (1.6 km), 5620 ft (1713 m). The spur ascending left (northwest) leads 0.3 mi (0.5 km) and 0.5 mi (0.8 km) to **vantage points** overlooking Fremont River Canyon and Fruita. They're worthwhile, but the scenery en route to Cassidy Arch is superior. Proceed northeast down Cohab Canyon.

Dip into the wash then rise to another signed junction at 1.1 mi (1.8 km), 5642 ft (1720 m). Left (east) arrives at Hickman Bridge trailhead on Hwy 24 in 0.6 mi (1 km). For Cassidy Arch and Grand Wash turn right (southwest) onto the **Frying Pan trail**.

After a moderate ascent, crest a broad, 5950-ft (1814-m) **saddle** nearly an hour from the trailhead. Visible north to northwest, on the far side of Fremont River Canyon, are the slickrock ledges ramping up to Navajo Knobs (Trip 37). Continuing to Cassidy Arch, follow cairns east toward a prominent **standing rock**, skirt left of it, then drop to a **second saddle** at 5895 ft (1797 m).

South, below this second saddle, is a deep, wide chasm. Visible left (southeast) are the sheer walls of Grand Wash. Study the far wall of the chasm. You'll soon be traversing that wall, ascending from left to right, ultimately cresting the gap just left of the knob directly south.

But first you must plunge into the chasm. From the second saddle, descend the sandy trail / cairned route generally southeast. Bottom-out in the wash at 5685 ft (1733 m), cross south, then begin a long ascent following cairns generally south-southwest among piñon and juniper on Kayenta sandstone ledges.

Top-out on the ridgecrest at 3.5 mi (5.6 km). This is the Frying Pan trail's 6450-ft (1966-m) **highpoint**. The panorama comprises countless sandstone

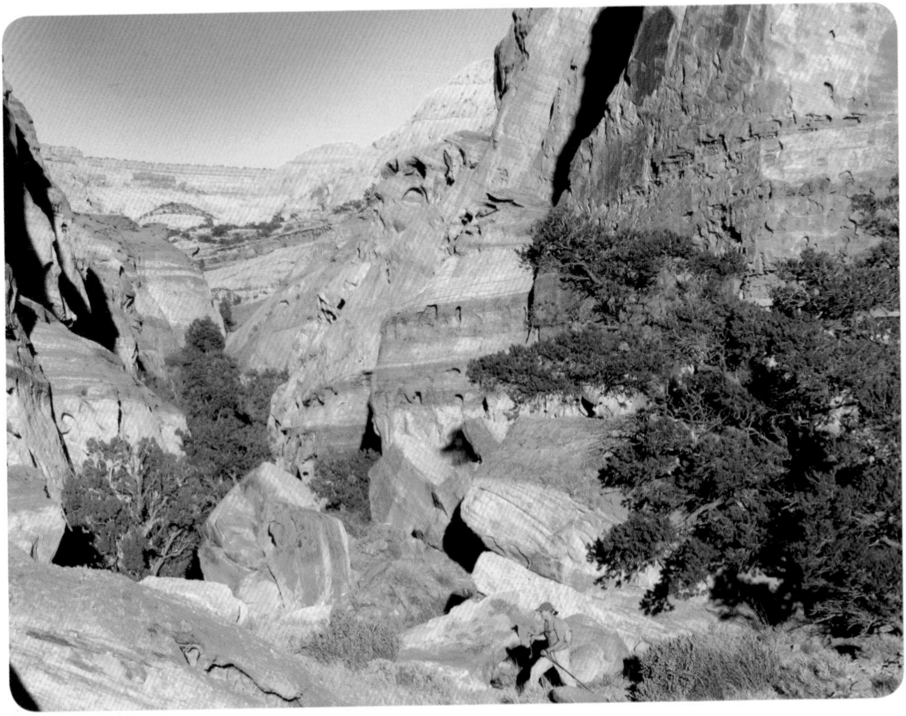
Cohab Canyon

domes. Fern's Nipple is southeast. Boulder Mtn is southwest. Thousand Lakes Plateau is northwest. The ensuing descent gradually curves east.

The route approaches a cliff at 4 mi (6.4 km). Visible 600 ft (183 m) below is the road in Grand Wash. At 4.2 mi (6.4 km), 5980 ft (1823 m), reach a signed junction. Straight (east) continues descending to Grand Wash. Right (southwest) detours to Cassidy Arch.

The 0.8-mi (1.3-km) round trip to **Cassidy Arch** takes only about 20 minutes. From the main trail, follow the cairned spur across slickrock to where the arch spans a 200-ft (61-m) deep cavity.

Back on the main trail, either turn left (west) to retrace your steps back to the Fruita trailhead and complete a round trip, or turn right and descend east into Grand Wash to complete a one way trip.

Resuming the eastward descent, soon skirt the rim and peer 360 ft (110 m) into Grand Wash. After swerving left (north), the trail curves right (southeast). Ledges and switchbacks eventually deliver you to the 5400-ft (1646-m) floor of **Grand Wash** at 5.3 mi (8.5 km), or 6.1 mi (9.8 km) including the arch detour.

If you're ending your one-way hike at the **Grand Wash / Scenic Drive** trailhead, go right (south) 0.2 mi (0.3 km) to the parking lot at 6.3 mi (10.1 km).

If you're continuing through Grand Wash, go left (north-northeast) and proceed deeper into the canyon, where the Navajo sandstone walls rise 600 to 800 ft (183 to 244 m).

At 6.9 mi (11.1 km) enter **The Narrows**—a 0.5-mi (0.8-km) corridor only 20 ft (6.1 m) wide. Beyond, the canyon broadens and the walls diminish. Reach the **Grand Wash / Hwy 24 trailhead**, where your one-way hike ends, at 8.1 mi (13 km), 5200 ft (1585 m).

TRIP 39

GOLDEN THRONE

LOCATION	Capitol Reef National Park
ROUND TRIP	4 mi (6.4 km)
ELEVATION GAIN	700 ft (213 m)
KEY ELEVATIONS	trailhead 5400 ft (1646 m) trail's end 6100 ft (1860 m)
HIKING TIME	1½ to 2½ hours
DIFFICULTY	easy
MAP	Trails Illustrated *Fish Lake North / Capitol Reef*

OPINION

Capitol Reef National Park enshrines a long, narrow, north-south trending, dramatically tilted sandstone swell: the Waterpocket Fold. Pioneers called it a "reef" because it impeded travel much the way barrier reefs obstructed sailors. And one of the reef's prominent geologic features is a golden-white slickrock dome resembling the U.S. Capitol building's rotunda. Hence the name *Capitol Reef.*

Within the park, however, are dozens of features as distinctive as Capitol Dome. One is the Golden Throne—a flaxen-hued, horizon-dominating, smooth-walled monolith jutting 1000 ft (305 m) skyward from its sandstone base. Like everything else in canyon country, it's the result of intense erosion. The Throne was originally part of a spacious plateau, which the elements whittled down to a mesa then further chiseled into a solitary butte.

The Golden Throne trail is short, not terribly steep, but fascinating to hike. En route to a superb vantage of the Throne, it climbs atop the Waterpocket Fold and grants vistas across a magnificently contorted wilderness.

The optimal time to be here is late afternoon, when the Throne is most photogenic. That's also when Scenic Drive, which leads to the trailhead, is likely to fulfill its promise. The sun, sinking in the west, bathes the nearby escarpments in low-angle light that intensifies their red, pink, mauve, orange, and mustard tones.

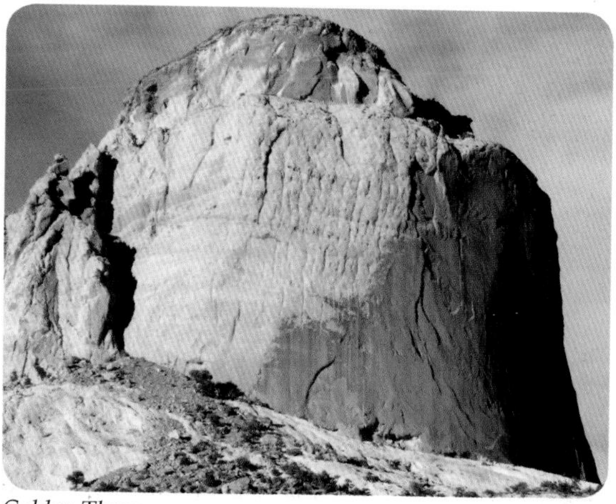

Golden Throne

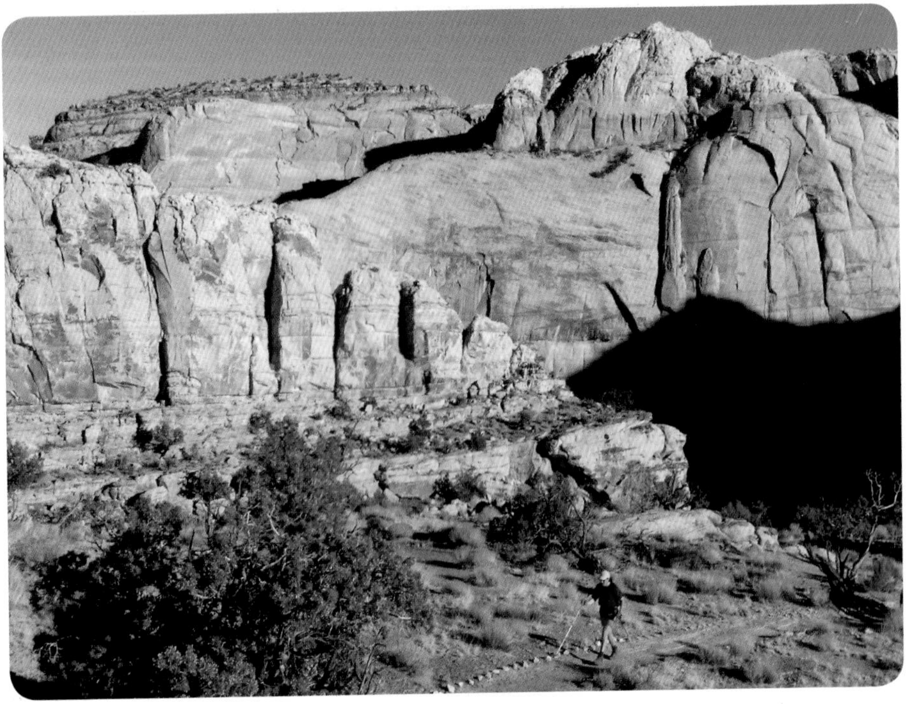

En route to Golden Throne

FACT

BY VEHICLE

From Torrey, drive Hwy 24 east into the national park. At 11 mi (17.7 km) turn right (southeast) onto Scenic Drive.

From Hanksville, drive Hwy 24 west. Reset your trip odometer to 0 when you pass the Notom road (left / south) and enter the national park. At 8.7 mi (14 km) turn left (southeast) onto Scenic Drive.

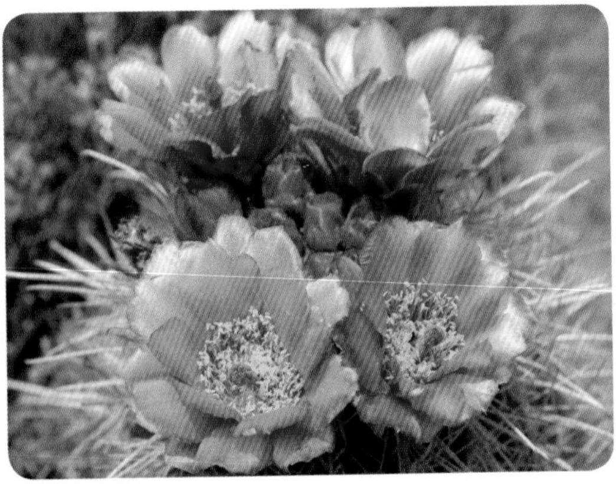

Fishhook cactus, April

From either approach, drive 7.8 mi (12.6 km) past the visitor center and turn left (west) onto the unpaved spur. Proceed 2.2 mi (3.5 km) to the Capitol Gorge trailhead parking area at road's end. Elevation: 5400 ft (1646 m).

ON FOOT

The trail departs the west end of the parking area and ascends beneath overhanging

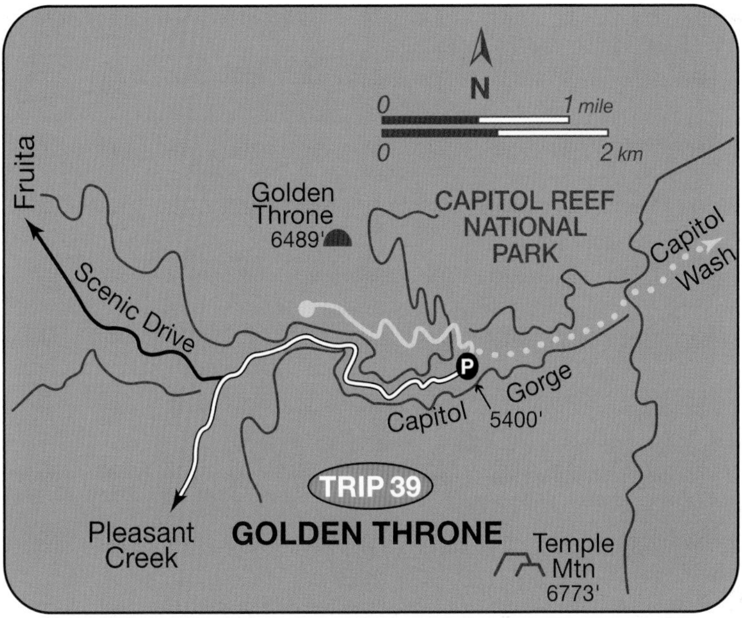

Kayenta sandstone. Across slickrock, it's lined with stones.

About five minutes along, at 5600 ft (1707 m), curve right (north) into the first of three tributary drainages. Piñon pine and juniper grace the rocky ledges. At 1 mi (1.6 km), turning into the third drainage, the Golden Throne's southeast face is visible. Switchback out of the third drainage to cross a low ridge and head northwest. Boulder Mtn is visible west.

At 2 mi (3.2 km), 6100 ft (1860 m), about 45 minutes along, the trail ends 0.5 mi (0.8 km) shy of the **Golden Throne**, which soars 1000 ft (305 m) from its sandstone base. Capitol Gorge is visible below. The Henry Mtns dominate the eastern horizon.

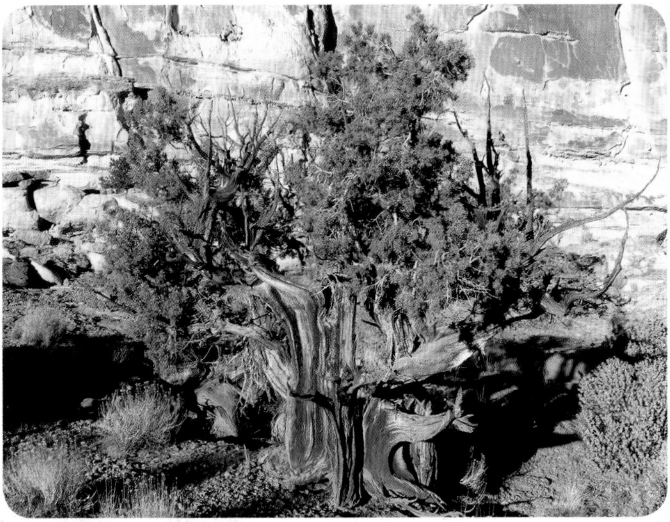

Utah juniper

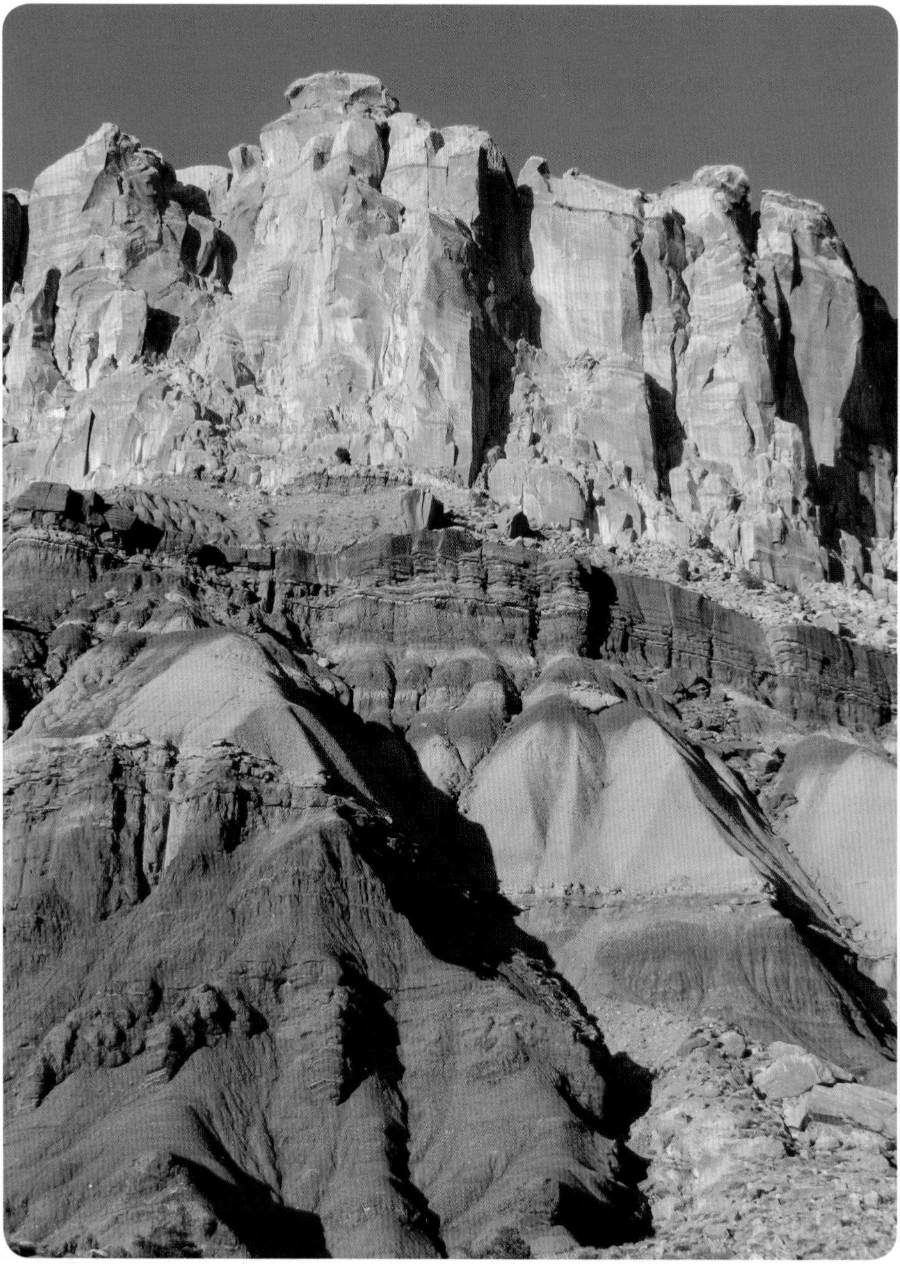

Capitol Reef National Park

TRIP 40

SHEETS GULCH

LOCATION	Capitol Reef National Park, Notom Road
ROUND TRIP	4 mi (6.4 km) or more
ELEVATION GAIN	250 ft (76 m)
KEY ELEVATIONS	trailhead 5200 ft (1585 m) one-hour turnaround point 5450 ft (1662 m)
HIKING TIME	2 hours or more
DIFFICULTY	moderate
MAPS	Trails Illustrated *Capitol Reef National Park* USGS *Sandy Creek Benches*

OPINION

The less you know, the more adventure.

Tossed against that rock-hard truth, guidebooks fall to the ground in a flutter of useless paper. They do make hiking less adventurous. It's also true, however, that few of us are capable of grappling with that hairy, merciless beast *The Unknown*. So we turn to guidebooks as a way of attacking it in short, easy-to-win skirmishes rather than a single, savage battle we're sure to lose.

Use guidebooks enough, and you'll develop the skills and confidence to forge your own route into the wilderness and, more important, find your way out again—with all your parts intact.

So a truly helpful guidebook should, upon escorting you to trail's end, sometimes point you beyond. And, at a few opportune moments, it should throw away the tether, withhold the bread crumbs, turn you loose, and simply say "That way."

Here's one of those moments.

The east side of the extraordinary Waterpocket Fold (see Trip 38 for a detailed description) has numerous slot-like, Navajo sandstone defiles. Though trail-less, all invite freelance exploration and will reward even a short, tentative inquiry. Just follow them into the Fold, then continue along the wash or atop the slickrock ledges as far as you please.

Where a pool, muddy quagmire, pouroff or chokestone prohibits passage, look for an up-and-out bypass. Skirt the obstacle, then seek a route back into the ravine. Just stay within your comfort zone. If you're deeply hesitant, trust your instinct: turn back. But first, stop, sit, and appreciate the tranquility and complexity surrounding you.

We recommend you start with Sheets Gulch. Consider probing it the evening before or the morning after you hike nearby Upper Muley Twist (Trip 35).

FACT

BEFORE YOUR TRIP

Stop at the Capitol Reef National Park Visitor Center. Check the current weather report, ask about the condition of the Notom Road, and see if they have a recent field report on Sheets Gulch.

All deep, narrow canyons, regardless how easy to enter, are dangerous. Even distant rain can cause an overwhelming volume of water to suddenly rush through them. Hike here only during a period of sunny weather, when there's little risk of a flashflood.

Sheets Gulch might be dry but will likely contain muddy pools, so amphibious footwear is preferable. Wear technical sandals designed for hiking, or fabric hiking boots you don't mind dunking. Insulating neoprene socks will ensure wet feet ≠ frigid feet.

Even if Sheets Gulch contains water, it will require filtering and / or purifying. Spend your time exploring instead. Carry all the drinking water you'll need.

BY VEHICLE

From the Capitol Reef National Park Visitor Center, drive Hwy 24 east 8.7 mi (14 km). From Hanksville, at the junction of Hwys 95 and 24, drive Hwy 24 west 28.4 mi (45.7 km).

From either approach, upon reaching the junction of Hwy 24 and the Notom Road, at the signed east entry to Capitol Reef National Park, turn south onto the Notom Road and reset your trip odometer to 0.

Pavement ends at 5 mi (8.1 km). Cross Burro Wash at 7.8 mi (12.5 km), Cottonwood Wash at 9 mi (14.5 km), and Fivemile Wash at 10 mi (16.2 km).

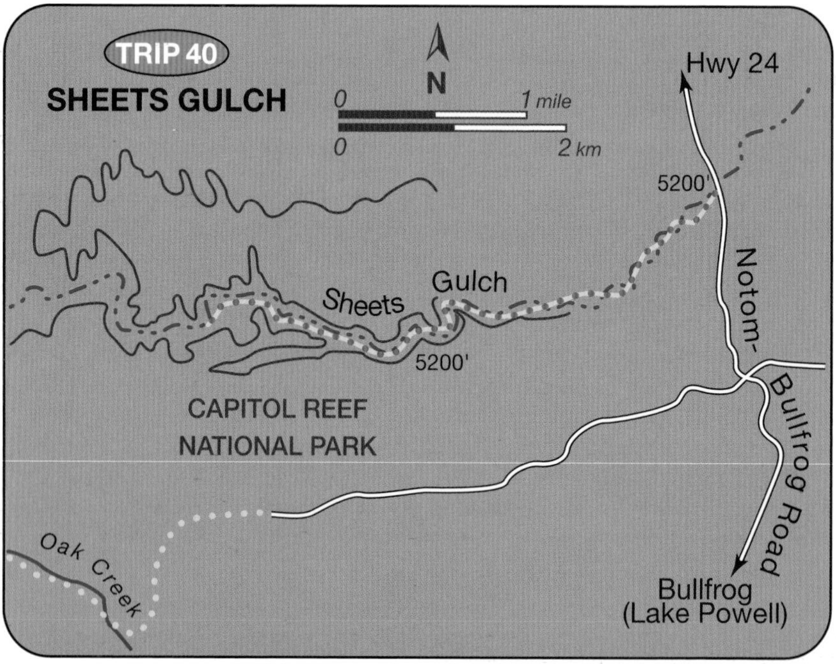

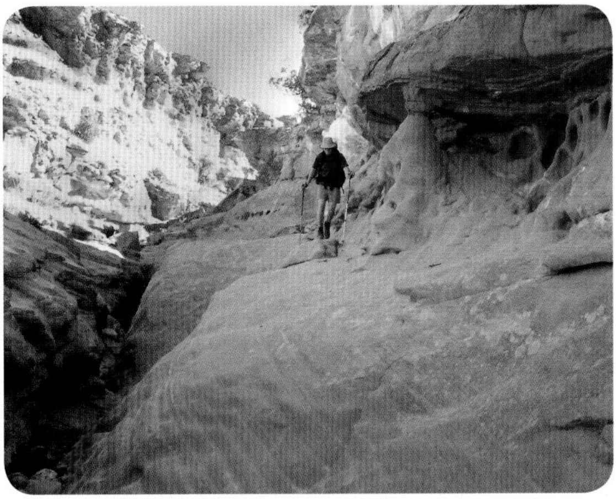
Sheets Gulch

At 13.2 mi (21.2 km) cross the wash draining Sheets Gulch. There's no traihead parking area, so pull off the road nearby, at 5200 ft (1585 m).

ON FOOT

Following the primary wash, hike west, toward the Reef. At 1 mi (1.6 km), 5260 ft (1604 m), about 25 minutes along, the wash forks. Left leads southwest. Go right (west) into the deeper drainage rimmed by hanging ledges. A minute farther, bypass a pool by ascending left, onto a ledge, then resume in the wash.

Shortly beyond, the wash slots up, will likely contain a muddy pool, and ahead is blocked by a chokestone. Cairns (left / south) suggest a bypass route via broken ledges. Above, follow the dirt path 30 seconds to a rounded, slickrock ledge allowing re-entry. Carefully descend, then resume in the wash.

After hiking about 50 minutes from the Notom Road, you should be near 1.75 mi (2.4 km), 5420 ft (1652 m). Here the gravel-floored wash is about 25 ft (8 m) wide and 60 ft (18 m) deep, but it soon constricts again.

Proceed up Sheets Gulch—along the wash and/or above the rim—as far as curiosity, energy, time, and ability allow. Most hikers will probably reach at least 2 mi (3.2 km), 5450 ft (1662 m), which is about a two-hour round trip from the Notom Road.

At 3.5 mi (5.6 km), it's necessary to negotiate a significant pouroff. A competent scrambler can manage it unaided, but it's safer and easier if two or more help each other.

At 4.5 mi (7.2 km) arrive at a high pouroff in a cavernous chamber. Bypass it by retreating 110 yd (100 m) and exiting the left (south) side of the wash. Ahead, the walls of Sheets Gulch change from white Navajo sandstone to red Wingate sandstone.

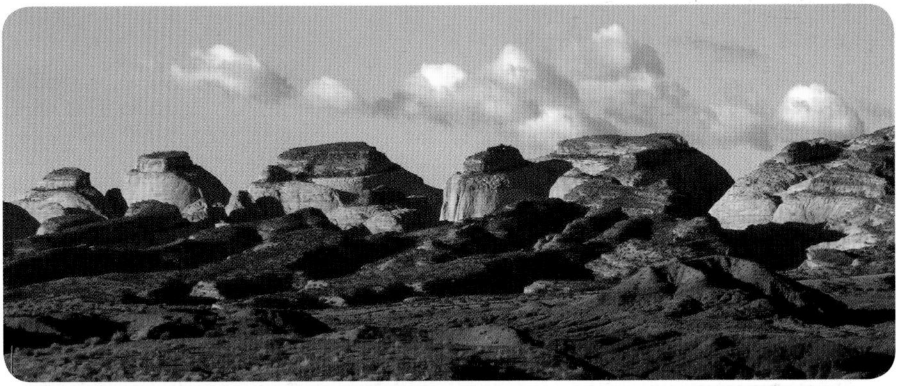
Capitol Reef National Park, from the Notom Road

TRIP 41

GOBLIN VALLEY

LOCATION	southwest of Green River, north of Hanksville
DISTANCE	3-mi (4.8-km) loop for Entrada & Curtis 1.5-mi (2.4-km) loop for Molly's & Carmel 8 mi (13 km) for both plus recommended extensions
ELEVATION GAIN	275 ft (84 m) for both loops plus recommended extensions
KEY ELEVATIONS	trailhead 5200 ft (1585 m), Curtis Bench 5280 ft (1610 m) Goblin Valley floor 5150 ft (1570 m) Molly's Castle viewpoint 5155 ft (1572 m)
HIKING TIME	1 to 5 hours
DIFFICULTY	easy
MAP	Goblin Valley State Park brochure (free, available at entry station)

OPINION

When Utah was an inland sea, 170 million years ago, debris washed down from highlands and accumulated on a vast tidal flat. After the sea retreated, rain and wind gradually sculpted the debris into thousands of bizarre, spherical shapes.

But we don't call this place "Debris Lands," or "Ancient Tidal Flat," or "Entrada Sandstone Valley" after the primary component of the debris. Though geologically correct, such a name would be worse than boring. It would disavow the magic that's afoot here.

Even the pedantic state legislators agreed to call it "Goblin Valley," enshrining not the scientific reality of the place but instead an imaginative interpretation of it. So let your right brain rule while visiting Goblin Valley State Park. Trust your most creatively inspired response to what you see.

Our response? These aren't boulders that resemble living beings. They're living beings that resemble boulders. Halloween fantasy goblins? Nah. That's prosaic. These are genuine golems.

According to Jewish legend, a golem is a creature made of clay, brought to life by an incantation from a holy person, someone intimately close to God. A golem lacks the gift of speech and possesses only a simple mind fixated on performing whatever task its creator requests of it.

Too outrageous? Okay, here's a more practical yet still lively explanation: This is Utah's boulder hatchery. The state's wilderness-area authorities come here to choose whatever size and shape boulders they need for the lands they manage. No matter how many they haul away, the valley just keeps giving birth to more.

Ponder your unique vision of Goblin Valley while hiking the short trail network or wandering at will, preferably both.

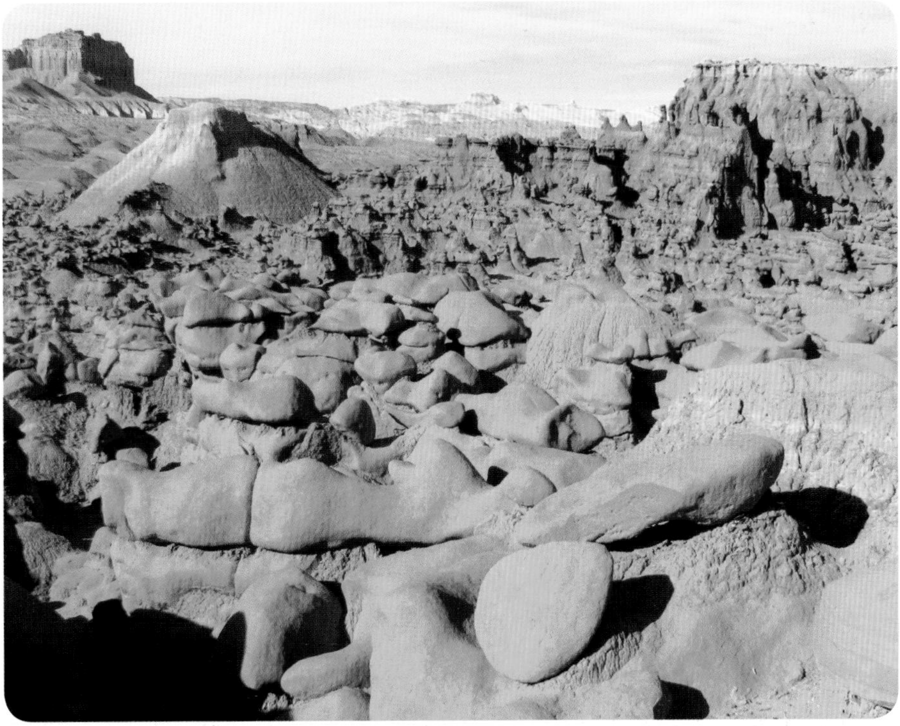

Goblin Valley. Wild Horse Butte distant left.

The Entrada Canyon trail follows a shallow, serpentine drainage (dramamine anyone?) beneath intriguing formations. It intersects the Curtis Bench trail, which grants a panorama of the goblins then funnels you into their midst. These two trails form a loop, but you can and should detour off it for some fun, easy, very rewarding cross-country exploration.

The Molly's Castle / Carmel Canyon trail veers away from the goblins. It affords a close look at the castle-like sandstone mountain that guards them, invites you to investigate the surrounding desert, then leads to a narrow ravine that wiggles back up to the trailhead.

The optimal Goblin Valley hike begins on the Entrada Canyon trail and continues on the Curtis Bench trail. After a tantalizing overview of the goblins, fork off the bench and descend into the valley proper. Then, before looping back to the trailhead, roam south among the goblins.

The map in the state-park brochure suggests there are three Goblin valleys. It labels them 1, 2, and 3. The truth is, there's only one valley, and it's relatively small. You can, however, mentally divide it into three sections: upper (near the Observation Point trailhead parking lot), middle (which you can descend into from Curtis Bench), and lower (the south end of the valley, farthest from the trailhead).

There are no established trails in the valley proper. That's because they're unnecessary and would curtail your enjoyment. The valley is so short and shallow that the trailhead is often visible from the upper and middle sections. Only in the valley's lower reaches will you lose sight of the trailhead for long. Stay alert to your surroundings and you're unlikely to get lost. Losing your way should be impossible if you carry a compass; simply follow the level valley floor north until the trailhead is again in sight.

In general, while exploring the south end of the valley, work your way up the drainages toward the vertical eastern wall. Go as far as your curiosity and the topography allow, then exit the way you entered. Countless route possibilities will keep enthusiastic explorers intrigued for hours.

After returning to the trailhead, if you're keen to sample more of the area, hike the Molly's Castle / Carmel Canyon loop. It's short, scenic, interesting, but the Entrada / Curtis / Goblins hike is superior.

FACT

BEFORE YOUR TRIP

The Goblin Valley campground is excellent: isolated, picturesque, surprisingly well-equipped. It even has hot showers. And each campsite has a sheltering ramada. Base yourself here for Trips 42, 43, and 44, all of which are nearby.

BY VEHICLE

From Green River, drive I-70 west 11.2 mi (18 km). Turn south onto Hwy 24 and continue another 23.6 mi (38 km). From Hanksville, drive Hwy 24 north 19 mi (30.6 km). From either approach, turn west at the sign for Goblin Valley State Park (near milepost 136) and reset your trip odometer to 0.

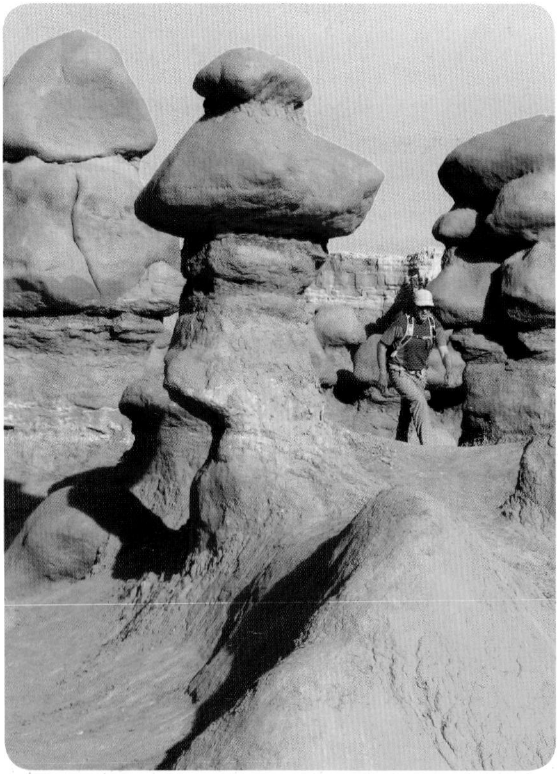

Hoodoos in Goblin Valley

Reach a junction in 5 mi (8.1 km). Straight (northwest) leads to Crack and Chute canyons (Trips 43 and 44) in the San Rafael Swell. For Goblin Valley, turn left (southwest).

Pass the park boundary sign. Reach a junction at 11 mi (17.7 km). The unpaved road right (southwest) leads to Bell and Little Wild Horse canyons (Trip 42). For Goblin Valley, bear left (southeast) on pavement.

Stop and pay the entry fee at 11.3 mi (18.2 km). Reach a T-junction at 11.8 mi (19 km). Right leads to the campground. Go left. (Though the Curtis Bench trail is signed here, this is not where you should access it.)

At 12.4 mi (20 km), 5200 ft (1585 m), enter the road's end trailhead parking lot and reach Observation Point.

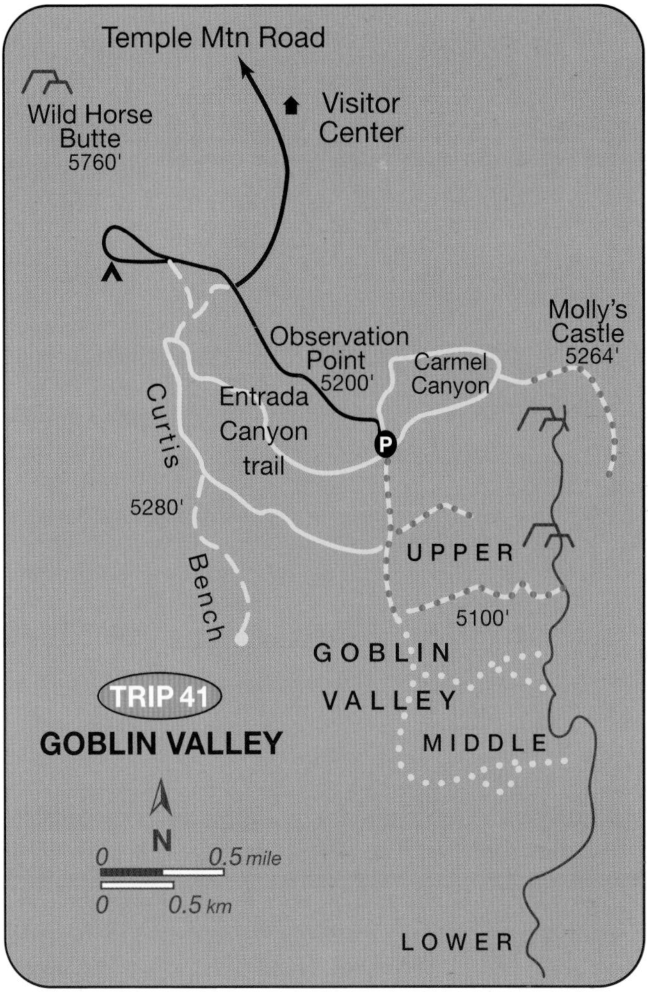

ON FOOT

Entrada Canyon

The signed trail departs the northwest side of the parking lot, between the entrance and the toilets. It initially descends left (southwest) between mounds of pinkish, hardened mud or, to be precise, Entrada sandstone.

The narrow, winding passage between steep slopes is intriguing for the first 15 minutes because it passes numerous goblins.

Within 30 minutes, at 1.2 mi (1.9 km), 5280 ft (1610 m), follow the trail out of the drainage and intersect a signed, unpaved, **service road**. Straight (north-northwest) continues to the campground. Go left (southwest).

Just 50 yd/m farther, fork left (east-southeast), off the road, onto the signed **Curtis Bench trail**.

Curtis Bench

Departing the unpaved service road, initially hike east-southeast. The sandy, rolling terrain is blanketed with tufts of fragile, filament-like Indian ricegrass, and hardy, dark-green, spindle-branched Mormon tea bushes. The Henry Mountains dominate the southern horizon.

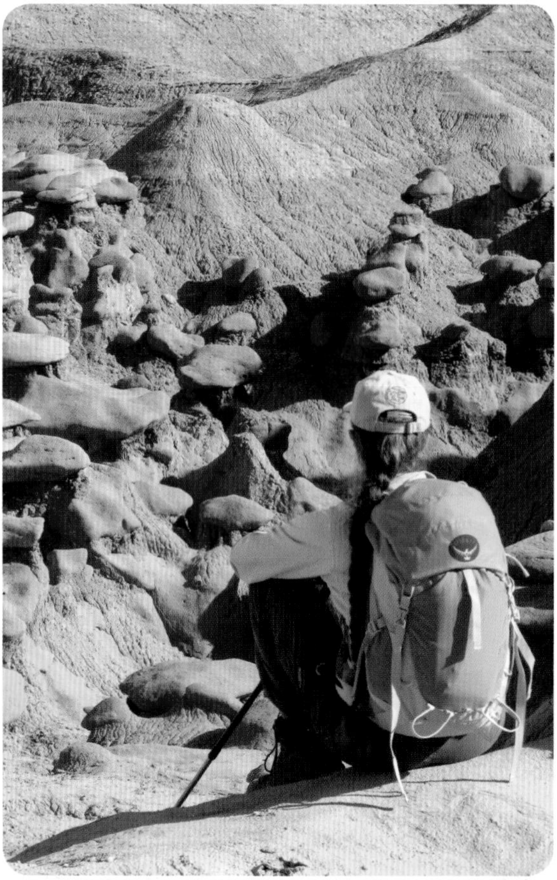
Goblins, from Curtis Bench

In about five minutes, the heart of Goblin Valley is visible east. About ten minutes farther, the trail curves east to a signed **junction** at 1.9 mi (3.1 km), 5280 ft (1610 m). The parking lot is also now in view. A nearby, spacious rock slab invites you to rest and survey the goblin multitudes from an aerial perspective.

From the 1.9-mi (3.1-km) junction, the Curtis Bench trail continues right (southeast) but the scenery does not improve in that direction. Instead, go left (east-southeast) and begin descending to see the goblins up close.

About 20 minutes after departing the 1.9-mi (3.1-km) junction, reach the **floor of Goblin Valley** at 5150 ft (1570 m). You've now hiked 2.6 mi (4.2 km) from the trailhead via Entrada Canyon and Curtis Bench. The parking lot is visible left (north), just 0.4 mi (0.6 km) distant.

Go left (northeast) here to circle back to the parking lot through upper Goblin Valley and complete a 3-mi (4.8-km) loop. Or, ideally, continue hiking south into middle Goblin Valley and perhaps farther south into lower Goblin Valley.

If you proceed into the middle or lower sections of the valley, you'll be freelancing, wandering at will, letting curiosity be your guide. Frequently turn around and note prominent landmarks, so you're always oriented. Stay within your comfort zone. If you get anxious about finding your way back, it's time to head home.

Molly's Castle & Carmel Canyon

The signed trail departs the northeast end of the parking lot (far left as you enter). Initially follow it northeast along a narrow ridge.

Because the trail is convoluted, watch for cairns; they're easier to follow than a written route description. If you don't see a cairn, look for the path bootbeaten into the dirt by the hikers who've preceded you.

In a few minutes, behind the first monolith, turn left (northwest) and descend. Soon reach a **T-junction** in a wash at 5155 ft (1572 m). Left (northwest) leads to Carmel Canyon. For now, go right to reach **Molly's Castle viewpoint** and the end of official trail at 0.75 mi (1.2 km).

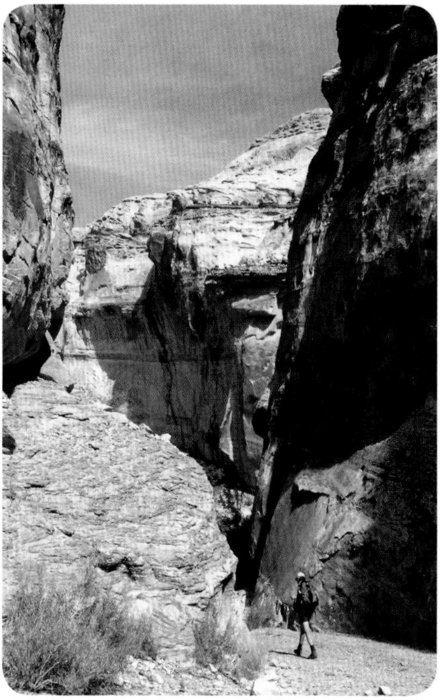

Entering Bell Canyon

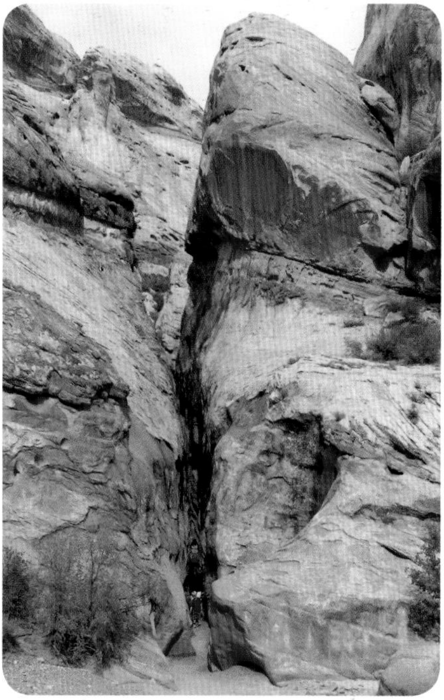

Exiting Little Wild Horse Canyon

If the area's uranium mining history interests you, however, detour left and follow the road west-northwest about eight minutes to an abandoned cabin at the site of the 1950s **Cistern Mine**.

Resuming toward Little Wild Horse Canyon, the road ascends generally north-northeast along the back of the San Rafael Reef. The colors of the eroded layers of rock include charcoal, moss green, mustard, and red.

At 3.5 mi (5.6 km) reach the 5660-ft (1726-m) **highpoint** between canyons, at the far (north) end of the circuit. Here the road curves right (east-southeast) around the end of a mauve-and-purple slope beneath a towering cream-and-salmon promontory.

Cross a tributary wash at 4.1 mi (6.6 km). Abandon the road, which ascends out of the wash and curves left (north). Bear right and hike southeast in the wash. Reach the **north end of Little Wild Horse Canyon** at 4.8 mi (7.7 km), 5450 ft (1661 m), about two hours from the trailhead.

The canyon gradually deepens. Pass between giant boulders. Soon enter the **narrows**—a slender sandstone groove so convoluted that, looking ahead, it appears there's no way forward. But each twist leads to another. Where the slot widens, the walls rise to 350 ft (107 m).

At 8.1 mi (13 km), 5030 ft (1534 m), after hiking nearly three-and-a-half-hours, reach the **confluence** with Bell Canyon. You're now on familiar ground. Turn left (southeast) and retrace your steps about 15 minutes to reach the **trailhead** at 8.7 mi (14 km).

TRIP 43

CRACK CANYON

LOCATION	southwest of Green River, north of Hanksville near Goblin Valley State Park
ROUND TRIP	7 mi (11.3 km)
ELEVATION CHANGE	260-ft (79-m) loss and gain
KEY ELEVATIONS	trailhead 5460 ft (1665 m), lowpoint 5200 ft (1585 m)
HIKING TIME	3½ to 4½ hours
DIFFICULTY	easy
MAP	Trails Illustrated *San Rafael Swell*

OPINION

The San Rafael Swell is a tsunami of solid rock. It stretches more than 40 mi (64 km) across the desert. Crack Canyon is one of several intriguing chasms slicing through the Swell's southeast edge—the San Rafael Reef—allowing you to dive into a sandstone sea.

The canyon's colorful, textured walls, three exceptionally narrow passages, and a few minor obstacles requiring gymnastic effort make for an engaging hike.

If you seek answers, you can ponder the mystery of *taffoni*—the holes, pockets and tiny alcoves peppering the canyon walls. If you prefer mystery, you can laugh at such arcane study (taffoni? baloney!) and instead respond imaginatively to nature's whimsical display.

Ideally, explore Crack Canyon and neighboring Chute Canyon (Trip 44) the same day. Car camping near the trailheads here on the back (northwest) side of the Reef is a convenient option.

FACT

BEFORE YOUR TRIP

All slot canyons, regardless how easy to enter, are dangerous, because even distant rain can cause an overwhelming volume of water to suddenly rush through them. Hike here only during a period of sunny weather, when there's little risk of a flashflood. Check the forecast at nearby Goblin Valley State Park.

BY VEHICLE

From Green River, drive I-70 west 11.2 mi (18 km). Turn south onto Hwy 24 and continue another 23.6 mi (38 km). From Hanksville, drive Hwy 24 north 19 mi (30.6 km). From either approach, turn west at the sign for Goblin Valley State Park (near milepost 136) and reset your trip odometer to 0.

Reach a junction in 5 mi (8.1 km). Left (southwest) leads to Bell and Little Wild Horse canyons (Trip 42) and Goblin Valley (Trip 41). Proceed straight (northwest) on Temple Mtn Road. Pavement soon ends.

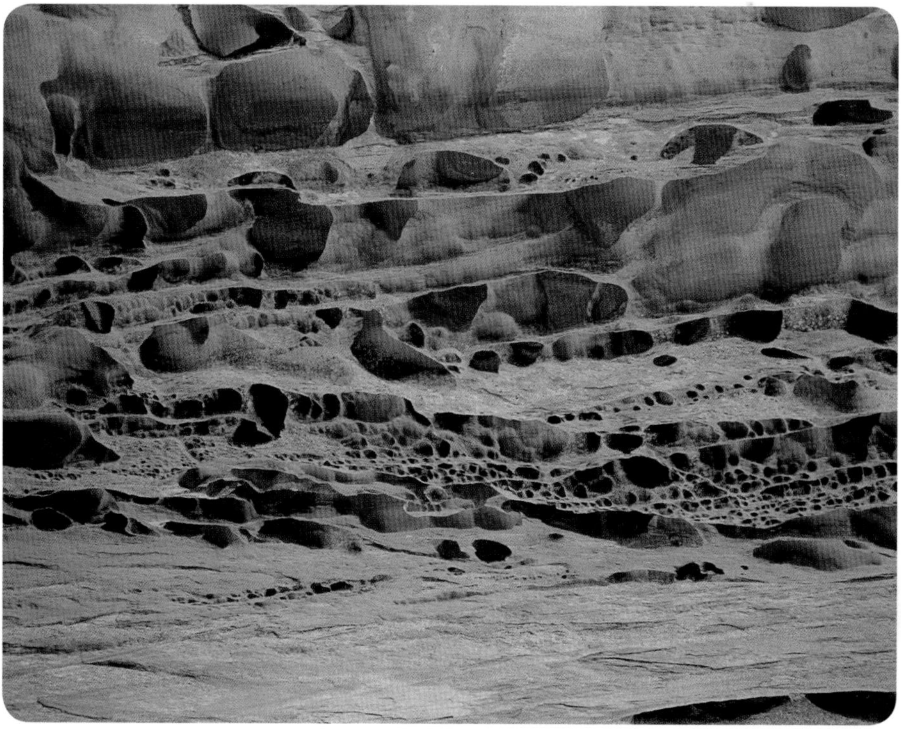

Taffoni in Crack Canyon

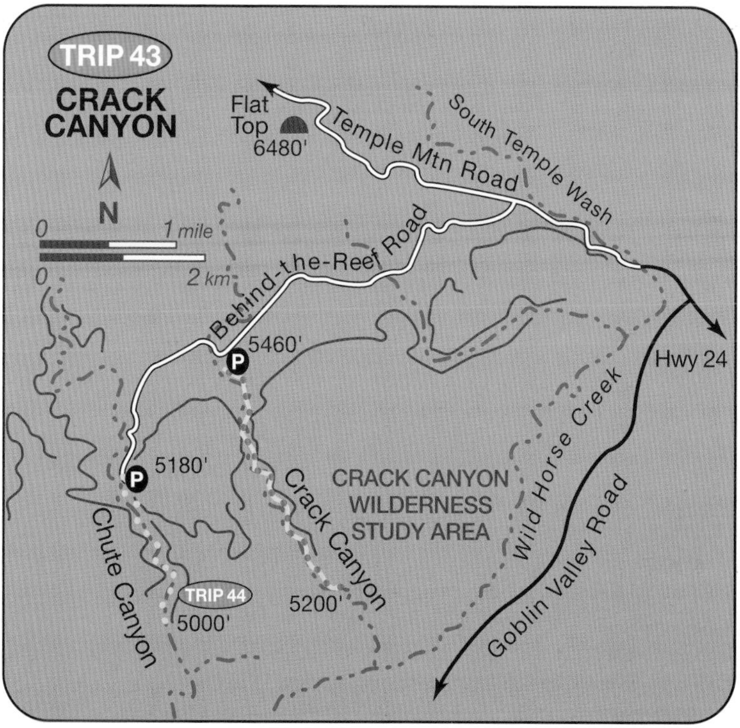

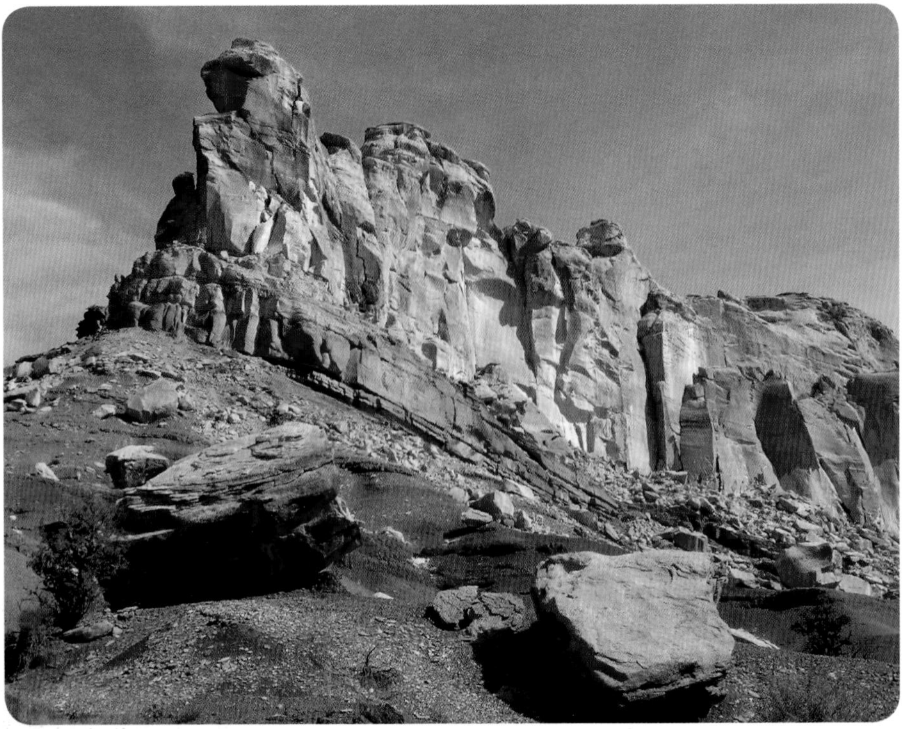

San Rafael Reef, from Behind-the-Reef Road

The sandstone domes ahead (left / west, beyond and above the spacious pullout) afford a couple hours of enjoyable, freelance slickwalking.

At 7 mi (11.3 km), just after the cliffs recede, turn left (southwest) onto Behind-the-Reef Road. At 11.5 mi (18.5 km), where the road bends sharply right, reach the mouth of Crack Canyon. Park here, at 5460 ft (1665 m).

ON FOOT

Go left, in the wash, following a 4WD spur generally south toward the Reef.

At 0.4 mi (0.9 km), about seven minutes along, ignore the ascending right fork. Proceed down-canyon. Cross the rocky wash several times, gradually descending south-southeast.

At 1.6 mi (2.6 km), 5420 ft (1652 m), about 30 minutes along, enter Crack Canyon Wilderness Study Area. Follow the wash into the constricting, deepening canyon. Soon reach a 6-ft (2-m) **pouroff**. It's easy to scoot down the three tiers.

After hiking about 50 minutes, reach a 10-ft (3-m) high chute at 5280 ft (1610 m). It leads to the narrow, **inner gorge** of Navajo sandstone. In this undercut section, the ceiling overhangs the channel 5 to 7 ft (1.5 to 2 m) on each side.

The canyon widens then contracts into a **second narrows**. The **third narrows** is deeper, darker, with towering vertical walls rising above a sand-and-gravel floor.

After 3 mi (4.8 km) the **canyon opens** but continues snaking 0.75 mi (1.2 km) through Kayenta sandstone fins and domes.

Most hikers turn around within 1¾ hours, near 3.5 mi (5.6 km), 5200 ft (1585 m), rather than continue into the featureless San Rafael Desert.

TRIP 44

CHUTE CANYON

LOCATION	southwest of Green River, north of Hanksville near Goblin Valley State Park
ROUND TRIP	4.5 mi (7.2 km)
ELEVATION CHANGE	180-ft (55-m) loss and gain
KEY ELEVATIONS	trailhead 5180 ft (1579 m), lowpoint 5000 ft (1524 m)
HIKING TIME	2 to 3 hours
DIFFICULTY	easy
MAP	Trails Illustrated *San Rafael Swell*

OPINION

Chute Canyon could have been designed by a 17th century European artist. It's positively baroque. Most canyons appear sculpted, which they were. This one is so rich with ornate filigree you might imagine it was decorated instead.

Unlike neighboring Crack Canyon (Trip 43), Chute poses no obstacles. It constricts but doesn't remain astonishingly narrow for long. You can hike through it: traversing the San Rafael Reef, exiting into the San Rafael Desert, perhaps looping back via Crack. But the terrain between the canyons is dull. Probing them individually—on short, in-and-out forays—is quicker, easier, more rewarding.

Thoroughly exploring both Chute and Crack can take most of a day, so consider spending the night here on the back (northwest) side of the Reef, perhaps near the Chute trailhead. It's a peaceful place to car camp, which is ironic given that during the 1940s nearby Temple Mtn was a key source of uranium for one of the most peace-shattering events in human history: the Manhattan Project.

FACT

BEFORE YOUR TRIP

All slot canyons, regardless how easy to enter, are dangerous, because even distant rain can cause an overwhelming volume of water to suddenly rush through them. Hike here only during a period of sunny weather, when there's little risk of a flashflood. Check the forecast at nearby Goblin Valley State Park.

BY VEHICLE

From Green River, drive I-70 west 11.2 mi (18 km). Turn south onto Hwy 24 and continue another 23.6 mi (38 km). From Hanksville, drive Hwy 24 north 19 mi (30.6 km). From either approach, turn west at the sign for Goblin Valley State Park (near milepost 136) and reset your trip odometer to 0.

Reach a junction in 5 mi (8.1 km). Left (southwest) leads to Bell and Little Wild Horse canyons (Trip 42) and Goblin Valley (Trip 41). Proceed straight (northwest) on Temple Mtn Road. Pavement soon ends.

The sandstone domes ahead (left / west, beyond and above the spacious pullout) afford a couple hours of enjoyable, freelance slickwalking.

At 7 mi (11.3 km), just after the cliffs recede, turn left (southwest) onto Behind-the-Reef Road. At 11.5 mi (18.5 km), where the road bends sharply right, pass the mouth of Crack Canyon (Trip 43). At 14 mi (22.5 km) the road deteriorates. Park here, near the cottonwoods, at 5180 ft (1579 m).

ON FOOT

Proceed south on the road. Within 0.5 mi (0.8 km) it gets rougher.

Bear left. Follow the wash generally southeast into the Reef, working around mauve-and-purple Chinle outcrops toward the inner canyon.

In about 20 minutes, the intricately sculpted **canyon constricts** to just 6.5 ft (2 m). Enter Crack Canyon Wilderness Study Area. Pass a sign stating vehicles are prohibited.

In about 45 minutes, reach another short **narrows** where the canyon walls are 12 ft (3.7 m) apart. Continue as far as your energy and curiosity dictate, then retrace your steps.

Most hikers turn around in about one hour, near 2.25 mi (3.6 km), 5000 ft (1524 m), rather than continue through the Reef into the featureless San Rafael Desert.

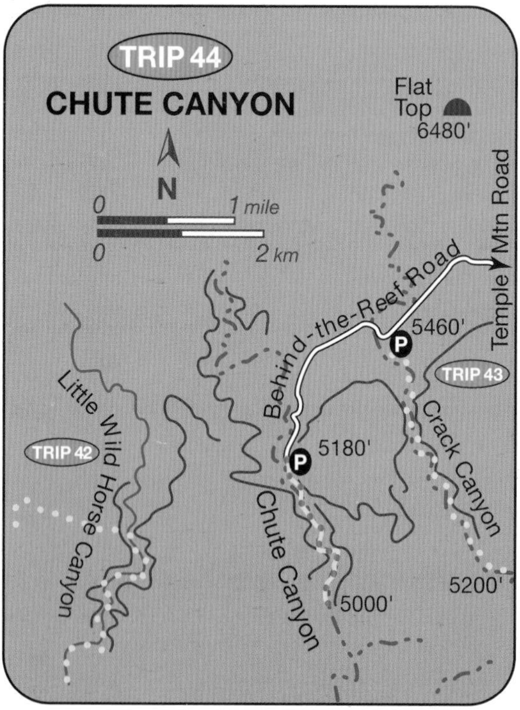

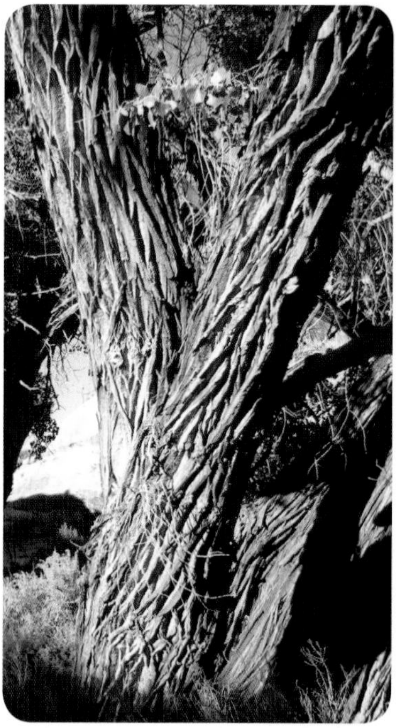

Cottonwood

Chute Canyon

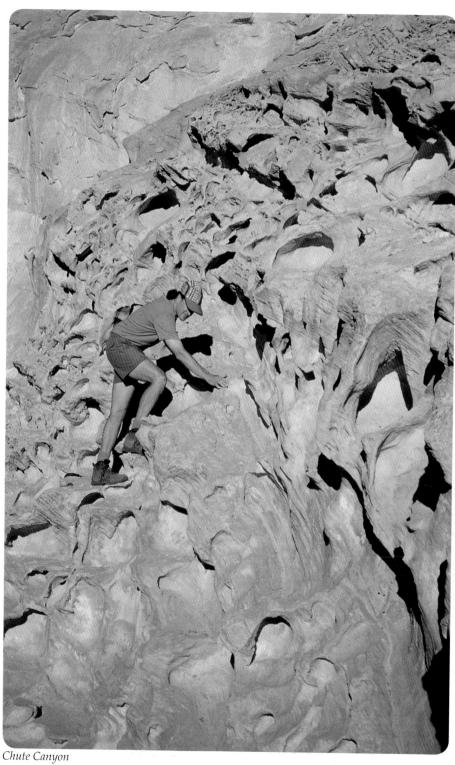

TRIP 45

CHUTE OF MUDDY CREEK

LOCATION	Muddy Creek Wilderness Study Area San Rafael Swell, south of I-70
DISTANCE	one way: 18 mi (28.9 km) round trip: 16 to 18 mi (25.8 to 28.9 km)
ELEVATION CHANGE	one way: 450-ft (137-m) loss, 150-ft (46-m) gain round trip: 250-ft (76-m) loss and gain
KEY ELEVATIONS	Tomsich Butte trailhead 5100 ft (1555 m), south end of the Chute 4850 ft (1478 m), lowpoint beneath Chimney Canyon trailhead 4650 ft (1417 m), Chimney Canyon trailhead 4800 ft (1463 m)
HIKING TIME	7 to 9 hours one way or round trip
DIFFICULTY	challenging due to length
MAPS	Trails Illustrated *San Rafael Swell* USGS *Tomsich Butte, Hunt Draw*

OPINION

It's a big job being curious. In Utah alone there are thousands of canyons to inspect. But this one should be near the top of your list. The Chute of Muddy Creek is fantastic.

The disheartening name is apt. Muddy Creek is even more turbid than most canyon-country watercourses. Drink it, and you'll be chewing before you swallow. So don't. Just walk through it, into the San Rafael Swell's deepest canyon. You'll be chewing on the experience long after.

The canyon, known as *the Chute,* is a classic slot, with colorful, towering, vertical, Coconino-sandstone walls only a few feet apart. Yet this slot poses none of the intimidating technical challenge that spawned the adventure known as *canyoneering*. Here, you don't need a helmet, rope, or climbing skills. All you need is stamina.

It's a long hike—9 mi (14.5 km) to be exact—to the heart of the Chute from either of two trailheads. So whether you arrange a shuttle and hike one way, or opt for an in-and-out round trip, your total distance will be 18 mi (28.9 km). You can shorten that slightly on a round trip, but not much, or you'll miss seeing the canyon's climactic segment.

Following our directions, which begin at the Tomsich Butte trailhead, north of the Chute, it's 6 mi (9.6 km) to where the canyon begins constricting dramatically. The narrows continue 4 mi (6.4 km). So a 16-mi (25.8-km) round trip is the minimum requirement to be fully compensated for your effort.

That's not to say the 6-mi (9.6-km) approach is boring. The canyon is scenic from the start, as you'll see upon arriving at Tomsich Butte. Even the drive *to* the

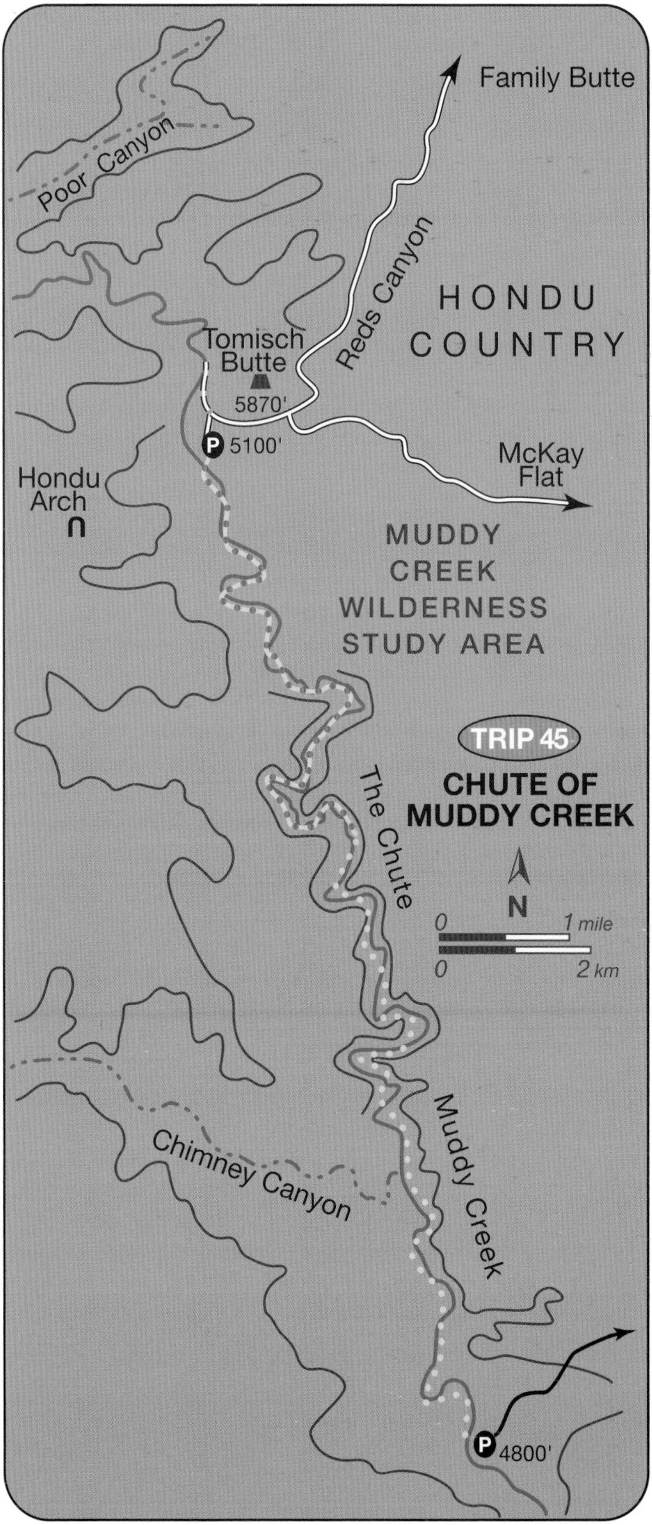
Family Butte
Poor Canyon
Reds Canyon
HONDU COUNTRY
Tomisch Butte
5870'
5100'
McKay Flat
Hondu Arch
MUDDY CREEK WILDERNESS STUDY AREA
TRIP 45
CHUTE OF MUDDY CREEK
The Chute
N
0
1 mile
0
2 km
Muddy Creek
Chimney Canyon
4800'

TRIP 46

BLACK DRAGON

LOCATION	San Rafael Reef, west of Green River northwest of the I-70 / Hwy 24 junction
ROUND TRIP	6.4 mi (10.3 km)
ELEVATION GAIN	1400 ft (427 m)
KEY ELEVATIONS	trailhead 4500 ft (1372 m), highpoint 5800 ft (1768 m)
HIKING TIME	2½ to 3½ hours
DIFFICULTY	moderate
MAP	Trails Illustrated *San Rafael Swell*

OPINION

At some point on every hike in this book you'll set foot on slickrock. It's sandstone, usually Wingate, Kayenta, Navajo, or Entrada. Most canyon-country hikes entail long stretches of slickrock. Many are almost entirely on slickrock. These we call *slickwalks*.

Slickwalking inspires a rapturous sense of freedom. With no vegetation to shunt you this way or that, you can follow your bliss. The rock's gritty surface ("slick" is actually a misnomer) grants extraordinary traction, enabling you to negotiate steep pitches with Spiderman confidence. And the colorful, sensuous, monolithic terrain underfoot, coupled with the constant, unhindered views, make it a beautiful experience.

Opportunities to go slickwalking are unlimited in Utah canyon country, because slickrock is everywhere. Trails? Unnecessary. Trailheads? They're wherever you think you can clamber onto the stone and keep hiking far enough and high enough to be rewarded for the effort. If we documented all the freelance slickwalks we've enjoyed, they'd fill a separate guidebook.

But guiding is contrary to the independent spirit of slickwalking. It's also unnecessary. Desire, curiosity and creativity are your slickwalk guides. Daylight, gravity and energy are your only limitations.

Just as fishermen driving riverside roads glance at the water wondering where a stealthy presentation might land a lunker, Utah hikers driving canyon-country roads scan for opportunities to scurry onto a slickrock finger and roam toward the horizon. Both, however, always welcome a tip from a friend. And here's one for you: Black Dragon.

The Black Dragon pictograph panel is well known. The slickwalk above it is not. The panel is enshrined in a colossal alcove on a soaring wall within Black Dragon Canyon—a short, deep passage through the San Rafael Reef. Intent on admiring the rock art, seeing nothing to divert their attention to hiking, most people spend only about 30 minutes here. Now that you know what to look for, you'll be astounded at what they miss.

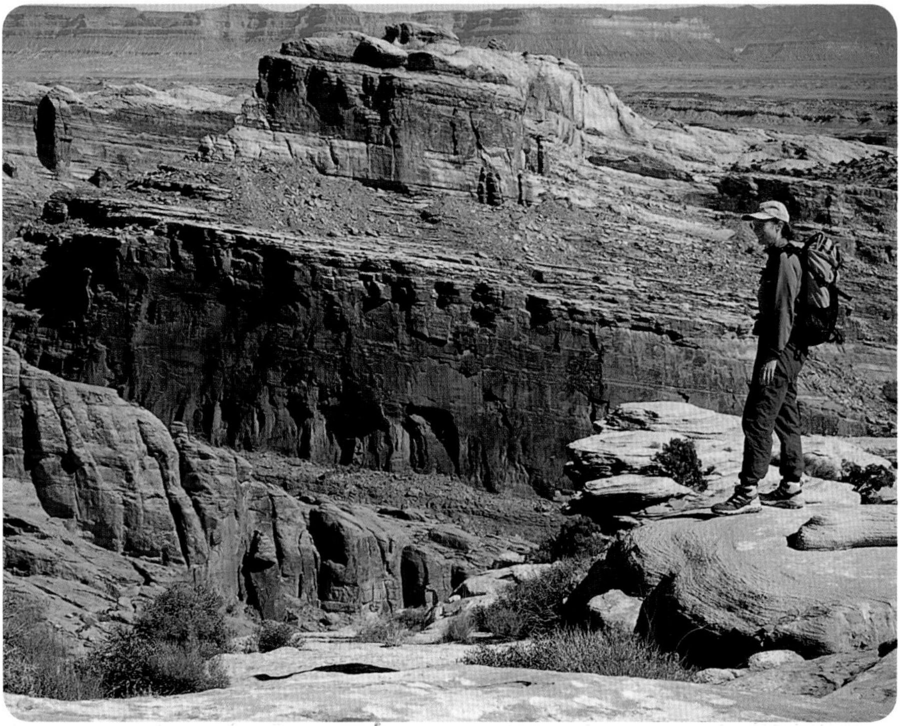

Overlooking San Rafael River Canyon, from Black Dragon slickwalk

FACT

BY VEHICLE

From Salina, drive I-70 east. Take exit 149 for Hwy 24. At the stop sign, turn left (north). Pass over I-70, turn left (west), reset your trip odometer to 0, and proceed west.

From Green River, drive I-70 west. Reset your trip odometer to 0 on the middle of the overpass at the Hwy 24 junction. Proceed west.

From either approach, slow down where I-70 crosses the San Rafael River at 1.1 mi (1.8 km). Pass milepost 145 at 1.5 mi (2.5 km) and slow way down. Turn right (north) at 1.8 mi (2.9 km) onto an unsigned, unpaved road. Reset your trip odometer to 0.

Pass through the wire gate and proceed north. At 1.9 mi (3.1 km) cross a shallow wash. At 2.4 mi (3.9 km) ignore a left spur leading to the reef and Double Arch. At 2.8 mi (4.5 km) turn left. Just ahead is a BLM sign in a large parking area near the mouth of Black Dragon Canyon, at 4500 ft (1372 m).

ON FOOT

To see the Black Dragon pictograph panel, follow the road five minutes up-canyon to the huge alcove (right / northeast).

To begin the Black Dragon slickwalk, enter the wash paralleling the right side of the road and hike northwest. In a couple minutes, bear right (north), out

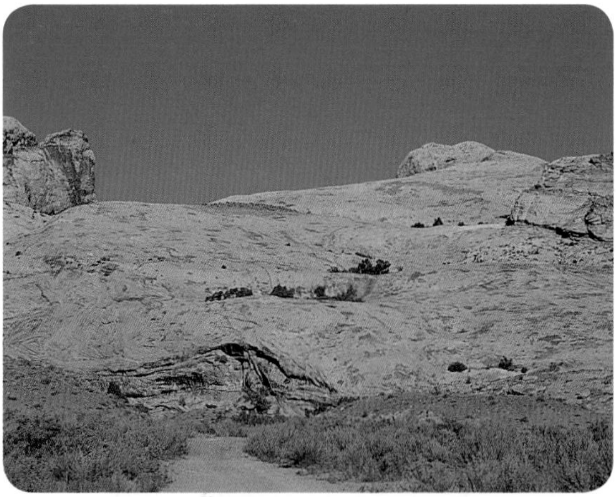
Ascend the gentle sandstone out of Black Dragon wash.

of the wash, toward the slickrock slope that soars above the alcove harboring the pictograph panel. It's less steep, therefore easier to mount, farther right.

Once atop the slickrock, ascend northwest. From here on, you're navigating cross-country. Just keep climbing. Flow upward on the gentlest slopes, avoid sharp drop-offs, stay within your comfort zone. If the slickrock steepens to the point of exposure, back off, seek another way forward. Ascending to 5800 ft (1768 m) is easy and safe if you're patient, observant, and cautious.

Attempting to precisely guide you across untracked slickrock by means of a written description would be laborious for us and tedious for you. Why burden you with detail only to sap your experience of joy? So instead of directions, we offer the suggestions below. Like a highway guard rail, they're probably unnecessary but conceivably helpful.

Angling left, you'll approach the edge of the canyon directly **above the pictograph alcove** (see inside back cover). Ascend the slickrock ramp to the dome-shaped knob at 5060 ft (1543 m), just northwest of the alcove below. From here you can see Black Dragon Canyon is very short. Its red Wingate cliffs rapidly diminish to the west.

Working your way north, gain 50 ft (15 m) to the next knob, drop 40 ft (12 m) into a sandy basin, and crest a smooth dome at 5180 ft (1580 m). Then drop northwest into a juniper-clad depression.

Cross a couple northwest-trending slickrock defiles. Ascend a smooth, white-gray ramp. Reach the edge of the **San Rafael River Canyon** at 5360 ft (1707 m), about 1½ hours from the trailhead. The river is visible north, 900 ft (274 m) below. The La Sal Mountains (beyond Moab) are southeast. The San Rafael Reef extends south toward Goblin Valley (Trip 41).

Bear left (west), ascending slabby benches. About two hours along, overlook Lower Black Box (northwest), which resembles the inner gorge of the Grand Canyon. North of it, the river wraps tightly around 6393-ft (1949-m) Mexican Mtn. At about 3.2 mi (5.2 km), having hiked 2½ hours, reach the slickrock massif's 5800-ft (1768-m) **highpoint**.

The low, stair-stepping cliffs to the west are the Jackass Benches. Northwest, at the base of tan cliffs, is the road to Swaseys Leap. Beyond it, above distant Wingate cliffs, Cedar Mtn is on the northwest horizon.

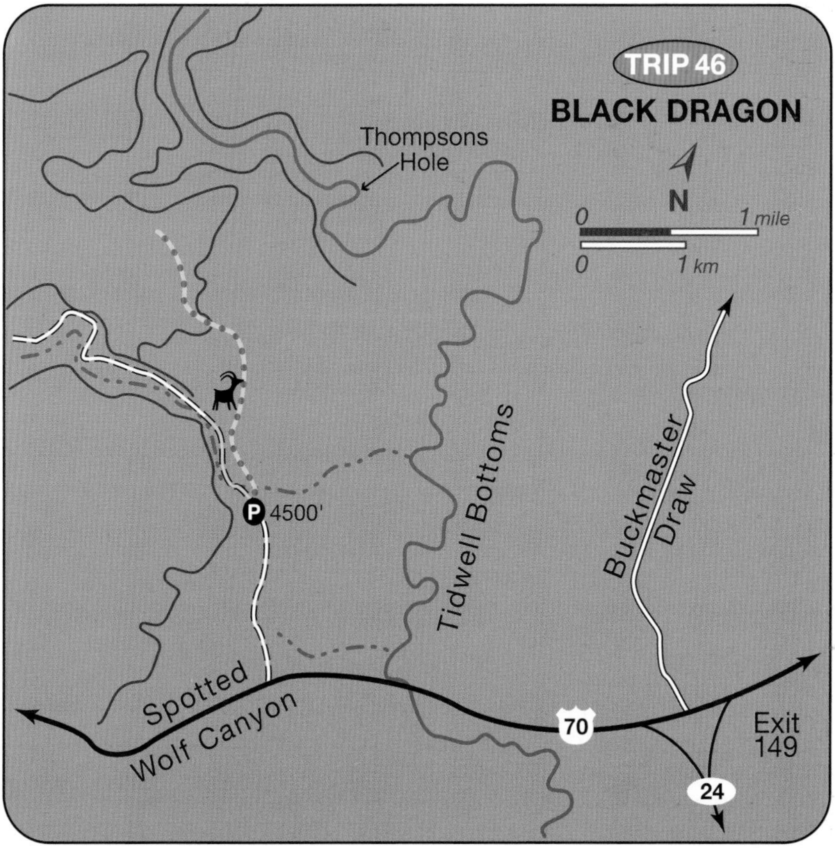

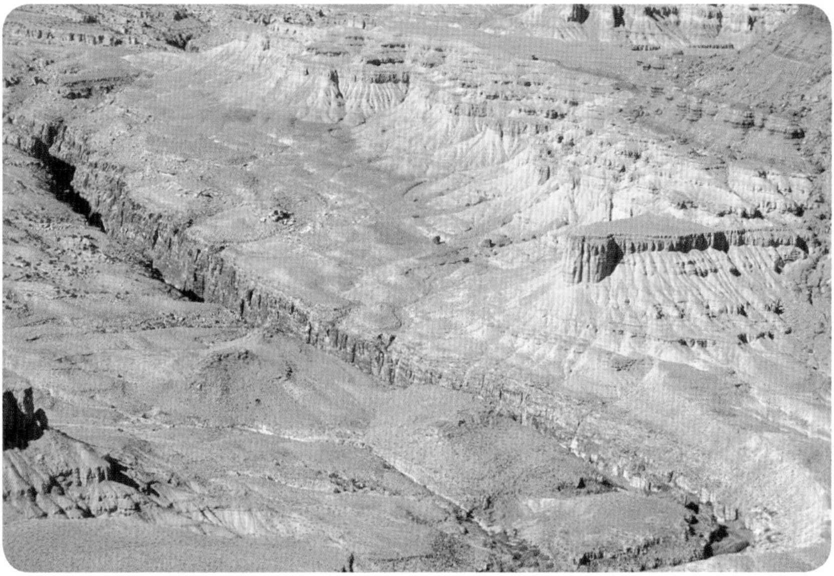

Overlooking Lower Black Box of the San Rafael River, from Black Dragon slickwalk

TRIP 47

DEVILS GARDEN

LOCATION	Arches National Park
LOOP	7.7 mi (12.4 km) including all recommended digressions
ELEVATION GAIN	650 ft (198 m)
KEY ELEVATIONS	trailhead 5180 ft (1579 m) highpoint at Black Arch overlook 5510 ft (1679 m) lowpoint in Fin Canyon 5100 ft (1554 m)
HIKING TIME	3½ to 4 hours
DIFFICULTY	easy
MAPS	Trails Illustrated *Arches National Park* Latitude 40 *Classic Moab Trails*

OPINION

Devils Garden, in Arches National Park, harbors the highest concentration of significant natural arches on earth. Among them is Landscape Arch—an impossibly slender ribbon of stone longer than a football field. It ranks among our planet's greatest natural wonders.

For notoriety, Landscape Arch competes with nearby Delicate Arch (Trip 49). Both are composed of Entrada sandstone. But because Landscape Arch is horizontal, it's not as photogenic as Delicate Arch, whose compact, vertical profile fits stylishly on Utah postage stamps and license plates and has thus become emblematic of the American southwest.

Landscape is the world's longest natural arch. It's a smidge longer than the runner-up, Kolob Arch (Trip 2) in Zion National Park. Landscape is also incomparably elegant, which is why most observers consider it a more astounding sight than Kolob. It's certainly easier to reach. Viewing Kolob necessitates a 14-mi (22.5-km) round-trip dayhike. Landscape is a mere one mile from the trailhead.

And what a trailhead it is: 150 paved parking stalls, all of which are frequently occupied because this is the most popular trail in the park. "Trail," however, is initially a euphemism. A broad, smooth, pedestrian highway leads to Landscape Arch. Beyond, it diminishes to an actual trail, then tapers to what the park calls a "primitive" trail. So most visitors—unfit, unambitious, unprepared for a genuine hike, and incurious—turn around after ogling Landscape, allowing you to continue in relative tranquility.

The crowd always misses the finer points, of course. What they miss here is the longest maintained trail in the park—a loop revealing numerous arches less miraculous than Landscape but equally beautiful and enthralling. Because these arches are sequestered, they tend to be in unexpected, intimate settings, so you're apt to feel an exhilarating sense of discovery when you finally clap eyes

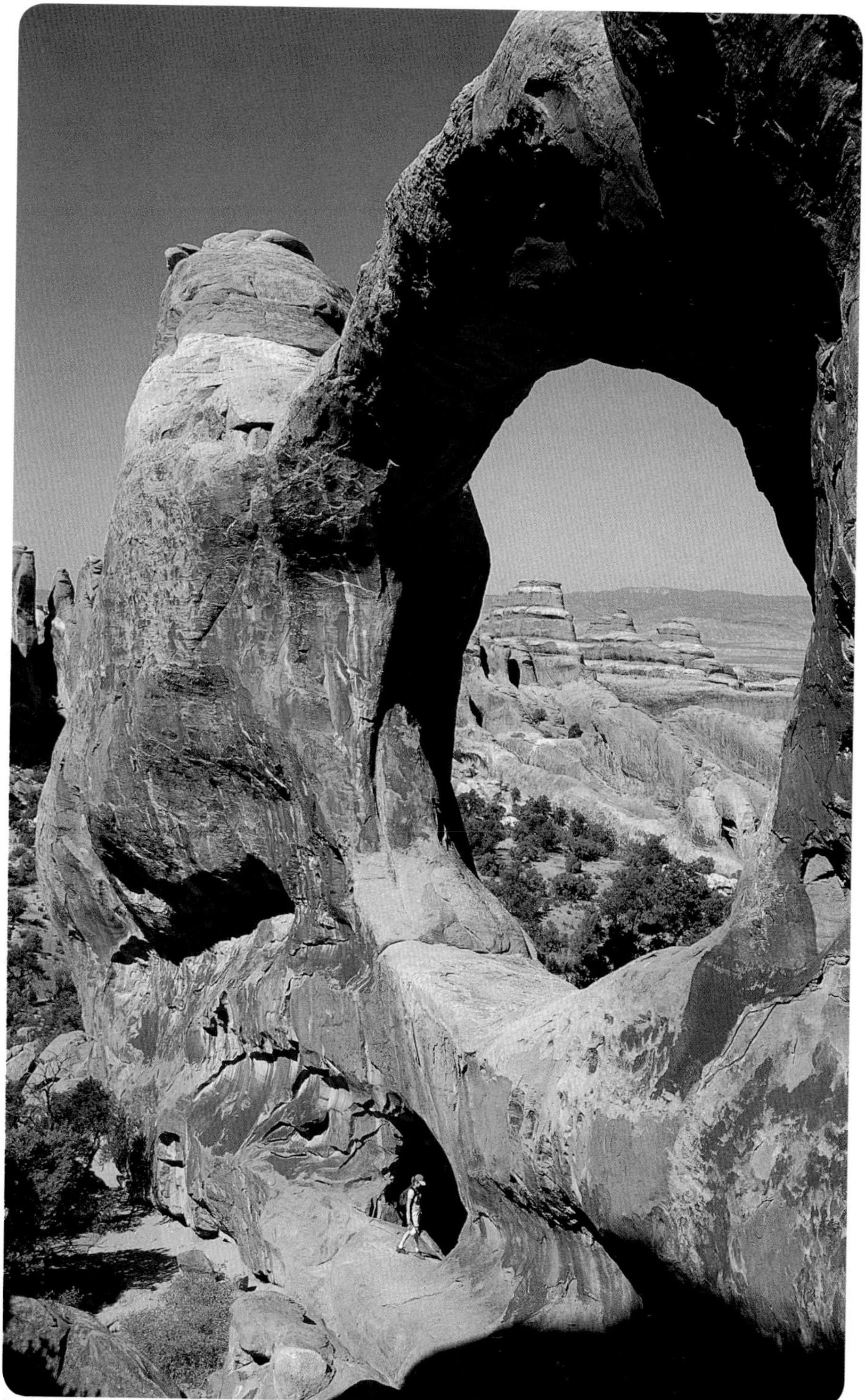

Double-O Arch

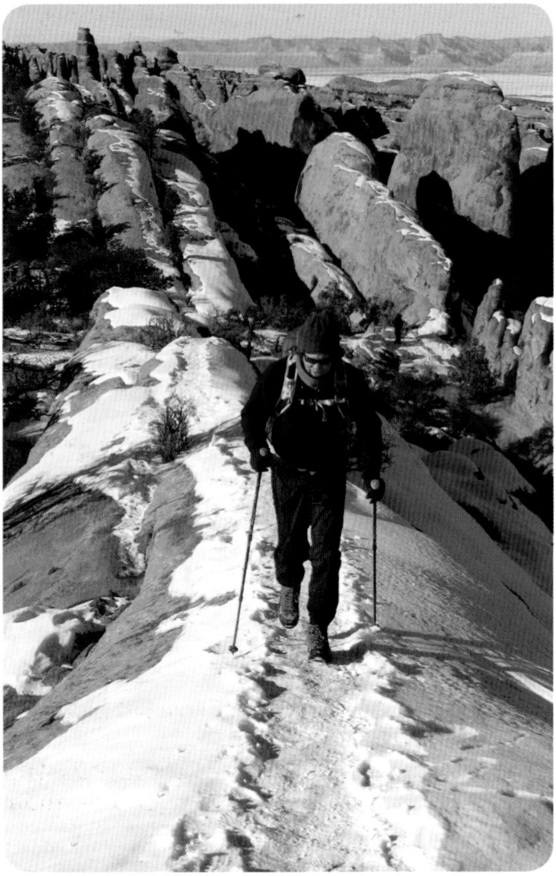
Returning from Double-O Arch, late December

on them. With luck (boost yours by hiking very early or late in the day), solitude will enrich your experience.

The Devils Garden hike reveals but a fraction of the national park's more than 2,000 cataloged arches. They range in size from a three-foot opening—the minimum to be considered an arch—to the implausible, taffy-pull expanse of Landscape Arch. Though all are solid stone, and many appear stalwart, they're impermanent, even fragile. Created by 100 million years of erosion (wind, water, ice) and weathering (decomposition), they will eventually succumb to the same forces that created them and the inexorable pull of gravity. Likewise, new arches are slowly being created. So the art here is constantly changing, just as it does in any gallery.

While admiring the more horizontal arches, particularly Landscape Arch, you might wonder: "Is it really an arch? Or is it actually a bridge?" Though somewhat arbitrary, there is a distinction—enough to justify the name *Natural Bridges National Monument* for another of Utah's scenic treasure troves, farther south. An arch is formed by weathering and/or a combination of erosional forces. A natural bridge is a type of natural arch, but one primarily formed by flowing water.

FACT

BEFORE YOUR TRIP

If you're intent on photographing Landscape Arch in optimal light, begin hiking early in the morning, when the sun will illuminate the arch from behind you.

BY VEHICLE

From the junction of Hwys 191 and 128, beside the Colorado River bridge just north of Moab, drive Hwy 191 northwest. Cross the bridge. At 2 mi (3.2 km) turn right (north) to enter Arches National Park.

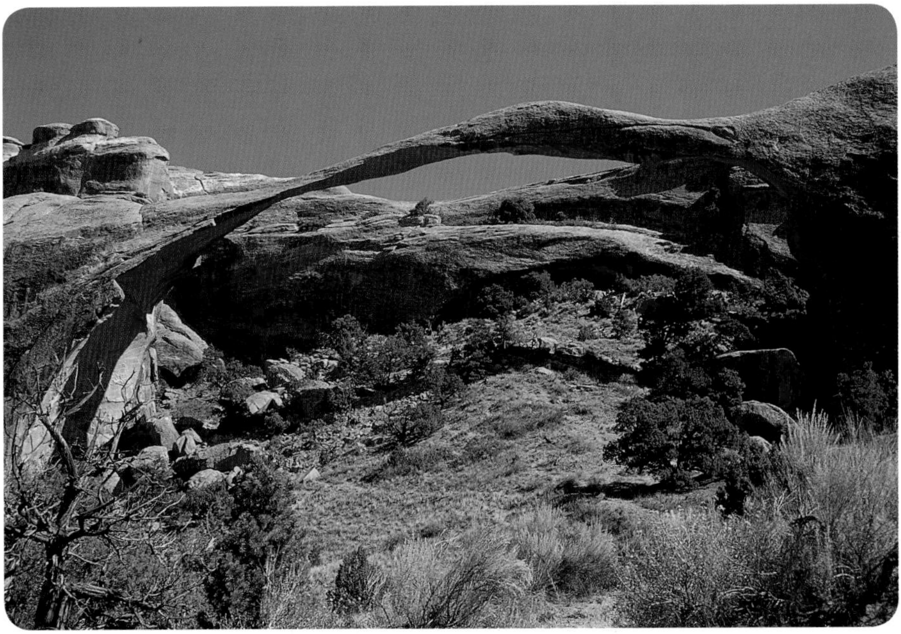

Landscape Arch

From I-70, drive Hwy 191 southeast. At 26.4 mi (42.5 km) turn left (north) to enter Arches National Park.

From the visitor center, stay on the main park road another 17.2 mi (27.8 km) to its north terminus at the Devils Garden trailhead parking lot. Elevation: 5180 ft (1579 m).

ON FOOT

Follow the road-width, gravel trail northwest through slickrock fins. Within five minutes begin a moderate ascent on steps.

These fins formed when the earth rose beneath a solid layer of sandstone, which fractured into long, parallel, vertical ridges that allowed the arches to develop.

At 0.3 mi (0.5 km) a right spur affords a 0.6-mi (1-km) round-trip digression to **Pinetree and Tunnel arches**. Both are relatively young, in other words small, but they're a fitting prelude to the exceedingly old arch you'll see next.

Resuming northwest on the main trail, reach a fork at 0.9 mi (1.4 km), 5230 ft (1594 m). Right, heading generally north-northwest, is the so-called Primitive trail. You'll return that way if you follow our suggested loop, so for now proceed left (northwest).

Landscape Arch is visible left (west) at 1 mi (1.6 km). Roughly 306 ft (93 m) long and 105 ft (32 m) high, it narrows to an astonishingly scant 11 ft (3.4 m). Judging by the first known photo of Landscape Arch, taken in 1896, it has changed very little during the intervening years. Nevertheless it could collapse at any time. Since 1991, portions of the arch have broken off and fallen to the ground, which is why walking beneath it is now prohibited.

Continuing northwest on the main trail, briefly follow cairns across slickrock while ascending between fins. Soon pass **Wall Arch** (right / northeast). Beyond, begin climbing moderately to steeply on sand and slickrock.

At 1.3 mi (2.1 km), 5450 ft (1661 m), a left (southwest) spur affords a 0.7-mi (1.1-km) round-trip digression to **Navajo Arch and Partition Arch**. Both are compelling sights in secretive locations. Navajo, rooted in smooth gravel, is graceful despite its hefty girth. Partition comprises two, nearly round arches—separated by a stone "partition"—in one wall.

Back on the main trail, resume hiking west-northwest. Soon enjoy expansive views. Walk over slickrock and atop fins to reach the next junction at 2.2 mi (3.5 km), 5510 ft (1679 m)—the loop highpoint. Right (north) quickly ends at a viewpoint overlooking **Black Arch** in Fin Canyon. Go left (west) for Double-O Arch.

A few minutes farther, **Double-O Arch** is visible left. Proceed to the foot of the arch by descending northwest atop a slickrock fin then curving left (southwest) among large piñon pines. Double-O comprises a big arch directly above a smaller one. To appreciate it fully, scramble into the lower arch, immediately turn left and ascend a slickrock ramp southeast, then curve right until you're directly south of the arches, at a height midway between them. That's the optimal viewpoint.

Immediately below (northeast of) Double-O, near the end of the fin it occupies, is a junction at 2.3 mi (3.7 km). Left (west) is a spur affording a 1-mi (1.6-km) round-trip digression to a desert-varnished spire called **Dark Angel**—a solitary remnant of an ancient fin. The views en route are vast, but the spire itself is underwhelming. Go right (northwest) to loop back to the trailhead via the **Primitive trail**.

The name "Primitive" and a sign warning of "difficult hiking" ahead are intended to discourage neophytes. Experienced, intermediate hikers who are reasonably cautious and keep to this smaller yet distinct trail will face no obstacles of note—*if* the slickrock is not icy.

The Primitive trail gently descends into a dry wash and curves northeast between fins. Reach a junction at 2.7 mi (4.3 km), 5290 ft (1612 m). The right (southeast) spur affords a 0.4-mi (0.6-km) round-trip digression to **Private Arch**. Hidden among nearby fins, this massive-yet-sensuous arch is an engaging spectacle.

Continuing the loop, the trail itself soon commands attention and keeps you entertained as it descends via slickrock ramps and ledges, past magnificent piñon trees, to the sandy floor of **Fin Canyon** at 5100 ft (1554 m)—the loop lowpoint.

Be alert. At the sign *Main Trail* (arrow pointing right), turn right and begin a brief ascent out of the canyon. The trail levels again, heading generally south-southeast. The La Sal Mountains are visible left (southeast).

Reach a T-junction at 4.4 mi (7.1 km), 5230 ft (1594 m). You're now on familiar ground. Right (northwest) leads 0.1 mi (0.2 km) to Landscape Arch. Turn left and hike southeast 0.9 mi (1.4 km) back to the trailhead parking lot.

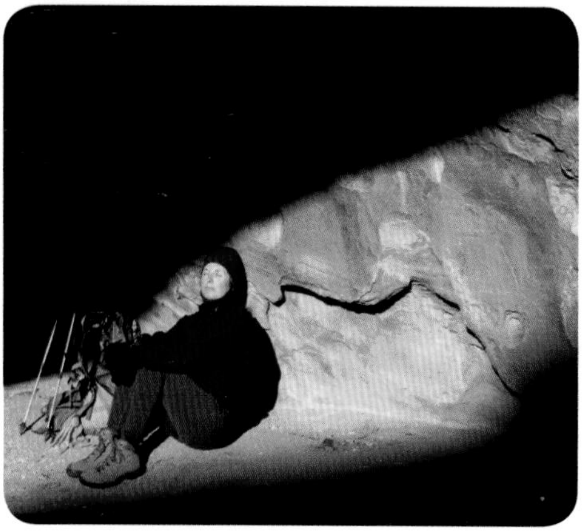

Winter warmth at Navajo Arch

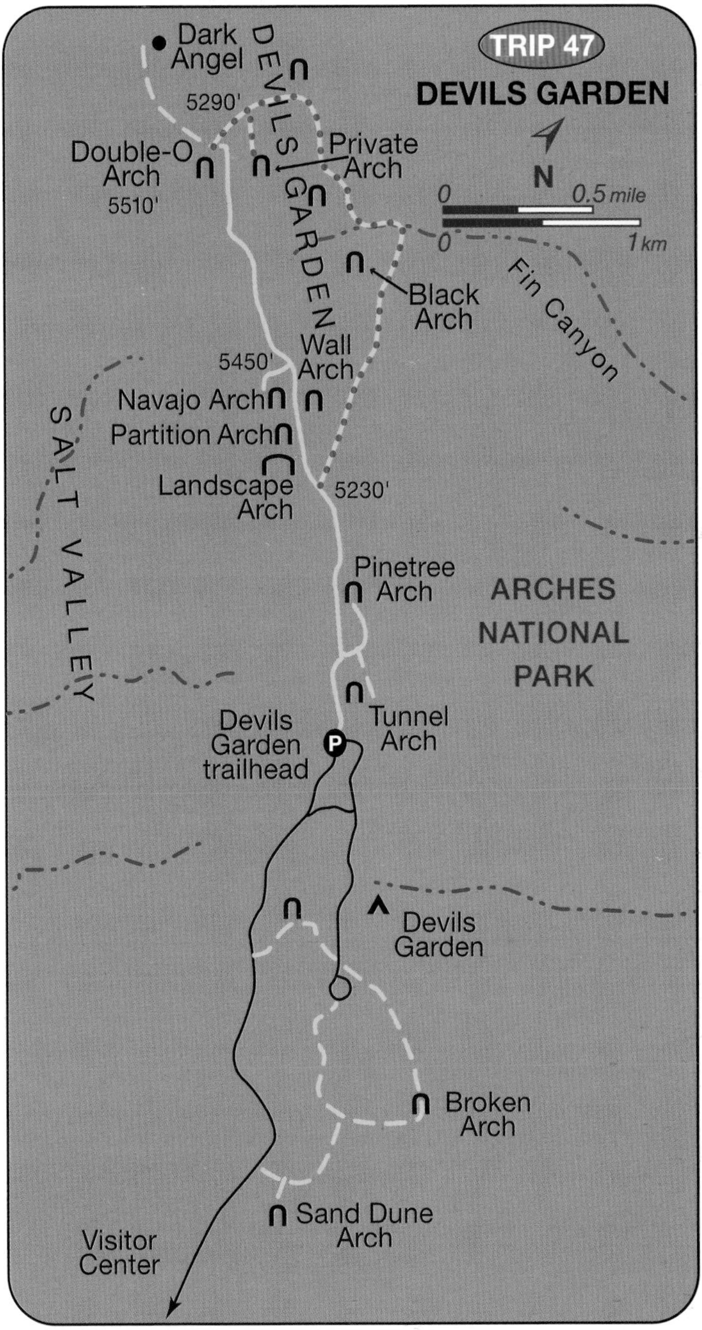
TRIP 47
DEVILS GARDEN
N
0 0.5 mile
0 1 km
Dark Angel
DEVILS GARDEN
5290'
Double-O Arch
5510'
Private Arch
Black Arch
Fin Canyon
Wall Arch
5450'
Navajo Arch
Partition Arch
Landscape Arch
5230'
SALT VALLEY
Pinetree Arch
ARCHES NATIONAL PARK
Tunnel Arch
Devils Garden trailhead
P
Devils Garden
Broken Arch
Sand Dune Arch
Visitor Center

TRIP 48

FIERY FURNACE

LOCATION	Arches National Park
LOOP	2 mi (3.2 km)
ELEVATION GAIN	200 ft (61 m)
KEY ELEVATIONS	trailhead 4650 ft (1417 m), highpoint 4850 ft (1478 m)
HIKING TIME	2 to 3 hours
DIFFICULTY	easy hiking, moderate routefinding
MAP	Trails Illustrated *Arches National Park*

OPINION

The Fiery Furnace is to canyon country what espresso is to coffee: a small serving, but highly concentrated.

It's essentially a compact squadron of lofty, redrock fins creating a phalanx of tightly constricted canyons. Though the name suggests heat, the Furnace is relatively cool because the fins keep the canyons in perpetual shade. What's fiery is the color. The sandstone, especially at sunset, is reminiscent of glowing embers.

The Furnace is so strange, beautiful and fascinating, it would be a popular destination no matter how obscure its location. But because it's a quick stroll from a paved trailhead within a national park, it's famous. Too famous.

Most park visitors are new to canyon country. New even to hiking. And the Furnace is wildly convoluted terrain devoid of directional signage. It poses routefinding challenges only experienced desert rats can comfortably handle. It also requires light scrambling.

Plus, the Furnace harbors fragile cryptogamic soil in such tight quarters that neophytes are likely to trample it, along with other rare plant species that have found refuge here.

As a result, the Park made the wise decision in 1994 to restrict visitation to the Furnace. You may enter on your own, but only if you obtain a permit. To do that, you must watch an educational film at the visitor center, then prove yourself capable by passing a test. Otherwise you must troop along behind a ranger on one of the regularly scheduled group tours.

The Furnace is a maze, but it's not an inscrutable labyrinth. If you're a competent cross-country navigator and have faithfully served your canyon-country apprenticeship, take the test. Get your permit. Go. But go slowly, remain wary, note landmarks, be certain you can reverse out if you don't complete the loop. When in doubt, look for bootprints in the sand or scuff marks on the slickrock.

Within the chasms, among the towering walls, you'll find alcoves, grottoes, arches, even a small, natural bridge. Aptly named *Skull Arch*, with its airy eye sockets, is particularly striking. Be alert for wildlife, too. The Furnace is the only place we've ever encountered a midget-faded rattlesnake.

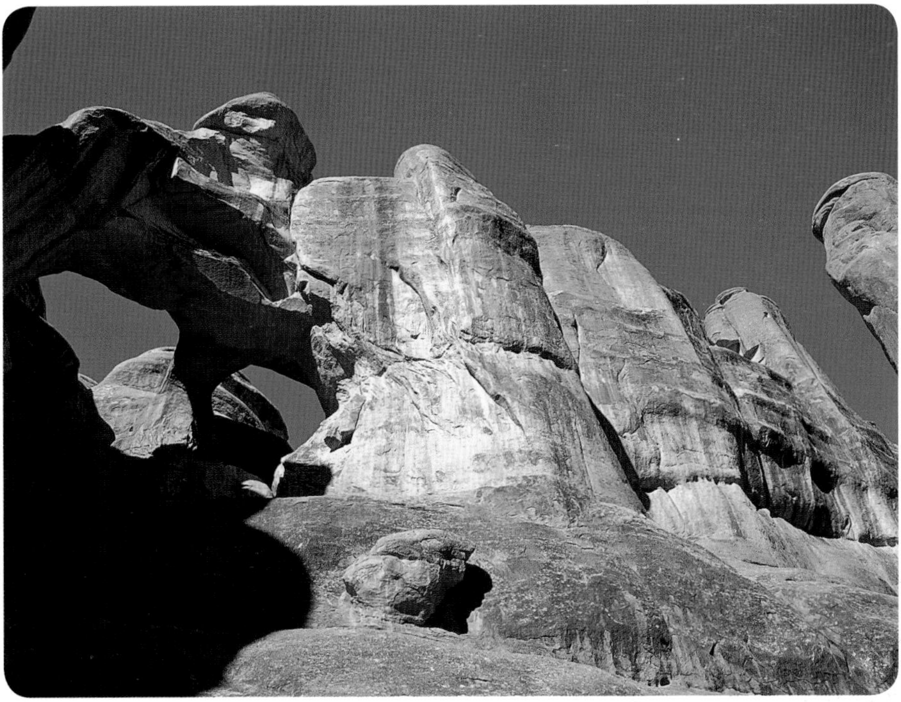

Skull Arch

If you hope to find tranquility in the Furnace, time your entry to avoid the ranger-led hike. If you think the Furnace might overtax you, it probably will. Join the group. You'll still have an extraordinary experience. And you're sure to appreciate aspects of the Furnace that independent hikers fail to notice.

FACT

BEFORE YOUR TRIP

Stop at the visitor center. Ask about obtaining a permit to hike on your own in the Fiery Furnace. Or make reservations and purchase a ticket for a guided tour. Tours begin at 9 a.m. and 1:30 p.m. daily, April through October. Maximum group size is only ten people, so tours are usually booked full a couple days ahead. You can make reservations up to a week in advance. Whether hiking alone or with a ranger, carry more water than you think you'll need.

BY VEHICLE

From the junction of Hwys 191 and 128, beside the Colorado River bridge just north of Moab, drive Hwy 191 northwest. Cross the bridge. At 2 mi (3.2 km) turn right (north) to enter Arches National Park.

From I-70, drive Hwy 191 southeast. At 26.4 mi (42.5 km) turn left (north) to enter Arches National Park.

From the visitor center, follow the main park road another 13.5 mi (21.7 km) generally north-northeast to a signed right spur leading east-southeast to the Fiery Furnace trailhead parking lot at 13.7 mi (22 km), 4650 ft (1417 m).

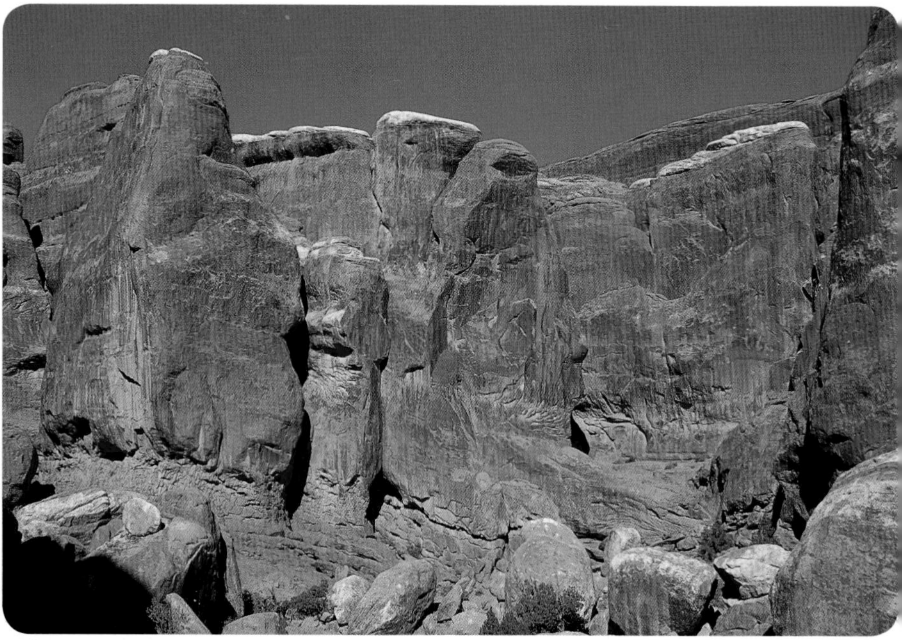

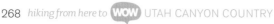

Walls of the Fiery Furnace

ON FOOT

Two paths depart the trailhead. Both enter the Fiery Furnace. Start on one, loop back on the other. Or hike in and out on either one. The Furnace itself is so complex that trying to follow a written route description would be a tedious, pleasure-sapping chore, like reading the assembly directions for a complete set of Ikea kitchen cabinets. Only if you can guide yourself are you capable of hiking here independently. Most people should opt for a ranger-led group tour.

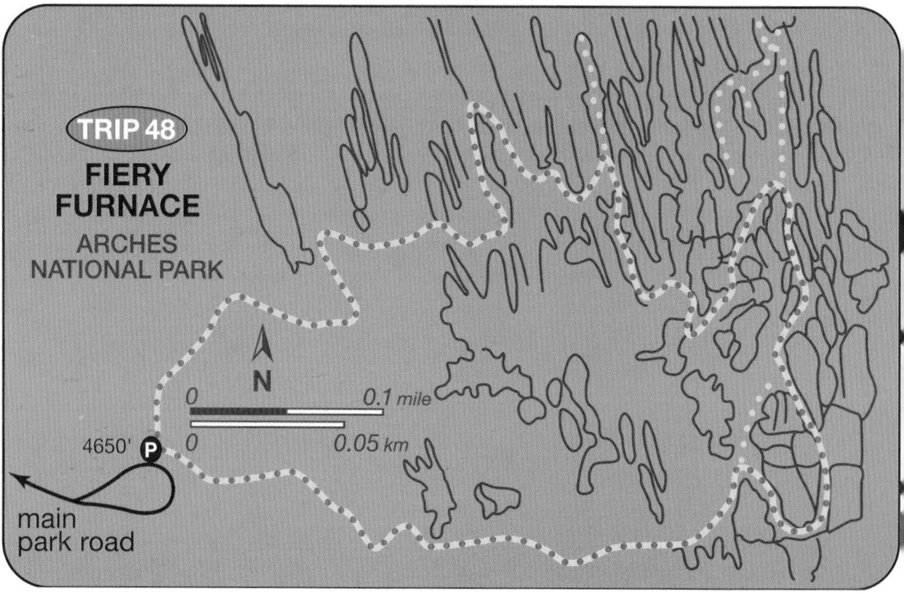

TRIP 49

DELICATE ARCH

LOCATION	Arches National Park
ROUND TRIP	3 mi (4.8 km)
ELEVATION GAIN	560 ft (171 m)
KEY ELEVATIONS	trailhead 4280 ft (1305 m) Delicate Arch 4840 ft (1475 m)
HIKING TIME	1½ to 2 hours
DIFFICULTY	easy
MAPS	Trails Illustrated *Arches National Park* Latitude 40 *Classic Moab Trails*

OPINION

After seeing a thousand images of Delicate Arch (and you will, because it's on nearly every Utah license plate), the real thing is still astounding. It ranks among the most impressive of our planet's natural wonders, and it's perhaps the most iconic of all.

It's also unspeakably beautiful.

The hike to Delicate Arch, however, is lackluster. The initial stretch is on a broad, dirt, pedestrian highway. Beyond, where it becomes a cairned route ascending a slickrock swell, views improve and the trip becomes more engaging.

Actually, this isn't a hike so much as a pilgrimage. Expect to share the quest with others. Lots of them. Regardless when you're here. They depart the trailhead before sunrise, laden with camera lenses as long as your arm. Undeterred by summer heat or winter cold, they set up their tripods beneath the arch every day of the year. They return after sunset, wearing headlamps or groping along in the dark.

Because the trip is so brief, and because the optimal (least crowded yet most scenic) times to view the arch are early morning and late evening, it's possible to come here on a day you devote to another Moab-area hike.

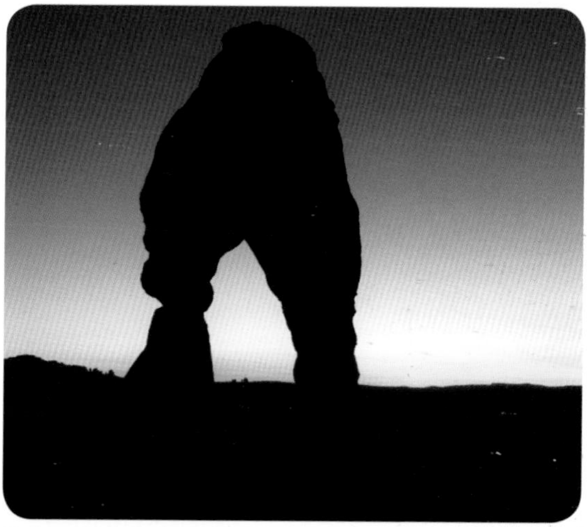

Delicate Arch at sunset

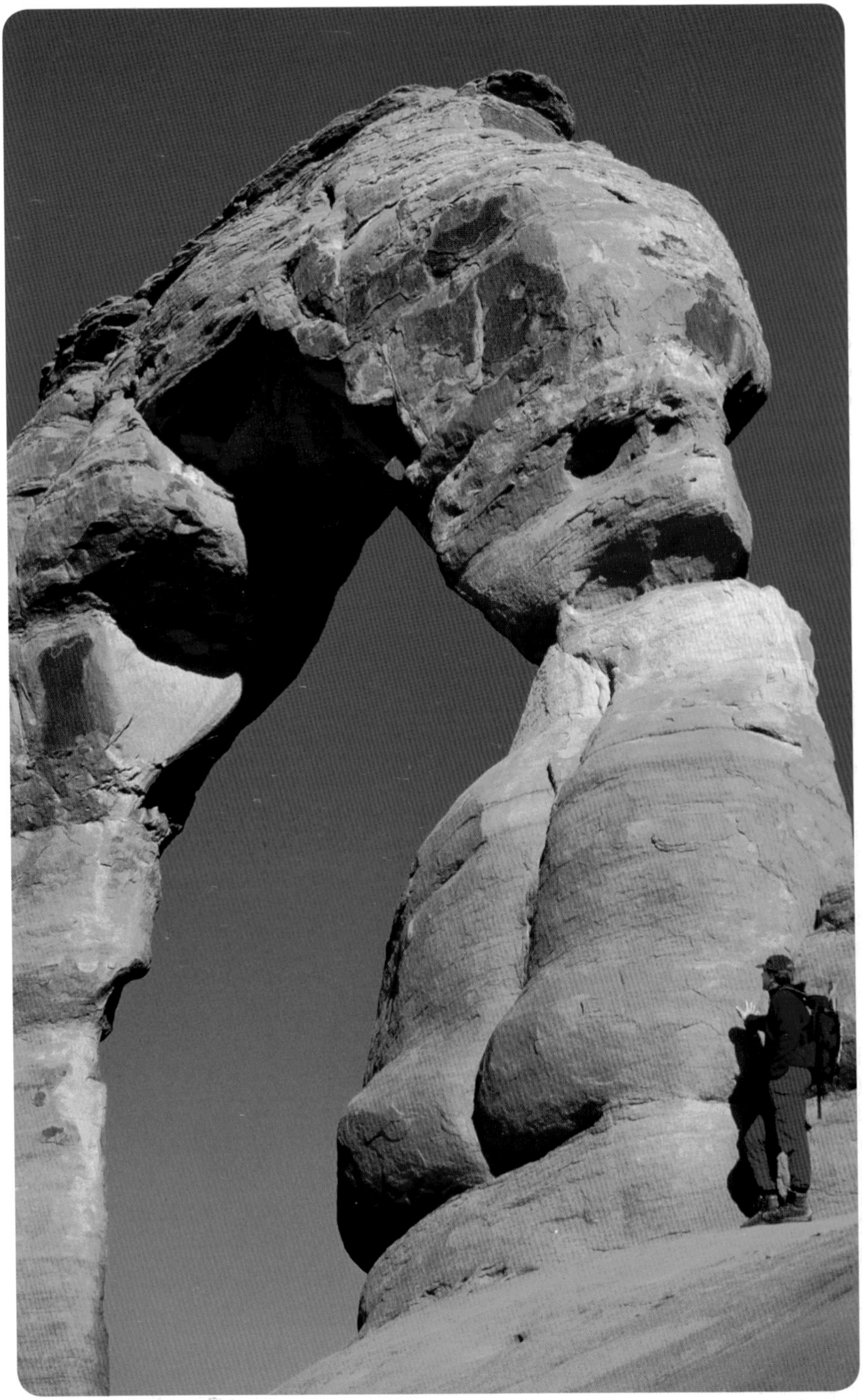

Delicate Arch

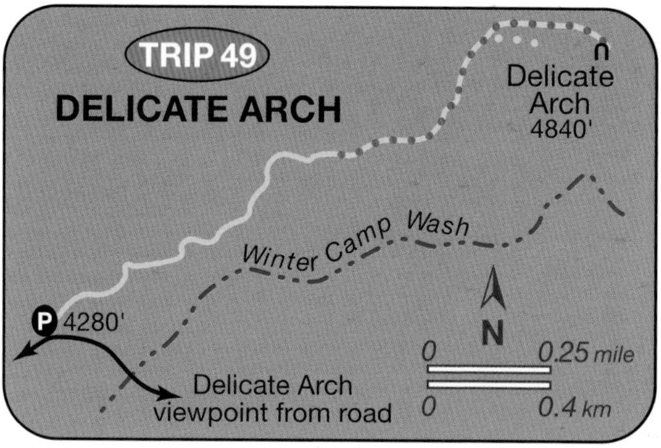

FACT

BEFORE YOUR TRIP

Pack a couple full water bottles per person. An alarming number of unprepared people succumb to heat exhaustion here. In summer, it happens almost daily. If it's still dark, or soon will be, don't even consider hiking without a reliable headlamp. And be prepared for a carnival atmosphere. Wear a smile. Expect to share the optimal camera angles with others.

BY VEHICLE

From the junction of Hwys 191 and 128, beside the Colorado River bridge just north of Moab, drive Hwy 191 northwest. Cross the bridge. At 2 mi (3.2 km) turn right (north) to enter Arches National Park.

From I-70, drive Hwy 191 southeast. At 26.4 mi (42.5 km) turn left (north) to enter Arches National Park.

From the visitor center, follow the main park road another 11.3 mi (18.2 km) generally north-northeast. Turn right at the sign for Delicate Arch and Wolfe Ranch. Continue northeast 1.2 mi (1.9 km) to the trailhead parking lot, on the left, at 4280 ft (1305 m).

ON FOOT

Your general direction of travel will be northeast all the way to the arch. Just beyond the trailhead, cross a bridge spanning Salt Wash, then continue on a broad, dirt path.

Immediately before the first noticeable ascent, where the trail veers left then switchbacks above, watch for a signed left spur to a Ute Indian **pictograph panel**. It's one of only two easily accessible rock-art sites in the park.

Above the switchback, the trail becomes a cairned route ascending slickrock. Views are vast, yet the celebrated arch remains hidden.

The final approach is on a ledge blasted out of the left (north) side of a sandstone fin. Reach **Delicate Arch** at 1.5 mi (2.4 km), 4840 ft (1475 m), perched above an enormous bowl. The distant La Sal Mountains complete the famous scene.

Wondering about the monolith's dimensions? It stands 45 ft (14 m) high, and the span between abutments is 33 ft (10 m).

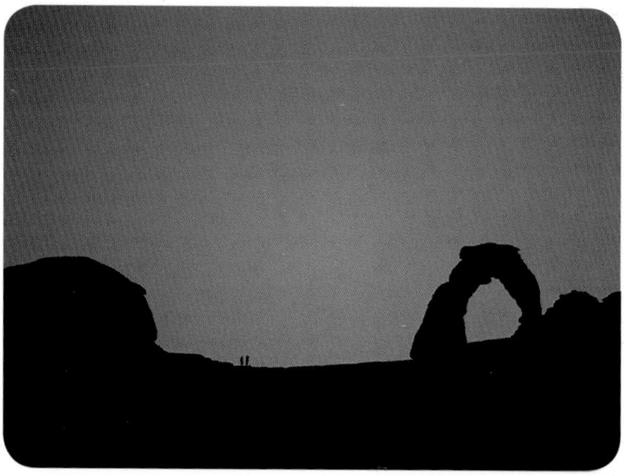

Delicate Arch at sunrise

TRIP 50

CORONA ARCH

LOCATION	Potash Road, west of Moab
ROUND TRIP	3 mi (5 km)
ELEVATION GAIN	556 ft (170 m)
KEY ELEVATIONS	trailhead 4000 ft (1220 m), Corona Arch 4396 ft (1340 m)
HIKING TIME	1½ to 2½ hours
DIFFICULTY	easy
MAPS	Trails Illustrated *Moab South* Latitude 40 *Classic Moab Trails*

OPINION

The most impressive arch in southeast Utah—excluding those enshrined in nearby Arches National Park—is Corona. A testament to its extraordinary size and beauty is that Corona is sometimes called "Little Rainbow Bridge." It does resemble the famous natural bridge on an inlet of Lake Powell, but Corona is unique.

From Moab, the Corona trailhead is closer than that of any arch in the national park. Yet you'll find Corona less crowded, because reaching it requires a 45-minute hike—a fun romp, mostly on slickrock.

Corona is mammoth: 140 ft (43 m) high, with a span of 335 ft (102 m). Its setting is equally impressive: on the wall of Bootlegger Canyon, in a huge amphitheatre also containing Bowtie Arch.

Bowtie is a bonus sight. It appears that a haywire missile from a passing spacecraft blasted through the back wall of its deep alcove. If so, perhaps one of the alien pilot's many appendages accidentally bumped the ship's controls while all of his eyes were ogling Corona Arch.

FACT

BY VEHICLE

From the junction of Hwys 191 and 128, beside the Colorado River bridge just north of Moab, drive Hwy 191 northwest. Cross the bridge. At 1.6 mi (2.5 km), turn left (southwest) onto Hwy 279 (Potash Road). It soon parallels the river. Continue through the canyon mouth known as *The Portal*. At 11.2 mi (18 km) turn right (east) into the trailhead parking lot. Elevation: 4000 ft (1220 m).

ON FOOT

The trail departs the south end of the parking lot. Switchback upward for a couple minutes, then hike generally northeast. Cross the railroad tracks. Soon curve right (east), then left (northeast).

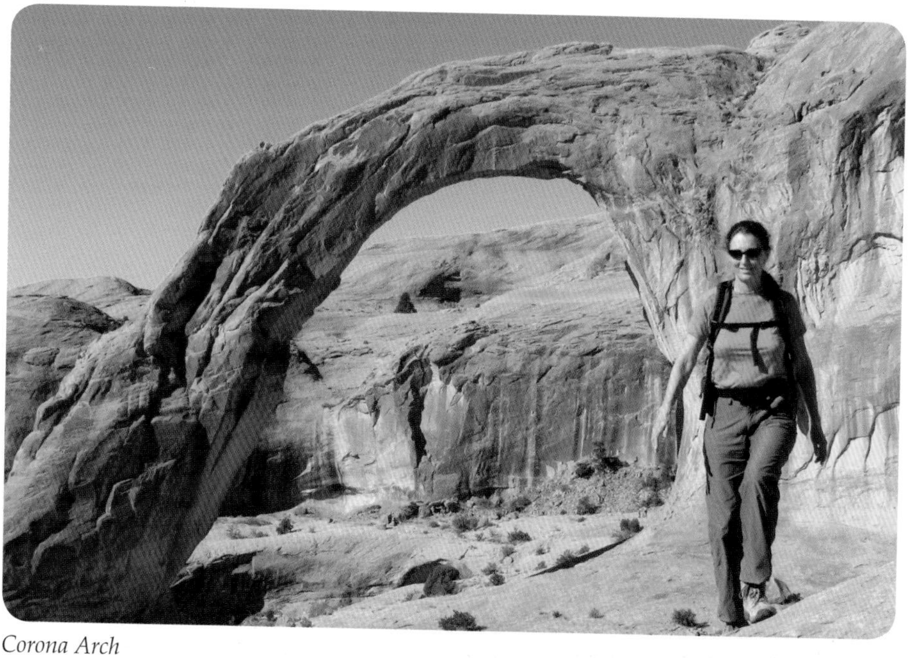

Corona Arch

After a very short rough stretch, the trail levels above and the view expands. Look left (north-northeast) for **Pinto Arch** high on the canyon wall. It's right (east) of two deep alcoves. Resume a gradual ascent for about eight minutes, following cairns across slickrock then continuing on the sandy trail.

About 30 minutes from the trailhead, reach 4280 ft (1305 m). After a short descent east to 4200 ft (1280 m), the remainder of the hike is a carined slickrock route. Reach a fixed, horizontal cable where the terrain steepens.

Around the next corner, **Bowtie Arch** is visible left (north-northeast) in the roof of a deep alcove. But much larger Corona Arch—northeast, at the far end of the amphitheater—is the dominant sight.

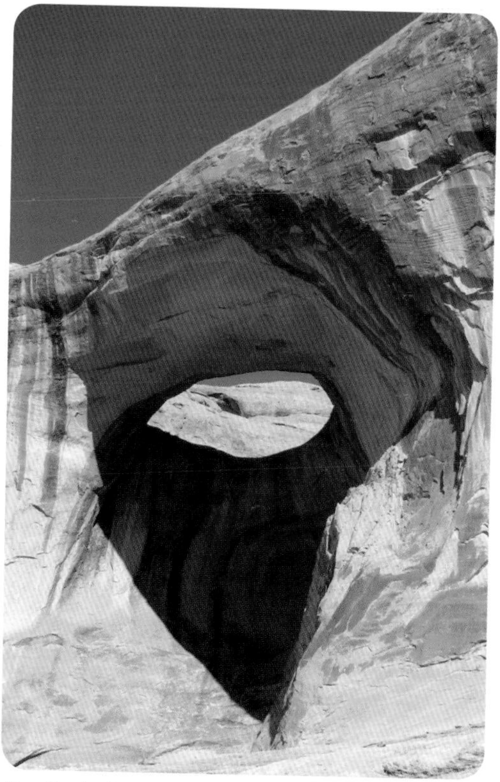

Bowtie Arch

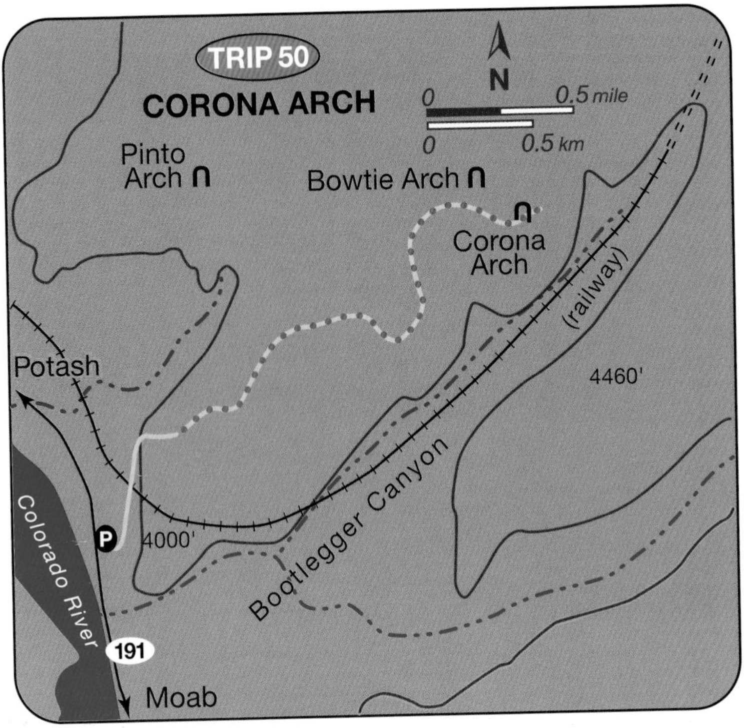

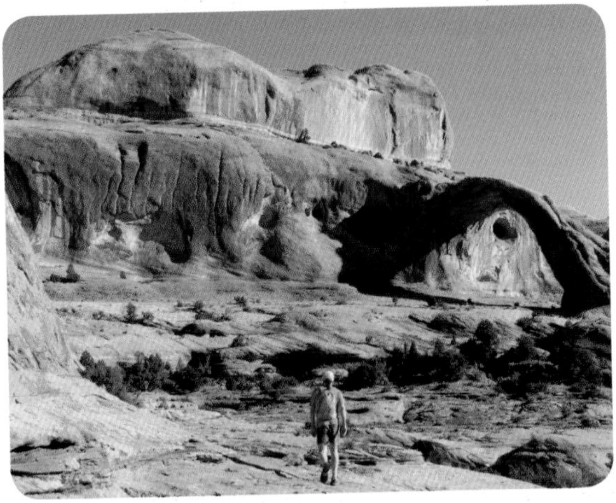
En route to Corona Arch

Arrive at a vertical cable and a crude-but-effective staircase cut into the sandstone. Then climb a short ladder to complete the ascent onto a slickrock terrace. The way forward is now obvious: simply follow the cairns as you contour through the amphitheater.

You're hiking along the northwest wall of **Bootlegger Canyon**. Gradually curve right (east) along the slickrock terrace. Reach **Corona Arch** at 1.5 mi (2.4 km), 4396 ft (1340 m). Continue beneath and beyond the arch to fully appreciate the impressive setting.

Yes, that's a railroad track you see below. It exits upper Bootlegger Canyon through a tunnel. The train carries potash from the mine down river.

TRIP 51

DRAGONFLY CANYON

LOCATION	Potash Road, west of Moab
ROUND TRIP	3.2 mi (5.2 km) to Jeep Arch viewpoint 6 mi (9.7 km) to Gold Bar Rim
ELEVATION GAIN	887 ft (270 m) to Jeep Arch viewpoint 1300 ft (396 m) to Gold Bar Rim
KEY ELEVATIONS	trailhead 4000 ft (1220 m), spire 4707 ft (1435 m) Jeep Arch viewpoint 4887 ft (1490 m) Gold Bar Rim 5300 ft (1615 m)
HIKING TIME	2 hours for Jeep Arch viewpoint 4 to 5 hours for Gold Bar Rim
DIFFICULTY	moderate
MAPS	Trails Illustrated *Moab South* Latitude 40 *Classic Moab Trails*

OPINION

Wandering is to hiking what scat singing is to music. When you wander, you're improvising an instrumental jazz solo with your feet instead of your voice: *bippity-bippity-doo-wop-razzamatazz-skoobie-doobie-bee-bop-a-lula-shabazz*. And the optimal place to wander near Moab is Dragonfly Canyon.

Also known as Culvert Canyon, it's at the bottom of a vast, stony, multiple-wash drainage gradually sloping 1300 ft (396 m) from Gold Bar Rim down to the Colorado River. The upper edge of the rim is the long, steep wall paralleling the southwest side of Hwy 191 northwest of Moab.

The scenery in Dragonfly is engrossing. Attempting to precisely guide you through the complex, trail-less terrain by means of a written description, however, would be laborious for us and tedious for you. Why burden you with detail only to sap your experience of joy?

There's no established trail here. We can do little more than point you in the right direction and enthusiastically suggest you go. Dragonfly is a canyon made for wandering. Let the wandering begin.

Stuff your pack with everything you might conceivably need, including extra food and clothing—just in case. Bring two or three quarts (liters) of water per person. Carry a compass and refer to it frequently to help you stay oriented.

Remember, covering a prescribed distance is not the point here. Nor is clapping eyes on a particular sight. Yes, Jeep Arch is remarkable, but the slickrock playground surrounding it is fascinating. Don't fixate on the arch. Aim to just have fun. You'll find beauty everywhere you look. Whether you go for one hour or all day, a big grin means you win.

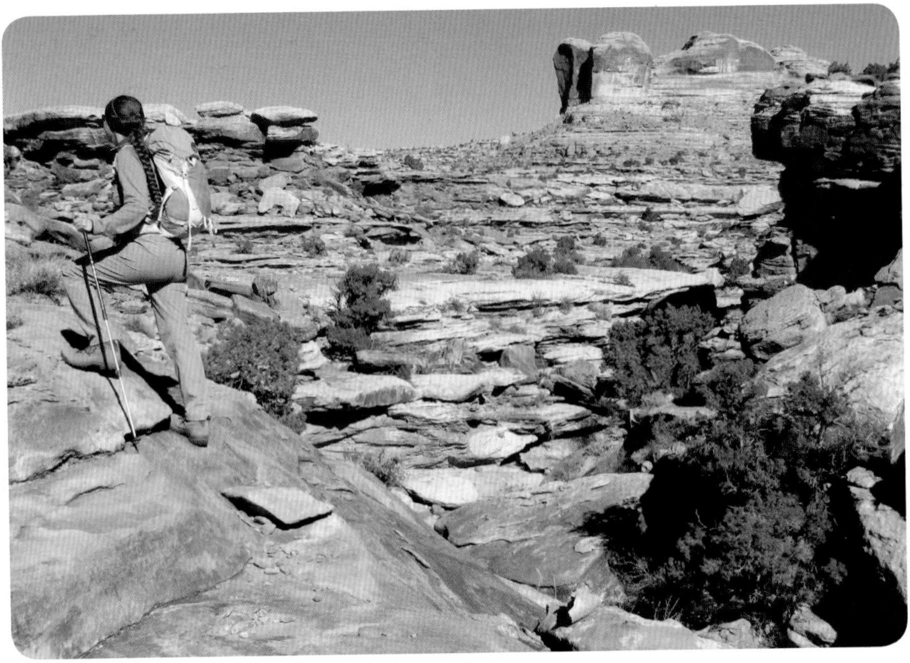

Dragonfly Canyon

FACT

BY VEHICLE

From the junction of Hwys 191 and 128, beside the Colorado River bridge just north of Moab, drive Hwy 191 northwest. Cross the bridge. At 1.6 mi (2.5 km) turn left (southwest) onto Hwy 279 (Potash Road). It soon parallels the river. Continue through the canyon mouth known as *The Portal*. At 11.2 mi (18 km) pass the trailhead for Corona Arch. Slow down. Park on the right (east) side of the road at 11.5 mi (18.5 km), 4000 ft (1220 m).

ON FOOT

Pass beneath the railroad tracks via the large culvert. Proceed north on the canyon floor. Bypass (on the right) **three pouroffs** within fifteen minutes. Continue in the wash bottom on a lavish expanse of **bedrock** at 4133 ft (1260 m), then ascend **slickrock ledges** above either side (your choice). Depending on route, you can gain 1000 ft (305 m) in an hour of vigorous up-canyon meandering.

Frequently turn around and note prominent landmarks, so you're always oriented. Stay within your comfort zone. If you get anxious about finding your way back, it's time to head home. No one expects you to graduate from Sacajawea* University during a single afternoon of wandering.

You insist on a destination? Oh, alright. Aim for Gold Bar Arch. It has an uncanny resemblance to a 4WD vehicle, so it's also known as *Jeep Arch*. Roughly, here's how to find it.

Above the three pouroffs, ascend left. Near the **first bay** on the canyon's left (northwest) wall, pick up a cairned, bootbeaten path on a ledge. Follow it north toward a butte with dual, stubby horns. Watch left (north-northwest) for a spire in a saddle. The path, though sketchy, ascends to the base of that spire via its right side. Avoid the impassable cul-de-sac left of and below the spire.

Reach the **base of the spire** at 1.2 mi (1.9 km), 4707 ft (1435 m). You've earned an impressive view. The La Sal Mountains are east-southeast. The Moab Rim and Behind The Rocks are southeast. The Colorado River is south. The Abajo Mountains are on the southern horizon.

Though it's inviting, the broad slickrock bench continuing directly north is not the way to Jeep Arch; it ends in 220 yd (200 m) at another vantage. From the spire, hike northwest on flatter terrain toward the next pass. Take care to avoid the profuse cryptogamic soil.

Just five minutes beyond the spire, **Jeep Arch** is visible right, in a southwest-facing wall. Five minutes farther, you'll be directly across from it and can appreciate its full jeepness. You've now hiked 1.6 mi (2.6 km) in about one hour. The elevation here is 4887 ft (1490 m).

It's possible to contour around the amphitheater, scramble into the arch, walk through it, descend the far side of the fin, and wander—mostly on slickrock—generally northeast up to the crest of **Gold Bar Rim** at approximately 5300 ft (1615 m), 3 mi (4.8 km). If you do that, however, you'll be probing the darker origins of the name *Jeep Arch*: the Gold Bar region is wildly popular with four-wheelers. You'll likely see them and (worse) hear them.

Another option after piercing the arch and descending the far side of the fin is to complete a circuit by working your way—in a southward arc—back down to the mouth of Dragonfly Canyon. Happy wandering.

*Sacajawea was the Shoshone woman who assisted Meriwether Lewis and William Clark while they explored western North America.

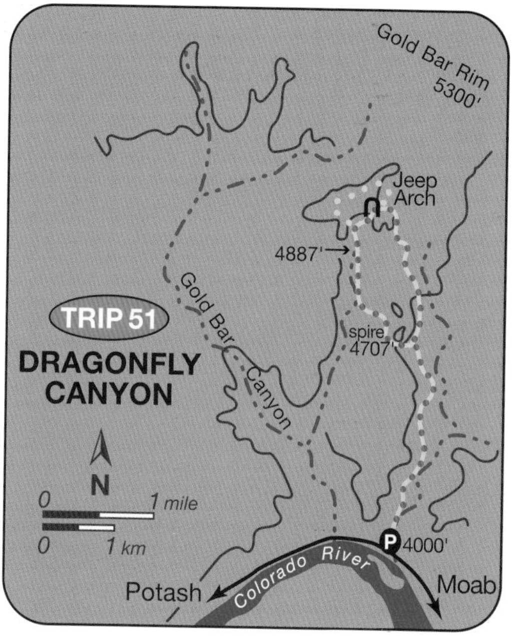

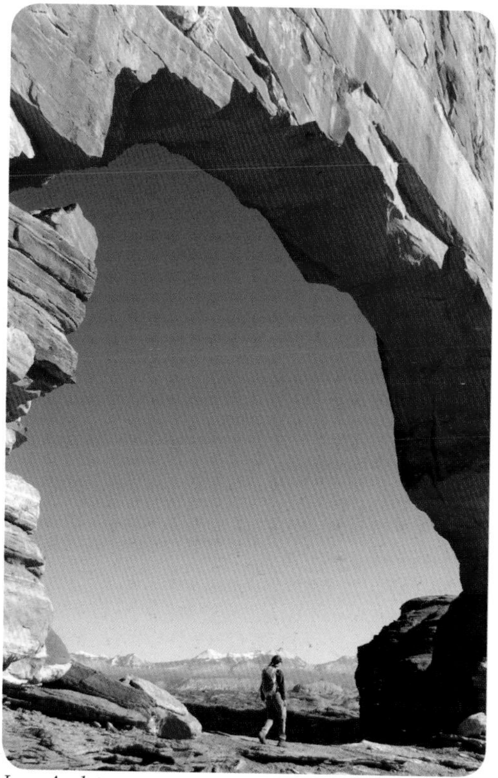

Jeep Arch

TRIP 52

SLICKROCK TRAIL

LOCATION	northeast edge of Moab
CIRCUIT	10.5 mi (16.9 km)
ELEVATION GAIN	approximately 760 ft (232 m)
KEY ELEVATIONS	trailhead 4642 ft (1415 m), Shrimp Rock 4598 ft (1402 m) highpoint near Swiss Cheese Ridge 4838 ft (1475 m)
HIKING TIME	3½ to 4½ hours
DIFFICULTY	moderate
MAPS	Sand Flats Bike Trails brochure (free, available at trailhead), Latitude 40 *Classic Moab Trails* Trails Illustrated *Moab South*

OPINION

"Rubber on wheels is faster'n rubber on heels" sang blues man Lightnin' Hopkins. And that's about as lucent an explanation as you'll hear for why, in Moab, mountainbiking is vastly more popular than hiking.

Whatever the reason, if you're a hiker, be glad. Two-wheeled travel is prohibited or impossible on many hiking trails, so you don't have to share them with legions of bikers. But you can, and should, stride a few of their bike routes, especially the most famous of all: the Moab Slickrock Trail. Advanced biking skills are necessary to safely, enjoyably ride it. On foot, anyone in reasonable physical condition will find it manageable yet thrilling.

Yes, a mere walk can be thrilling. That's certainly true on slickrock. With no vegetation to shunt you this way or that, you can follow your bliss. And the rock's gritty surface ("slick" is actually a misnomer) grants extraordinary traction, enabling you to negotiate steep pitches with gecko-like aplomb.

A *slickwalk*, where much of the way is on sandstone, inspires a rapturous sense of freedom. And the colorful, sensuous, monolithic terrain underfoot, coupled with the constant, unhindered views, make it a beautiful experience.

On this particular slickwalk, the distant scenery includes the towering, often snow-covered La Sal Mountains, the immense Moab Rim, the deep, sinuous Colorado River Canyon, and the rarely visited nether regions of Arches National Park.

You'll also see mountainbikers, of course. It can be an entertaining diversion. But you don't want to see too many, or you'll be constantly scuttling out of their way. Nor should you impede their progress since this is, by dint of majority rule, their trail, not yours. So hike here only when fat-tire season is at low ebb: late November to early March.

The weather in Moab can be surprisingly mild in mid-winter. Yet it's possible to be here alone then, despite the Slickrock Trail's international renown. That's prime time for novice slickwalkers to test the limits of this exotic medium. Just do it in sturdy hiking boots. Ankle support prevents injury on severe grades. Shock absorption lessens impact on your joints. Slickrock *is* rock, after all.

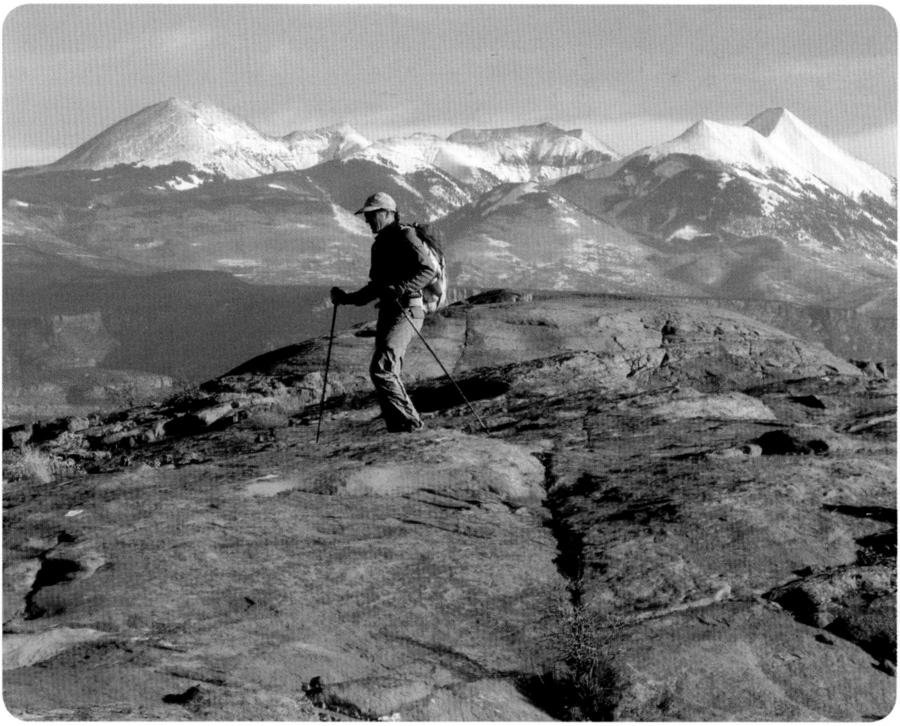

The La Sal Mountains, from the Slickrock Trail, early December

Though we offer detailed directions below, they're really just a handrail: necessary only if you falter. Simply follow the route (white rectangles, resembling a highway center line) painted on the rock.

Bear in mind, the Slickrock Trail was established in 1969 by motorcyclists. Though mountainbikers now predominate, crotch rockets are still allowed. If you hear one coming, yield the route. And try not to do it begrudgingly. Remember: whoever's wearing that Marvel-comic superhero costume atop that clamorous machine is a member of the clan who pioneered the trail. Stand aside and tip your hat in appreciation.

FACT

BY VEHICLE

From the Moab Info Center, at the corner of Main and Center streets, drive south on Main. Turn left (east) onto 300 South. Proceed four blocks to a T-junction and turn right (south) onto 400 East. Two blocks farther, turn left (east) onto Millcreek Drive. Follow it to a stop sign at a 3-way junction. Go straight (east) up the hill on Sand Flats Road. Continue 1.6 mi (2.6 km) to the toll booth at the Sand Flats Rec Area boundary. Purchase a daily, weekly or annual pass. Continue 0.7 mi (1.2 km) to the trailhead parking area, on the left, at 4642 ft (1415 m).

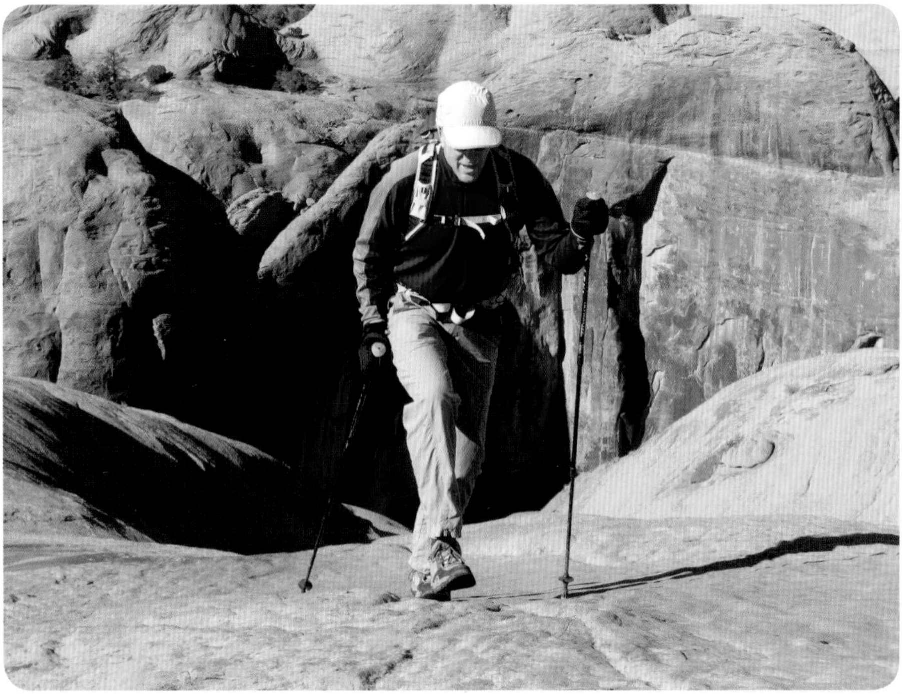
Above Abyss Canyon

ON FOOT

The entire trail is marked with white dashes painted on the rock. At junctions, words painted on the rock clearly spell out your options. Alternate routes and spurs (most of which we neither recommend nor describe) are marked with white dots. Yellow flame symbols indicate the Hell's Revenge 4WD route, which crosses the Slickrock Trail several times.

At the north end of the parking lot, right (east) of the toilets, pick up a free map then follow the trail north-northeast. In one minute, go left through a barbed-wire fence, but don't keep descending into the sand. Immediately turn sharp right (north-northeast) onto slickrock. The trail soon curves left (north).

Reach a junction at 0.3 mi (0.5 km), 4664 ft (1422 m). Right (north-northeast) is the cyclists' practice loop. Proceed straight (northwest) on the main trail.

At 0.8 mi (1.3 km), 4592 ft (1400 m), reach another junction. Right north is the practice loop. Go left (west) on the main trail.

Skirt the upper (southwest) end of **Abyss Canyon** at 1.6 mi (2.6 km). It's a tributary of Morning Glory Canyon (Trip 56), which is visible northeast. Ascend north over slickrock domes.

About 45 minutes from the trailhead, reach a **junction** at 2.3 mi (3.7 km), 4642 ft (1415 m). Left (west-southwest) is the easiest direction for cyclists. But since the difficulties don't apply to hikers, turn right (northeast) and begin a counter-clockwise loop. You'll find the scenery builds to a more satisfying climax in this direction. Plus, if you encounter cyclists, they won't ambush you from behind; you'll see them ahead.

If you notice a right fork at about 3 mi (4.8 km), follow it north to overlook **Icebox Canyon**. This short detour loops back to the main trail within ten minutes, where you should bear right and continue generally north.

After hiking about 1¼ hours from the trailhead, crest a rise affording a grand view north to the Windows Section of Arches National Park. Just beyond, at 3.8 mi (6.1 km), 4598 ft (1402 m), the trail pirouettes around the small-but-singular butte known as **Shrimp Rock**. The Colorado River Canyon is immediately below (north).

From here, the trail briefly swings west, away from the canyon rim, then veers northwest, grazing the rim yet again. Soon reach the trail's **northernmost point**, where it finally curves left and begins meandering southward.

Reach the next major fork at 6.3 mi (10.1 km), 4805 ft (1465 m). Total hiking time: a little over two hours. The right spur detours 0.6 mi (1 km) northwest to Panorama Viewpoint near Updraft Arch. Skip it. The scenery doesn't improve; you'll just be closer to the noise from Hwy 191. Go left and proceed generally south on the main trail.

At 6.5 mi (10.5 km) another right spur detours northwest. This one leads 0.2 mi (0.3 km) to Portal Viewpoint. Ignore it for the same reasons you blew off the last one. Go left, continuing generally southeast on the main trail.

Soon enjoy a virtually level stretch at about 4838 ft (1475 m)—the trail's **highpoint**. You're hiking parallel to and just below **Swiss Cheese Ridge**. The Hell's Revenge 4WD route follows the ridgecrest.

After leaving the ridge and curving through a long, broad, sensuous, slickrock wash, the trail drifts north, then wiggles east to reach a **junction** at 8.2 mi (13.2 km), 4642 ft (1415 m). Total hiking time: about 2½ hours. This is where you previously began the counter-clockwise loop. You're now on familiar ground. Turn right, descend, and begin retracing your steps. Just 45 minutes farther, reach the trailhead and complete the 10.5-mi (16.9-km) circuit.

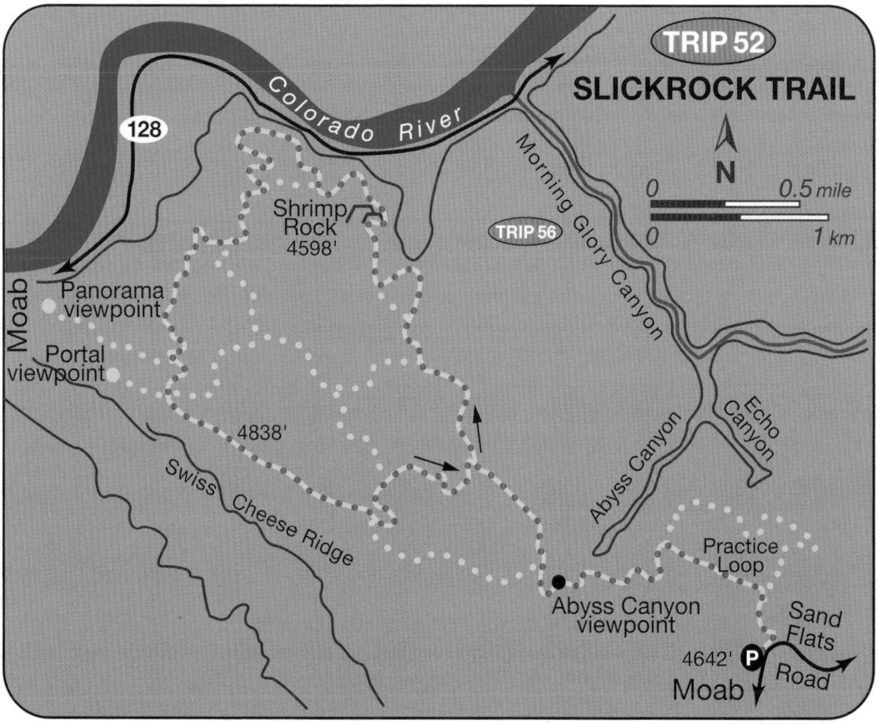

TRIP 53

MILL CREEK CANYON

LOCATION	east edge of Moab
ROUND TRIP	2 to 8 mi (3.2 to 12.9 km)
ELEVATION GAIN	250 to 550 ft (76 to 168 m)
KEY ELEVATIONS	trailhead 4429 ft (1350 m) rock-art site between pools 4576 ft (1395 m) Rill Creek confluence 4730 ft (1442 m)
HIKING TIME	1 to 5 hours
DIFFICULTY	easy
MAPS	Trails Illustrated *Moab South* Latitude 40 *Classic Moab Trails*

OPINION

A perennial stream in a desert canyon is cause for celebration. This one is conveniently located on the edge of Moab, between soaring Navajo-sandstone walls harboring some exceptional prehistoric rock art. Cascades and swimming holes heighten its appeal.

But those attributes ensure you won't find solitude in the lower reaches of Mill Creek Canyon. You might find a crowd. You're certain to hear noise from Hwy 191 a half hour or more beyond the trailhead.

The consensus seems to be this isn't a serious hike. It's a place to cool off and relax, splash along in your Tevas, eat a big, fat burrito, stretch out on a comfy ledge, and bask in the sun. We concede. So instead of enshrining Mill Creek Canyon among our favourite Moab trails, we're simply giving it an honorable mention.

Though very easy, an 8-mi (12.9-km), 5-hour round trip along Mill Creek's north fork to the confluence with Rill Creek Canyon would be exceptionally ambitious compared to most people's indolent agendas. Nearly everyone turns around well before, yet it's possible to go much farther.

The creek can be ankle-to knee-deep, and you'll be rockhopping or fording repeatedly, so amphibious footwear is preferable. Technical sandals designed for hiking are ideal. Fabric hiking boots you don't mind dunking are fine, too. A pack towel is also a good idea—to dry off at rest stops, or in case you swim.

FACT

BY VEHICLE

From the Moab Info Center, at the corner of Main and Center streets, drive east on Center. In four blocks, turn right (south) onto 400 East. In 0.75 mi

(1.2 km), at Dave's Corner Market, turn left onto Millcreek Drive. Just ahead, turn right at the stop sign. Take the next left (east), at 1.7 mi (2.8 km), onto Powerhouse Lane. It's paved only a short distance. Continue to the road's end trailhead parking lot at 2.4 mi (3.8 km), 4429 ft (1350 m), wreathed by Kayenta sandstone cliffs.

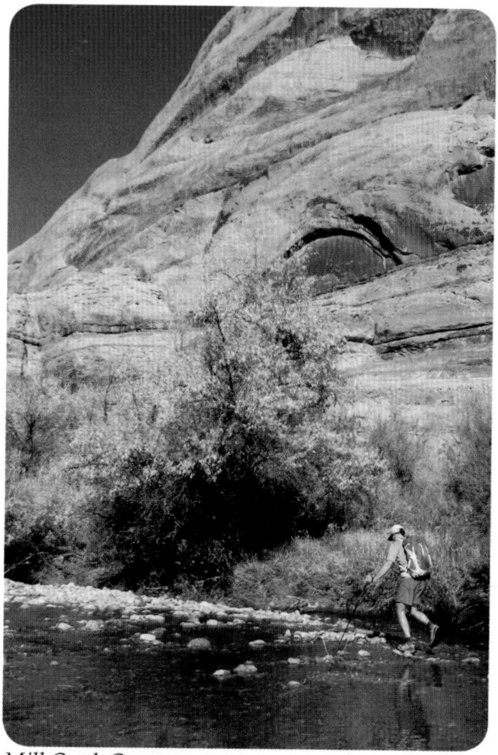
Mill Creek Canyon

ON FOOT

Before setting out, look up-canyon (east) from the parking lot. A shallow, eye-shaped depression is visible on the left (north) wall, near where the canyon's north and south forks split. You'll find rock art along the bottom of that depression.

The trail departs the northeast corner of the parking lot. Follow it east. Pass right of a **cement weir**—the remains of a 1950s electricity-generating dam that was immediately KO'd by a silt-laden flashflood. Clamber along a rock shelf at the edge of the creek, then proceed on sandy trail.

Pass the eye-shaped depression in about eight minutes. Just beyond, bear left (east) to probe the steeper-walled **north fork of Mill Creek Canyon**. Right (south-southeast) is the south fork.

Following the path of least resistance—either in the water or along the bootbeaten trail through brush and over ledges—work your way upstream on the canyon floor.

Within 20 minutes, reach a **huge pool beneath an impassable cascade**. Circumvent it by going back about 165 ft (150 m), turning right, and ascending the canyon's north wall, then proceeding up-canyon on a comfortable shelf.

About 35 minutes after leaving the trailhead, look up left (north) for a **boulder-riddled pocket**.

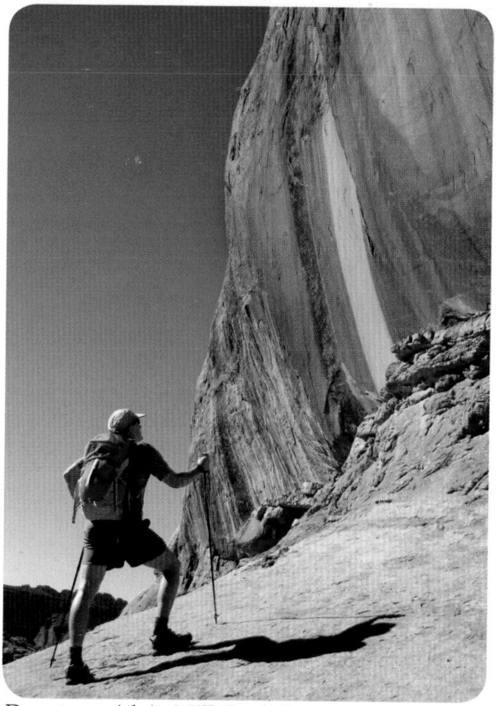
Desert varnish in Mill Creek Canyon

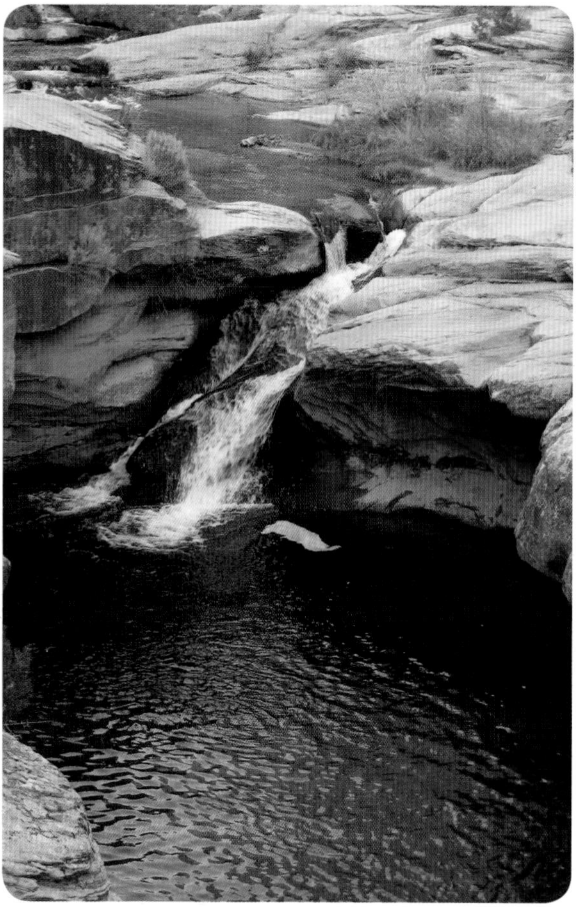

Mill Creek

A long stretch of the canyon wall here is slightly overhung and strewn with rock art. Ascend a steep slickrock slope to the base of the sheer sandstone at 4576 ft (1395 m). You'll find art all along the wall and on many boulders whose flat surfaces face the wall.

After descending from the bay, proceed up-canyon on sandy trail across a brushy bench. About ten minutes farther, encounter a **second deep pool**. Either swim it, or circumvent it by hiking down-canyon a couple minutes, ascending slickrock on the canyon's north wall, then resuming up-canyon progress. The shelf narrows dramatically for a short stretch but poses no actual exposure. The aerial view of the canyon is impressive.

A bootbeaten path descends to the treed, brushy, canyon floor. Few hikers continue beyond, so the trail is faint and sporadic. Proceed up-canyon whichever way seems easiest. Take care not to crush the prolific cryptogamic soil.

Pierce a stand of charred, dead-standing cottonwoods. Just past the mouth of an impassable tributary drainage, the trail rises onto a bench along the canyon's right (south) wall.

After hiking about 2½ hours from the trailhead, reach the **confluence of Mill and Rill creeks** at 4 mi (6.4 km), 4730 ft (1442 m). Rill is left (northeast). Mill Creek's north fork continues right (east-southeast). Rill has only a seasonal stream. Most hikers will find this an acceptable turnaround point.

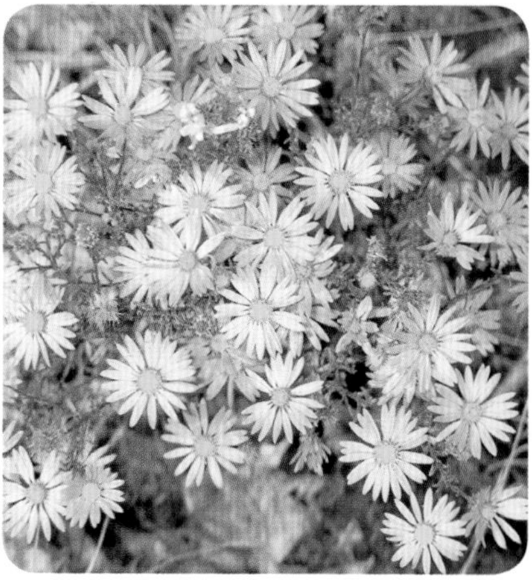

Daisies

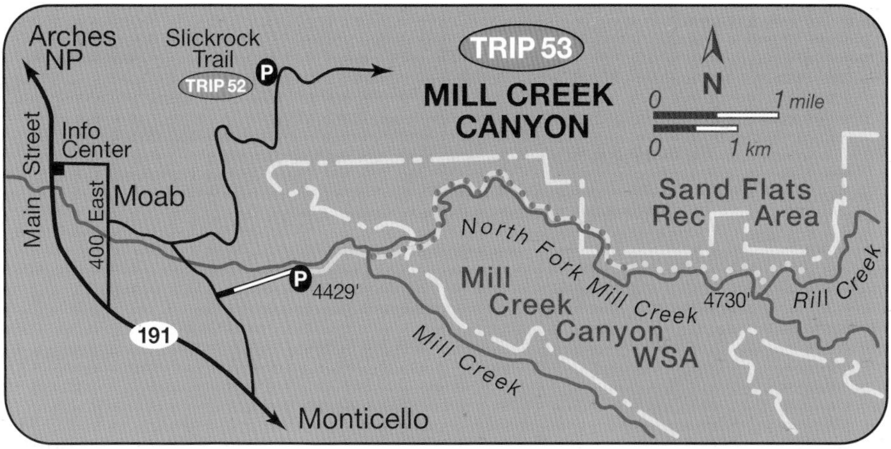

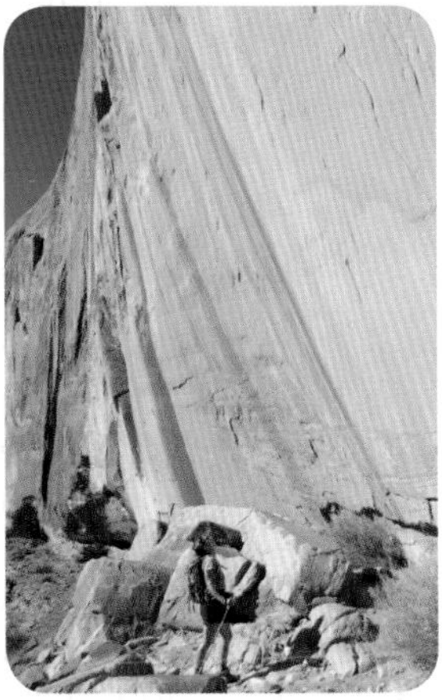

Examining rock art in Mill Creek Canyon

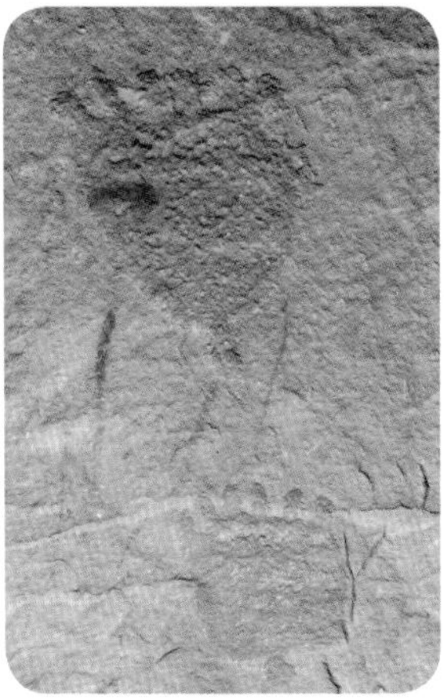

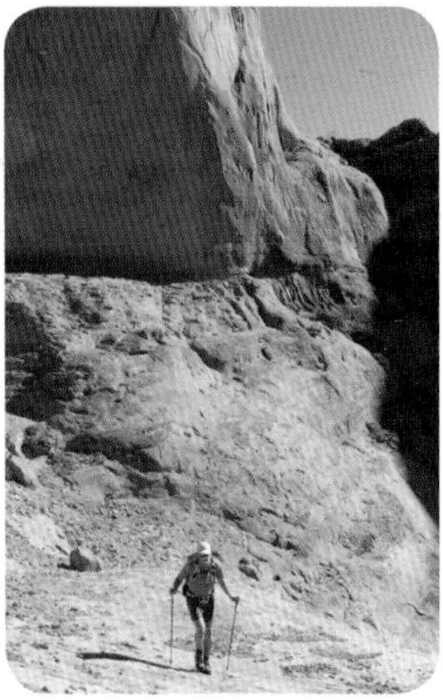

Rock-art alcove in Mill Creek Canyon

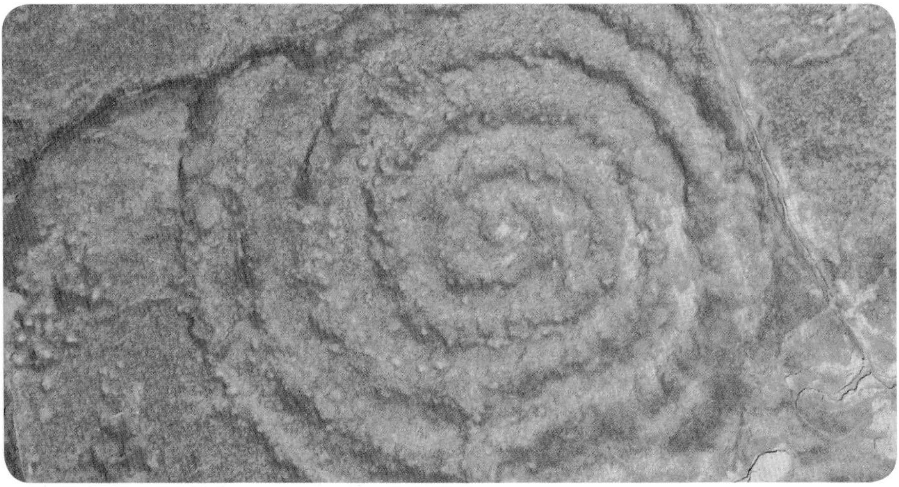

Swirl petroglyph in Mill Creek Canyon

TRIP 54

BEHIND THE ROCKS

LOCATION	immediately southwest of Moab
DISTANCE	4.8-mi (7.7-km) round trip for Hidden Valley 5-mi (8.1-km) round trip for Moab Rim 6.8-mi (10.9-km) one-way trip from Rim to Valley
ELEVATION GAIN	754 ft (230 m) for Hidden Valley 1400 ft (427 m) for Moab Rim 1620 ft (494 m) for Rim to Valley
KEY ELEVATIONS	Hidden Valley trailhead 4560 ft (1390 m) Moab Rim trailhead 4030 ft (1228 m) Rim-to-Valley highpoint (rock-art site near pass) 5314 ft (1620 m)
HIKING TIME	2½ hours for Hidden Valley 2½ hours for Moab Rim 4 hours for Rim to Valley
DIFFICULTY	moderate for all three options
MAPS	Trails Illustrated *Moab South* Latitude 40 *Classic Moab Trails*

OPINION

Look southwest from anywhere in Moab, and the dominant sight is the Moab Rim. It walls off the town, in fact all of Spanish Valley, from the BLM Wilderness Study Area known as *Behind The Rocks*—an intriguing chaos of sandstone fins, walls and domes.

Here you can slickwalk for long stretches, admire ancient rock art, stride through fields of wildflowers (in spring), and enjoy sweeping views. You'll see the Colorado River Canyon and the spectacular, red-rock desert beyond: from Dead Horse Point State Park to Canyonlands National Park.

A trail—actually a 4WD route for most of its length—hugs the Moab Rim and dances along the northeast edge of Behind The Rocks. One end, known as the *Moab Rim trail*, starts beside the Colorado River, near The Portal, west of town. The other end, known as the *Hidden Valley trail*, starts at the southeast end of town.

Each end affords a distinctly different round trip. Both are short, however, so if a longer hike probing more of Behind The Rocks appeals to you, make this a one-way journey. The only drawback to this third option is that it necessitates a vehicle shuttle.

trip 54a - Moab Rim

Ascending slickrock slabs and ramps can be a giddy experience. Here's a convenient place to do it near Moab. The route immediately overlooks the Colorado River and quickly leads to grand views of the town, Spanish Valley, the Moab Rim, and Behind the Rocks.

PETROGLYPHS ABOVE HIDDEN VALLEY

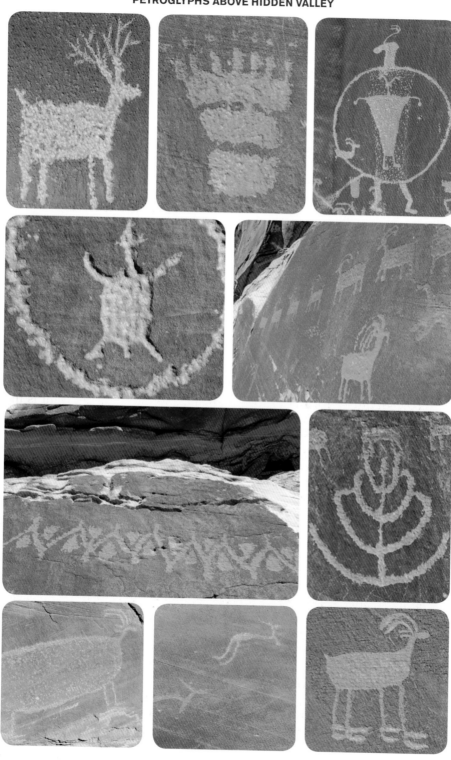

Be prepared to share the route with 4WD vehicles. It's possible you won't see any, but if you do, try thinking of them as a curiosity rather than an annoyance. You might be entertained. What those motorheads do in their rock crawlers *is* amazing.

trip 54b - Hidden Valley

Valley? Not quite. It's actually two hanging terraces. You'll reach them via a short, steep, rough ascent on a genuine trail. (Traffic on Hwy 191 is loud, but you'll encounter no 4WD vehicles and few if any mountainbikers.)

After striding through the terraces, reach a fork atop a pass. The main trail descends into Behind The Rocks and broadens into a 4WD road, while a bootbeaten path detours along the base of a sandstone wall bearing a superb rock-art gallery.

The petroglyphs include herds of pronghorn antelope, a Jewish menorah-shaped image, leaping deer, six- and seven-toed bear paws, a horned toad or tortoise (you decide), and a group of hand-holding peaceniks.

trip 54c - Rim to Valley

After ascending the Moab Rim slickrock route, continue along the back of the rim through Behind The Rocks, stop to inspect numerous petroglyph panels near a pass, then descend via Hidden Valley to a trailhead just off Hwy 191, at the southeast end of Moab.

By linking the two out-and-back hikes into a one-way trip, you'll enjoy a more complete, satisfying experience. You'll also need a second vehicle and comrades willing to arrange a shuttle. Your other option is to engage the services of a local shuttle company. Try Coyote (259-8656), Roadrunner (259-9402), or Porcupine (260-0896).

FACT

BY VEHICLE

Moab Rim trailhead

In Moab, from the junction of Main (Hwy 191) and Center streets, drive south on Main 0.6 mi (1 km). Just before McDonald's, turn right (north) onto Kane Creek Blvd. Bear left at 1.4 mi (2.3 km). At 3.1 mi (5 km) cross the first cattleguard. Reach the trailhead parking lot, on the left, at 3.3 mi (5.3 km), 4030 ft (1228 m).

Hidden Valley trailhead

In Moab, from the junction of Main (Hwy 191) and Center streets, drive south on Main. In 4 mi (6.4 km), at the small, brown, BLM sign *Hidden Valley Trail*, turn right (southwest) onto Angel Rock Road. Reach a T-junction at 4.3 mi (6.9 km). Turn right onto Rimrock Lane. It curves left and pavement ends at 4.5 mi (7.2 km). Reach the trailhead parking lot at 4.6 mi (7.4 km), 4560 ft (1390 m).

ON FOOT

trip 54a **Moab Rim**
round trip **5 mi (8.1 km)**
elevation gain **1400 ft (427 m)**
hiking time **2½ hours, mostly on slickrock.**

Depart the northeast end of the trailhead. Pass right of the huge, split boulder. Ascend generally northeast on ramps of Kayenta sandstone. Unfortunately, white painted rectangles, brown plastic BLM posts, tire marks, and oil stains indicate the way.

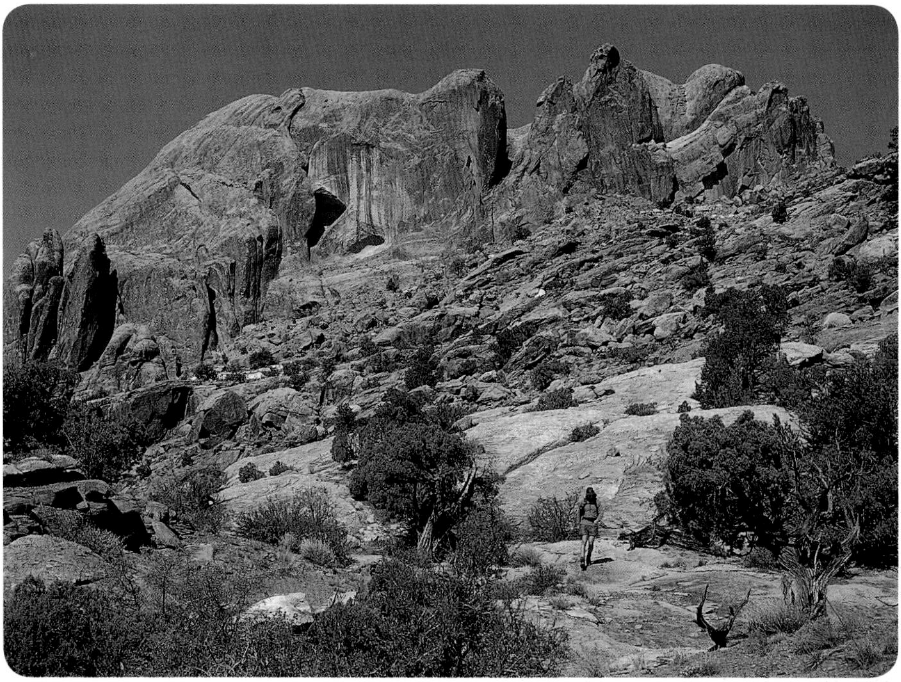

Behind the Rocks

In about 25 minutes, at 4936 ft (1505 m), curve right (southeast) at a wood fence near the **crest of the Moab Rim**. At 1.1 mi (1.8 km), 4970 ft (1515 m), you've completed the initial, steep ascent. Detour left (northeast) for a climactic panorama.

The town is below. Arches National Park (Trips 47-49) is north-northeast. The Slickrock Trail (Trip 52) is northeast. Mill Creek Canyon (Trip 53) is east. The La Sal Mountains are east-southeast.

Resume southeast. A sign indicates you're entering Behind The Rocks WSA. Pass a second left spur to a viewpoint. Gradually curve right (south) between massive **Navajo sandstone domes**. The route—occasionally in sand, often on slickrock—remains an obvious 4WD road.

Descend to 4855 ft (1480 m), then ascend southwest. Look left (south) and you'll see a road in a sandy wash below. That's the way you *don't* want to hike and will soon have the option to avoid.

Reach a **signed fork** at 1.8 mi (2.9 km), 4855 ft (1480 m), about 50 minutes from the trailhead. Left (south-southeast) descends into the viewless, sandy wash you overlooked. Go right (southwest)—the easier, higher, more scenic route. White painted rectangles indicate the way forward.

Still heading generally southwest, descend to 4725 ft (1441 m). At one hour, curve southeast. A few minutes farther, at 4820 ft (1470 m), begin ascending over a **slickrock dome**. Top out at 2.5 mi (4 km), 4936 ft (1505 m), about 1¼ hours from the trailhead.

The view is grand. The Moab Rim is nearby, behind you (northeast, east, and southeast). Ahead, just across the Colorado River Canyon, is Poison Spider Mesa (west). Immediately beyond it is Amasa Back (Trip 55). On the horizon are Dead Horse Point State Park (west-southwest) and Canyonlands National Park (southwest).

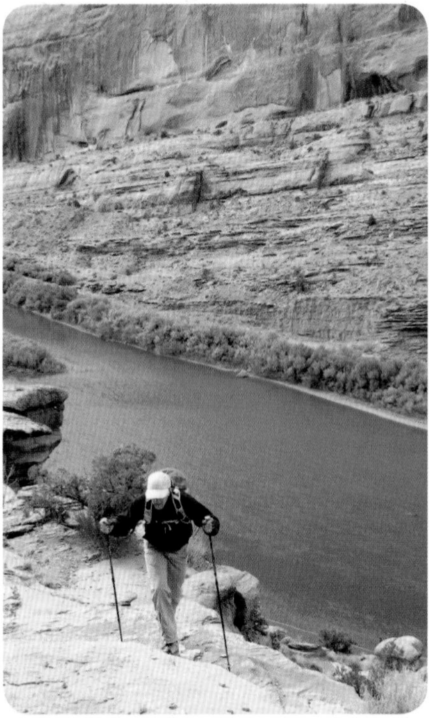

Moab Rim trail above the Colorado River

For a short round trip, turn around here, on the slickrock dome. Return the way you came. You intend to make this a one-way hike exiting via Hidden Valley? Skip below to Trip 54c, where directions resume.

trip 54b	**Hidden Valley**
round trip	**4.8 mi (7.7 km)**
elevation gain	**754 ft (230 m)**
hiking time	**2½ hours, plus an hour to admire the rock art**

The trail departs the south corner of the parking lot. Follow it south. Soon begin a rocky, switchbacking ascent, gradually curving northwest.

At 0.5 mi (0.8 km), 5070 ft (1545 m), you've vanquished most of the elevation gain. Fit hikers will approach the **first terrace**, behind the rim's outer barrier, in about 20 minutes. Proceed northwest.

After a long, level, grassy stretch, the trail briefly ascends then levels again in the **second terrace**. At the far end, curve left and crest an east-west **pass** at 2 mi (3.2 km), 5271 ft (1607 m).

The main trail descends northwest then west into Behind the Rocks, soon widening into a 4WD road. But to see the rock art, veer right (north) onto a bootbeaten path. It skirts the right (east) side of a standing rock in the pass, ascends to 5314 ft (1620 m), then forks. Go left (west) and begin a gradual descent along the base of the **south-facing wall**.

The first rock-art panel is only a minute farther. Panels continue sporadically the entire length of the wall, nearly to the 4WD road in the wash below. They end where the bootbeaten path disappears on grey bedrock, at 2.4 mi (3.8 km). Return the way you came.

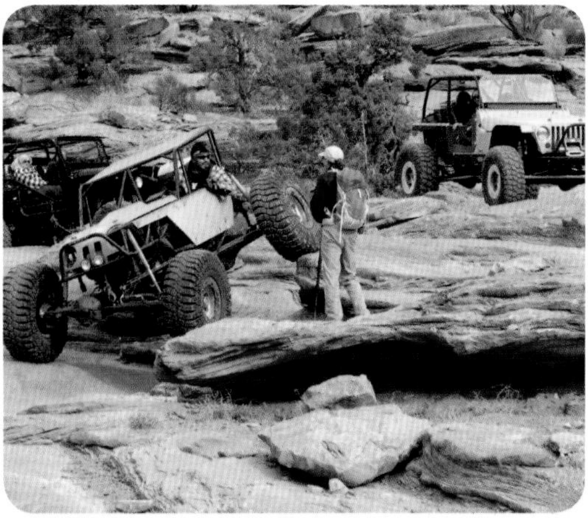

Friendly encounter with motorheads, Moab Rim trail

trip 54c	**Rim to Valley**
one-way trip	**6.8 mi (10.9 km)**
elevation gain	**1620 ft (494 m)**
hiking time	**4 hours, plus an hour to admire the rock art**

Having followed the directions in trip 54a, you've hiked about 1¼ hours from the Moab Rim trailhead. You're now atop the **slickrock dome** at 2.5 mi (4 km), 4936 ft (1505 m).

Before continuing generally southeast toward Hidden Valley, pause to survey the terrain ahead.

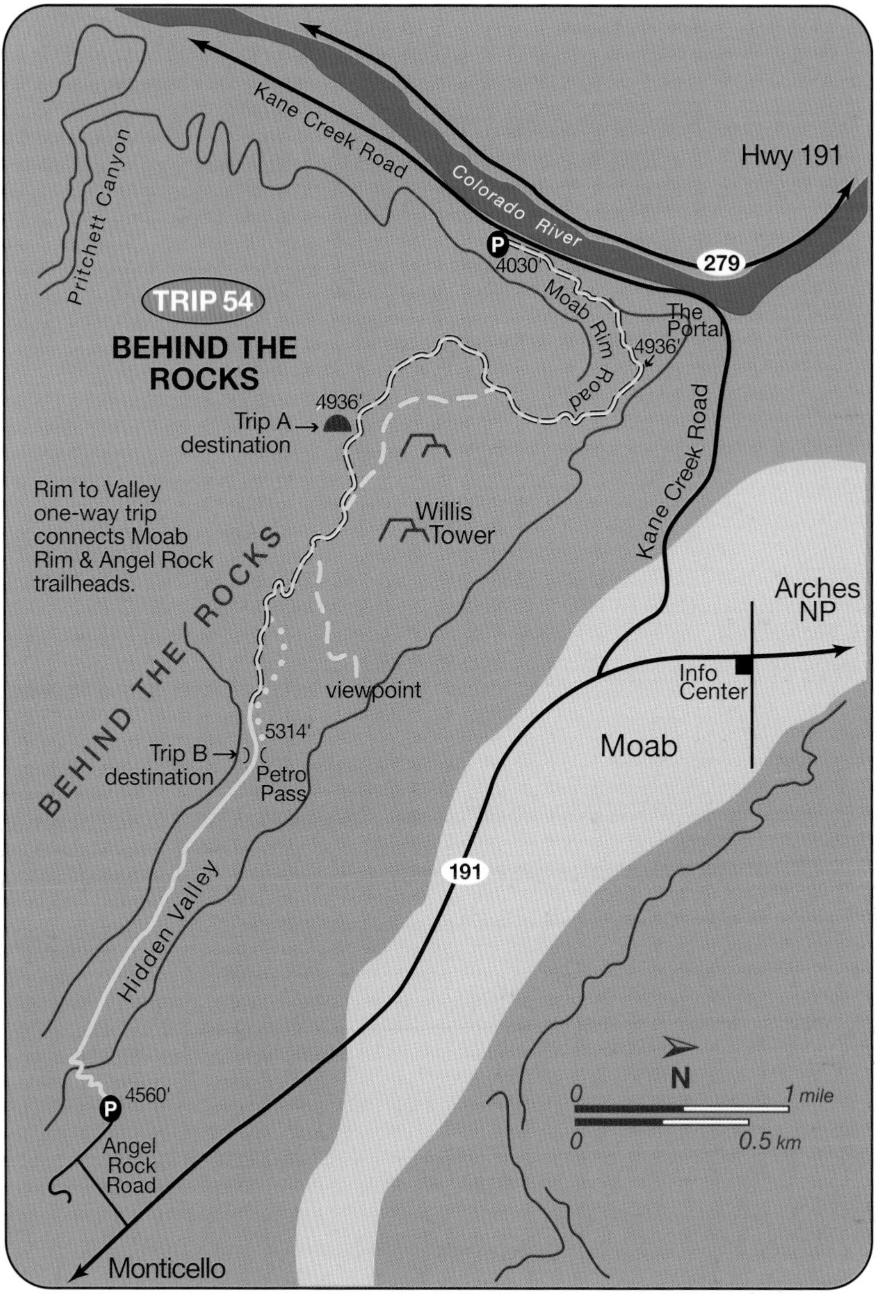

Specifically, look east-southeast. Two roads are visible. Both ascend to gaps in the Moab Rim. The left one is a spur that ends near the crest. The right one leads to the pass through which you'll descend into Hidden Valley.

Onward. Follow the white painted rectangles over the dome's 4960-ft (1512-m) summit and down the far side. About 12 minutes beyond the dome, at 3.1 mi (5 km), 4936 ft (1505 m), reach a **junction**.

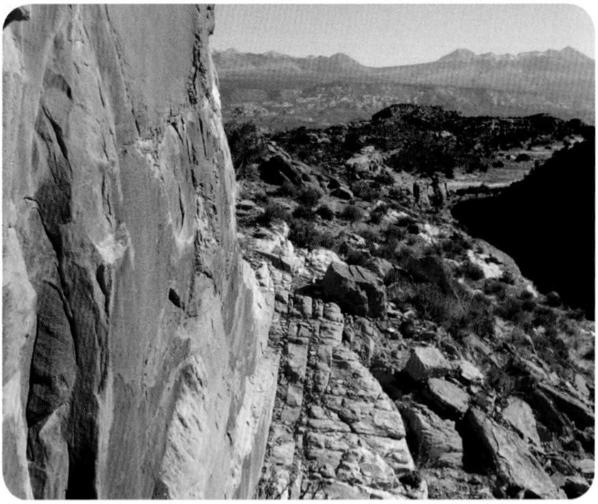
Overlooking Hidden Valley from rock-art site. La Sal Mountains in distance.

Left (northeast) descends, returning via the viewless, sandy wash to the signed fork at 1.8 mi (2.9 km), 4855 ft (1480 m), about 50 minutes from the trailhead, where you previously opted for the easier, higher, more scenic route. Proceed straight (east), descending gradually.

About 15 minutes beyond the dome, ignore the rockier fork. Continue straight on the main road. About 25 minutes beyond the dome, reach a **junction in a wash** at 3.5 mi (5.6 km), 4953 ft (1510 m).

The two roads you saw from atop the slickrock dome split here. For Hidden Valley, ascend right (east-southeast). Left dips north, immediately curves right, and ascends generally east. It ends in 0.8 mi (1.3 km) at a 5305-ft (1617-m) vantage atop the Moab Rim—a worthwhile detour if you have time and energy.

En route to Hidden Valley, about five minutes past the 3.5-mi (5.6-km) junction, reach a **fork** at 5085 ft (1550 m). Left ascends east-southeast. Go right, descending south.

Soon curve sharply left (southeast) into a **slickrock wash**. The road vanishes here. Ascend left (east) following cairns across slickrock. The road resumes about 15 minutes farther. Continue following it generally east.

The road drops to and crosses a tributary drainage, rises, then drops into a **second tributary drainage** at 4.5 mi (7.2 km), 5133 ft (1565 m). Stop. Decision time. The road continues ascending to the pass visible just ahead (east). That's the quick, direct exit via Hidden Valley, but it skirts an impressive rock-art site.

To see the art, turn left (north-northwest) and leave the road. Descend this second tributary drainage, then ascend onto the grey bedrock and continue up to the **south-facing wall** that's about 55 yd (60 m) from the road. Pick up a bootbeaten path gradually ascending east along the base of the wall.

Petroglyph panels continue sporadically the entire length of the wall. Follow it upward. At the east end of the wall, having ascended to 5314 ft (1620 m), you've concluded your art walk. The road is visible in the wash below. It parallels the wall, dwindles to trail, and rises to an east-west pass.

Descend the path right (south) to intersect the road/trail in the **pass** at 4.8 mi (7.7 km), 5271 ft (1607 m). From here, the trail curves southeast bisecting two **terraces** (mistakenly known as a "valley") where wildflowers bloom in May.

At 6.3 mi (10.1 km), 5070 ft (1545 m), begin a rocky, switchbacking descent, gradually curving north. Reach the **Hidden Valley trailhead** at 6.8 mi (10.9 km), 4560 ft (1390 m), beneath the Moab Rim, near the southeast end of town.

TRIP 55

AMASA BACK

LOCATION	Kane Creek Road, southeast of Moab
ROUND TRIP	7 to 9.2 mi (11.3 to 14.8 km)
ELEVATION GAIN	1444 to 1644 ft (440 to 501 m) including ups and downs
KEY ELEVATIONS	trailhead parking 4000 ft (1219 m) actual trailhead 4200 ft (1280 m) Kane Creek 3950 ft (1204 m), ridge 4722 ft (1439 m) spur viewpoint 4700 ft (1433 m) bighorn panel 4900 ft (1494 m)
HIKING TIME	3½ to 4½ hours
DIFFICULTY	moderate
MAPS	Trails Illustrated *Moab South* Latitude 40 *Classic Moab Trails*

OPINION

Viewed from above, the Colorado River's wildly sinuous course is as inscrutable as a Rorschach test. So maybe your impression of it reveals something about yourself.

Does the waterway appear aimless? Confused? As predictable as a staggering drunk? Maybe it strikes you as a curious wanderer, eagerly exploring every intriguing sight. Or perhaps you think it's like human nature: flowing wherever resistance is least, just as people usually do.

Formulate your interpretation while hiking Amasa Back—a steep-walled, finger-like peninsula, one of thousands stubbornly denying the Colorado a straight course. On top, the trail traverses the peninsula's narrow isthmus, granting you two distinctly different yet equally enthralling aerial views of the river and its magnificent, snaking canyon, plus the most striking perspective you'll likely ever attain of Behind The Rocks—the fascinating sandstone chaos immediately southwest of Moab Rim.

The Amasa Back trail, like many in Utah, is an old road, more popular with mountainbikers, four-wheelers and motorcyclists than with hikers. That's because most people's attitude is "Why walk when you can ride?" The snappy answer to that stupid question is "Because if you want to engage the earth directly, rather than be preoccupied with a machine, walking is more enjoyable and fulfilling than riding."

At least you won't feel like you're hiking a road here, because this one is rougher than the average trail. It's certainly not an eyesore. As for sharing it, a few mountainbikers won't detract from your hiking experience. And most motorheads are friendly people piloting surprisingly quiet vehicles. Watching them attempt a road like this is engrossing.

An off-road motorcycle, however, is hellishly noisy, even if ridden by a saint. But if you hike Amasa Back midweek, especially late fall or early spring, dirtbikers will be as rare as snowflakes. Uninterrupted tranquility is more likely.

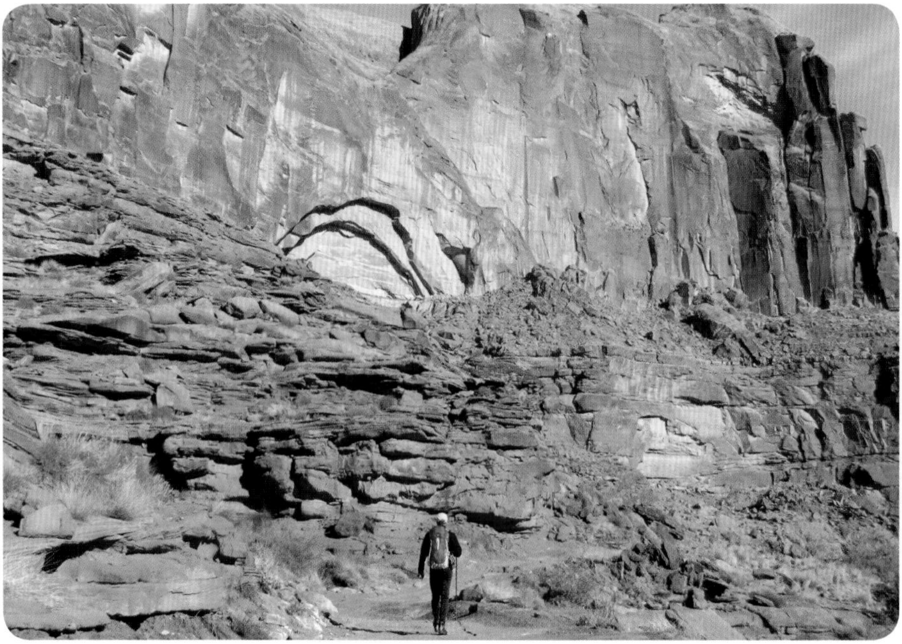

En route to Amasa Back

You'll ascend Amasa Back by zigzagging through ledgy canyon terrain: slickrock ramps, scattered boulders, pockets of sandy dirt punctuated by juniper trees. The hike is engaging the entire way, initially because of the immediate surroundings, later because of the panoramic vistas.

Atop Amasa Back, after attaining the first ridgetop vantage, most hikers will choose to cross the peninsula's narrow isthmus, following a spur to a second viewpoint. Here you can relax on slickrock slabs at the canyon's edge, meditate on the river's unceasing, languorous flow, and perhaps see mountainbikers or four-wheelers ascend the popular Poison Spider trail. Or, if you have time and energy for a longer exploration, you can pass the isthmus and continue out the peninsula where yet more slickrock awaits.

When you return to your vehicle at the trailhead parking area, don't leave. Not until you see the nearby rock-art site. It's on the canyon wall, just above the road—a mere 15-minute round trip. The numerous images include a superb Kokopelli sans flute.

FACT

BY VEHICLE

From the junction of Hwys 191 and 128, beside the Colorado River bridge just north of Moab, drive Hwy 191 southeast 1.2 mi (2 km). Just south of Motel 6, turn right (south) onto 500 West. (Denny's restaurant is on the southwest corner.) Cross 400 North and continue south. At 2.6 mi (4.2 km) reach a Y-junction. Turn sharply right onto Kane Creek Blvd. Reset your trip odometer to 0.

From the junction of Main (Hwy 191) and Center streets in Moab, drive south on Main 0.6 mi (1 km). Just before McDonald's, turn right (north) onto Kane Creek Blvd. Bear left at 1.4 mi (2.3 km). Reset your trip odometer to 0.

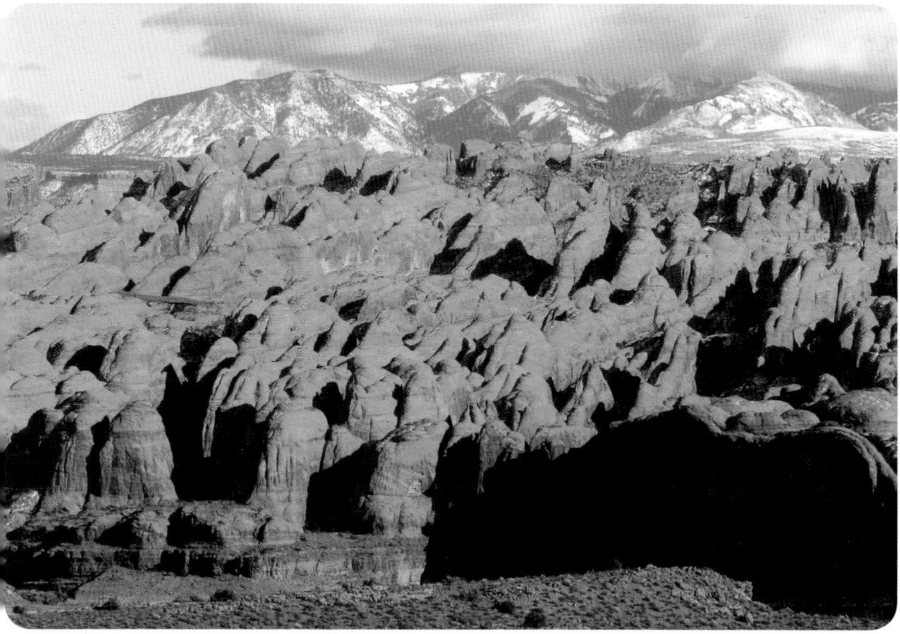

Behind the Rocks backed by the La Sal Mountains

From either approach, follow Kane Creek Blvd. west, then south-southwest along the Colorado River. It soon becomes Kane Creek Road. Pass the Moonflower petroglyph panel on the left at 2.3 mi (3.7 km). (Worth a stop. It's on the right/south side of the parking area.) At 3.4 mi (5.5 km) pass a campground near the mouth of Pritchett Canyon. (Mediocre hiking to impressive Pritchett Natural Bridge.) At 3.8 mi (6.1 km) pavement ends. Reach the **trailhead parking area**, on the right, at 4.4 mi (7.1 km), 4000 ft (1219 m).

ON FOOT

The trail does not begin at the trailhead parking area. Leave your vehicle here and walk back onto Kane Creek Road. Turn right (south). Follow the unpaved road south, then west. In about 10 minutes, at 0.6 mile (1 km), reach the **actual trailhead,** where there's no room to park safely. It's signed, on the right, at 4200 ft (1280 m).

The trail is a 4WD road. It begins with a sharp descent north. (See the tire marks? Four-wheelers negotiate these rock obstacles. Hard to believe unless you witness it.) Soon reach **Kane Creek**, at 3950 ft (1204 m). Rockhop to the northwest bank, then ascend left (southwest).

About ten minutes farther, reach an apparent fork. Left (south-southwest) rises to the canyon edge, where it ends abruptly on slickrock. Go right (west) to enter a **cove**. Circle back right (north-northeast), then curve left (west) and traverse above the cove.

Continue generally south, mostly on ledges, ascending gradually above **Kane Creek canyon**. The road is easy to recognize, because it's the only passage wide enough for a vehicle. It also bears frequent evidence of the many tires that have preceded you.

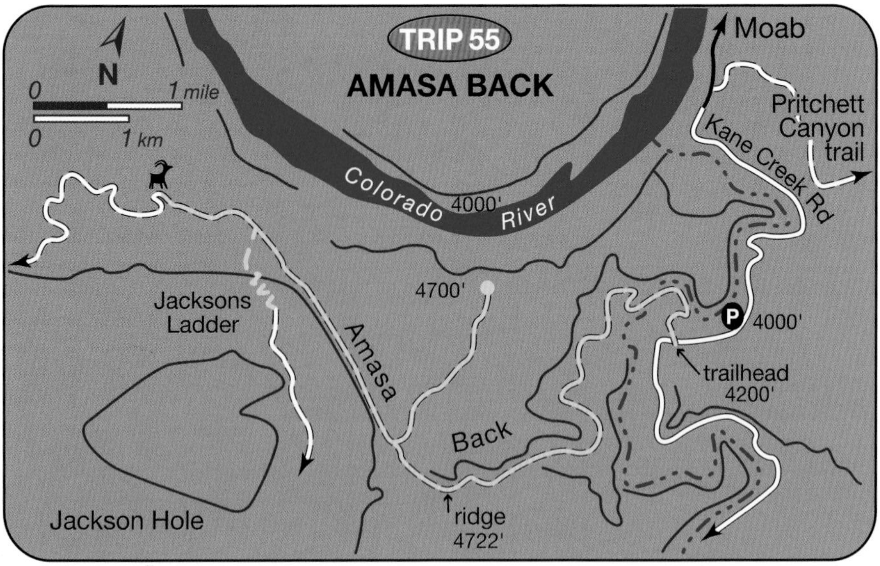

Visible east and southeast is a concentration of sandstone fins in the wilderness study area known as *Behind the Rocks*. Beyond are the La Sal Mountains. The view improves as you ascend, of course. Look back frequently to enjoy what surely ranks among Utah's most spectacular scenes.

The road eventually curves right (west), departing Kane Creek canyon. Ascend a long, gentle slickrock ramp. After hiking 2.6 mi (4.2 km) from the parking area—a one hour task for strong hikers—crest a **ridge** at 4722 ft (1439 m).

Visible left (west-northwest) is **Jackson Hole**—a Colorado River Canyon bay punctuated by a lone butte. The river created the butte long ago by carving one side away from the canyon wall, then straightening its course and slicing off the other side. This left Jackson Hole dry, with a lone butte as its centerpiece. A mountainbike route now loops around the butte. North of Jackson Hole, is Amasa Back—a jumbled, rocky, bush-stippled peninsula defying the Colorado River, forcing it to take a circuitous oxbow detour.

From the ridgecrest, the road curves right (north) and descends slightly to a **junction** at 2.8 mi (4.5 km), amid sand, low bushes and broken rock. You now have two options:

(1) Turn right (northeast) onto a sandy **spur**. Within 15 minutes (brief ascent and descent, views east and southeast to Behind the Rocks and the La Sals) you'll cross the narrow Amasa Back isthmus and reach the **spur viewpoint** in 0.7 mi (1.1 km). Elevation: 4700 ft (1433 m). Distance from the parking area: 3.5 mi (5.6 km). Here you're on the edge of the Colorado River Canyon. The river is directly below. Amasa Back is visible left (northwest). The Poison Spider trail begins on the river's far bank, directly north.

(2) Bear left (north-northwest) on the **main road**. It descends then contours along the edge of the sheer canyon wall above Jackson Hole before proceeding generally northwest onto **Amasa Back**. The Potash industrial site opposite Jackson Hole, on the Colorado River's west bank, will be visible, but you'll lose sight of it if you continue. One destination (though it's possible to hike much farther out the peninsula) is the **bighorn petroglyph panel**.

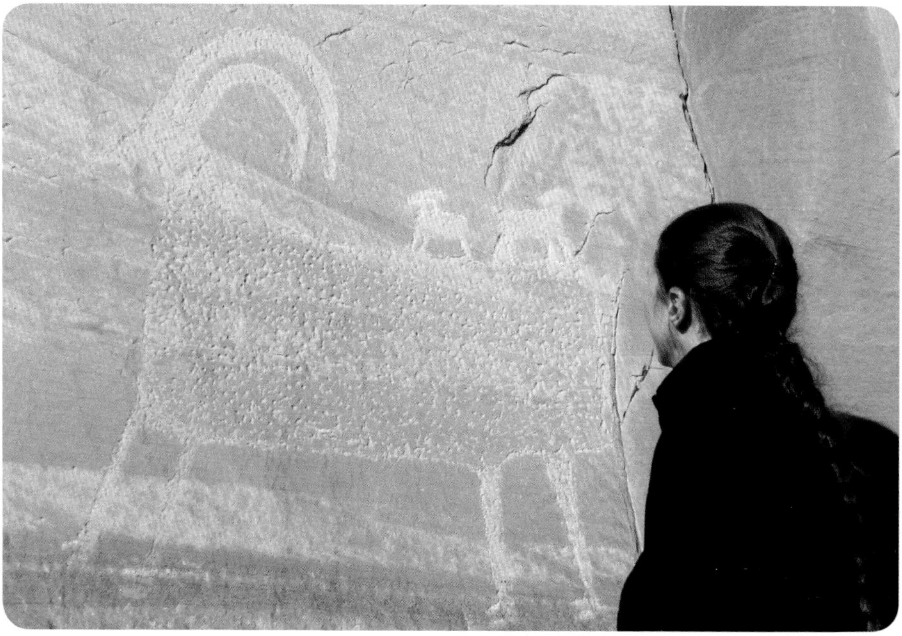

Bighorn petroglyph, Amasa Back

To reach the panel, keep following the main road northwest. Note the time when you pass beneath the power lines. Stay on the main road, ignoring left and right forks. Twelve minutes past the power lines, the road crosses a prominent, broad, circular, slickrock cascade. Distance from the parking area: 4.4 mi (7.1 km). Elevation: 4850 ft (1478 m).

Stop here and look west-northwest to the second (left and slightly more distant) of two promontories. At the base of its south-facing wall, near the right side, a large chunk of rock fell away exposing an angular section of white rock beneath a protective overhang. That's where you'll find a life-size petroglyph of a bighorn sheep with two smaller sheep riding on its back. Depart the road and hike directly toward it, arriving at 4.6 mi (7.4 km), 4900 ft (1494 m).

Trailhead Rock Art

A mere 15-minute round trip from the Amasa Back trailhead parking area will allow you to appreciate some impressive rock art. From the kiosk, cross to the northeast side of the road. Look for the low, hiker signpost. A trail, initially lined with rocks, ascends north-northeast. It soon steepens and begins switchbacking. Gain 150 ft (46 m) to the base of a lightly desert-varnished cliff. The trail then leads right, curving around to the cliff's south side, where you'll find the first petroglyphs. Contour along the cliff base another 40 yd/m to see bighorn sheep, a Kokopelli sans flute, a swirl, a snake, and various symbols.

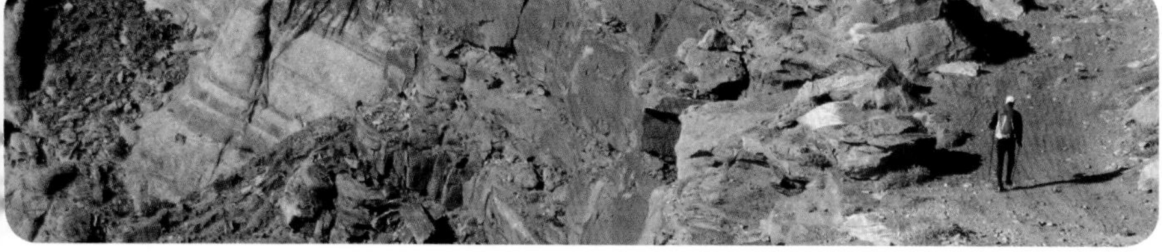

TRIP 56

MORNING GLORY CANYON

LOCATION	northeast of Moab
ROUND TRIP	4.6 mi (7.4 km) to Morning Glory plus at least 3 mi (4.8 km) exploring
ELEVATION GAIN	327 ft (100 m) to Morning Glory plus at least 345 ft (105 m) exploring
KEY ELEVATIONS	trailhead 4000 ft (1219 m) Morning Glory Natural Bridge 4327 ft (1319 m) hanging tributary drainage 4446 ft (1355 m) slickrock domes 4530 ft (1381 m)
HIKING TIME	2 hours for Morning Glory plus at least 2½ hours exploring
DIFFICULTY	easy to Morning Glory, moderate beyond
MAPS	Trails Illustrated *Moab South* Latitude 40 *Classic Moab Trails*

OPINION

You'll hear the name *Negro Bill* in reference to this canyon and the surrounding Wilderness Study Area. But that's the last you'll hear it from us.

Some names, regardless of historical origin, should be stricken from the record. Otherwise they reinforce attitudes now universally recognized as noxious, repugnant or just plain asinine—in this case all three.

The primary feature distinguishing the canyon is Morning Glory Natural Bridge, the sixth-longest rock span in the U.S. and an arresting sight. So BLM, take note: When you cease your interminable "study" and finally declare this a full-fledged Wilderness Area, change the insensitive name. We propose you officially call it *Morning Glory Canyon*.

Though big—243 ft (74 m) long, to be precise—the namesake bridge is difficult to appreciate until you're directly beneath it. But it's only 2.3 mi (3.7 km) from the trailhead. Besides, the canyon itself is beautiful, with bulging, soaring, sensuous, Navajo sandstone walls; a clear, perennial stream; lush vegetation including cottonwoods and gambel oaks; and abundant wildlife ranging from crayfish to hawks.

Plus the going is easy. The short, comfortable trail gains little elevation, so it's ideal for families with hikers-in-training, strong striders seeking a quick-but-scenic workout, or even non-hikers wanting to take a step in the right direction. During spring runoff, you might have to get your feet wet while crossing the stream (bring sandals), but most of the year it's possible to keep your boots dry by rockhopping.

"It's popular" is the worst thing you can say about Morning Glory. The canyon is simply too appealing and close to town to afford solitude. If you're

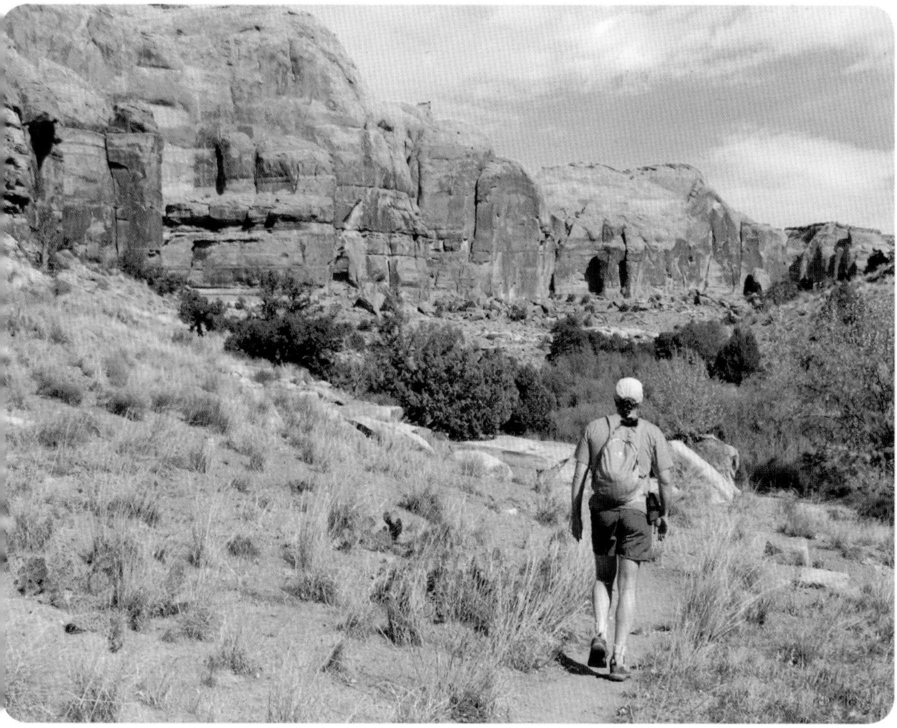

Beyond Morning Glory Bridge

here very early or late in the day, or when the weather's uncomfortably hot or cold, you'll of course see fewer people. But if you're here during prime time along with everyone else, ditch the crowd by out-hiking them.

Almost nobody ventures beyond the natural bridge, yet the canyon extends another eight miles. Our recommendation for experienced navigators, described below, is to briefly head upstream then veer into the intriguing expanse of slickrock above the canyon's north wall. You'll be there in a mere half mile. You can then decide to keep exploring cross-country all the way to overlook the Colorado River Canyon, or imitate the surrounding boulders by stopping, sitting, and silently absorbing the canyon atmosphere.

BY VEHICLE

From Hwy 191, at the northwest edge of Moab, turn east onto Hwy 128. Follow it 3 mi (4.8 km), paralleling the Colorado River.

From I-70, near Cisco, drive Hwy 128 generally south, then southwest. Continue 41.5 mi (66.8 km) to milepost 3.

From either approach, turn southeast into the trailhead parking area. Elevation: 4000 ft (1219 m).

ON FOOT

The trail departs the east side of the parking area, right (south) of the map kiosk. Initially lined with rocks, briefly atop slickrock, the trail soon becomes a sandy path heading generally southeast, following the creek upstream, on the left (northeast) bank.

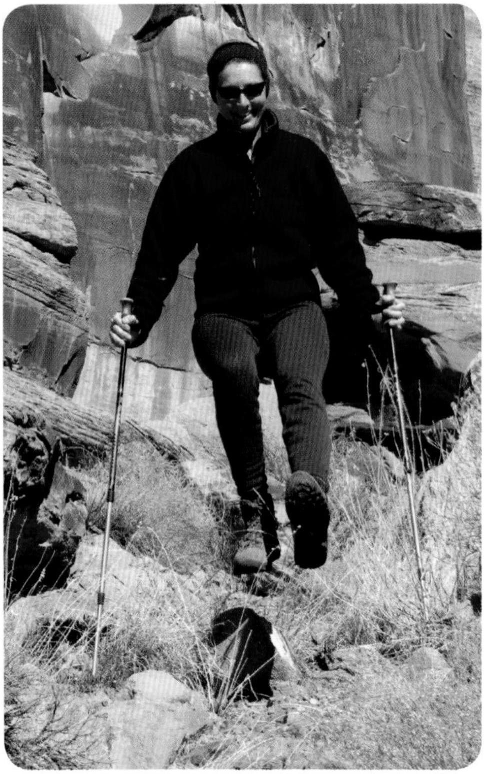

Flying through Morning Glory Canyon, mid-December

You'll cross the creek several times. Where to do so is always apparent thanks to directional signs, cairns, prominent stepping stones in the water, and the bootprints of previous hikers on the well-worn path.

At 1.3 mi (2.1 km) pass the mouth of a brushy tributary canyon on the right. Proceed on the sandy, main trail. A gentle ascent ensues. After descending back to the creek, cross to the north bank.

About 45 minutes from the trailhead, reach a **junction** at 1.9 mi (3.1 km), 4185 ft (1276 m), near the broad mouth of a second tributary canyon (right / south). The trail left (northeast) continues following the creek up the main canyon. For now, go right (south), cross the creek, and enter the tributary canyon.

The trail ascends steeply about eight minutes to a broad ledge at 4330 ft (1320 m). From here, **Morning Glory Natural Bridge** is visible southeast at the head of the tributary canyon. The optimal view is from directly beneath the bridge, at 2.3 mi (3.7 km), 4327 ft (1319 m).

The impressive size of the bridge is not its only merit. As natural bridges go, it's unusual. Most bridges were formed by a stream. That's what distinguishes them from arches, which were created by weathering and/or a combination of erosional forces. But Morning Glory was carved at the base of a waterfall. And the gap separating the bridge from the cliff over which the water cascaded is slim: only 15 ft (4.6 m) wide.

The falls seldom flows these days, but a seep spring near the bridge feeds **Morning Glory pool**. Itch alert: poison ivy is prolific here. It has shiny leaves (three per stem), each with serrated edges. Do not touch.

After returning to the tributary mouth, rockhop back to the junction on the creek's north bank. Then either turn left to retrace your steps to the trailhead, or turn right to explore up-canyon (northeast). It's brushy here, so the trail up-canyon might initially be obscure, but it soon becomes obvious again.

In a couple minutes, the trail rises onto a low ledge (left, above the creek), then drops and requires you to briefly tunnel through tamarisk. Soon pass a shallow, steep-walled bay on the left (north) wall of the canyon.

About 10 minutes from the junction, turn left into the second bay on the canyon's north wall. Follow the bootbeaten route. It soon ascends steeply among boulders. About seven minutes from the main canyon floor, reach the **hanging tributary drainage** above, at 4446 ft (1355 m).

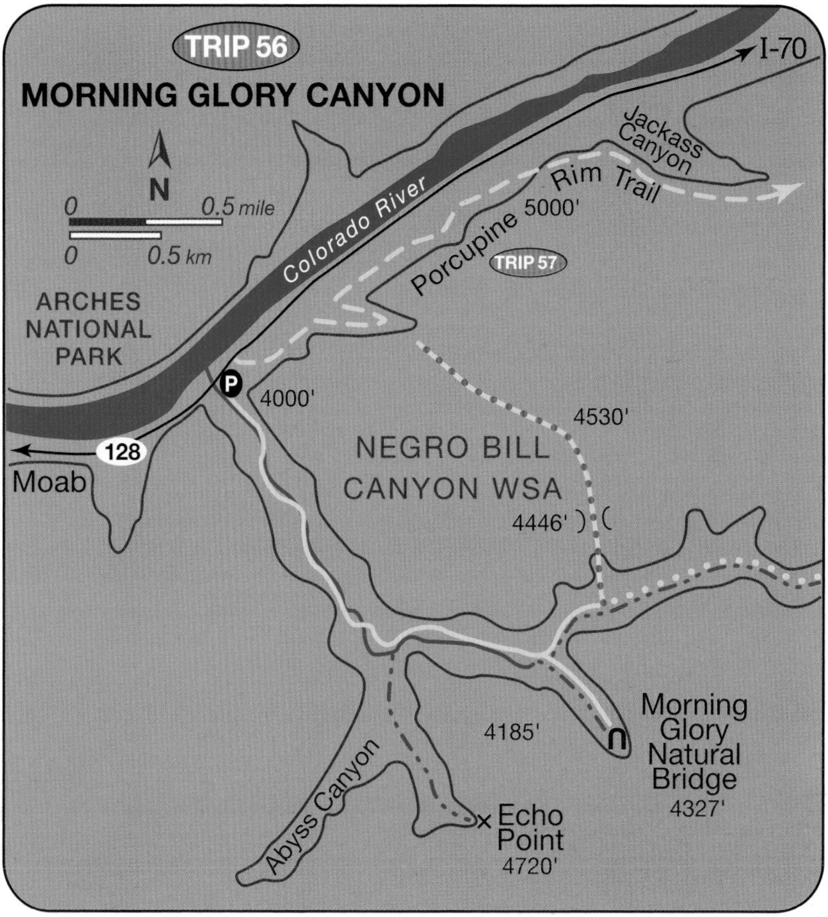

Voilà. Flat slickrock at the lip of the drainage invites you to sit, relax, admire the canyon below, and savor the tranquility. But if the intriguing domes farther north tug at your curiosity, keep going. Just be careful not to crush the cryptogamic soil.

In about 15 minutes, you can be atop those domes, gazing at the La Sal Mountains south-southeast. The elevation here is 4530 ft (1381 m). Total hiking distance: 3 mi (4.8 km).

Confident scramblers experienced at cross-country navigation can proceed northwest another 0.75 mi (1.2 km) to overlook the Porcupine trail (popular with mountain bikers) and the Colorado River. If you go, avoid stepping on the profuse cryptogamic soil by hiking on slickrock or in dry watercourses. Continually look back, so you stay oriented and can easily retrace your steps to the trailhead.

Having witnessed the canyon's beauty—ancient history wrought in stone—knowing a little about its recent human history will complete your experience. Here goes…

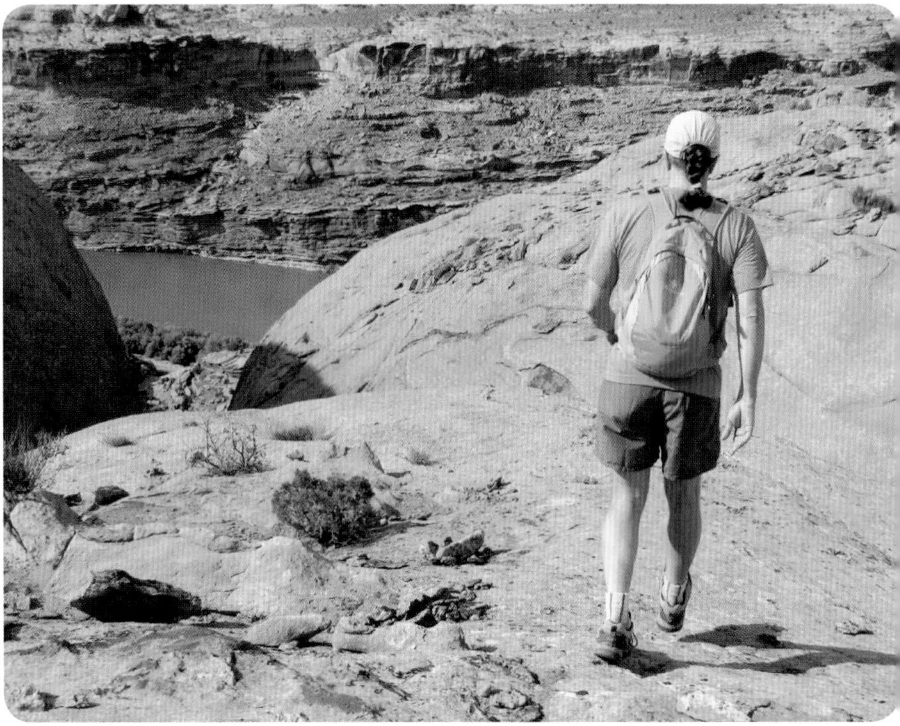

Exploring slickrock cross-country to Colorado River overlook.

The canyon's racist name derives from William Granstaff, a prospector and rancher who grazed cattle here during the late 1800s. Nearly a century later, the BLM initiated a study to determine if the canyon qualified for protection as a Wilderness Area. To prevent further damage by ORVs, they built a dirt barrier at the canyon mouth.

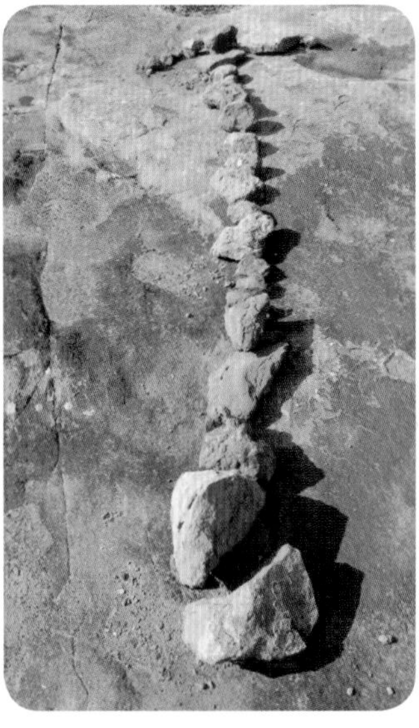

This incensed locals who believed the county, not the federal government, owned the canyon. They bulldozed the barrier. When the BLM rebuilt it, the irate, anti-fed, anti-enviro faction again demolished it. Then they spread gravel in the canyon, claimed it was an "improved road" and argued it no longer qualified as "roadless," which is a prerequisite for Wilderness status.

This Sagebrush Rebellion skirmish ended when the federal government filed suit in U.S. district court. The result was a negotiated settlement allowing the Wilderness Area Study to continue, which it supposedly still does.

TRIP 57

COLORADO RIVER CANYON

LOCATION	northeast of Moab
ROUND TRIP	6.4 mi (10.3 km)
ELEVATION GAIN	915 ft (279 m)
KEY ELEVATIONS	trailhead 4000 ft (1219 m) head of Jackass Canyon 4915 ft (1498 m)
HIKING TIME	2½ to 3½ hours
DIFFICULTY	easy
MAPS	Trails Illustrated *Moab South* Latitude 40 *Classic Moab Trails*

OPINION

It's curious to see how marginalized hiking is in Moab. Biking gets all the attention here, despite the fact that only on foot can you fully explore and appreciate canyon country.

But there's no reason you can't stride where bikers pedal. And several Moab-area "bike trails" afford excellent hiking, like this one starting beside the Colorado River and ascending toward Porcupine Rim.

Many mountainbikers actually find the Porcupine Rim trail—from end to end—overwhelming. It is to biking what the north shore of Oahu is to surfing: a challenge if you're skilled, a threat if you're not.

Even for hikers, however, we recommend only a short, out-and-back excursion on the Porcupine Rim trail's northwest end. Not because the rim-top terrain is difficult to walk, but because the reward-to-effort ratio diminishes beyond our suggested turnaround point: the head of Jackass Canyon.

What you'll enjoy en route are nearly constant views of the Colorado River Canyon: the mighty river itself as well as the sensational canyon walls. The trail ascends the canyon's southeast wall, so the scenery extends from micro to macro, from what's underfoot to the horizon.

Bear in mind that until the trail turns up Jackass Canyon, you'll be immediately above Highway 128. The pavement is only occasionally visible, but vehicles are constantly audible, so avoid hiking here when traffic is heavy: mid-March (Spring break) through September. That's also when you'd encounter the most mountainbikers.

The optimal time to hike here is between October and mid-March. You won't hear vehicle noise continually reverberating off the canyon walls then. Nor will you be constantly ceding the trail to bikers.

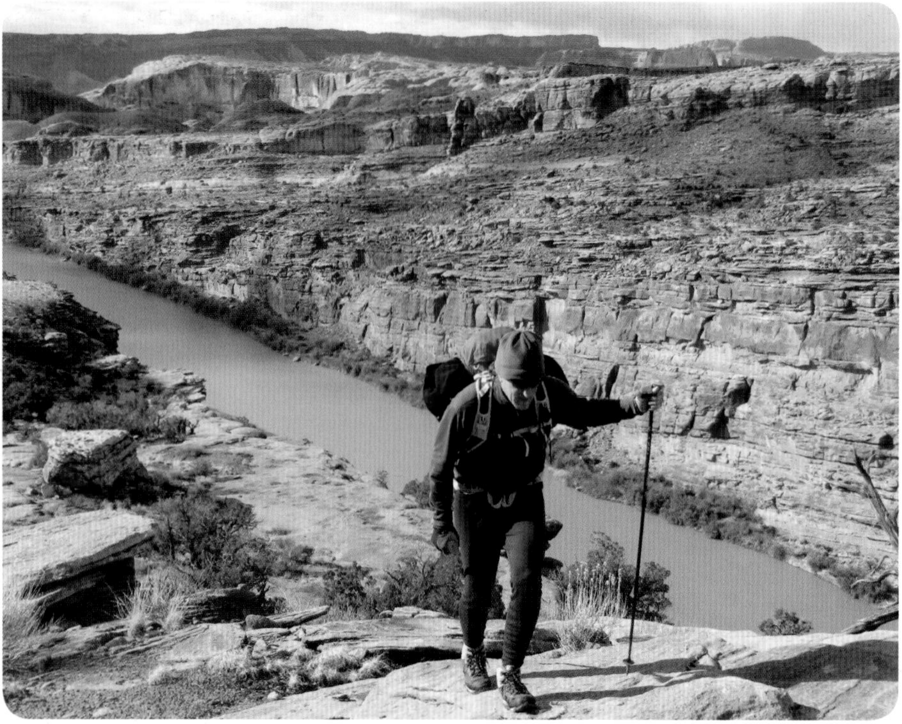

Porcupine Rim trail, above Colorado River Canyon

FACT

BY VEHICLE

From Hwy 191, at the northwest edge of Moab, turn right (east) onto Hwy 128. Follow it 3 mi (4.8 km), paralleling the Colorado River. Pass the paved trailhead parking lot for Morning Glory Bridge (Trip 56) on the right (southeast) and slow down. Just 200 yd (180 m) farther, turn sharp left (west) into the signed, unpaved, Porcupine trail parking area. Elevation: 4000 ft (1219 m).

ON FOOT

From the parking area, return to the highway, cross to the far side, turn left and walk about 90 paces north-northeast. Just past the culvert, veer right onto the dirt path covered with tire-tread prints and begin a gentle ascent northeast.

Soon turn right (east) into a short, **tributary drainage**. Contour the slope above it. The trail is visible on the opposite bench. Within ten minutes, you'll be back out at the mouth of the drainage, overlooking the Colorado River from 4170 ft (1271 m).

Continue an easy ascent northeast on a bench sprinkled with blackbrush. You'll lose sight of the river and road for a while. Arches National Park fills the horizon across the canyon. At 4515 ft (1377 m) the river is again in view. Domes near the Slickrock Trail are visible southwest above canyon walls.

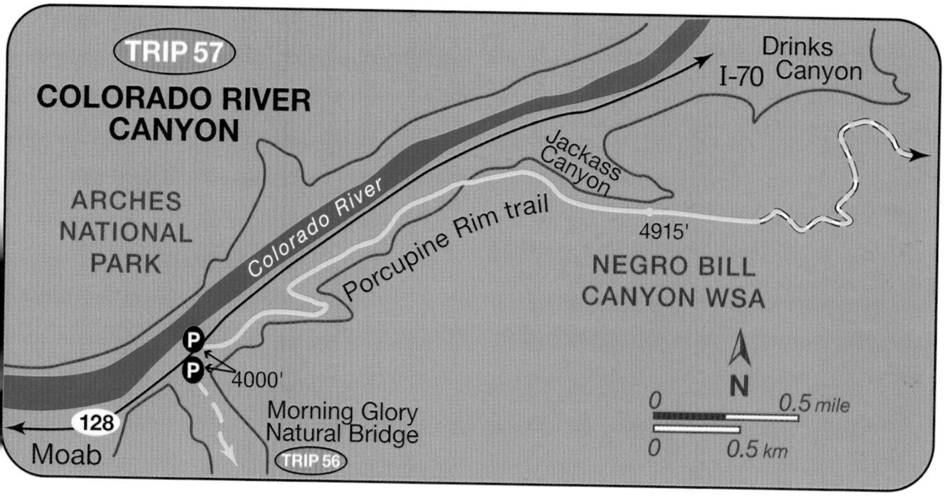

About one hour in, the trail curves right (east-southeast) and contours near 4740 ft (1445 m) above **Jackass Canyon**. The La Sal Mountains are southeast. At 3.2 mi (5.2 km), 4915 ft (1498 m), you're above a broad pouroff where the canyon's southeast end pinches into slickrock slabs. This is a good place for hikers to turn around.

Ahead, the terrain becomes less dramatic: a rolly, sandy, tree-scattered plateau. From the upper reaches of Jackass Canyon, the single-track trail soon broadens into a 4WD road. The crest of Porcupine Rim (overlooking Castle Valley) is about 7.1 mi (11.4 km) distant. The Porcupine Rim trailhead on Sand Flats Road (2WD) is about 4.4 mi (7.1 km) farther. That's *not* to suggest you should continue hiking in that direction, but simply to satisfy your curiosity.

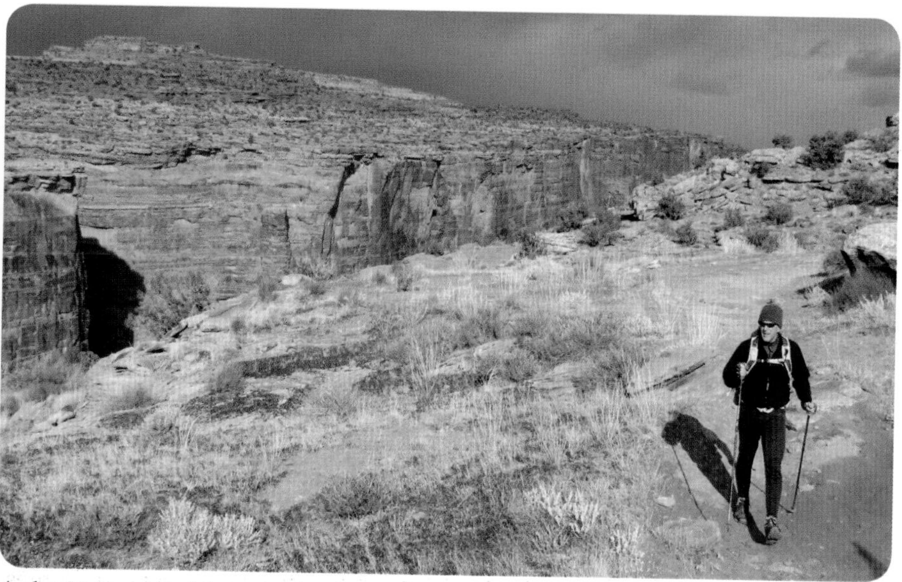

Arches National Park beyond Colorado River Canyon, from Porcupine Rim trail

TRIP 58

PROFESSOR CREEK & MARY JANE CANYON

LOCATION	northeast of Moab
ROUND TRIP	8.6 mi (13.8 km)
ELEVATION GAIN	410 ft (125 m)
KEY ELEVATIONS	trailhead 4335 ft (1322 m), highpoint 4745 ft (1447 m)
HIKING TIME	4 to 5 hours
DIFFICULTY	easy
MAP	Trails Illustrated *Moab North*

OPINION

Think of Moab as an acronym for *Moments Of Absolute Bliss.* Not the town itself, but the surrounding area, where a profusion of sublime trails keeps hikers elated. One of them is a short, easy jaunt, following Professor Creek into Mary Jane Canyon.

Less than an hour from the trailhead, you'll find yourself in a narrowing, deepening, sinuous, red-rock ravine. The walls amplify the creek's delicate water music, bathing you in omniphonic sound. You've entered a tiny wrinkle in the earth's skin and discovered a beautiful, soothing sanctuary.

If canyon-fired curiosity quickens your pace, another hour will bring you to where Mary Jane Canyon pinches shut, denying further exploration to all but commando canyoneers. Here, a dual-spouted waterfall gushes over a huge chokestone shaped like a snake's head. Time to stop, contemplate, absorb.

Succumb to mesmerism and you'll see the rock reptile's head is cocked to one side. His eyes are closed. His smile is that of a benevolent Buddha. He's a beatific beast, luxuriating in this cool, peaceful refuge, inviting you to commune with him.

By southern Utah standards, Mary Jane is a modest canyon. And Professor Creek, except during a rare, brief freshet, is a tame, meandering trickle. The water depth varies seasonally, according to how much snow is melting in Manti-La Sal National Forest and how much rain has recently fallen. It's usually ankle- to calf-deep. Despite their humble dimensions, however, the creek and canyon tantalize and ultimately enthrall.

FACT

BEFORE YOUR TRIP

The creek's generally low flow gives you a choice: wear sandals, slosh through, get wet; or wear boots and stay dry by rockhopping frequently with the aid of trekking poles. Base your decision on the air and water temperatures. On a hot day in desert canyon country, walking in water is exhilarating yet

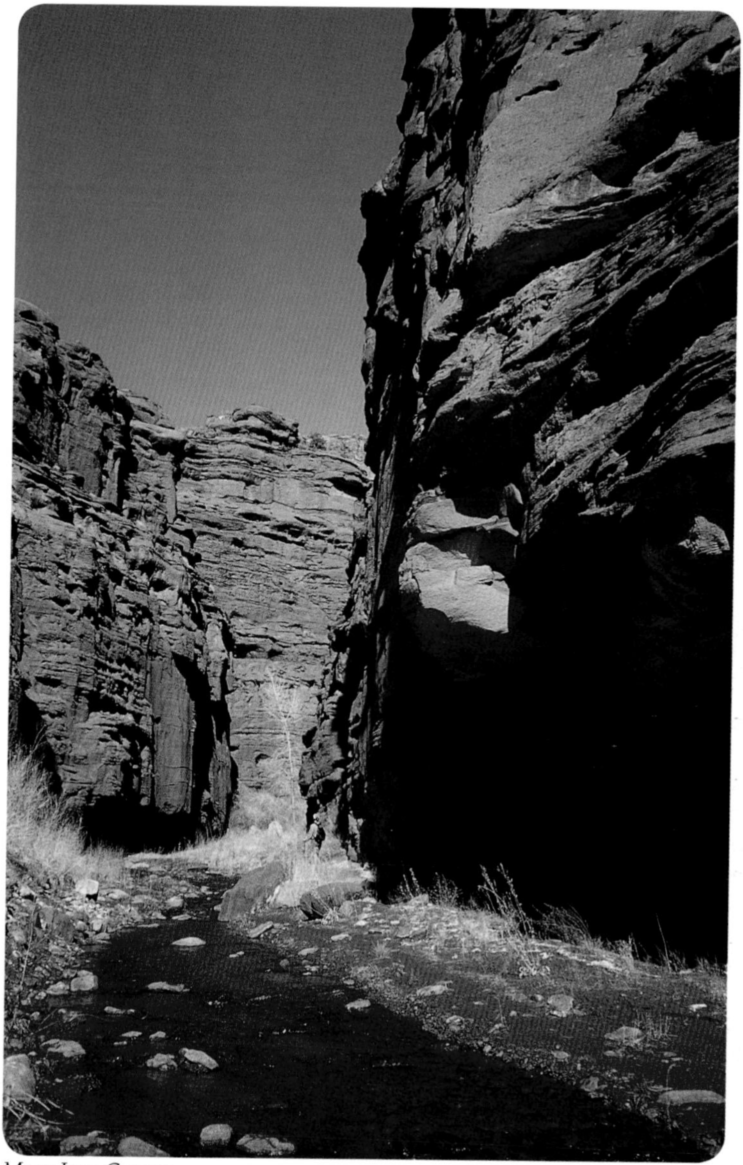

Mary Jane Canyon

soothing. Do it if possible. Opportunities like this a rare. Another water-walk near Moab is Mill Creek Canyon (Trip 53).

BY VEHICLE

From Hwy 191, at the northwest edge of Moab, turn east onto Hwy 128. Follow it 18.4 mi (30 km), paralleling the Colorado River. Just before milepost 19 and the sign *Onion Creek 2*, turn right (east-southeast) onto a dirt road signed *Ranch Road, Dead End.*

From I-70, near Cisco, drive Hwy 128 generally south 26.7 mi (43 km). Turn left (east-southeast) onto a dirt road signed *Ranch Road, Dead End.*

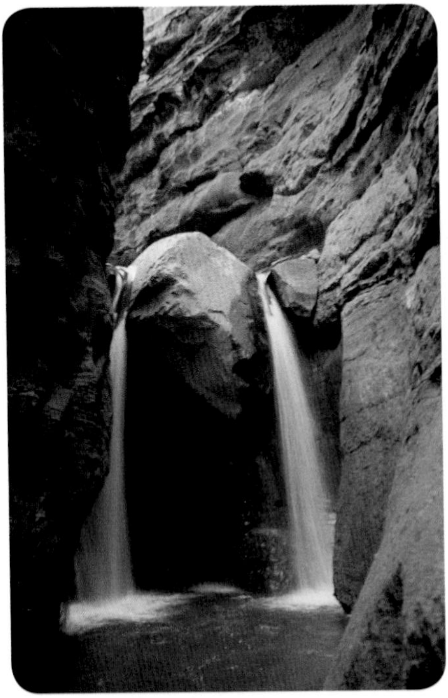

Professor Creek cascade where a chokestone halts hikers' progress in upper Mary Jane Canyon

From either approach, reset your trip odometer to 0 and proceed on the ranch road. At 1.6 mi (2.6 km), bear right (east-southeast). At 1.7 mi (2.7 km), continue straight where a road forks right. Curve right at 1.9 mi (3 km), passing a homesite on the left. At 2.1 mi (3.4 km) pass a fenced diversion dam on the right. At 3.5 mi (2.2 km), where the road bends right (southwest) toward Castle Rock and the Priest & Nuns formation visible on the horizon, park in a clearing on the left. Elevation: 4335 ft (1322 m).

ON FOOT

Drop to Professor Creek. Cross it, bear right, and hike upstream (southeast) along the bank. Southeast will remain your general direction of travel until trail's end.

Soon cross back to the right (south) bank. Cottonwood and juniper trees grace the initially very shallow drainage. The creek originates as creeklets draining Fisher Mesa (left / east) and Adobe Mesa (right / south-southeast).

If it's hot, and you're wearing sandals or footwear you don't mind soaking, then splash through the water. (Before plunging in, judge the water temperature. It can be frigid in spring and fall.) Otherwise, depending on the creek's depth, it's possible to keep your boots dry, but you'll have to cross and re-cross frequently to attain whichever bank affords easier hiking. Most of the way, a bootbeaten path is evident, suggesting where to switch to the opposite bank, or where to leave the creekbed and shortcut sandy benches.

About 30 minutes from the trailhead, the drainage walls are noticeably higher. You're entering **Mary Jane Canyon**. At this point, it's about 80 ft (24 m) wide and 65 ft (20 m) deep. Continue following the creek upstream, passing several side canyons—usually dry.

At about 2.3 mi (3.7 km), 4565 ft (1392 m), a little more than one hour from the trailhead, the canyon is 130 ft (40 m) to 180 ft (55 m) deep. Proceed through **narrows** for the next 2 mi (3.2 km).

A double-tongued **waterfall** flowing over a chokestone at 4.3 mi (6.9 km), 4745 ft (1447 m), halts upstream progress for most of us. Fast hikers will arrive here within two hours.

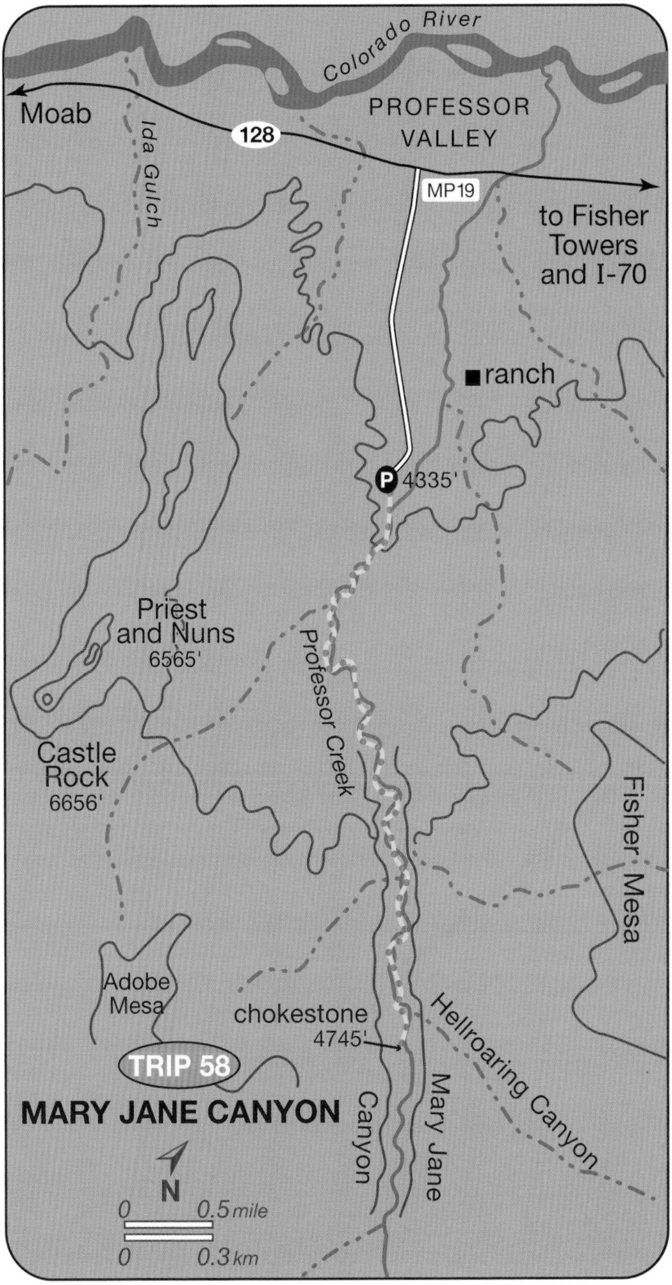
Colorado River
Moab
PROFESSOR VALLEY
128
Ida Gulch
MP19
to Fisher Towers and I-70
ranch
4335'
Priest and Nuns
6565'
Professor Creek
Castle Rock
6656'
Fisher Mesa
Adobe Mesa
chokestone
4745'
Hellroaring Canyon
TRIP 58
MARY JANE CANYON
Canyon
Mary Jane
N
0 0.5 mile
0 0.3 km

TRIP 59

FISHER TOWERS

LOCATION	Colorado River Canyon, northeast of Moab
ROUND TRIP	4.6 mi (7.4 km)
ELEVATION GAIN	1050 ft (320 m) including ups & downs
KEY ELEVATIONS	trailhead 4720 ft (1440 m) official trail's end 5430 ft (1655 m)
HIKING TIME	2½ to 3½ hours
DIFFICULTY	easy
MAPS	Trails Illustrated *Moab North* Latitude 40 *Classic Moab Trails*

OPINION

The phantasmagoria of southern Utah inspire imaginative comparisons. "That one looks like..." is the usual response. Which is always interesting. But if these formations were art—as indeed they are, every piece created by the master sculptor Erosion—your admiration wouldn't be limited to free associating. You would ask yourself, "What does it mean? What is it saying?"

The Fisher Towers look like the soaring, ornate, baroque architecture of Belgium, at Brussels' Le Grand Place, or Ghent's Michelmas. Or the ancient, fantastic, erotic shrines at Khajuraho, India, minus the shocking eroticism. But what do the lofty, incomprehensibly intricate Fisher Towers *say*? Perhaps their message is, "Don't endure a mundane existence. Unleash your wild mind. Think original thoughts. Act on them exuberantly. Be an iconoclast and celebrate it."

The trailhead is at the very base of these rippling, filigreed, hardened-mud monoliths. It's surprising how many people shuffle only a few steps from their vehicle, stare open-mouthed, then leave. But the trail winds intimately among the Fisher Towers, affording the hiker a consummately vivid, memorable encounter.

Despite frequent ups and downs, this short, out-and-back journey is easily galloped in a couple hours. Yet it packs as much scenic wallop as any hike anywhere. Sweeping vistas across the Colorado River Canyon and into the La Sal Mountains complement the reach-out-and-touch-'em views of the towers. Upon your arrival in the Moab area, even if it's late afternoon, come here to stretch your legs, jettison humdrum concerns, and disengage your duty-burdened brain.

Tallest of the towers, the 900-ft (274-m) Titan, was first summitted in 1962 by three Coloradoans. Climbing sandstone was dicey as space travel then but is less so now thanks to improved hardware. Climbers achieve an even greater affinity with the Fisher Towers than do hikers. It's the difference between peering into a kaleidoscope and being in one.

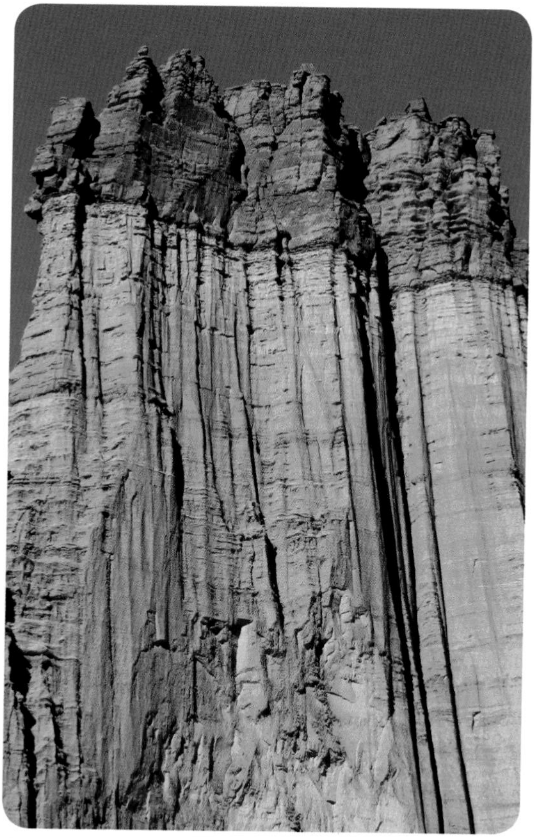

Fisher Towers

FACT

BY VEHICLE

From Hwy 191, at the northwest edge of Moab, turn east onto Hwy 128. Follow it 21 mi (33.8 km), paralleling the Colorado River. At milepost 21, turn right (east-southeast) onto unpaved Fisher Road, signed *Fisher Towers*.

From I-70, near Cisco, drive Hwy 128 generally south 23.5 mi (37.8 km). Turn left (east-southeast) onto unpaved Fisher Road, signed *Fisher Towers*.

From either approach, proceed 2.2 mi (3.5 km) to the trailhead parking area near the base of the towers. Elevation: 4720 ft (1440 m).

There's a small BLM campground here. It has pit toilets, tables, and fire pits, but no water. The chimney-like pinnacle of Castle Rock is visible south-southwest. Beyond it is Porcupine Rim.

ON FOOT

The trail departs the south-southwest corner of the parking area, between the metal register and the wood sign. Immediately descend a short staircase, curve left, then begin a gradual ascent generally south. Initially the trail is lined with rocks. In about six minutes, follow a sign directing you left, through a **cleft**, down into a wash.

In about 30 minutes, reach a level **shoulder** affording a sweeping view of intricate tower walls and odd sandstone formations. From here, the trail curves left (northeast) then gently ascends around another shallow gully. At 1 mi (1.6 km) reach the base of the 900-ft (274-m) **Titan**, tallest of the towers.

About 45 minutes from the trailhead, a 4-rung metal ladder helps you drop into a gully. Ascend the other side via short, accommodating ledges. Ten minutes farther, leave the tower alleyways and ascend to a level **saddle** on a peninsula, at 2.2 mi (3.5 km), 5430 ft (1655 m). It's possible to continue in two directions: briefly right, or farther left.

Right (south-southwest) from the saddle, the **main trail ends** within four minutes (mostly level) at an **overlook** above Onion Creek canyon. The distant view north-northwest is upstream into the Colorado River Valley. You've now hiked about an hour from the trailhead.

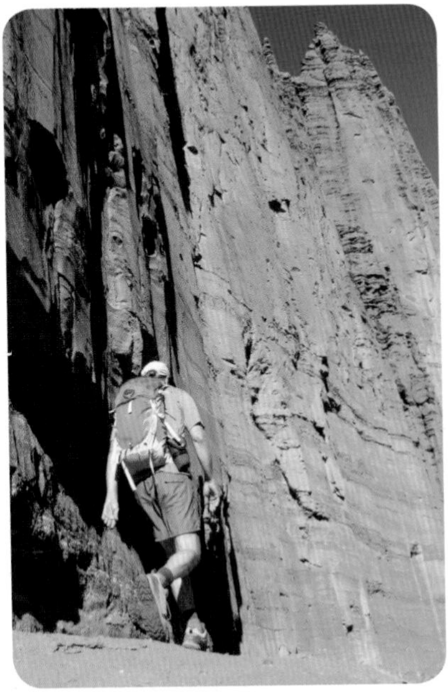

Fisher Towers trail

To proceed left (east) from the saddle, look right for bootprints revealing a short, narrow trough—the easiest way to step down. Then contour left (east), following more bootprints. Ascend between boulders.

About four minutes from the saddle, reach a fairly level **expanse of slickrock** affording a view north to the back of the towers and overlooking a startlingly deep drainage. From here it's possible to ramble 15 minutes or so farther—up and down the convoluted slickrock ridge—generally south. The edges are precipitous, but it's safe if you find the correct passage.

From the expanse of slickrock, turn your back to the towers and head south. Look right for a **small natural bridge**. Scramble beneath it to continue. Bear left (east). Bootprints in the sand will probably guide you.

Ascend over a promontory. On its left (east) side, skirt the edge of the 1000-ft (305-m) abyss. Be sure footed. Figure your way toward the final, **bulbous sandstone formation** where a sheer cliff halts progress. Onion Creek is visible below. Fisher Valley Ranch is southeast, backed by Manti - La Sal National Forest.

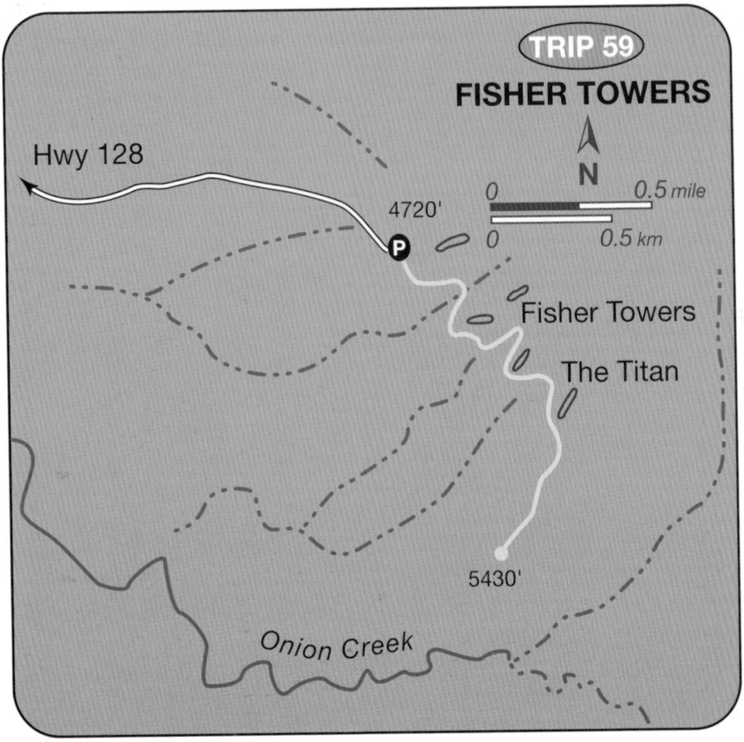

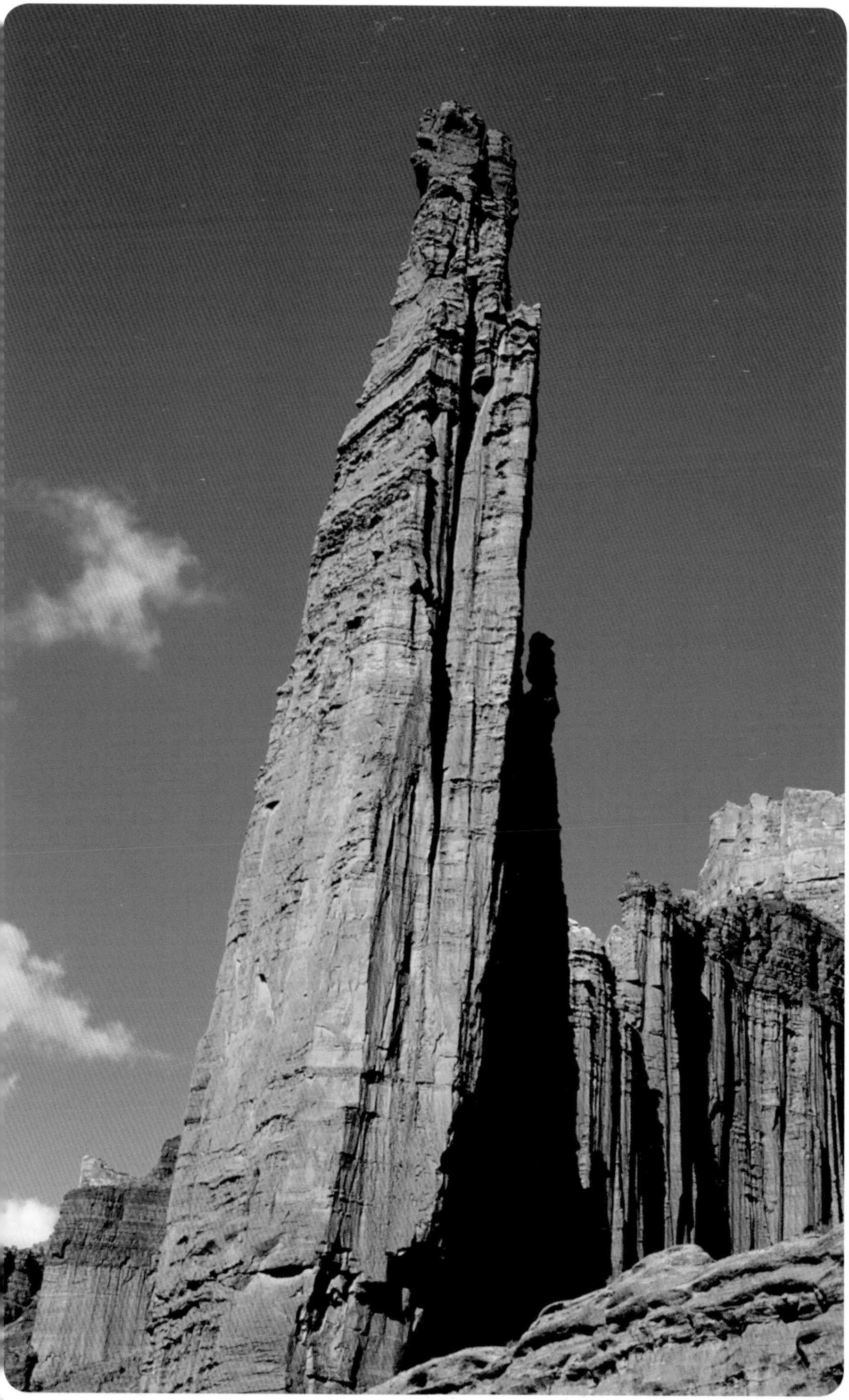

Titan Tower

TRIP 60

HORSESHOE CANYON

LOCATION	Canyonlands National Park, Maze District south of Green River, east-northeast of Hanksville
ROUND TRIP	7.4 mi (11.9 km)
ELEVATION CHANGE	700-ft (213-m) loss and gain
KEY ELEVATIONS	trailhead 5300 ft (1616 m), canyon floor 4700 ft (1433 m) Great Gallery 4800 ft (1463 m)
HIKING TIME	3 to 4½ hours
DIFFICULTY	moderate
MAP	Trails Illustrated *Canyonlands National Park: Maze District & NE Glen Canyon NRA*

OPINION

There are two keys to knowledge: your left foot and your right.

You can confidently say you know something only when you've walked the distance, experienced the context, observed it close enough to touch, hear, smell and taste it.

You've seen photos of the Golden Gate Bridge. You might even have driven over it. But when you ride your bicycle across it, you'll suddenly realize you knew little about it until then.

The same is true of the Great Gallery, in Horseshoe Canyon. Photos only suggest the soul-gripping power that emanates from this astonishing rock-art panel. You don't just hike here to see it. You hike here to *feel* it.

Hiking itself is part of the event. There's a reason pilgrims walk to Santiago de Compostela. It's humbling. It softens their hearts, opens their minds, makes them more respectful. It heightens the impact and meaning of the journey's climactic ending.

And hiking to the Great Gallery has the additional benefit of strengthening your affinity with the canyon's former inhabitants: lifelong hikers who expressed their deepest beliefs and hopes in the art you've come to admire and contemplate.

Not that you have a choice. Thanks to the national park service, hiking is now the only way to reach the Great Gallery. It ensures the atmosphere remains tranquil and decreases the likelihood of vandalism. An ORV would be as blasphemous in Horseshoe Canyon as it would in the Louvre.

The Great Gallery is the single greatest display of prehistoric rock art in North America. It's 15 ft (4.6 m) high and 200 ft (61 m) long. It bears more than 75 pictographs in dark red, brown, and white. They were painted 2,000 to 8,000 years ago by Desert Archaic Indians, predecessors of the Ancestral Puebloans.

The panel features life-size phantom-like figures in what is known as the *Barrier Canyon* style. The name originated here, because this is the most impressive display of its kind, and because the canyon itself was originally called *Barrier Canyon*. Today, only the creek within the canyon retains the name.

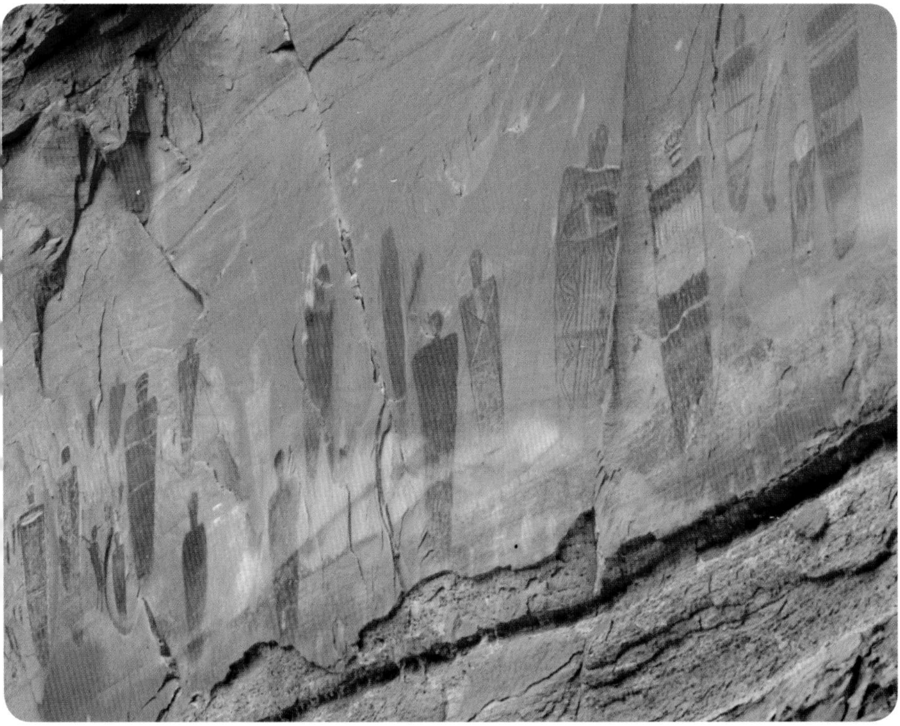

The Great Gallery, Horseshoe Canyon

It's the otherworldly aspect of the panel's central figures and their enormous size that make the Great Gallery so compelling. Chief among them is a 7-ft (2.1-m) tall, ethereal presence known as the *Holy Ghost*. It has huge, round, empty eye sockets, a head that appears to waver, and a streamlined, arm-less, leg-less body that seems to be rising upward. Surrounding it are six slightly smaller, less distinctive anthropomorphic figures. They too look like they're in perpetual vertical motion.

What's it all mean? Allow plenty of time to gaze at the Great Gallery and ponder that question.

Our answer, based only on a few hours of starring plus our subsequent reflection and conversation, is that the artists where shamans. They were trying to show, rather than merely describe, their spiritual journey of transformation from the human world to the realm of the spirit. Shedding their physicality, they must have felt weightless, hence the streamlined bodies. Departing for the unknown, they must have felt they were traveling, hence the skyward trajectory.

Perhaps they were saying to the tribe, "This was our experience. This is what is possible for our species." If so, it's a profound message, as meaningful today as it was then.

Whoever the artists were, and whatever they were communicating, they created paint by mixing finely-ground mineral pigments with vegetable juice or animal fat. Due to the arid climate and the gallery's sheltered location, the mineral coloring remains.

FACT

BEFORE YOUR TRIP

The Maze District of Canyonlands National Park is remote compared to the Needles and Island in the Sky districts. Reaching Horseshoe Canyon requires a 62.4-mi (100.5-km) round-trip drive on an unpaved road, which takes about an hour each way. For convenience, consider camping at the trailhead before or after your hike. The road should be passable in a 2WD car, but if wet it can be challenging even in a 4WD vehicle.

To learn more about ancient rock art, read a specialist's research: *Trance and Transformation in the Canyons—Shamanism and Early Rock Art on the Colorado Plateau*, by Polly Schaafsma.

BY VEHICLE

From Green River, drive I-70 west 11.2 mi (18 km). Turn south onto Hwy 24 and continue another 24.2 mi (38.9 km), just past the road to Goblin Valley State Park. From Hanksville, drive Hwy 24 north 18.4 mi (29.6 km). From either approach, turn east onto the unpaved road signed for Hans Flat Ranger Station. Reset your trip odometer to 0

0 mi (0 km)
Departing Hwy 24.

2 mi (3.2 km)
Bear right.

2.8 mi (4.5 km)
Proceed on the main road, ignoring forks. Ascend to a gap between buttes, then descend.

11 mi (17.7 km)
Bear right, ignoring the left fork to Dugout Spring. Soon ascend.

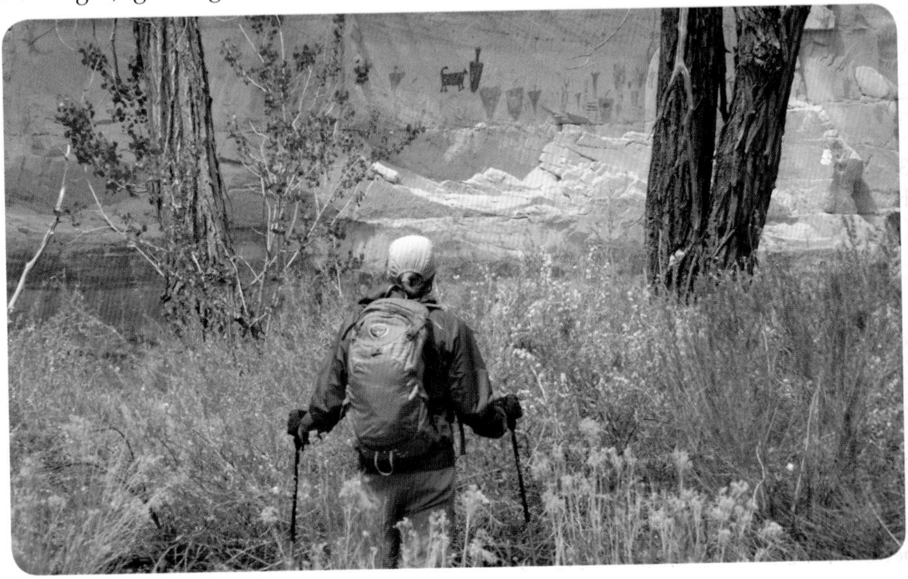

High Gallery, Horseshoe Canyon

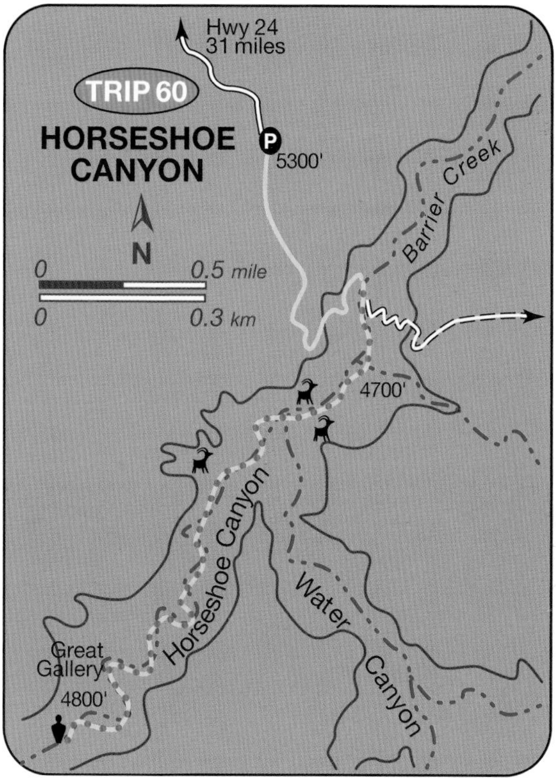

16 mi (25.8 km)
Proceed on the main road, ignoring a right fork.

24.2 mi (39 km)
Go left and descend. Right leads to Hans Flat Ranger Station.

29.5 mi (47.5 km)
Turn right onto a rough, rocky spur. Ascend.

31.2 mi (50.2 km)
Reach the trailhead parking lot, on the rim of Horseshoe Canyon, at 5300 ft (1616 m).

ON FOOT

The trail departs the south-southwest corner of the parking lot, behind the kiosk. Initially a defunct oil-exploration road, it affords views into Horseshoe Canyon. Cairns also indicate the way across bedrock and sand, but they're unnecessary because the old road is obvious.

In ten minutes pass a water tank built by cattle ranchers before the area was protected as a national park. Five minutes farther, at 0.5 mi (0.8 km), pass through a **hiker's maze**, which keeps cattle out of the canyon. The road ascending the far canyon wall is visible. Down-canyon, you can see broken Kayenta ledges beneath the Navajo sandstone cliffs.

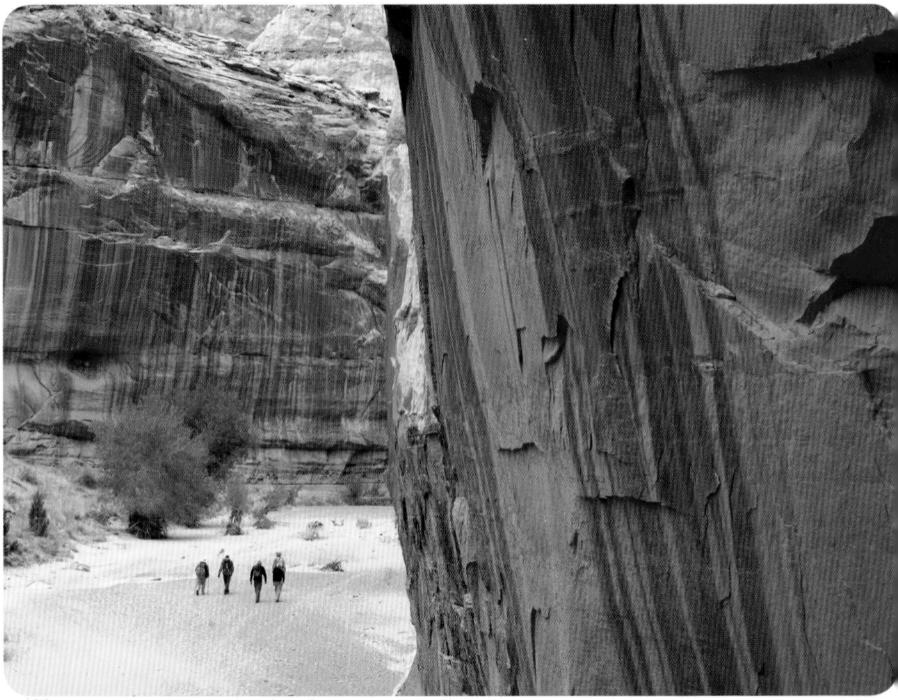
Horseshoe Canyon

Reach the **canyon floor** at 1.5 mi (2.4 km), 4700 ft (1433 m), about 30 minutes from the trailhead. Proceed straight (south), up the sandy canyon, along intermittent **Barrier Creek**. Pass the road that ascends the left (east) wall.

The canyon narrows. Cottonwoods appear, providing invaluable shade. At 2 mi (3.2 km), about 40 minutes along, a left spur leads to **High Gallery** on the southeast wall. It's a pictograph panel bearing several human figures and handprints.

Just two minutes farther up-canyon, a right spur leads to **Horseshoe Shelter** pictograph panel on the north wall. It has more drawings, including several ghost-like figures.

Resuming up-canyon, pass **Water Canyon** (left / southeast) about 45 minutes from the trailhead, or a mere two minutes beyond the last rock-art panel.

At 2.5 mi (4 km), about an hour along, reach **Alcove Gallery**. It's on the right (west) wall, at the base of the alcove. The pictographs are faint—defaced, as well as eroded. It's apparent the canyon floor is now lower than where the native artists once stood.

Continue past four southeast-trending bends in the canyon. At 3.7 mi (6 km), 4800 ft (1463 m), about 1½ hours from the trailhead, reach the **Great Gallery** beneath a protective overhang on the right (north) wall.

A national-park employee or volunteer is often on site to answer questions and ensure the rock art is not defaced. There might also be an ammo box here containing scholarly papers about the art.

About 0.2 mi (0.3 km) up-canyon from the Great Gallery are the tracks of a three-toed dinosaur that roamed here 50 to 100 million years ago. Where Barrier Creek flows over a small slab of flat, dark, hard sandstone, look near the right (west) bank. You'll see three footprints about 4 ft (1.2 m) apart. Each is about 10 inches (25 cm) in diameter.

TRIP 61

DEAD HORSE POINT STATE PARK

LOCATION	Dead Horse Point State Park, southwest of Moab
LOOP	9.1 mi (14.7 km) including overlook detours
ELEVATION GAIN	260 ft (79 m)
KEY ELEVATIONS	trailhead 6040 ft (1841 m) Dead Horse Point Overlook 5918 ft (1804 m)
HIKING TIME	3½ to 4½ hours
DIFFICULTY	moderate
MAPS	Latitude 40 *Classic Moab Trails*, Dead Horse Point State Park brochure (free, available at entry station)

OPINION

"Shall we go to Dead Horse Point, or Island in the Sky?"

Not a tough decision, if all you know about the two places are their names. And if it occurs to you that the land of equine corpses only merits state-park status while the heavenly atoll earns top honors as a national park, well then, no contest. Like most visitors, you'll proceed into Canyonlands, motoring past the boneyard or glue factory, or whatever the heck is out on that point, without even a sideways glance.

But *Dead Horse* is only a name, and it's boundaries are geopolitical fiction. The land itself is actually part of Canyonlands. The views it affords are as dazzling as any in southern Utah. And the nearly-level Dead Horse rim-route trail is more stroll than hike. If you complete our recommended loop, including

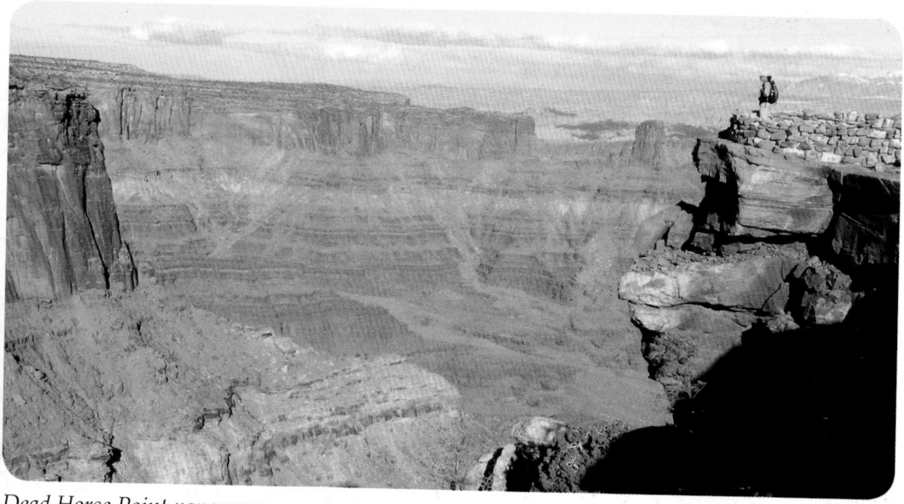

Dead Horse Point panorama

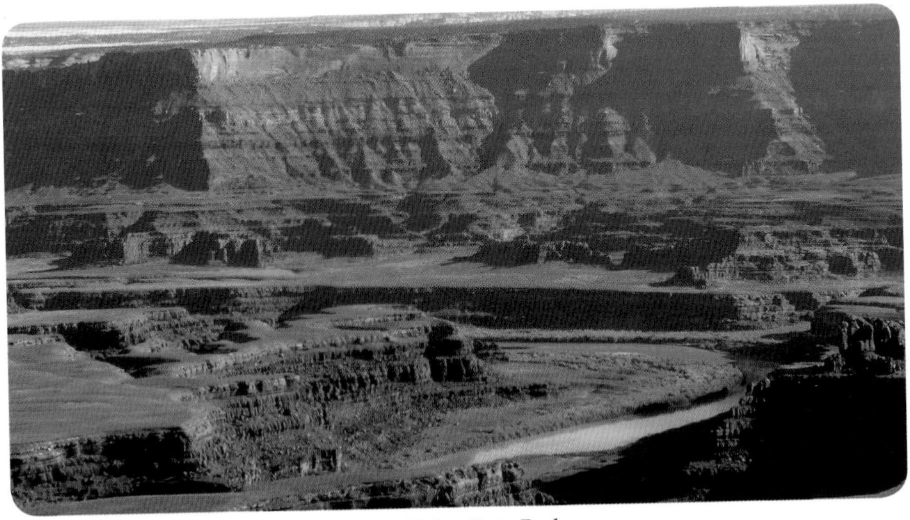

Colorado River Canyon, from Dead Horse Point State Park

detours to Basin, Dead Horse Point, Meander, Shafer Canyon, Rim, and Big Horn overlooks, your total distance will be a substantial 9.1 mi (14.7 km). But you can also shorten that considerably, tailoring the experience to fit your time, energy or curiosity. Spectacle overload, however, should be your only limitation.

Dead Horse Point is a high, cliffbound promontory. Because it's relatively narrow, hikers frequently, quickly, easily attain new views of the Colorado River Canyon 2000 ft (610 m) below and sculpted canyon country stretching to the snow-capped La Sal Mountains on the horizon. So why isn't it named *Bird's-Eye Point?* Because of a persistent cowboy legend.

Long ago, mustangs ran wild here. Cowboys would herd them to the tip of the promontory, then corral them by fencing off the slender isthmus. They led away the best horses and left the "broomtails," the inferior ones, behind. But before the cowboys departed, did they open the corral so the remaining horses could wander away? Nobody knows. But apparently the broomtails either felt trapped or were trapped. They died of thirst. When the promontory was declared a state park in 1959, it was named after the legendary dead horses.

FACT

BY VEHICLE

From Hwy 128, at the northwest edge of Moab, drive Hwy 191 northwest 8.6 mi (13.8 km) and turn left. From I-70, drive Hwy 191 southeast 20.3 mi (32.7 km) and turn right. From either approach, reset your trip odometer to 0 and drive southwest on Hwy 313 signed *Canyonlands, Island in the Sky*.

At 14.5 mi (23.4 km), where straight (south) proceeds into Canyonlands National Park, turn left (east). At 18.7 mi (30.1 km) enter Dead Horse State Park (entry fee required). Reach the visitor center and trailhead parking lot at 21.2 mi (34.1 km), 6040 ft (1841 m). Begin hiking here. At 22.5 mi (36.2 km) the road ends upon reaching Dead Horse Point Overlook.

ON FOOT

From the northeast corner of the visitor center, near the rim, follow the paved path east to begin a clockwise loop.

After heading south about 0.8 mi (1.3 km), detour left (east) to **Basin Overlook**. Upon returning to the main trail, go left (south).

Continue along **The Neck**, a narrow isthmus. About 0.5 mi (0.8 km) farther reach **Dead Horse Point Overlook**—the end of the peninsula—at 5918 ft (1804 m).

Resuming the clockwise loop, hike generally north to **Meander Overlook**. The trail gradually curves left (northwest). Soon detour left (west) to **Shafer Canyon Overlook**.

Farther north along the loop is a short detour left (northwest) to **Rim Overlook**. After returning to the main trail, go left (east).

Soon reach another junction. Left (north) is **Big Horn Overlook**—a 2.4-mi (3.9-km) round-trip detour. Straight (east) quickly reaches the **visitor center**, where your total distance will be 9.1 mi (14.7 km) including all the overlook detours.

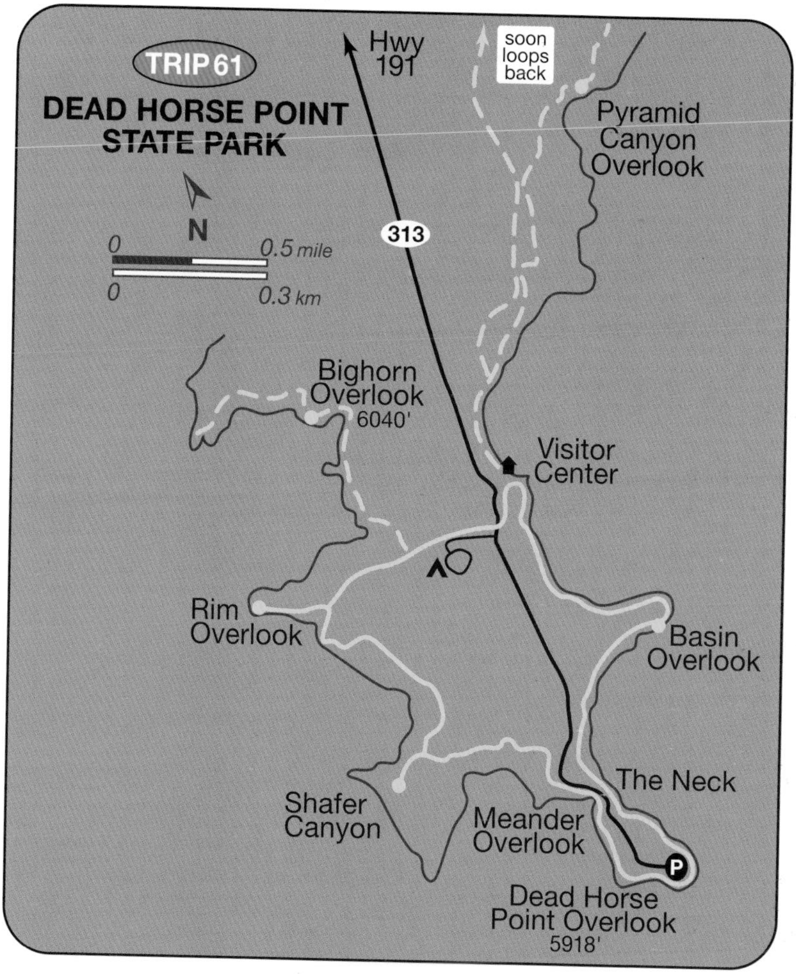

TRIP 62

LATHROP CANYON

LOCATION	Canyonlands National Park, Island in the Sky District
ROUND TRIP	5.6 mi (9 km) to head of upper Lathrop Canyon 11 mi (17.7 km) to White Rim Road 18.4 mi (29.6 km) to Colorado River
ELEVATION CHANGE	515-ft (157-m) loss and gain for upper Lathrop Canyon 1815-ft (533-m) loss and gain for White Rim Road 2215-ft (675-m) loss and gain for Colorado River
KEY ELEVATIONS	trailhead 5985 ft (1825 m), mesa rim 5870 ft (1790 m) head of upper Lathrop Canyon 5700 ft (1738 m) White Rim Road 4400 ft (1340 m) Colorado River 4000 ft (1220 m)
HIKING TIME	2½ hours for head of upper Lathrop Canyon 5 hours for White Rim Road, 8 hours for Colorado River
DIFFICULTY	easy to challenging
MAPS	Trails Illustrated *Moab South*, Latitude 40 *Moab West*

OPINION

Flowing out of the Rockies, the Colorado River conducts itself in a socially acceptable manner. Then, suddenly, near the Utah border, it abandons all sense of decorum and indulges in a furious canyon-cutting orgy. The result is both shocking and glorious, as you'll see while hiking off the Island in the Sky, into Lathrop Canyon, perhaps continuing all the way to the lusty river's edge.

Other trails in this book afford sweeping vistas, but none quite compare to this one. Even Murphy Hogback (Trip 63) and Upheaval Canyon/Syncline Valley (Trip 64), both of which immediately leap off the Island in the Sky, don't reveal as vast and compelling a swath of canyon country.

Yet the Lathrop trail asks that you be more patient, because it starts 2.5 mi (4 km) from the mesa edge. That's a 5-mi (8-km) round trip in which you won't, for the most part, be stretching your eyeballs. Still, it's worth it, even if you don't continue over the mesa edge, because what you'll see from there is comparable to the scenery along the south rim of the Grand Canyon.

But try to keep going. The trail itself soon snatches your attention away from the views because it slyly negotiates all-but-impassable terrain via a miraculous route. After completing the Houdini-esque feat of conveying you safely down the cliffs, it intersects the White Rim Road, where most hikers turn around.

This is the only Island in the Sky trail, however, that accesses the Colorado River, so continuing beyond and below the White Rim is an option. Don't pursue it, however, unless (a) you're strong and fast, (b) you start early, (c) you're carrying plenty of water, and (d) you're willing to hike that final 7.4-mi (11.9-km) round-trip leg strictly for the accomplishment or simply to satisfy curiosity, because the scenery diminishes.

The compelling sight here isn't the river itself, it's what the river's *done*. And you'll have seen plenty of that by the time you arrive at the White Rim Road.

FACT

BY VEHICLE

From Hwy 128, at the northwest edge of Moab, drive Hwy 191 northwest 8.6 mi (13.8 km) and turn left. From I-70, drive Hwy 191 southeast 20.3 mi (32.7 km) and turn right. From either approach, reset your trip odometer and drive southwest on Hwy 313 signed *Canyonlands, Island in the Sky*.

At 14.5 mi (23.4 km), pass the road to Dead Horse Point State Park (left / east). Shortly beyond, Navajo Mtn and the Henry Mountains are visible on the horizon (right / west).

At 19.2 mi (30.9 km) enter Canyonlands National Park. At 21.6 mi (34.8 km) arrive at the visitor center. Continue south across The Neck, passing Shafer Canyon overlook. At 23.4 mi (37.8 km), between mileposts 9 and 10, park in the pullout on the left (southeast) at 5985 ft (1825 m).

ON FOOT

The sandy trail leads south-southeast across Grays Pasture, where spring wildflowers include orange globemallow. You might also see broom snakeweed and Uinta groundsel, both of which have small yellow blossoms.

Within 25 minutes, a slight ascent leads to a 6100-ft (1860-m) **hilltop** where the view encompasses the mesa rim ahead, canyon walls southeast and east beyond the Colorado River, the La Sal Mountains east-northeast, the Book Cliffs distant north-northeast, and the San Rafael Swell distant northwest.

After descending, continue on Navajo sandstone at 6065 ft (1850 m), about 30 minutes along. Cairns and logs guide you left (east-southeast) back onto a sandy path. Just 10 yd/m farther, the route is again on **slickrock**, heading northeast, paralleling the mesa rim.

Visible directly south is 5812-ft (1772-m) Airport Tower. Below and left of it (south-southeast) is the Colorado River. Beyond are the Abajo Mountains.

The slickrock route drops among broken rock slabs. Sandy trail continues descending south. Within 45 minutes, attain views into Lathrop Canyon. The trail below the rim is visible, descending a talus slope and sweeping out across the drainage.

Cairns lead east, across a flat dotted with blackbrush, toward the rim. Drop into a wash and follow it southeast. Reach the **mesa rim** at 2.5 mi (4 km), 5870 ft (1790 m). Even if you're inclined to turn around here, continue 15 minutes farther to appreciate the ingenious descent route.

The trail leads southeast to a point, contours northwest, then slips through the red-orange Wingate formation. Here, at 5700 ft (1738 m), you're at the head of **upper Lathrop Canyon**. Below (southeast) is the White Rim Road. Southwest are fragments of an old uranium-exploration road snaking along the Chinle and Moenkopi formations.

A steep, southward descent ensues. Cairns indicate the route zigzagging across ledges, through a rockslide. Intersect an eroded exploration road at 4950 ft (1509 m). Follow it, descending east, then switchback west on a lower spur. Signs warn not to enter the abandoned mine shafts, which were excavated during the 1950s uranium boom.

Still on road, cross Lathrop Canyon wash, contour above it, then curve around a ridge. Soon depart the road and descend southeast to intersect the **White Rim Road** at 5.5 mi (8.9 km), 4400 ft (1340 m). (Maps and park signs disagree on this distance. Having studied them all and hiked the trail, this is our best estimate.)

Continuing the descent? Turn right and follow the White Rim Road south 0.1 mi (0.2 km). Then turn left (east) onto the badly-eroded road dropping through **lower Lathrop Canyon** 3.6 mi (5.8 km) generally south-southeast to the **Colorado River** at 9.2 mi (14.8 km), 4000 ft (1220 m).

Camping in the lower canyon and along the river is prohibited. There are, however, four backcountry campsites clustered near the base of Airport Tower, about 1 mi (1.6 km) south of where the Lathrop trail intersects the White Rim Road.

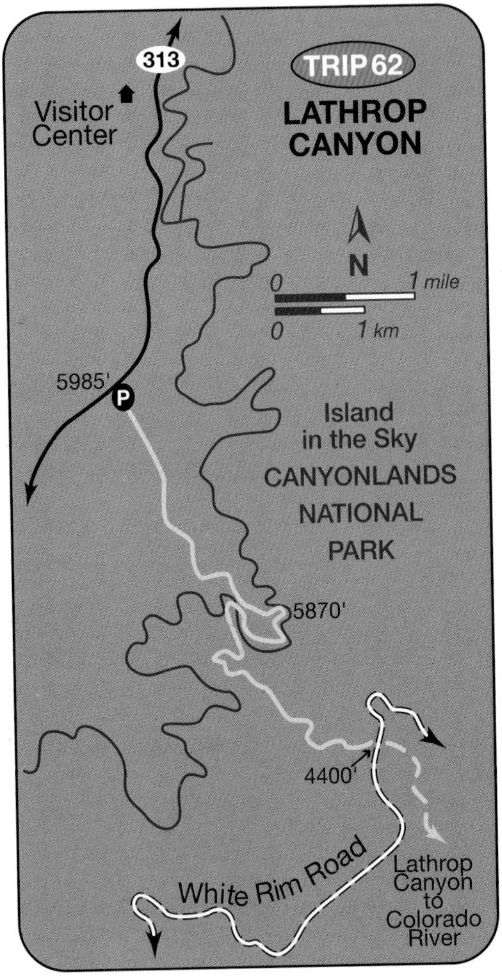

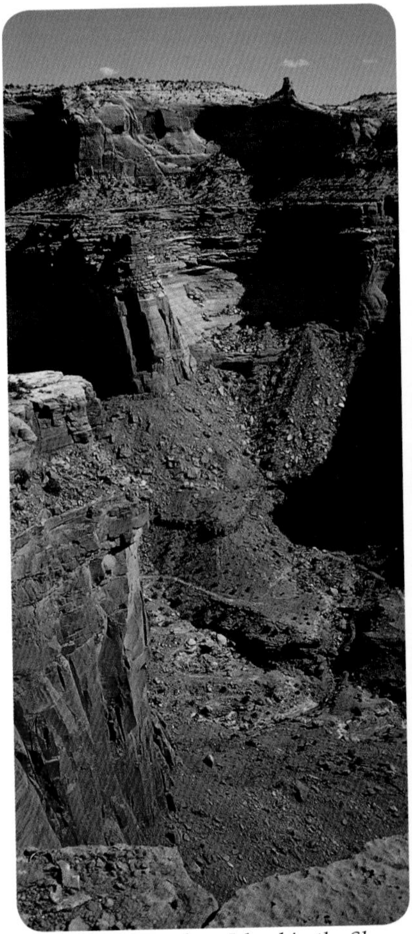
Lathrop Canyon, from Island in the Sky

TRIP 63

MURPHY HOGBACK

LOCATION	Canyonlands National Park, Island in the Sky District
CIRCUIT	10.8 mi (17.4 km)
ELEVATION CHANGE	1240-ft (378-m) loss and gain
KEY ELEVATIONS	trailhead 6120 ft (1866 m), base of canyon rim 5170 ft (1576 m), White Rim Road 4880 ft (1488 m)
HIKING TIME	4½ to 6 hours
DIFFICULTY	moderate
MAPS	Trails Illustrated *Canyonlands National Park / Needles & Island in the Sky*, Trails Illustrated *Moab South*

OPINION

From airy vantages in southern Utah, gazing across canyon country is like staring up at a clear night sky. The baffling, dizzying, overwhelming complexity of the earth's surface is as unfathomable as an infinite, star-filled universe. The Island in the Sky District of Canyonlands affords many such spectacles. And the Murphy Hogback trail invites you to leap into one.

It's not an easy invitation to accept. After quickly spurting from trailhead to canyon edge, the trail performs a swooping 1240-ft (378-m) dive onto the White Rim. "Whoa. Why give up this view to trudge all the way down there and back?" you wonder. Well, for the same reason you don't just stare at an artfully presented gourmet meal. You devour it. Hard to believe now, but only after the hike will you fully appreciate the view. Because only then will it be enriched with understanding and accomplishment.

Specific reasons to take the plunge: Astounding passages are thrilling to hike, and this is certainly one. Yet it's not dangerous, despite how unnerving it might be to watch your companions negotiate the skinny ledges. You'll marvel at the daring or desperate Murphy brothers who in 1918 contrived this unlikely cattle route down sheer cliffs of Wingate sandstone, and crumbling, sliding, Chinle formation talus slopes. (Imagine their pathetic beasts, bug-eyed with fright.)

There are vistas down there you can't see, or even imagine, from above. Hiking the hogback—a narrow ridge with a level top—you'll enjoy distant views left and right. If you've ever considered biking the famous White Rim Loop, here's your chance to grok it in a single day, on foot.

Granted, the wash you'll follow en route to the White Rim Road gradually loses its intrigue, but the rest of the journey more than compensates. Even the wash is rewarding to observant hikers who notice the colorful blend of stones underfoot, admire the artful erosion patterns of the maroon and lavender Moenkopi formation, and remember to glance back at the looming Island in the Sky.

Oh yeah, and what about that dreaded return ascent? Quit worrying. Hardened hikers do it in 25 minutes or less.

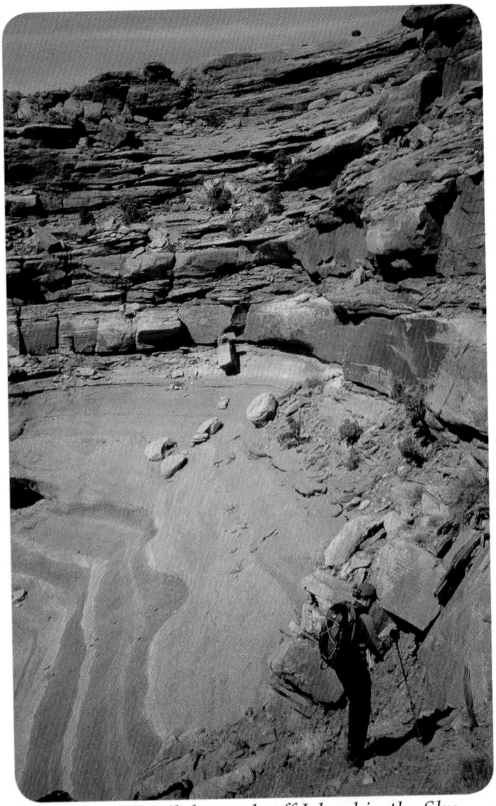
The Murphy trail descends off Island in the Sky.

A couple reminders before you go. Shade is nil, so save this trip for a cool day. You'll find no water en route, so pack more than you think you'll need, and leave a full bottle in your vehicle for when you return.

FACT

BEFORE YOUR TRIP

Consider camping at Murphy Point, a mere 1.8 mi (2.9 km) from the trailhead. It's the park's only backcountry campsite on the canyon rim, where the panorama is spectacular. You'll need a permit, but it ensures you'll be the sole residents for the night.

BY VEHICLE

From the junction of Highways 191 and 128, at the northwest edge of Moab, drive Hwy 191 northwest 8.6 mi (13.8 km) and turn left. From I-70, drive Hwy 191 southeast 20.3 mi (32.7 km) and turn right. From either approach, reset your trip odometer to 0 and drive southwest on Hwy 313 signed *Canyonlands, Island in the Sky*.

At 14.5 mi (23.4 km), pass the road to Dead Horse Point State Park (left / east). Shortly beyond, Navajo Mtn and the Henry Mountains are visible on the horizon (right / west).

At 19.2 mi (30.9 km) enter Canyonlands National Park. At 21.6 mi (34.8 km) arrive at the visitor center. At the 27.7-mi (44.6-km) junction, go left for Murphy Point.

At 30.1 mi (48.5 km) turn right (west) into the unpaved trailhead parking lot at 6120 ft (1866 m).

ON FOOT

A former road (unpaved, eroded) now serves as the initial 0.5 mi (0.8 km) of trail. Follow it southwest for about seven minutes to a signed fork. Right continues southwest 1.3 mi (2.1 km) to Murphy Point (see *Before your trip*). Go left (south-southwest) onto the trail signed *White Rim 4.3 miles*. Our directions lead to the White Rim via the wash and return via the hogback.

The trail is initially a level, narrow, sandy trough beelining through piñon and juniper forest. Brief slickrock sections are cairned. Approach the **canyon rim** at 1.25 mi (2 km), just ten minutes past the fork. Logs placed by rangers funnel you to where the trail drops over the edge: south, then sharply left (east) through a break in the rim.

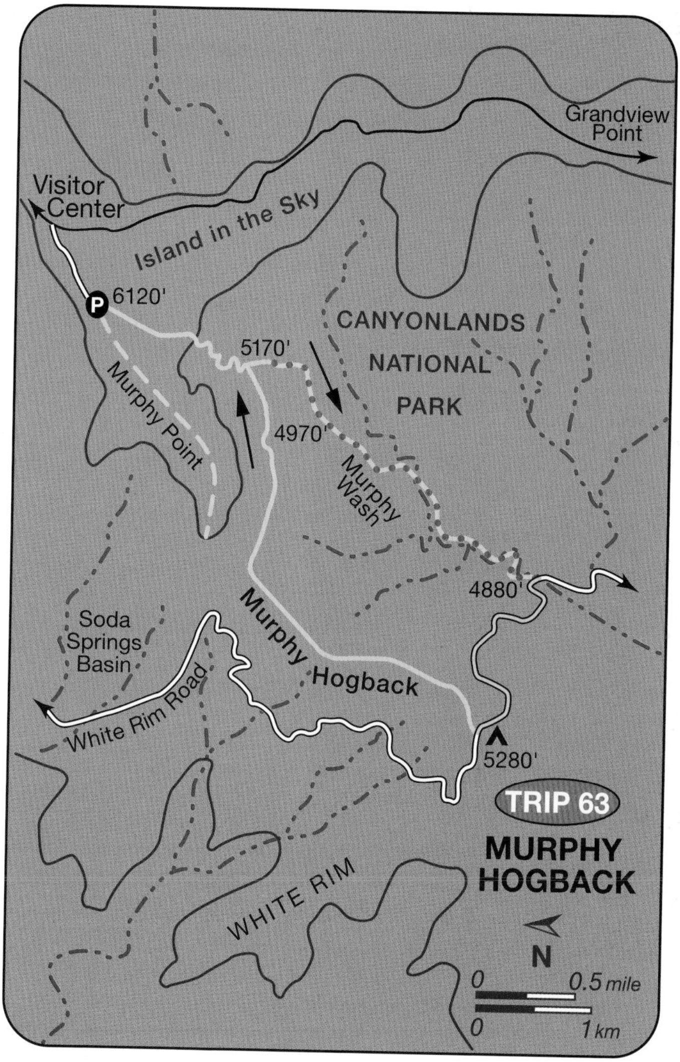

Ledges on the upper canyon wall afford a surprisingly gentle, switchbacking descent. About five minutes down, reach a talus slope of broken rock and boulders. Tight zigzags ensue. Then longer switchbacks resume. A sturdy, wood bridge enables the trail to traverse a sheer rock face.

At 2 mi (3.2 km), 5170 ft (1576 m), reach a **signed junction** near the bottom of the talus. You've hiked about an hour from the trailhead and descended 950 ft (290 m) from the rim. Surrounded by boulders and junipers, this is a secluded, peaceful setting where you can gaze up at the rim and out at deepening canyons beyond.

The trail forks here. Both options lead to the White Rim Road. Right (southwest) runs along Murphy Hogback. Left (south-southeast) descends via the wash. The two trails meet at Murphy Camp. Go either way. If you turn left, following our directions, you'll loop clockwise and appreciate Murphy Point's dramatic, red cliffs on the return.

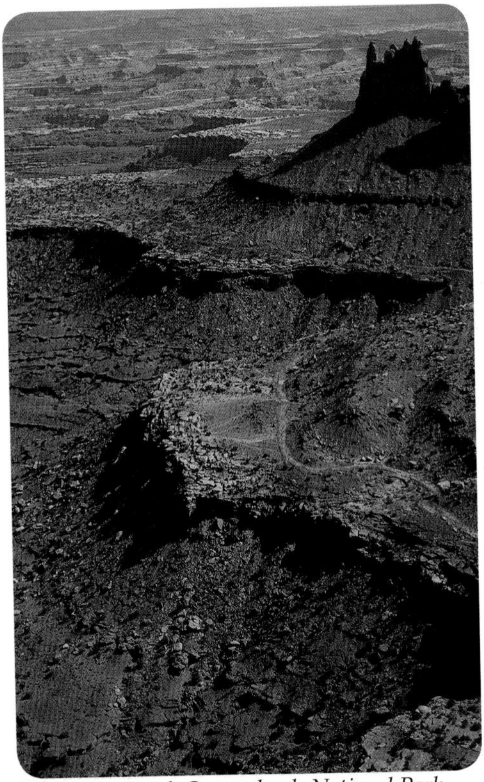
White Rim Road, Canyonlands National Park

Turning left (south-southeast) at the junction, begin a gentle descent into the **wash**. Soon leave trees behind. Within 15 minutes, the wash is about 20 ft (6 m) deep. Boulders diminish as it broadens. The bottom becomes sandy and level. Notice where overhangs have collapsed due to deep undercutting of the banks: obviously an imprudent place for a shady rest. Pass a cow pen—crudely made, long-ago abandoned. The elevation here is 4970 ft (1515 m).

Reach the **White Rim Road** at 4.7 mi (7.6 km), 4880 ft (1488 m). Turn right and follow it uphill, curving west-northwest. About 25 minutes farther, at 5030 ft (1534 m), near a sharp boulder on the right, the road begins climbing steeply.

Surmount **Murphy Hogback** at 6 mi (3.7 km), 5280 ft (1610 m). Immediately ahead is Murphy Camp A, with a panoramic view. It has tent sites and a pit toilet, but no water and no trash cans. Pack out everything you packed in.

From Camp A, proceed generally north on the road a couple minutes farther. After passing Camp B, but before the road swings left (west), look for a **trail forking right** (northeast), signed *Murphy Trailhead*. Depart the road and follow this sandy path through scrub. It will soon be apparent you're hiking atop a narrow ridge—the Murphy Hogback.

About five minutes from the road, detour left (northwest), off trail, to the edge of the hogback and a commanding **vista**. About 425 ft (130 m) below is the White Rim Road. You can see it plunge off the hogback, then wiggle north into Soda Springs Basin. A short stretch of the Green River is visible west/northwest, where it enters Stillwater Canyon after wrapping around a butte called Turks Head (northwest).

Reach the **base of Murphy Point** about 30 minutes after leaving Murphy Camp. Here, at 5200 ft (1585 m), cairns indicate where the trail curves right (east) to exit the hogback and skirt the **red cliffs**.

About 25 minutes farther, having hiked 8.8 mi (14.2 km), arrive at the **signed junction** you previously encountered upon descending from the rim. You've now completed the loop and are on terra cognita. All that remains is the ascent.

Fast hikers regain the **rim** in 25 minutes. The view is still astounding yet now intimately familiar. Stride 10 minutes through P-J forest to the end of the former road at 10.3 mi (16.6 km). Follow the road seven minutes back to the trailhead, where your total circuit distance is 10.8-mi (17.4-km) circuit.

TRIP 64

UPHEAVAL CANYON & SYNCLINE VALLEY

LOCATION	Canyonlands National Park, Island in the Sky District
LOOP	8 mi (12.9 km)
ELEVATION CHANGE	1480-ft (451-m) loss and gain
KEY ELEVATIONS	trailhead 5740 ft (1750 m), lowpoint at Upheaval/ Syncline confluence 4260 ft (1300 m)
HIKING TIME	4½ to 6 hours
DIFFICULTY	moderate
MAPS	Trails Illustrated *Canyonlands National Park / Needles & Island in the Sky*, Trails Illustrated *Moab South*

OPINION

"I have a surprise for you," the Earth says. And she always fulfills that promise, everywhere, but not with the frequency and hallucinatory variation that she does in canyon country.

For much of the way along most of the trails in this book, the Earth's shapes, colors and textures change with every few steps you take. It's startling yet entrancing. Desert rats unanimously cite this when attempting to explain the mystical allure of canyon-country hiking. And you'll experience it in Upheaval Canyon and Syncline Valley.

Not only is the terrain varied here, but you'll be hiking a loop—forward ever, backward never. And in addition to all the other little surprises along the way, you'll encounter two big ones: abrupt changes in elevation. Early on, the trail plummets off the Island in the Sky, into Upheaval Canyon. Later it surges out of lower Syncline Valley, conniving and muscling its way up a gorge that appears impassable. This intensifies the challenge but makes the journey more interesting.

Be prepared for a hike as demanding as it is dramatic. Expect the initial descent and subsequent ascent to be steep and rugged, though both are brief. The ascent is on a particularly rough route, mildly exposed in two places where a burst of gymnastic effort is necessary to avoid an injurious fall. Alleviate these difficulties—plus gain the benefit of some timely, post-exertion shade—by looping clockwise, as described below. The counter-clockwise hikers we've met here were distressed, admitting the trip was more time-consuming and arduous then they'd anticipated. Which also suggests this shouldn't be your first-ever canyon-country outing; work up to it.

What you'll be looping around is called Upheaval Dome. It's actually a crater. The dome collapsed eons ago—perhaps when struck by a meteor, according to one theory. About midway along the loop, a spur probes the jumbled, eroded moonscape within the crater. It's mildly engaging, but the loop is long enough without adding this 2-mi (3.2-km) round trip. Skip it, unless you're a geologist eager to theorize.

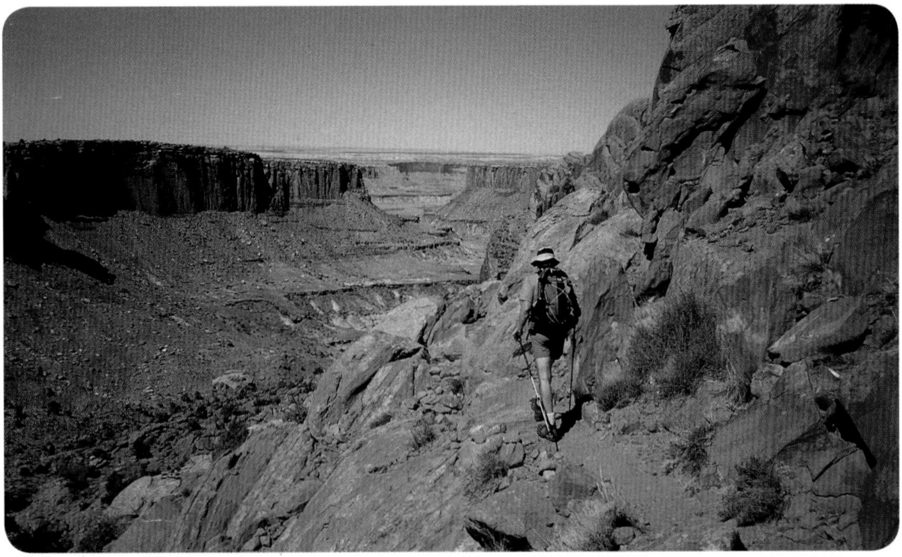

Descending into Upheaval Canyon

Loopsters also have the option of hiking lower Upheaval Canyon to the White Rim Road—a 7-mi (11.3-km) round trip. The canyon quickly broadens and loses its intrigue. Just up the road from the canyon mouth is Upheaval campground, but it's reserved for four-wheelers. And the Green River is just a few minutes down-canyon from the road, but it's a placid, unimpressive sight. So skip this excursion too.

Do, however, hike the Upheaval Dome / Crater View spur—an easy, rewarding, 2.5-mi (4-km) round trip. There's little elevation gain or loss. It's mostly on slickrock, so it's fun. The views—of the huge crater below, and the canyons and mesas beyond—are marvelous. And the bird's eye perspective of the crater will satisfy your curiosity, allaying any compulsion to hike into it from the bottom. Ideally, dash out here before starting the Upheaval / Syncline loop. Even the first viewpoint, a mere 0.5-mi (0.8-km) round trip, will enhance your subsequent appreciation of the area.

Though a gratifying hike, Upheaval / Syncline lacks the chief attraction of the Island in the Sky: panoramic vistas. So if you can devote but one day to this district of Canyonlands Park, choose a different trip.

The quick, 0.5-mi (0.8-km) Mesa Arch loop (too short to qualify as a "hike," therefore not in this book) affords a stellar view. The loop begins near the 27.7-mi (44.6-km) junction described in the *By Vehicle* section below. Do it. Then you'll know. If that kind of sweeping, Grand-Canyon-like scenery is your desire, hike the Murphy Hogback (Trip 63) rather than Upheaval / Syncline.

FACT

BY VEHICLE

From the junction of Hwys 191 and 128, at the northwest edge of Moab, drive Hwy 191 northwest 8.6 mi (13.8 km) and turn left. From I-70, drive Hwy 191 southeast 20.3 mi (32.7 km) and turn right. From either approach, reset your trip odometer and drive southwest on Hwy 313 signed *Canyonlands, Island in the Sky*.

At 14.5 mi (23.4 km), pass the road to Dead Horse Point State Park (left / east). Shortly beyond, Navajo Mtn and the Henry Mountains are visible on the horizon (right / west).

At 19.2 mi (30.9 km) enter Canyonlands National Park. At 21.6 mi (34.8 km) arrive at the visitor center. At the 27.7-mi (44.6-km) junction, go right, toward Upheaval Dome. Reach road's end (picnic tables, toilets, paved trailhead parking area) at 32.5 mi (52.3 km), 5740 ft (1750 m).

ON FOOT

Begin on the signed trail at the west end of the parking area. In one minute, arrive at a four-way **junction**. Straight (northwest) is the Upheaval Dome / Crater View trail, described below. The Syncline trail goes left (west) and right (northeast). Turn left to hike the loop clockwise; it's easier that way. Upon completing the loop, you'll return to this junction.

Heading west, the trail ascends gently for about five minutes, then descends gradually. Within 30 minutes, the trail grants an **overview** of the descent route into Upheaval Canyon. On the left is a bulbous sandstone wall with a cleft down the middle.

An earnest descent begins. Tight switchbacks plunge into a boulder-strewn gully. About 45 minutes from the trailhead, pass a **pouroff** at 4965 ft (1514 m). Bear right (northwest) following cairns up through a small gap. On the other side, resume the steep descent. Your immediate goal, the canyon floor, still looks surprisingly distant. The trail zigzags off ledges, then careens down another bouldery slope.

About an hour from the trailhead, reach the **wash bottom in Upheaval Canyon**, at 4590 ft (1400 m). The wash is usually dry. The trail heads downstream (north-northwest) on sand and gravel, among cottonwoods and junipers. It crosses the wash frequently. Because the wash has cut into the Chinle formation, its banks vary in color: initially rose and steel-blue, later yellow and gray. High above the talus slopes are red-orange Wingate cliffs.

Reach a signed **junction** at 3.2 mi (5.2 km), 4260 ft (1300 m), about 1½ hours from the trailhead. This is the **confluence** of Upheaval Canyon and Syncline Valley. Left (west) follows broad, sandy, brushy Upheaval Canyon generally northwest. It intersects the White Rim Road in 3.5 mi (5.6 km), at 3980 ft (1213 m). It ends 0.25 mi (0.4 km) farther at the Green River. Turn right (north-northeast) into **Syncline Valley** and continue looping around Upheaval Dome. The trail remains on the wash bottom.

Just two minutes from the Upheaval / Syncline confluence junction, the **wash forks** left (northeast) and right (southeast). In both directions, formidable pouroffs are immediately ahead. Proceed between them (directly east), onto a sandy bank. Ascend a steep, manmade **staircase** of pale yellow stone. Attain the bench above.

About eight minutes from the Upheaval / Syncline confluence junction, the trail forks at another signed **junction**. Right (southeast) leads 1.5 mi (2.4 km) into Upheaval Dome crater. Go left (north-northeast) and continue looping around Upheaval Dome.

The trail soon begins ascending boulder-strewn slopes, probing a deep, narrow **gorge** within Syncline Valley. The looming walls and more intimate environment are an intriguing, welcome change.

At 4 mi (6.4 km), about 30 minutes from the Upheaval / Syncline confluence junction, the trail begins climbing steeply over sandstone ledges. Gain 360 ft (110 m) in the next 0.3 mile (0.2 km). This is the exhilarating section of the loop; savor it. At 4700 ft (1433 m) cross to the north-northwest side of the gorge.

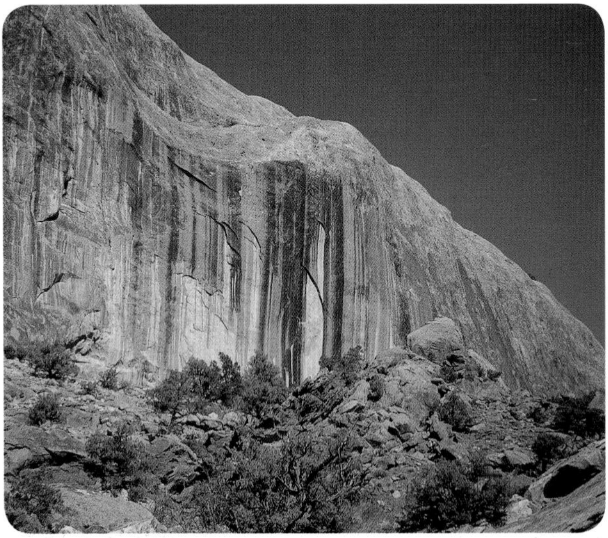
Desert varnish on walls of Syncline Valley

An **aggressive ascent** ensues among huge boulders. To follow the easiest route, stay attentive.

About five minutes after crossing the gorge, reach a **cable** bolted to a rock wall. It provides a secure handhold, enabling you to swing your leg over a precipice. Two minutes farther, spider-walk up an 8-ft (2.4-m) expanse of **smooth, tilted stone**. The exposure here will unnerve some hikers. Be calm and stable to avoid falling.

Having overcome the gorge's two minor difficulties, follow cairns to skirt a large **pouroff**. Regain the wash bottom at 4880 ft (1488 m)—above the pouroff and the gorge below. The going is easy again. The trail heads east, through the **wash**, beneath 500-ft (152-m) walls. During spring or fall afternoons, the walls shade the trail—a relief after an athletic ascent in the sun-exposed gorge. Continue following occasional cairns leading generally northeast.

About an hour from the Upheaval / Syncline confluence junction, the terrain flattens. The trail, now on packed sand, rolls gently through blackbrush. This area is lush in spring, sustaining long grass, wildflowers and creosote bushes. Soon the **canyon forks**. Left (southeast) is impassable. Go right (south) into a narrow, walled channel.

Rise through a rocky section onto a **slickrock cascade**. The trail resumes on loose rock and dirt among boulders left of the slickrock, but it's more fun to keep ascending the long cascade. Where the slickrock finally pinches out, go up, left, onto the cairned trail. Follow it generally southeast. The imposing, sheer wall left (northeast) of the trail is a spectacle in low-angle, late-afternoon sunlight.

The trail ascends very gently now, through **broad, shallow washes**, amid piñon and juniper forest. It gradually curves south, then southwest. The final stretch of trail parallels the road, which is visible left (south). Keep following cairns over short ledges to arrive at the four-way **junction** where you started the Syncline loop. Right (northwest) is the Upheaval Dome / Crater View trail, described below. Turn left to reach the trailhead parking area in one minute.

Upheaval Dome / Crater View

round trip	2.5 mi (4 km)
elevation gain	300 ft (91 m)
hiking time	15 minutes to 1 hour
difficulty	easy

Begin on the signed trail at the west end of the parking area. In one minute, intersect the Syncline Loop, described above. At this four-way **junction**, go straight (northwest).

About 6 minutes farther, reach a **junction** at 5858 ft (1786 m). Right (north) ends shortly above, at 0.25 mi (0.4 km). This is the **first viewpoint**, atop a small slickrock dome, near the crater's south rim.

Proceed left (northwest) from the first viewpoint junction. Follow cairns across slickrock about another 8 minutes. At 0.75 mi (1.2 km) reach a **junction**. Ascend right (north), soon topping out at the **second viewpoint**. It's the most impressive, so turn back now if you're short on time or interest.

Continue left (west) from the second viewpoint junction. Descend, curving northwest, beneath the edge of an escarpment. Below, stone steps lead to a **rock-lined trail** across slickrock and gravel. Soon turn right (northeast), rise 5 ft (1.5 m), then drop to the **third viewpoint**. It's behind a pink metal fence, at 5678 ft (1731 m). Having hiked about 20 minutes from the trailhead, you're now on the southwest rim. The crater is 1200 ft (366 m) deep, 1 mi (1.6 km) wide).

From where you last turned to reach the third viewpoint, a **bootbeaten route** continues generally northwest. Follow it 10 minutes farther on red dirt, among piñon and juniper, left of a pale-rose slickrock convolution. Clamber on broken rock to gaze northwest toward the confluence of Syncline Valley and Upheaval Canyon. You're now 1.25 mi (2 km) from the trailhead. Return the way you came.

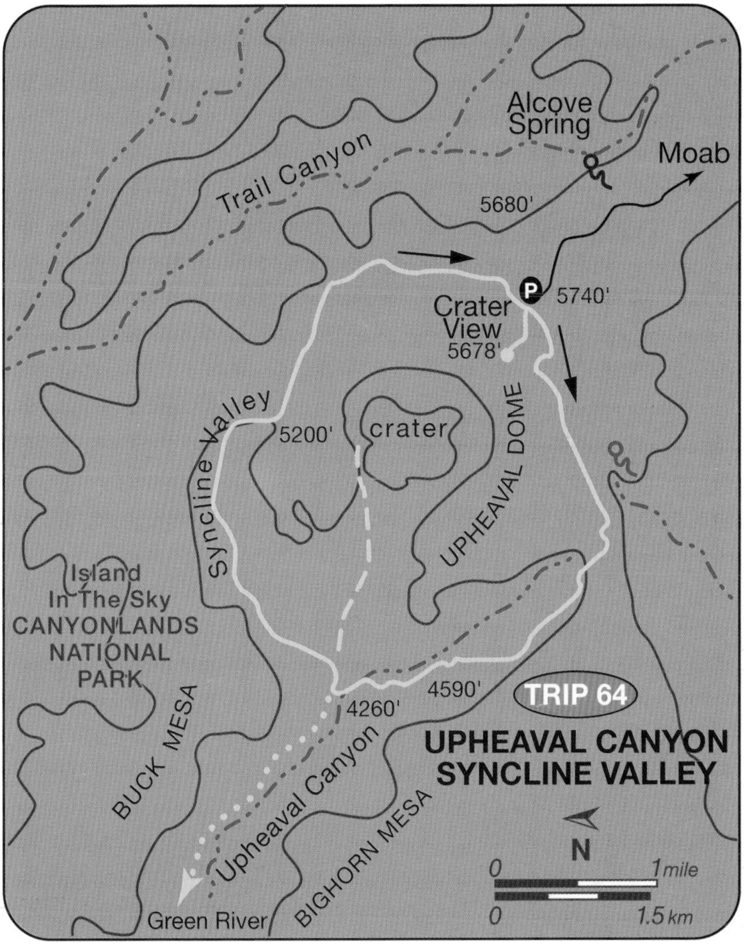

TRIP 65

BIG SPRING & SQUAW CANYONS

LOCATION	Canyonlands National Park, Needles District
LOOP	7.5 mi (12.1 km)
ELEVATION GAIN	430 ft (131 m)
KEY ELEVATIONS	trailhead 5180 ft (1580 m), slickrock saddle 5560 ft (1695 m)
HIKING TIME	3 to 3½ hours
DIFFICULTY	easy
MAP	Trails Illustrated *Canyonlands National Park / Needles & Island in the Sky*

OPINION

Problems ooze from every facet of life, often squirting into our faces when least expected. Why are solutions so scarce and reclusive, skulking in crevices until yanked out by their ears? At least this hike is an exception: a brilliant solution generously presents itself precisely when needed.

You'll hike up Big Spring Canyon, down Squaw Canyon. It's a short, easy, tantalizing preview of the loop and circuit dayhiking available on the 60-mi (96.6-km) trail network in Canyonlands' Needles District. These two particular canyons are separated in their upper reaches by an imposing slickrock wall. To hikers nearing the wall, it looks insurmountable. Proceed. The way will appear. But not until you're upon it. So the approach is an intriguing mystery. And the climax—a welcoming passageway amid steep, complex slickrock—feels like a gift.

Before and after breaching this concealed crux, you'll walk through beautiful high-desert environs: piñon and juniper forest, sandy washes, mushroom buttes, slickrock ridges, red-rock canyons. Only the culminating, 400-ft (122-m) high wall, however, is striking. Elsewhere along this trail, the immediate topography averages a mere 100 ft (30 m) high—impressive if you're new to canyon country, piddling compared to the soaring sides of Paria Canyon near Kanab, Spring Canyon in Capitol Reef Park, and many others.

Warning: The route linking Big Spring and Squaw canyons is briefly precipitous—ascending and descending. It might make acrophobes anxious.

Encouragement: Even if it's afternoon when you arrive in the Needles District, scamper around this loop. It will lend a sense of accomplishment to your day. The final 1.1 mi (1.8 km) is straightforward, easy to follow at dusk.

FACT

BEFORE YOUR TRIP

If you intend to dayhike in the area for a few days, try to camp at Squaw Flat. The campground has water (spring through fall) and toilets. The 26 sites, each with picnic table and fire pit, are available first come, first served. If the

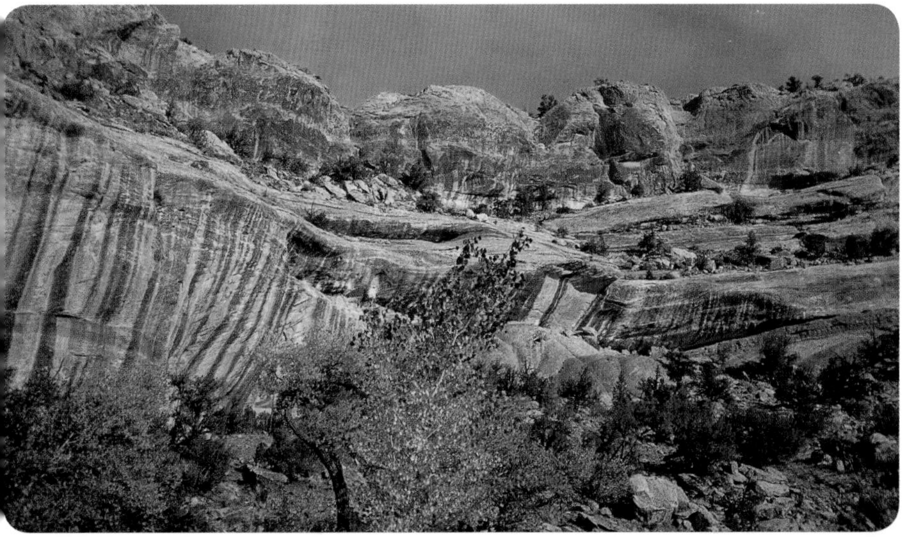

Desert varnish on walls of Big Spring Canyon

campground's full—which it usually is during peak season—arrive by 10 a.m., watch for someone to leave, then claim their vacated site.

BY VEHICLE

From Moab, drive Hwy 191 south 38.5 mi (62 km). Or, from Monticello, drive Hwy 191 north 13.5 mi (21.7 km). From either approach, turn west onto Hwy 211, signed *Canyonlands National Park, Needles District*. (A few miles north of this junction is a road west signed *Needles Overlook*, which is *not* your destination.)

Heading west on Hwy 211, pass Newspaper Rock—a must see—at 12 mi (19.3 km). Reach the visitor center at 33.5 mi (54 km). Continue about 2.5 mi (4 km) generally southwest following signs for Squaw Flat campground. Turn left to enter campground loop A. The paved trailhead parking area is just ahead. Shortly before the road ends, park on the left, near the toilets. Elevation: 5180 ft (1580 m).

ON FOOT

A sandy path departs the trailhead, near the toilets. Follow it south. Reach a **fork** within two minutes. Left (southeast) leads to Squaw Canyon and the Peekaboo trail (Trip 66). You'll return that way. For now, go right (southwest) toward Big Spring Canyon.

The trail soon crosses a small slickrock **ridge**. The Needles are visible west-southwest. About ten minutes from the trailhead, reach another **junction**. Right (north) returns to Squaw Flat Campground loop B. Go left (southwest) for Big Spring Canyon.

At 1.2 mi (1.6 km), having hiked about 20 minutes, arrive at an important **junction** in Big Spring Canyon. Right (southwest) leads to Chesler Park in 3.7 mi (6 km) and Druid Arch in 6.2 mi (10 km). Go left (south) to proceed into Big Spring Canyon and loop back to Squaw Flat Campground in 6.3 mi (3.8 km). Left also leads to Druid Arch in 7.2 mi (11.6 km). So the Druid circuit returns to this junction; see Trip 70 for details.

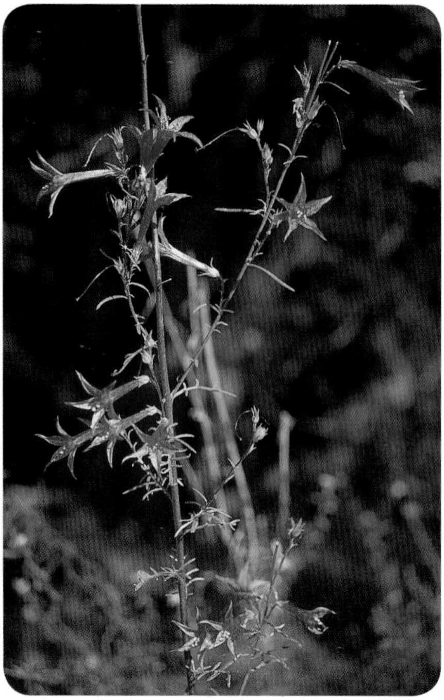

Scarlet gilia

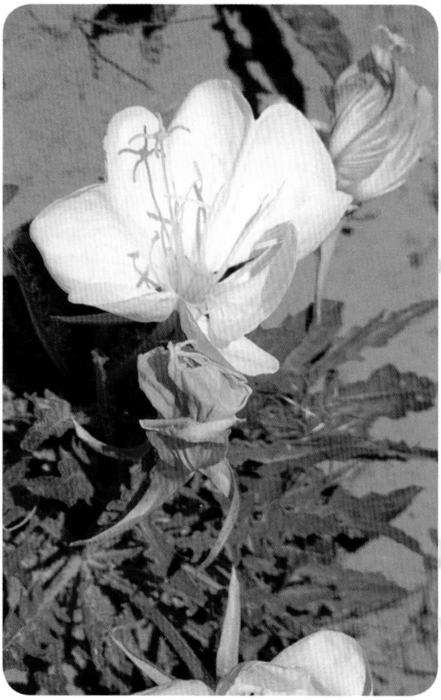

Evening primrose

Proceeding left (south) into **Big Spring Canyon**, pass backcountry campsite BS2 at 5180 ft (1580 m), about 40 minutes from the trailhead. Shortly beyond, the sandy trail goes left and launches onto a cairned slickrock **bench**. Gain 60 ft (28 m) in the next 10 minutes, cross the **creekbed**, then ascend left (southeast) following cairns.

Head south through a 20-ft (6-m) wide **wash** full of rock slabs. Soon, at a huge **wall**, the route rises onto a bench and becomes fascinating. Swift hikers will be here in 1¼ hours.

Climb slickrock steps beneath huge mushroom-shaped rocks to your left. Follow cairns over the slickrock **saddle**. Left of the huge wall, a **passageway**—concealed from below—is now apparent. Top out at 5560 ft (1695 m) and savor the view before dropping southeast. Below (northeast) is Squaw Canyon. Distant west-northwest are two singular pinnacles: North and South Six-shooter peaks. Chesler Park is west. North-northwest is Island in the Sky—the evocatively named mesa dominating the north half of Canyonlands Park (Trips 62 and 63).

From the saddle, descend 140 ft (42 m) on slickrock. Reach a signed **junction** on the edge of the slickrock, at 3.8 mi (6.1 km). Right (east-southeast) along the slickrock ridge leads 2.1 mi (3.4 km) to Elephant Canyon—potential access to Druid Arch and Chesler Park. Go left (northeast) along the slickrock ridge in the opposite direction, heading for Squaw Flat Campground, 3.7 mi (6 km) distant.

About 20 minutes from the saddle, reach a **junction** at 4.7 mi (7.6 km), 5220 ft (1590 m). Right (south) leads 5.7 mi (9.2 km) to Peekaboo Camp, via Lost Canyon. Go left (east) in **Squaw Canyon**. It has 100-ft (30-m) walls and a sandy floor shaded by cottonwood and oak trees.

The trail briefly crosses a grassy "park" before reaching a junction at 6.4 mi (10.3 km). Right (southeast) is the Peekaboo trail (Trip 66), an extraordinary slickwalk. Go left (northwest). Soon traverse two, small slickrock **bluffs** separated by sand. After descending the second bluff, a level, sandy path leads 300 yd (330 m) to Squaw Flat campground and the completion of your 7.5-mi (12.1-km) loop.

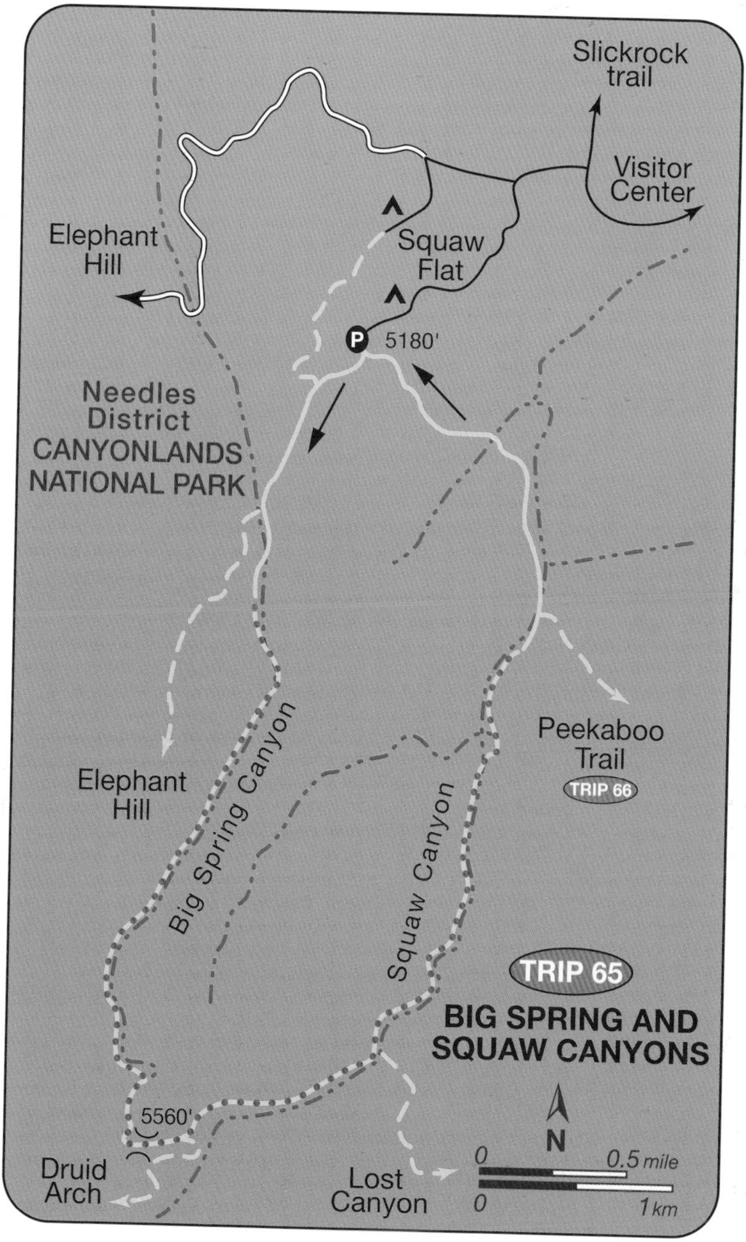

TRIP 66

PEEKABOO

LOCATION	Canyonlands National Park, Needles District
ROUND TRIP	10 mi (16.2 km)
ELEVATION GAIN	940 ft (287 m)
KEY ELEVATIONS	trailhead 5180 ft (1580 m), highpoint 5360 ft (1634 m) lowpoint in Salt Creek Canyon 5070 ft (1546 m)
HIKING TIME	5 to 6 hours
DIFFICULTY	moderate
MAP	Trails Illustrated *Canyonlands National Park / Needles & Island in the Sky*

OPINION

Many other canyon-country hikes are longer, wilder, lonelier, more challenging, more scenic. But the Peekaboo trail gets straight A's: amusing, amazing, awakening. It's the pièce de résistance of slickwalks. Think roller coaster, on foot. It ramps up, runs along ridges, nips over saddles, wraps around fins, hops onto bluffs, contours through drainages, slides into chutes, fakes left, veers right, even pops through a tiny window to earn its name. About the only thing it doesn't do is lose you along the way.

Fantastically tortuous terrain like this is common in southern Utah canyon country. But much of it would bamfoozle even a champion orienteer. What distinguishes the Peekaboo trail is that it's clearly indicated on maps and precisely cairned by national park rangers, allowing the average hiker to confidently follow its sinuous course. And unlike many slickrock areas near Moab, only hikers are allowed on Peekaboo. No mountain bikes. No motorcycles. No jeeps.

Although the national park refers to it as a trail, most of it is actually a route with nothing but the occasional cairn to indicate the way. You can follow a trail mindlessly. A route, especially a slickrock route, and this one in particular, requires you to be fully engaged. Often, the way forward is a mystery until your boots are upon it. Twice, there wouldn't *be* a way forward if not for strategically placed ladders. This is land you must grapple with mentally and emotionally, as well as physically. That's why Peekaboo is an extraordinarily fulfilling hike.

Rejuvenating is another way to describe it. Parents are forever going on about the pleasure of seeing life through their children's eyes. Well, hiking can top that easily. It can *make* you a kid again. Surprise, discovery, wonder and delight are impossible to suppress while giddily romping the Peekaboo. Ultimately, the experience transcends even the innocence of childhood, offering a sense of grace, of sanctification.

Which begs a question. Was it really just the mechanical processes of geology that aimlessly wrinkled this land? Or was there intent? The intent to inspire play and elicit joy among all creatures who wander here?

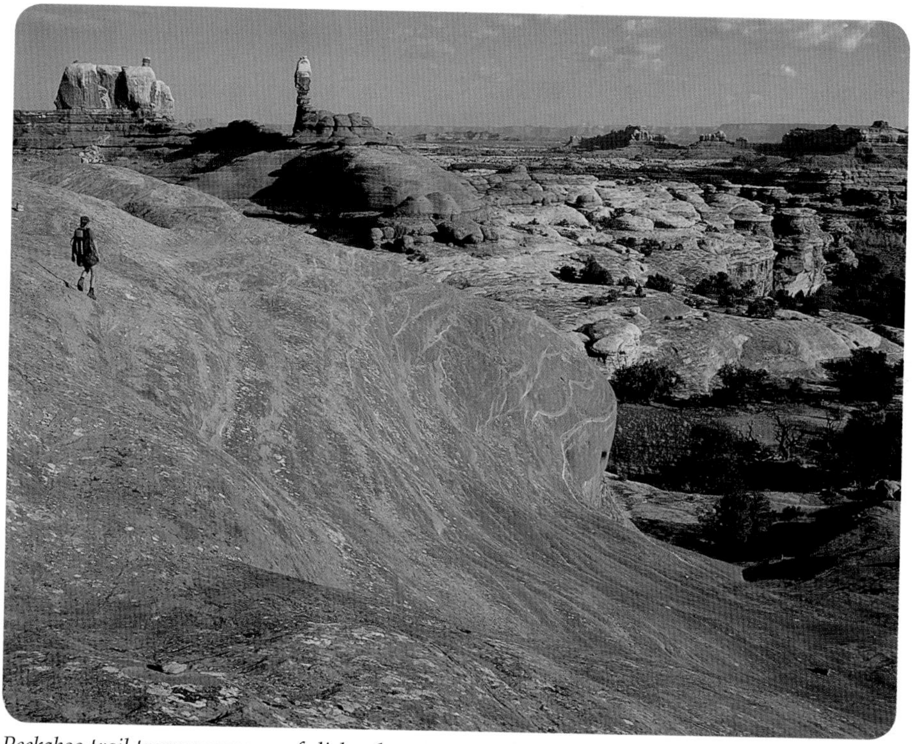

Peekaboo trail traverses waves of slickrock.

FACT

BEFORE YOUR TRIP

If you intend to dayhike in the area for a few days, try to camp at Squaw Flat. The campground has water (spring through fall) and toilets. The 26 sites, each with picnic table and fire pit, are available first come, first served. If the campground's full—which it usually is during peak season—arrive by 10 a.m., watch for someone to leave, then claim their vacated site.

BY VEHICLE

From Moab, drive Hwy 191 south 38.5 mi (62 km). Or, from Monticello, drive Hwy 191 north 13.5 mi (21.7 km). From either approach, turn west onto Hwy 211, signed *Canyonlands National Park, Needles District*. (A few miles north of this junction is a road west signed *Needles Overlook*, which is *not* your destination.)

Heading west on Hwy 211, pass Newspaper Rock—a must see—at 12 mi (19.3 km). Reach the visitor center at 33.5 mi (54 km). Continue about 2.5 mi (4 km) generally southwest following signs for Squaw Flat campground. Turn left to enter campground loop A. The paved trailhead parking area is just ahead. Shortly before the road ends, park on the left, near the toilets. Elevation: 5180 ft (1580 m).

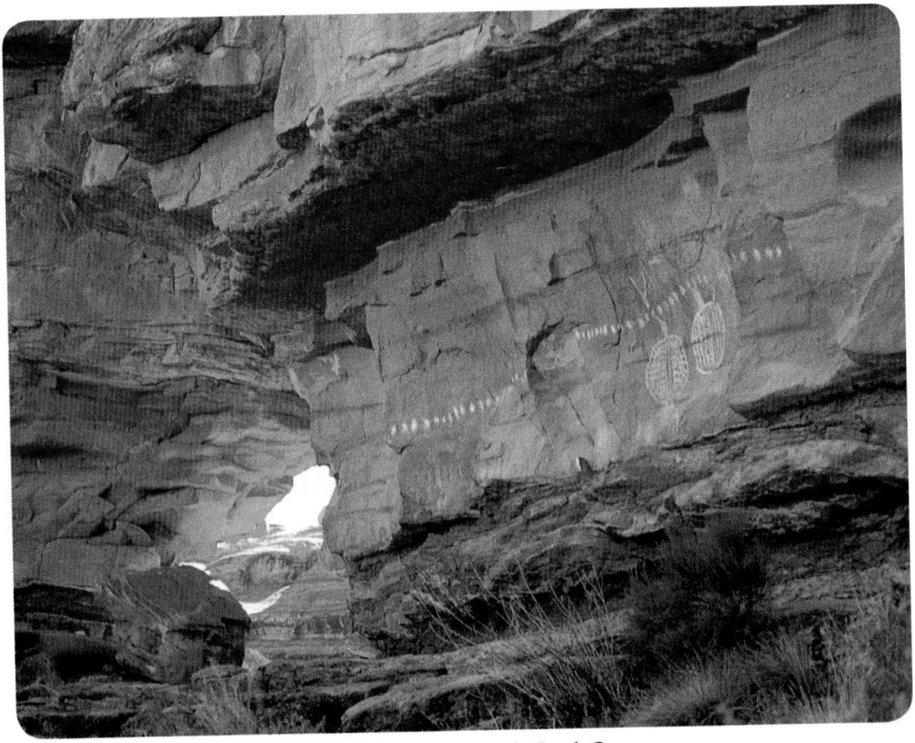

The Peekaboo trail ends near a pictograph panel in Salt Creek Canyon.

ON FOOT

A sandy path departs the trailhead, near the toilets. Follow it south. Reach a **fork** within two minutes. Right (southwest) leads to Big Spring Canyon (Trip 65) and Druid Arch (Trip 70). Go left (southeast) toward Squaw Canyon.

In 330 yd (300 m) ascend over a small slickrock **bluff**. After a sandy stretch, traverse another, similar **bluff**. About 20 minutes from the trailhead, reach a **junction** at 1.1 mi (1.8 km). Right (south) probes Squaw Canyon (Trip 65). Go left (southeast) on the Peekaboo trail, soon among gambel oaks.

About 40 minutes from the trailhead, ascend slickrock to 5240 ft (1598 m). Then drop 40 ft (12 m) and curve left (east) following cairns. Descend from red slickrock to white, to yellow, to black. Curve right (south) to where a metal **ladder** grants passage over a ledge.

Even with the ladder, the descent requires awareness. From there, go left (south-southeast) on white-and-tan slickrock. The route then drops into a sandy **wash** and becomes a trail among cottonwoods, juniper and piñon.

Heading southeast, the trail rises out of the wash onto sage flats. Reach a **junction** at 2.6 mi (4.2 km), 5060 ft (1542 m), about 1½ hours from the trailhead. Right (south) enters sandy **Lost Canyon** and loops 6.1 mi (9.8 km) back to the trailhead via Squaw Canyon. Continue straight (east-southeast) across the wash, to follow the Peekaboo trail.

After ascending over boulders onto yellow slickrock at 5250 ft (1600 m), the trail heads south and is once again a slickrock route, which it remains until just before the turnaround point at Peekaboo camp. Wooden Shoe Arch is visible northeast.

Cross a minor **saddle**. Contour right (south-southeast) on red slickrock. Following cairns, curve around the head of a drainage. Then turn left (north) to another **saddle** between knobs—about 15 minutes from the previous, minor saddle. North and South Six-shooter peaks are visible east-northeast.

Cairns lead right (east), descending slightly. Curve into an increasingly astonishing rockscape. The route goes right (south) through a 15-ft (4.6-m) wide **gap**. Descend a chute. Ahead is a towering wall.

Again curving around the head of a slickrock drainage, the route briefly traverses a **very steep slope**. This sharply angled section is short—just a few yards (meters)—but falling here would cause severe injury. Neophytes and acrophobes will be unnerved. If you're hesitant, turn back. Experienced canyon hikers who enjoy friction-walking on precipitous slickrock will proceed—aware but unworried.

Follow cairns curving right to the head of another drainage. Contour north-northeast until reaching the Peekaboo trail's namesake **window**, at 5360 ft (1634 m). Actually a hole in a fin, the window is just big enough for an adult to scrunch through.

On the other side, curve right (south), then left (east), contouring around the head of yet another drainage. Tall cottonwoods are now visible below (east) in Salt Creek Canyon. Soon, Peekaboo camp (a backcountry site frequented by four-wheelers) will be visible southeast.

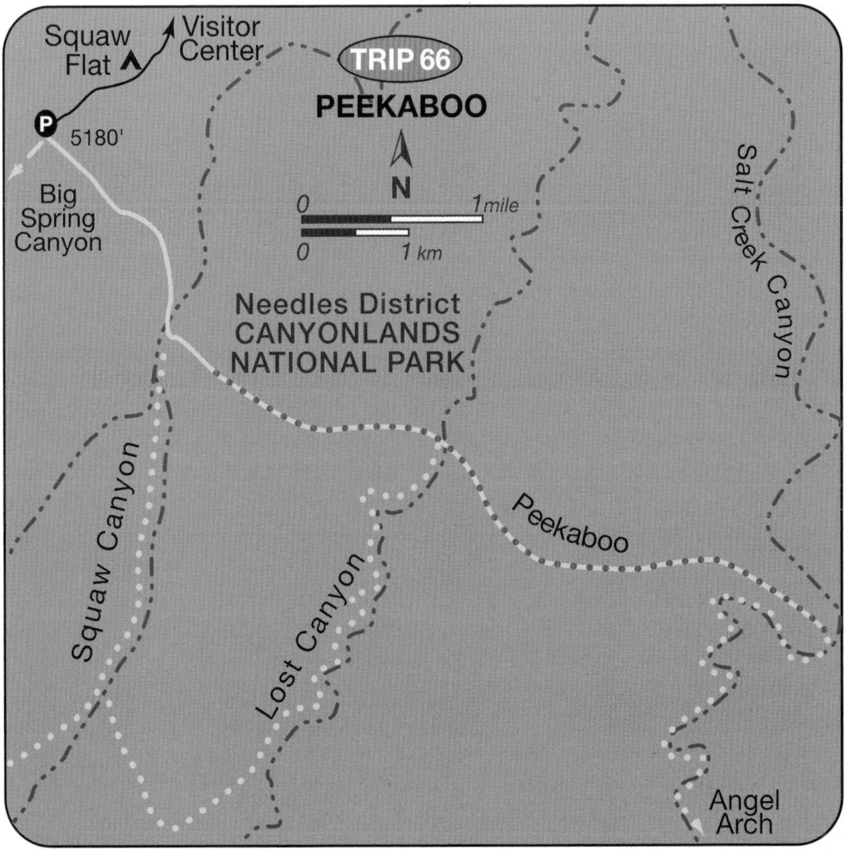

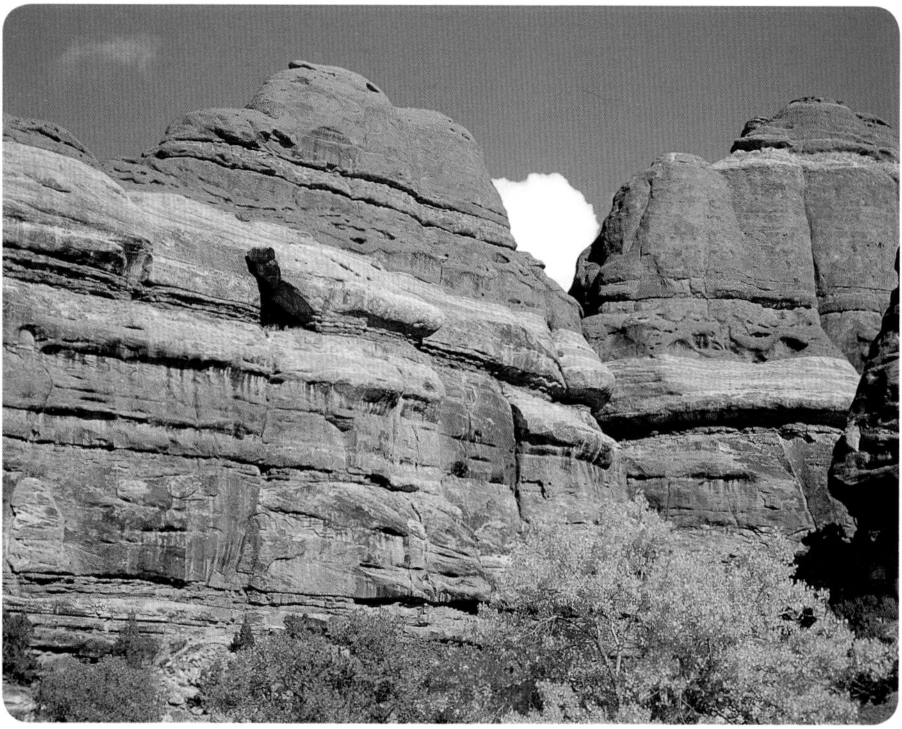

Salt Creek Canyon

Having hiked about 2½ hours from the trailhead, you're now on a slickrock **arm** that juts into the canyon but is still high above it. Ahead, the route will descend to the canyon floor. Don't turn around to avoid re-ascending. It's worth continuing to see the ancient rock-art panel near Peekaboo camp.

Hike northeast along the center of the arm, aiming for its end. Angle right, dropping toward the canyon. Near the bottom of the arm, follow a cairn right (south-southeast). Cairns then lead northeast. Still on slickrock, pass low trees to walk under a shallow, 10-ft (3-m) high **overhang**. Follow cairns down into a **joint**, where a 15-ft (4.6-m) **ladder** facilitates the final, sheer, 20-ft (6-m) descent.

Immediately beneath the ladder, curve right (southwest) to reach dirt in **Salt Creek Canyon**, at 5070 ft (1546 m). Don't drop the remaining 50 ft (16 m) to the wash bottom. Instead, contour right. Follow a path near the edge of the crumbling, **undercut bank**.

Just before Peekaboo camp, and slightly above it, there's a large **window** in the canyon wall (right / west). Right of the window is an impressive **rock-art panel** bearing Fremont shield-figure petroglyphs and handprint pictographs.

Peekaboo camp, at 5 mi (8.1 km), is just 2 minutes farther, but it holds no attraction for dayhikers. After appreciating the rock art, return the way you came, enjoying the Peekaboo slickwalk again.

TRIP 67, 68, 69, 70

THE NEEDLES, CHESLER PARK, THE JOINT, DEVILS KITCHEN, DRUID ARCH

LOCATION	Canyonlands National Park, Needles District
ROUND TRIP	5.6 mi (9 km) to 15.3 mi (24.6 km)
ELEVATION GAIN	770 ft (235 m) to 1430 ft (436 m)
KEY ELEVATIONS	trailhead 5200 ft (1585 m) Chesler Park overlook 5730 ft (1747 m) campsite north of Devils Kitchen 5500 ft (1677 m) base of Druid Arch 5840 ft (1780 m)
HIKING TIME	3 hours to all day
DIFFICULTY	easy to moderate
MAP	Trails Illustrated *Canyonlands National Park / Needles & Island in the Sky*

OPINION

Until you can vacation on distant planets, there's always Canyonlands National Park—a land as other-worldly as it gets without requiring a space suit to step out of your vehicle. This group of hikes penetrates the Needles—a concentration of fantastic redrock formations (pinnacles, fins, domes, hamburger buns, mushrooms, flying saucers) dominating the park's southern half.

Though the Needles are solid rock, their incomprehensible complexity gives the appearance of movement, vibration, dance. Perhaps because they keep your eyes darting from one implausible shape to the next. Perhaps because each intricate detail flows seamlessly, endlessly into another. Perhaps because you're indeed witnessing earth's living drama—a slower episode than a waterfall, a storm, or a volcanic eruption, but equally dynamic. Gazing at the Needles is like watching a jazz dance troupe writhing on stage: it's impossible to see every nuance, yet you try, because it's all so fascinating.

These four hikes begin at Elephant Hill trailhead. It's a busy place. A 4WD road departs here, and—despite all the hiking options—there's initially just one trail. But the 4WD road immediately veers in the opposite direction, and the trail soon branches into a web allowing hikers to disperse. It's possible to see it all—light and fast—in two or three dayhikes. The various round trips and circuits accommodate any schedule or energy level.

Trip 67 The Needles, Chesler Park Overlook

As its name suggests, Chesler Park is a broad, level expanse of desert grasses. The surrounding Needles make it special. The park's north side abuts the Needles' most intense concentration. Very near that north side is a pass affording a superb view. And the canyonscape en route to the pass is captivating. Round trip: 5.6 mi (9 km).

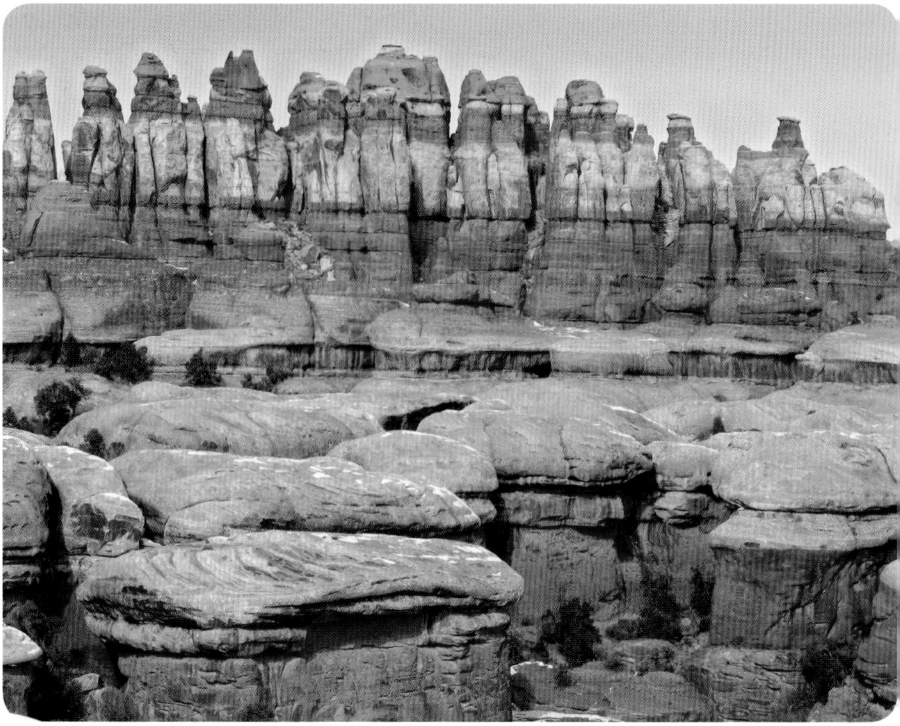

The Needles

Trip 68 The Needles, Chesler Park, The Joint

Continue through the pass overlooking Chesler Park, then loop around the park's outer edge. You'll visit the Joint—a slim corridor through fractured rock, where you can imagine yourself on Arrakis, trekking with the Zensunni wanderers. And you'll return immediately beneath the Needles' most bizarre cluster. Circuit: 11.1 mi (17.9 km).

Trip 69 The Needles, Chesler Park, The Joint, Devils Kitchen

After rounding the north edge of Chesler Park, beneath the Needles' most outrageous upsurge, return via Devils Kitchen. The Kitchen has a 4WD-accessible campground, so it's not a destination for hikers but merely a waypoint on the journey. The entire trek is through enthralling Needles scenery. Circuit: 10.5 mi (16.9 km).

Trip 70 Druid Arch

Druids were members of an ancient Celtic priesthood. In Irish and Welsh sagas and Christian legends, druids appear as magicians or wizards. The name *Druid Arch* is wildly inventive, yet bang on. The arch, strongly evocative of Stonehenge, feels like the work of a primeval, esoteric cult. The trail to this natural monument probes the slabby wash of Elephant Canyon. It culminates with a short, vigorous scamper onto the canyon's sandstone benches. Round trip: 10.8 mi (17.4 km). Strong hikers can vary the return and see more new terrain by cutting over to Chesler Park, visiting the Joint, and completing a 15.3-mi (24.6-km) circuit.

FACT

BEFORE YOUR TRIP

If you intend to dayhike in the area for a few days, try to camp at Squaw Flat. The campground has water (spring through fall) and toilets. The 26 sites, each with picnic table and fire pit, are available first come, first served. If the campground's full—which it usually is during peak season—arrive by 10 a.m., watch for someone to leave, then claim their vacated site.

BY VEHICLE

From Moab, drive Hwy 191 south 38.5 mi (62 km). Or, from Monticello, drive Hwy 191 north 13.5 mi (21.7 km). From either approach, turn west onto Hwy 211, signed *Canyonlands National Park, Needles District*. (A few miles north of this junction is a road west signed *Needles Overlook*, which is *not* your destination.)

Heading west on Hwy 211, pass Newspaper Rock—a must see—at 12 mi (19.3 km). Reach the visitor center at 33.5 mi (54 km). Continue about 2.5 mi (4 km) generally southwest following signs for Squaw Flat campground.

Bear right where left enters campground loop A. Shortly beyond, stay straight where left enters campground loop B. Proceed another 3 mi (5 km) on an unpaved but well-maintained 2WD road to the Elephant Hill trailhead parking area, at 5200 ft (1585 m).

ON FOOT

Trip 67 The Needles, Chesler Park Overlook

The trail departs the southwest side of the parking area, left of where a technical 4WD road begins climbing. Follow the trail generally south. Ascend stone **stairs** through a **cleft** to reach 5360 ft (1634 m). Proceed on the now sandy, gravelly trail among peculiar sandstone formations. Pass left of redrock walls. About 30 minutes from the trailhead, a 40-ft (12-m) high slickrock **bench** at 5420 ft (1652 m) offers a superb view of the Needles just 300 yd (330 m) ahead.

After a gentle descent, reach a **junction** at 1.5 mi (2.4 km) among piñon, juniper and rabbitbrush. Left (east-southeast) leads 3.5 mi (5.6 km) to Squaw Flat campground. Go right (southwest) to reach Chesler Park in 1.4 mi (2.3 km) and Druid Arch in 3.9 mi (6.3 km).

The trail hops onto slickrock, progressing between fins on slickrock buttes. Slip through a joint in the rock. Drop into an inner, redrock canyon alive with twisted juniper. Reach a **junction** at 2.1 mi (3.4 km), 5300 ft (1616 m), in **Elephant Canyon**. Left (south), up the canyon wash, leads 3.3 mi (5.3 km) to Druid Arch. For this trip, however, cross the wash and follow the trail right (west).

A moderate ascent weaves among boulders and juniper. Reach another **junction** at 2.7 mi (4.3 km), 5570 ft (1698 m), amid impressive pinnacles and fins rising 500 ft (152 m). Straight (north-northwest) leads 2.3 mi (3.8 km) to Devils Kitchen; you'll return that way on Trip 69. For this trip, go left (southwest).

A steep ascent, gaining 170 yd (155 m) on loose rock and slickrock in a gully between fins, climaxes at a small, 5730-ft (1747-m) **pass**. Having hiked 2.8 mi (4.5 km) from the trailhead, you're now smack against the Needles' east end, overlooking Chesler Park—a plain of sand, grass, and rabbitbrush. Southwest are sandstone mushrooms and buns, and a scattering of standing stones. The sandy trail drops to a junction below, on the edge of Chesler Park, but for this trip descend just part way. Drop your pack, relax on the slickrock, nosh your rye crisp and Emmenthal cheese, and devour the view. Return the way you came. Your total round-trip distance will be 5.6 mi (9 km).

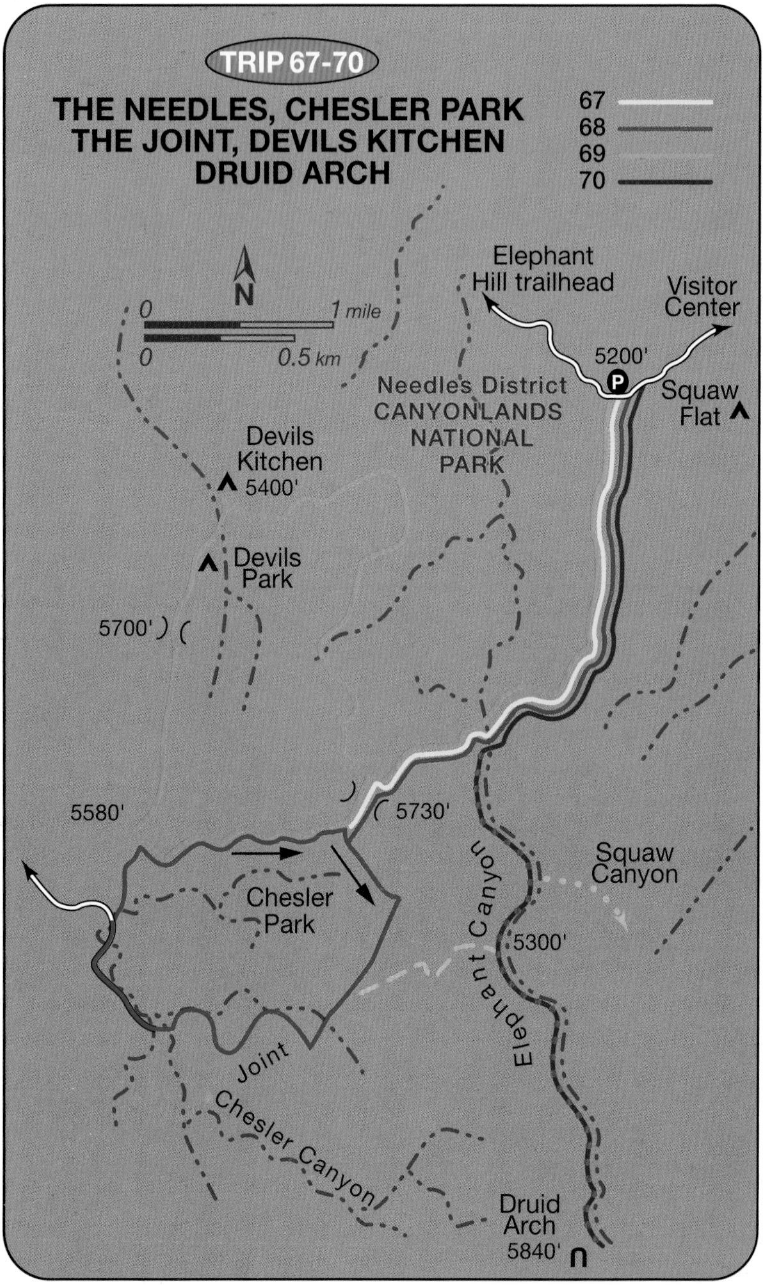

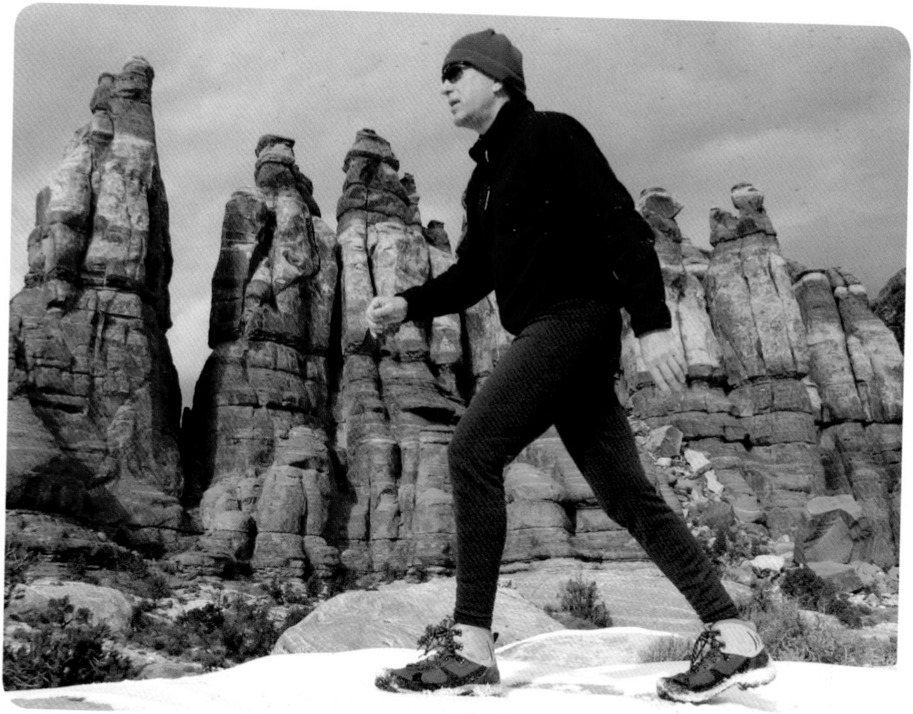

Near Chesler Park

Trip 68 The Needles, Chesler Park, The Joint

Follow the directions for Trip 67. From the **pass** at 2.8 mi (4.5 km), proceed down the sandy trail to the **junction** at 2.9 mi (4.7 km), on the edge of Chesler Park. Right (west-southwest) grazes the south edge of the Needles, en route to Devils Kitchen (Trip 69). For this trip, however, turn left (southeast) and begin looping around Chesler Park.

Reach a **junction** at 4.2 mi (6.8 km). Left leads 1 mi (1.6 km) generally east to intersect the Elephant Canyon trail north of Druid Arch. Bear right (south-southwest).

Soon pass backcountry **campsite** CP2 (sheltered between giant boulders) and a spur right (northwest) accessing three more campsites. At 4.9 mi (7.9 km) approach **the Joint**. It's a fissure: deep, narrow, long, shady, cool. The trail inside is sandy and brush-free. Slipping through this rock-walled slot is fun for all but claustrophobes. Upon exiting, cairns lead right (northwest). Descend through more rock curiosities to a **4WD road** at 5.7 mi (9.2 km).

Follow the road northwest 0.5 mi (0.8 km)—about 15 minutes. At 6.2 mi (10 km) bear right (north-northeast) onto a **trail** signed *Devils Kitchen*. The sign is just off the road, near where the road curves left / west.

Ascend through sandstone lumps to a **junction** at 7 mi (11.3 km). Left (northwest) leads to Devils Kitchen (Trip 69). Go right (east), beneath the most concentrated section of the Needles.

At 8.2 mi (13.2 km) arrive at the **junction** immediately south of and below the pass, where you began looping around Chesler Park. You're now on familiar ground. Return the way you came. Your total circuit distance will be 11.1 mi (17.9 km).

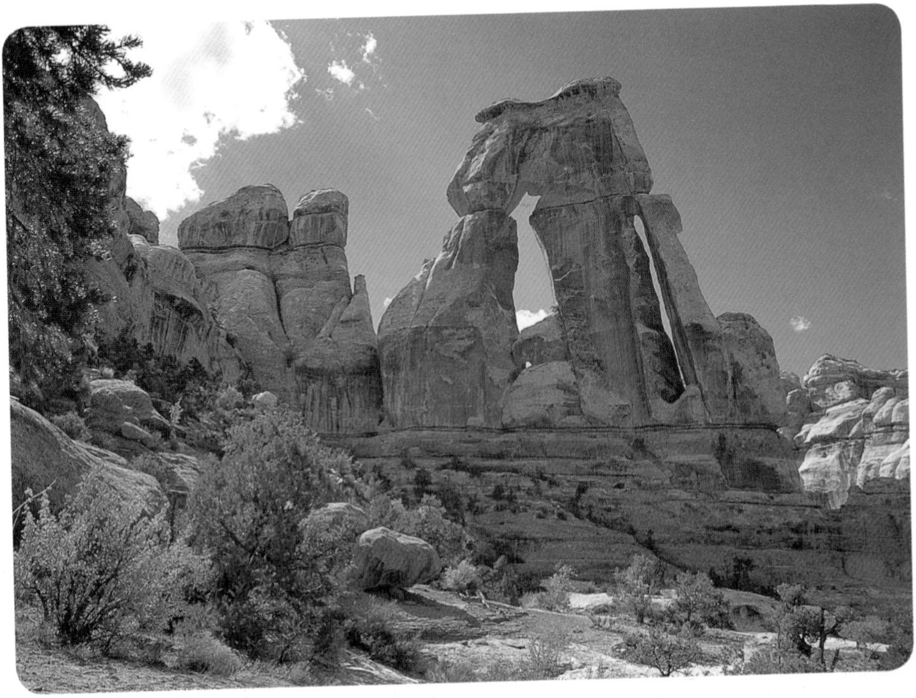

Druid Arch

Trip 69 The Needles, Chesler Park, Devils Kitchen

Follow the directions for Trip 67. From the **pass** at 2.8 mi (4.5 km), proceed down the sandy trail to the **junction** at 2.9 mi (4.7 km), on the edge of Chesler Park. Left (southeast) leads to the Joint (Trip 68). For this trip, however, go right (west-southwest), beneath the south edge of the Needles.

Reach a sandy **junction** at 4.1 mi (6.6 km), 5580 ft (1700 m). Left (south-southwest) is the return route from the Joint. Go right (northwest). Ascend a defile between walls. Continue on rock and sand to a small, 5700-ft (1738-m) **pass**.

Descend north—on rock stairs, then beneath an overhanging ledge. Enter Devils Park, a level, sandy area (similar to Chesler Park, but smaller) ringed by mushroom formations. About 30 minutes from the last junction, pass a right spur accessing backcountry **campsite** DP1, at 5500 ft (1677 m) behind a fin. Proceed generally north-northeast on the sandy, main trail, descending slightly, parallel to and left of a 100-ft (30-m) wall. At 5.5 mi (8.9 km), about 15 minutes from the campsite spur, arrive at **Devils Kitchen** backcountry campground, also accessible by 4WD. It has toilets, and a large, flat boulder shaded by a juniper—perfect for a lounging rest stop.

To resume, go around the juniper, keeping the toilet on your left. Ahead is a table beneath an overhanging boulder. The hiking trail leads east. Be sure you're not heading north on the 4WD road. Left of the trail are intriguing caverns in bulbous sandstone walls.

After ascending a slickrock pouroff, the trail rolls along on slickrock and sand, past juniper and piñon, through fins and pinnacles, to the head of another drainage. At 7.8 mi (12.6 km), about an hour from Devils Kitchen, reach a **junction** at 5570 ft (1698 m), amid impressive pinnacles and fins rising 500 ft

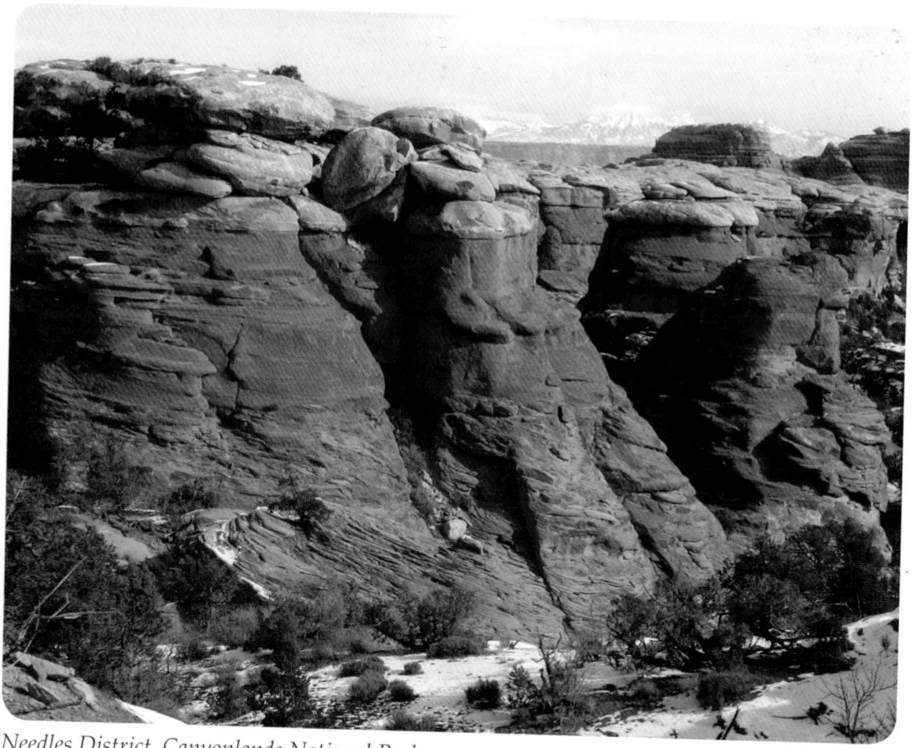

Needles District, Canyonlands National Park

(152 m). This is immediately northeast of and below the pass you crossed to enter Chesler Park. You're now on familiar ground. Go left (east-southeast) to return the way you came. Your total circuit distance will be 10.5 mi (16.9 km).

Trip 70 Druid Arch

Follow the directions for Trip 67 until the **junction** at 2.1 mi (3.4 km), 5300 ft (1616 m), in **Elephant Canyon**. Across the wash, right (west) leads to the Needles, Chesler Park, The Joint, and Devils Kitchen (Trips 67, 68, 69). For this trip, however, go left (south), up the canyon wash.

Reach a **junction** at 2.9 mi (4.7 km). Left (southeast) leads to Big Spring Canyon (Trip 65). Go right (south-southeast) for Druid Arch.

At 3.4 mi (5.5 km) reach another **junction**. Right leads 1 mi (1.6 km) generally west to a junction on the southeast edge of Chesler Park, near the Joint (Trip 68). Go left (southeast) for Druid Arch.

In a few minutes, at a convergence of washes, go left into the larger wash, toward higher canyon walls. The remaining 0.75 mi (1.2 km) is on a bench above the wash. Reach the base of **Druid Arch** at 5.4 mi (8.7 km), 5840 ft (1780 m). When the fin end of the stalwart 500-ft (152-m) high arch is visible, follow cairns ascending left onto a white rim. Climb a metal ladder. The fin is above you, immediately ahead. To attain the optimal viewpoint, the route ascends another 80 ft (24 m) above the rim. The going is rough but should pose no danger to sure-footed hikers.

Admire the arch while savoring your tuna-on-a-bagel sandwich, then return the way you came. Your total round-trip distance will be 10.8 mi (17.4 km).

TRIP 71

SALT CREEK CANYON

LOCATION	Canyonlands National Park, Needles District
DISTANCE	27.5 mi (44.3 km) one way
ELEVATION CHANGE	2050-ft (625-m) loss to Peekaboo camp plus 940-ft (287-m) gain to Squaw Flat
KEY ELEVATIONS	Cathedral Butte trailhead 7070 ft (2155 m) Big Pocket 5830 ft (1777 m), Upper Jump 5600 ft (1707 m) Angel Arch camp 5370 ft (1637 m) Peekaboo camp 5020 ft (1530 m) Squaw Flat trailhead 5180 ft (1580 m)
HIKING TIME	3 to 4 days
DIFFICULTY	moderate
MAPS	Trails Illustrated *Canyonlands National Park / Needles & Island in the Sky,* USGS *Cathedral Butte, Druid Arch South Sixshooter Peak*

OPINION

Do big things, or little things will do you.

The three or four days you don't spend backpacking in Salt Creek Canyon will likely be devoured by a ravenous swarm of insect-like chores, obligations and habits, then immediately forgotten. Devote that time here, and you'll gain momentum toward a more intrepid life.

That's a lot to expect of a backpack trip, but this one can shoulder the burden. It's a rousing adventure through raw wilderness; the most ambitious, remote trek in the Needles District of Canyonlands National Park.

Salt Creek Canyon showcases every nuance of the bizarre, fascinating topography distinguishing southern Utah: sheer cliffs, deep alcoves, bulbous domes, surreal arches, balancing boulders, stalwart towers, fragile spires, eccentric hoodoos.

You'll also be following in the footsteps of the Ancestral Puebloans who once wrested a living from this harsh land. Evidence of their tenure is abundant.

Big Ruin, the largest archaeological site in Canyonlands National Park, comprises 32 structures. All-American Man is a unique pictograph: a visage resembling a baseball, painted in red, white and blue. The Four Faces pictograph evokes... a matriarchal goddess-worshipping society? The blissful, hallucinogenic effects of datura? A tranquility cult? Allow yourself time to meditate on the Buddha-nature of these sweetly smiling, bejeweled beauties.

The south-to-north journey begins on the rim of Salt Creek Mesa, near Cathedral Butte. After plunging 1000 ft (305 m) into the canyon, you'll follow Salt Creek wash 22.5 mi (36.2 km) ever-so-slightly-downhill to Peekaboo camp. There you'll begin the arduous-but-thrilling slickwalk finale by mounting the Peekaboo trail (Trip 66) and following it 5 mi (8.1 km) generally northwest to Squaw Flat.

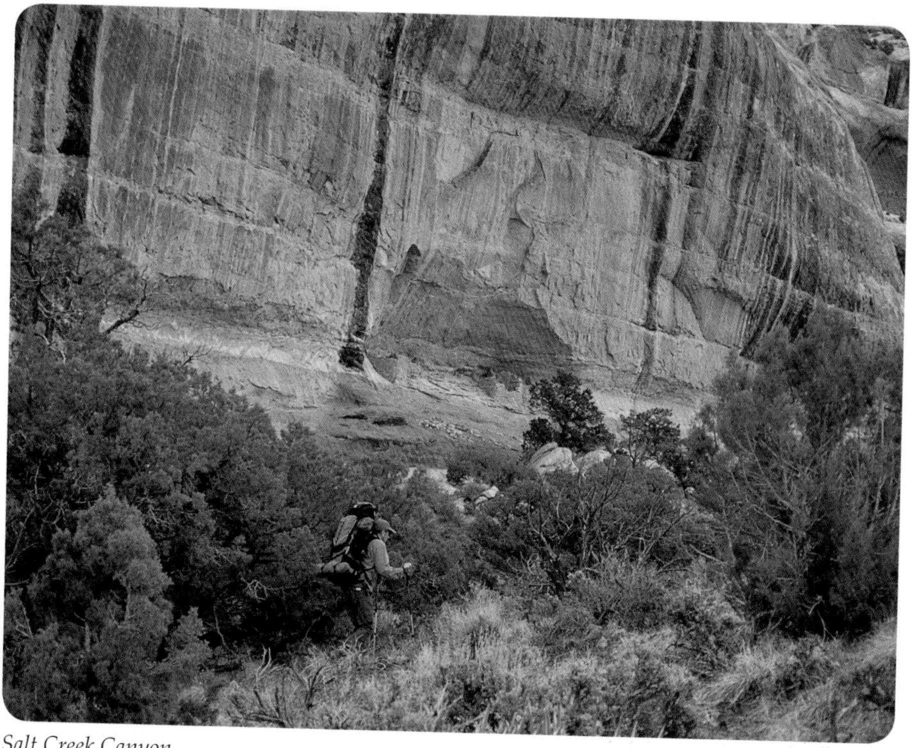

Salt Creek Canyon

Backpacking experience is a prerequisite for this challenging endeavor. Between Cathedral Butte and Angel Arch camp, the way forward is vague at times, requiring you to interpret the terrain with the aid of your map. Occasionally you must negotiate arroyos and push through riparian thickets. You'll be pitching your tent in austere campsites that meet the essential needs of a nomad but are not conducive to R&R.

The climax, between Peekaboo camp and Squaw Flat, is especially demanding. You'll find it safe and enjoyable only if you're (1) a bloodhound, able to navigate long stretches of convoluted slickrock route with only a few scattered cairns for guidance; (2) a mule, able to carry a full pack on wave-like terrain; and (3) a mountain goat, immune to acrophobia.

If you're not at least a strong, intermediate backpacker with a little routefinding under your boots, it would be wise to leave Salt Creek Canyon on your "someday" list. Meanwhile, try dayhiking the Peekaboo trail (Trip 66).

FACT

BEFORE YOUR TRIP

A round-trip in Salt Creek Canyon is unsatisfying. Arrange a vehicle shuttle, so you can hike one way, from south to north, and enjoy the optimal backpacking experience.

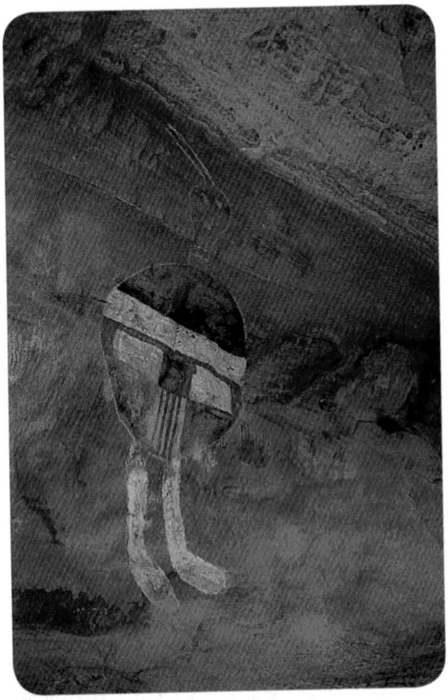

All American Man pictograph panel, Salt Creek Canyon

Get a backcountry camping permit from the Canyonlands National Park Needles District visitor center (see *Information Sources*). For details, visit www.nps.gov/cany, click on "Backcountry Permits," "Backpacking," and "Reservations."

When making reservations, be aware that campsite SC 1, at 4.3 mi (6.9 km), is bleak: a shadeless patch of hardpan affording no protection from wind or rain. Nearby campsite SC 2 is slightly more sheltered. Campsite SC 3, at 9.1 mi (14.7 km) is little better, though it offers a view of impressive cliffs and is closer to the canyon's celebrated rock-art sites. SC 4 and Angel Arch camp are a bit more hospitable.

Between Angel Arch Canyon and Peekaboo, at-large camping is allowed. Up to four permits are issued for this stretch each night. "At large" means wherever you want as long as you're (a) out of sight of the trail, (b) 1 mi (0.6 km) from anyone else's at-large campsite, and (c) 300 ft (91 m) from water sources. Peekaboo camp, at 22.5 mi (36.2 km), is exclusively for 4WDers, but hikers may camp 1 mi (0.6 km) south of it.

Late summer through fall, black bears are present in Salt Creek Canyon. They migrate from the Abajo Mtns to gorge on purple cactus pears, which ripen in early autumn. The bears are shy and relatively small but are potentially dangerous nonetheless. Ask at the visitor center for suggestions on how to avoid a serious encounter.

Cathedral Butte trailhead is on Salt Creek Mesa, just outside the national park boundary. It's a pleasant place to camp. Keep it in mind for the night before you begin hiking.

Water has historically been available in Salt Creek Canyon year round. But ask at the visitor center how much water to expect and where you'll likely find it.

BY VEHICLE

From Moab, drive Hwy 191 south 38.5 mi (62 km). Or, from Monticello, drive Hwy 191 north 13.5 mi (21.7 km). From either approach, turn west onto Hwy 211, signed *Canyonlands National Park, Needles District*. (A few miles north of this junction is a road west signed *Needles Overlook*, which is *not* your destination.)

Heading west on Hwy 211, pass Newspaper Rock—a must see—at 12 mi (19.3 km). At 20.2 mi (32.6 km) pass unpaved Beef Basin Road (left / southwest) which leads to the Cathedral Butte trailhead, where the one-way trip begins. Reach the visitor center at 33.5 mi (54 km). Continue about 2.5 mi (4 km) generally southwest following signs for Squaw Flat campground. Turn left to enter campground loop A. The paved trailhead parking area is just ahead. Leave your shuttle vehicle here, near the toilets, where the one-way trip ends. Elevation: 5180 ft (1580 m).

To reach Cathedral Butte trailhead, where the one-way trip begins, drive Hwy 211 east 13.3 mi (21.4 km) from the visitor center. Turn right (southwest) onto Beef Basin Road, reset your trip odometer to 0, and follow it generally south-southwest. Reach a fork at 9.2 mi (14.8 km). Go right (west). Soon curve left and resume generally south-southwest beneath Bridger Jack Mesa. After curving right (west) and approaching the rim of Salt Creek Canyon, the road curves left (south) around 7940-ft (2256-m) Cathedral Butte (left / east). Reach the unsigned trailhead parking area (right / northwest) at 17.1 mi (27.5 km), 7070 ft (2155 m). Start hiking here.

ON FOOT

Starting right of the map/sign and register, follow the trail left (west-southwest) one minute, then descend through P-J (piñon pine and juniper).

The grade is initially sharp, the terrain rocky. After dropping generally north-northwest, the trail veers left (west-northwest). The grade eases within 45 minutes.

Reach the **canyon floor** about 1000 ft (305 m) below the rim. Pass a barely recognizable **junction** with the sketchy Bright Angel trail (left /southwest). Bear right, enter the national park at 2 mi (3.2 km), and proceed northwest. The now level trail follows **East Fork Salt Creek** down-canyon amid sagebrush.

Cross a marshy area. Enter a stand of tamarisk. Briefly follow the canyon wall. Soon pass **Kirk Cabin** and a juniper-log corral. Rensselaer Lee Kirk worked an 80-acre ranch here for a decade, from 1895 to 1905.

About 70 yd (65 m) farther, at 4.3 mi (6.9 km), 5920 ft (1804 m), a signed right (east) spur quickly accesses **campsites SC 1 and 2**.

From the SC 1/2 spur, pass through an old, juniper fence and follow the main trail north-northeast. Ruins are visible in the alcoves ahead. At 4.7 mi (7.6 km) pass an accessible ruin in a southwest-facing alcove. Scan the left (west) horizon for **Kirk Arch** between and beyond two slickrock buttes.

At 5.7 mi (9.2 km), 5830 ft (1777 m), pass the mouth of **Big Pocket**—a broad tributary drainage (right / southeast)—and look left for **Big Ruin** on the canyon's west wall. Comprising 32 structures, the ruin is the largest archaeological site in Canyonlands National Park.

Detour to Big Ruin by looking right for a 30-ft (9-m) wide, diamond-shaped boulder with one point beneath the ground immediately north of Big Pocket. About 200 ft (61 m) farther, look left for a bootbeaten path. Follow it across Salt Creek to reach the ruin in about 15 minutes. Though the primary site occupies an inaccessible ledge, you'll gain a closer perspective and will see the ruins at the base of the cliff.

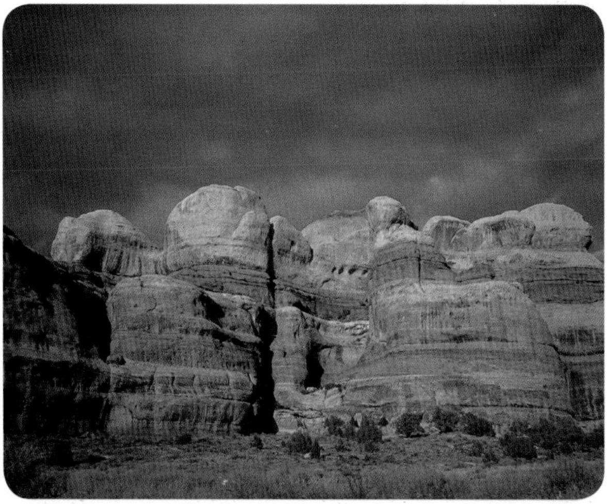

Salt Creek Canyon

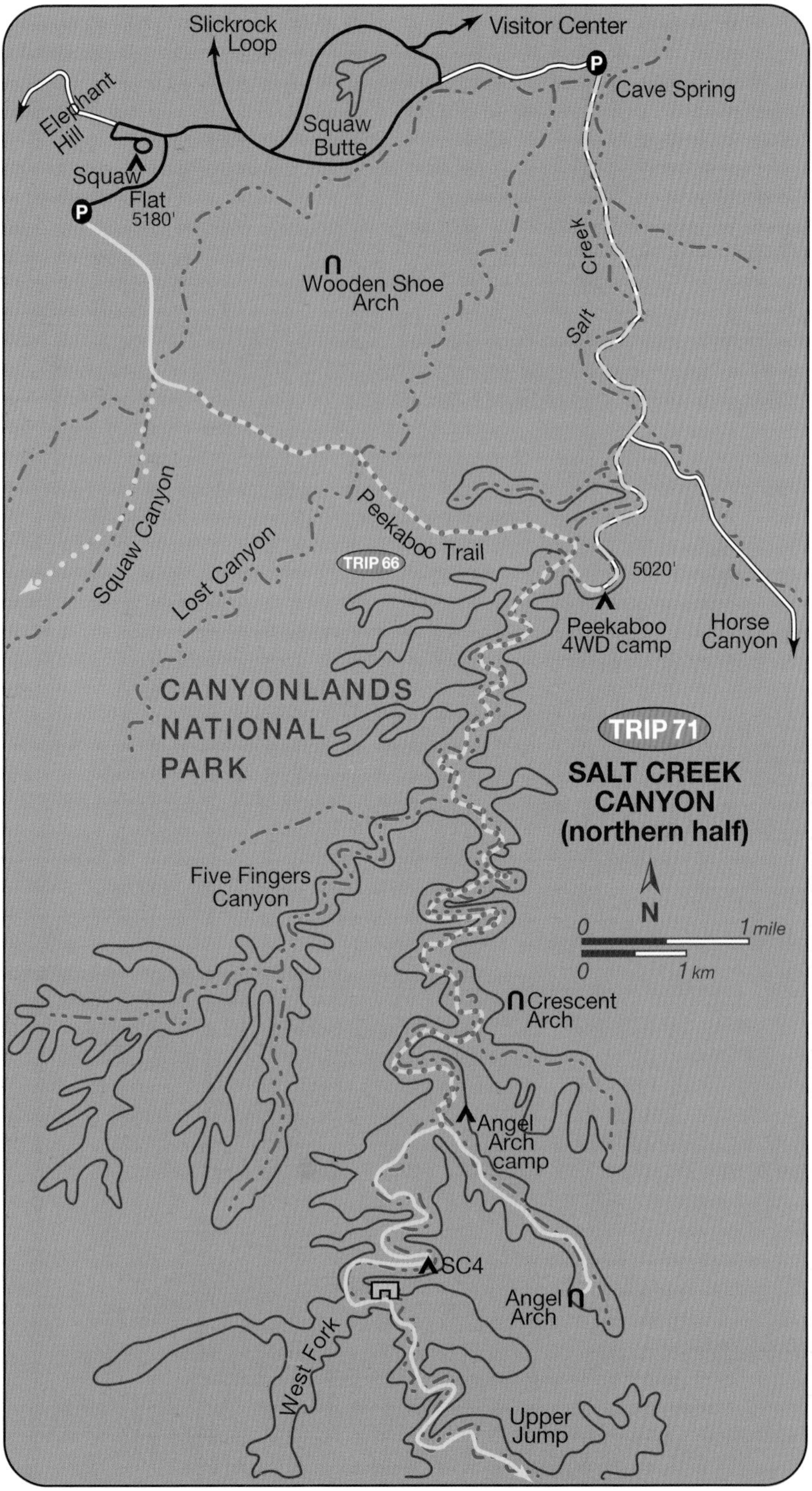
Slickrock Loop
Visitor Center
Elephant Hill
Cave Spring
Squaw Butte
Squaw Flat
5180'
Wooden Shoe Arch
Creek
Salt
Squaw Canyon
Lost Canyon
Peekaboo Trail
TRIP 66
5020'
Peekaboo 4WD camp
Horse Canyon
CANYONLANDS NATIONAL PARK
TRIP 71
SALT CREEK CANYON (northern half)
N
0
1 mile
0
1 km
Five Fingers Canyon
Crescent Arch
Angel Arch camp
SC4
Angel Arch
West Fork
Upper Jump

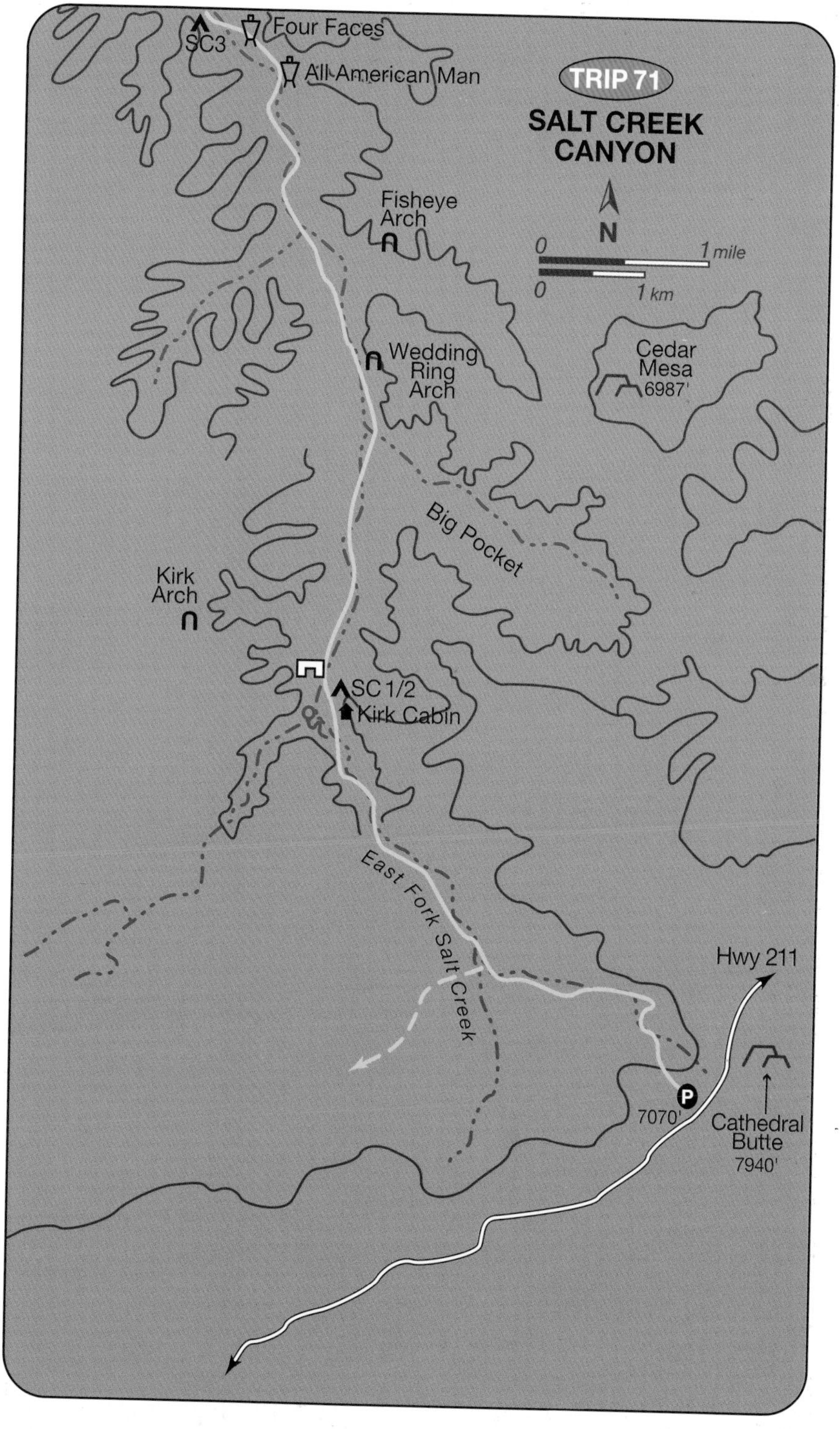
TRIP 71
SALT CREEK CANYON
N
0
1 mile
0
1 km
SC3
Four Faces
All American Man
Fisheye Arch
Wedding Ring Arch
Cedar Mesa 6987'
Big Pocket
Kirk Arch
SC 1/2
Kirk Cabin
East Fork Salt Creek
Hwy 211
P
7070'
Cathedral Butte 7940'

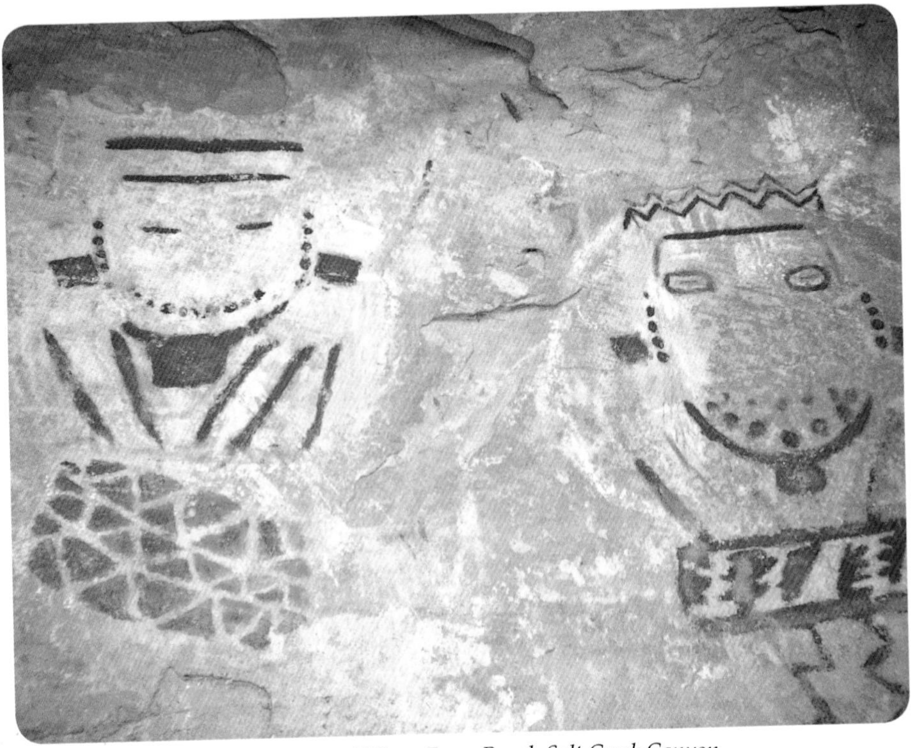

Two of the visages on the 700-year-old Four Faces Panel, Salt Creek Canyon

Big Pocket is not archaeologically rich, but it does harbor rock art and several ruins, including… (a) 260 yd (238 m) up-canyon (right / south), (b) 1.3 mi (2.1 km) up-canyon (right / south) in an east-facing alcove, and (c) 0.8 mi (1.3 km) northeast of the second ruin, in a south-facing alcove.

From Big Pocket, the main trail resumes north-northwest. Continually scan for ruins. At 6 mi (9.7 km), be alert for **Wedding Ring Arch** ahead (north). Though just right of the trail, it's easy to miss. Nearly as circular as the name suggests, it's about 200 ft (61 m) high and 150 ft (46 m) wide. A few minutes past it, a small, white-sandstone arch is visible ahead (right / north-northeast) near the rim.

At 7 mi (11.3 km) **Fisheye Arch** is visible on the right (east) rim. At 8.1 mi (13 km), nearly an hour from Big Pocket, the trail is near the canyon wall. Look right for a five-structure ruin in a small cave about 40 ft (64 m) above ground. Immediately beyond, at 8.2 mi (13.2 km), is one of the highlights of the journey: **All American Man**.

Resembling a red, white and blue baseball-shaped USA flag with legs, the ultrapatriotic man is about 6 ft (1.8 m) tall. The pictograph is in a small, dark cave, right of the trail, about 20 ft (6 m) above ground. Clamber up to see it clearly. But remember: touching rock art destroys it without deepening your appreciation.

The main trail then ascends about 150 ft (46 m) through a crack in a sandstone fin. It then resumes down-canyon, generally northwest, through dense willows.

About 20 minutes beyond All American Man, reach a clear, flowing spring at 8.9 mi (14.3 km). Immediately before the spring, look right (east). About 200 ft (61 m) off the trail is another premier archaeological site: **the Four Faces**. This astonishing pictograph panel is perhaps 700 years old. Below it is a ruin comprising several structures.

After crossing to the canyon's west side, the main trail resumes northwest. Within six minutes, at 9.1 mi (14.7 km), a left spur quickly accesses **campsite SC 3**.

Ahead, the main trail meanders to follow the canyon's gyrations but continues generally northwest. About fifteen minutes past SC 3, skirt left (west) of **Upper Jump**, a small waterfall at 9.7 mi (15.6 km), 5600 ft (1707 m).

The canyon soon narrows, deepening to 500 ft (152 m). Tall, dense, riparian vegetation becomes an obstacle. About ten minutes past Upper Jump, where you rise from the wash, look for a huge pictograph panel beneath an overhang.

From the panel, go right (east), around the bulging wall. On its other side, the trail veers left (west-southwest), on a bench, left (south) of the wash. Reach two deeply eroded gorges. The trail evades the first and drops into the second. It continues left of the main wash, not in it.

Curving (right) northeast, skirt another promontory. The bench diminishes, the canyon bends left (west) again, and you're forced back into the wash. After meandering generally north, the trail exits the willows, and rises to a bench right (northeast) of the wash.

Heading west now, it passes an accessible ruin comprising more than 15 structures. It's beneath bulbous cliffs, under a shallow overhang, on a south-facing, 150-yd (137-m) long ledge. Look for a pictograph of hand-holding figures at the far left (west) end of the site.

The canyon then curves from southwest to east, passing the mouth of **West Fork Salt Creek** (left / south) at 12.1 mi (19.5 km), 5500 ft (1676 m). A few minutes farther, reach **campsite SC 4** (right / south) on a bench, beneath cottonwoods, at 12.4 mi (20 km).

Continuing down-canyon from SC 4, northward progress is via circuitous meanders. Within 15 minutes look left (north-northwest) for a five-structure ruin beneath a blocky overhang with a nearly solid swath of black desert varnish on its right side. A few minutes farther, a spacious slickrock slab sloping into the creek invites you to stop and rest.

At about 14.5 mi (23.3 km), proceed along a **former 4WD road**. Unused for many years, it's initially faint. Farther down-canyon it becomes apparent but is not obtrusive. The road continues all the way north past Peekaboo camp to Cave Spring, near Hwy 211. Today, 4WD vehicles are allowed up-canyon only to Peekaboo, where you'll be departing Salt Creek Canyon.

Pass large, shallow pools in the broad creekbed just before reaching a junction at 15 mi (24.2 km), 5370 ft (1637 m). Right (southeast) is **Angel Arch Canyon**. Straight (north) 110 yd (100 m) down the main canyon is **Angel Arch camp** (right / east), on a flat, grassy clearing among cottonwoods.

Two ruins are visible within a couple minutes of the confluence of Salt Creek and Angel Arch canyons: (a) west, across Salt Creek, in a south-facing alcove, and (b) east, in the north wall of Angel Arch Canyon.

Detour to the impressive arch—the largest in Canyonlands National Park—by turning right (east) onto the former 4WD road entering Angel Arch Canyon. Follow it generally southeast about 35 minutes to road's end at 1.3 mi (2.1 km), 5500 ft (1676 m). A trail then leads right (south) 0.3 mi (0.5 km) to a viewpoint beneath the east side of **Angel Arch**. A cairned slickrock route continues 0.4 mi (0.6 km) to the base of the arch at 5950 ft (1814 m).

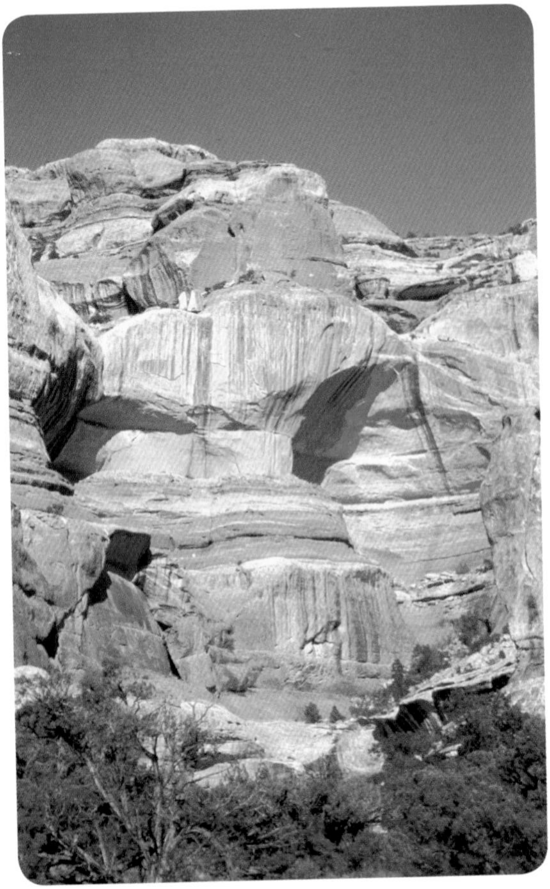
Angel Canyon

Resuming north in Salt Creek Canyon from Angel Arch camp, within 30 minutes Crescent Arch is visible high on the right (east) wall. Ahead, scan for other, small, unnamed arches and minor ruins.

At 19 mi (30.6 km), about two hours north of Angel Arch camp, pass **Five Fingers Canyon**, a major tributary drainage (left / west). It leads generally southwest. A boot-beaten path enters the mouth. Slickrock slabs to the right are a tempting place to rest. The namesake fingers at the end of the canyon warrant a full day of exploration. For a one-hour round-trip preview, hike 15 minutes to the first tributary (right / west), then continue left (south) another 15 minutes up the main channel to a great, overhanging wall where the ancient ones pecked a long string of dots.

From the mouth of Five Fingers, proceed north in Salt Creek Canyon. At 22.4 mi (36.1 km) the canyon bends right (southeast) to wrap around a protruding fin. At the base of the fin is a window. Turn left, depart the wash, and hike northeast through that window to reach **Peekaboo camp** on the other side of the fin, at 22.5 mi (36.2 km), 5020 ft (1530 m).

Though it's possible to conclude this trip by following the road in Salt Creek wash generally north 3.5 mi (5.6 km) to Cave Spring, it's an anticlimactic slog. Instead, follow the cairned Peekaboo trail (Trip 66) 5 mi (8.1 km) generally northwest to Squaw Flat.

To pick up the Peekaboo trail, do not drop from the window to Peekaboo camp on the northeast side of the fin. Stay above the wash. Bear left. Follow the path paralleling the wall. Pass an impressive **rock-art panel** bearing Fremont shield-figure petroglyphs and handprint pictographs.

Ahead on the left is a joint where a 15-ft (4.6-m) **ladder** facilitates a sheer, 20-ft (6-m) ascent. Reach slickrock above. Proceed beneath a shallow, 10-ft (3-m) high overhang. Pass low trees. Follow the cairns. You're now atop an arm jutting into Salt Creek Canyon. Your destination, Squaw Flat trailhead, is about 2½ hours distant.

Ascend along the center of the **slickrock arm**. Contour around the head of a drainage to the Peekaboo trail's namesake **window**, at 5360 ft (1634 m). Actually a hole in a fin, the window is just big enough for an adult to scrunch through. On the other side, contour left (south-southwest).

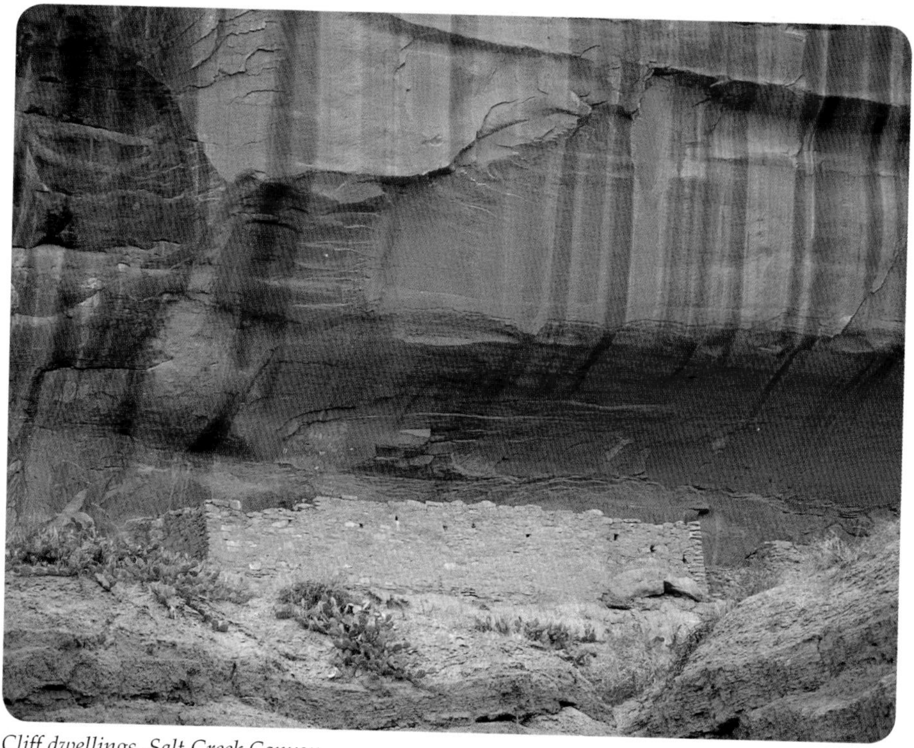

Cliff dwellings, Salt Creek Canyon

Ahead, the route briefly traverses a **very steep slope** to curve around the head of a slickrock drainage. The sharply angled section is short—just a few yards (meters)—but requires careful friction walking.

Ascend a chute. Go north through a 15-ft (4.6-m) wide **gap**. Continue following cairns. North and South Six-shooter peaks are visible east-northeast. Cross a **saddle** between knobs. Contour north-northwest on red slickrock. Cross a minor saddle. Wooden Shoe Arch is visible northeast.

From yellow slickrock, descend over boulders. Go west-northwest across a wash. Reach a **junction** at 24.9 mi (40.1 km), 5060 ft (1542 m), about one hour from Peekaboo camp. Left (south) enters sandy Lost Canyon. Proceed straight (west) across **sage flats**, curving right (west-northwest).

After following the trail among cottonwoods and P-J, rise from a sandy wash onto white-and-tan slickrock. Arrive at a **ladder** granting passage to the ledge above. Following cairns—north, curving west—ascend from black slickrock, to yellow, to white, to red. Top out at 5240 ft (1598 m).

Descend northwest. Proceed among gambel oaks. Reach a **junction** at 26.4 mi (42.5 km). Left (south) probes Squaw Canyon (Trip 65). Go straight, soon curving right (north).

Traverse a small slickrock **bluff**. After a sandy stretch, ascend over another, similar **bluff**. Just beyond, reach a junction. Left (southwest) leads to Big Spring Canyon (Trip 65) and Druid Arch (Trip 70). Go right (north).

Two minutes farther, reach the paved, **Squaw Flat trailhead** parking lot, near the toilets, at 27.5 mi (44.3 km), 5180 ft (1580 m).

TRIP 72

DARK CANYON

LOCATION	Glen Canyon National Recreation Area, Dark Canyon ISA Complex, south of Cataract Canyon and east of Hite Marina (Lake Powell)
ROUND TRIP	8 mi (12.9 km) or more
ELEVATION GAIN	1600-ft (488-m) loss and gain, or more
KEY ELEVATIONS	trailhead 5600 ft (1707 m), canyon rim 5280 ft (1609 m) canyon floor 4000 ft (1219 m)
HIKING TIME	8- to 9-hour dayhike, or two-night backpack trip
DIFFICULTY	challenging
MAPS	Trails Illustrated *Canyonlands National Park: Maze & NE Glen Canyon*, USGS *Indian Head Pass, Bowdie Canyon West*

OPINION

The difference between ascending a mountain and probing a canyon is the difference between the ego and the id.

Attaining a summit is celebratory. "Wahoo!" you say, "We made it!" Standing in the recesses of a canyon is meditative. "Whoa" you whisper, "This is cool."

The experience mirrors the topography, of course. Mountains are the earth's extroverts. Canyons are their opposite, the introverts.

Nowhere in canyon country, not even at the Grand Canyon, is this more evident than at the rim of Dark Canyon.

Hiking the Sundance trail, you anticipate the revelatory moment ahead. Yet you're startled when it arrives. Your breath falters. Aghast, you stare into the incredible depths.

When the shock subsides, you realize this great abyss isn't shaking its clenched fist in the air, defying the heavens, daring you to challenge it. Here, the earth is open, silent, submissive, patiently awaiting your entry.

Mountains talk, canyons listen.

Dark Canyon will grant you an audience after you've walked a mere one hour from the trailhead. Even if that's all you have time for, do it. The Sundance trail—actually a cairned route, largely on slickrock—is intriguing yet easy as far as the awesome vantage point on the canyon rim.

Reaching the inner sanctum, however, requires commitment. The descent is long, steep, rough, arduous. You'll be jousting with unstable rocks the whole way. Trekking poles are required safety equipment here.

Carrying only a daypack makes this a significantly easier hike. Start early, push the pace, and you *can* adequately sample Dark Canyon in a long day. Carrying a full backpack is a troublesome burden on the demanding ascent and descent, but to fully commune with the canyon you must sleep in its embrace. If that's you're intent, camp at least two nights. Otherwise you'll see nearly as much on an epic dayhike.

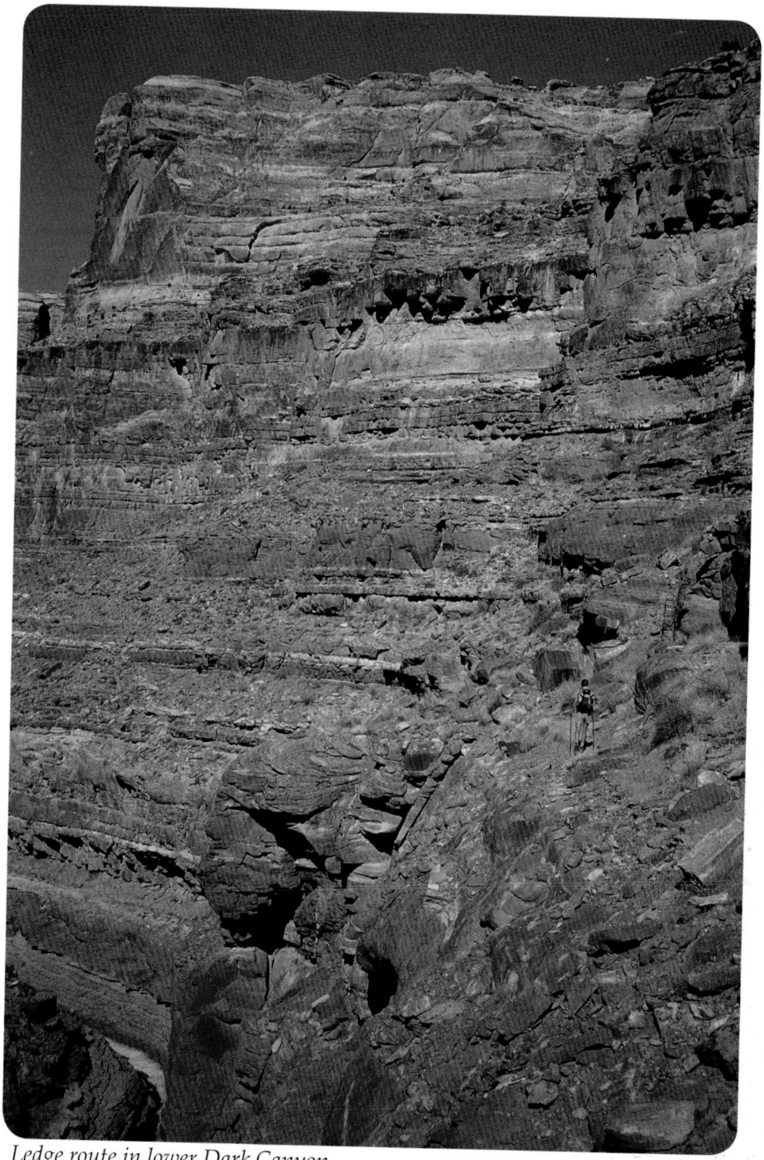

Ledge route in lower Dark Canyon

Say you're backpacking, and you've pitched your tent on a ledge above the perennial creek in Dark Canyon. On your first afternoon, wander downstream past Lean-To Canyon. Spend your second day exploring upstream past Lost Canyon to the mouth of Youngs Canyon.

If you're dayhiking, we recommend you continue downstream in Dark Canyon. Beyond Lean-To, the canyon floor becomes impassable, shunting you onto an exciting, airy ledge route where you can appreciate the canyon's immensity: average depth 1400 ft (427 m), average width 0.5 mi (0.8 km). In this direction you'll also soon encounter several huge pools where, on a hot day, you can reward yourself with a refreshing plunge.

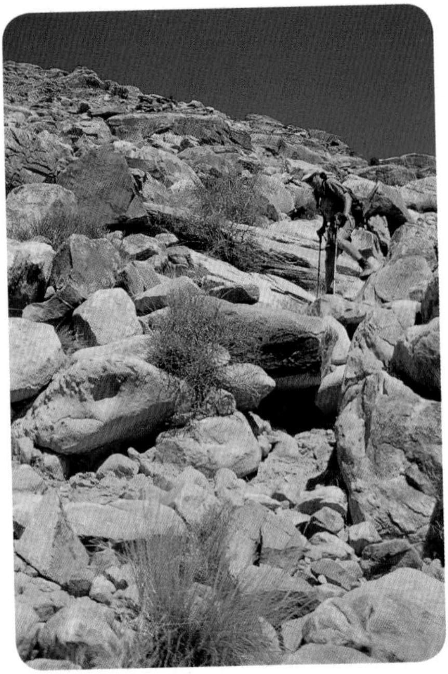

Sundance trail descends into Dark Canyon.

FACT

BY VEHICLE

When dry, the unpaved access road should be passable in a 2WD car, though high clearance is preferable. En route to the trailhead are numerous possible campsites: random, primitive, no fee.

From Hanksville, at the junction of Hwys 95 and 24, drive Hwy 95 south 26 mi (42 km) to the junction with Hwy 276 (access to Bullfrog). Set your trip odometer to 0 and continue southeast on Hwy 95. At 18.8 mi (30.3 km) cross the Dirty Devil River bridge. At 21 mi (33.8 km) cross the Colorado River bridge. At 22.3 mi (35.9 km) pass the entry to Hite Marina (right / west) and slow down. At 22.5 mi (36.2 km), near milepost 49, turn left (northeast) onto unpaved San Juan County Road 208A—Horse Tanks.

From the junction of Hwys 95 and 276 near Natural Bridges National Monument, drive Hwy 95 northwest. At 12 mi (19.3 km) pass Fry Canyon. Slow down after passing the Glen Canyon NRA sign. At 34.6 mi (55.8 km), near milepost 49, turn right (northeast) onto unpaved San Juan County Road 208A—Horse Tanks.

0 mi (0 km)
Departing Hwy 95, heading northeast.

0.25 mi (0.4 km)
Proceed straight, ignoring the fork ascending right.

4 mi (6.4 km)
Proceed straight (southeast) where a road forks right (west).

4.4 mi (7.1 km)
Continue straight on the main road.

6.6 mi (10.6 km)
Bear left, ignoring the fainter right fork.

7.3 mi (11.7 km)
Go right where a road forks left. Just ahead, cross a broad, gentle wash.

7.6 mi (12.3 km)
Turn left.

8.5 mi (13.7 km)
Stay left (northeast), ignoring the right (east-southeast) fork.

9.2 mi (14.8 km)
Continue straight where a rougher road forks left.

10.9 mi (17.5 km)
Turn left at the cairns, or park near here if the final approach appears too rough.

11.1 mi (17.9 km)
Reach the trailhead parking area, at 5600 ft (1707 m).

ON FOOT

Behind the trail register, cross the earthen dam of a stock pond. Look for the first cairn. Heading generally north-northeast, follow subsequent cairns on slickrock and sections of bootbeaten path through P-J (piñon and juniper) forest. The Henry Mtns are visible left (west).

About 30 minutes along, intersect a **sandy road**. Go left 22 paces, then resume right (east) on the cairned path. Ahead, the route proceeds north, then gradually curves right (east) and skirts the head of a tributary drainage. The way forward—either cairned or bootbeaten—remains evident. Negotiate terraces, ledges, short pouroffs, and easy friction pitches. Attain glimpses of Dark Canyon.

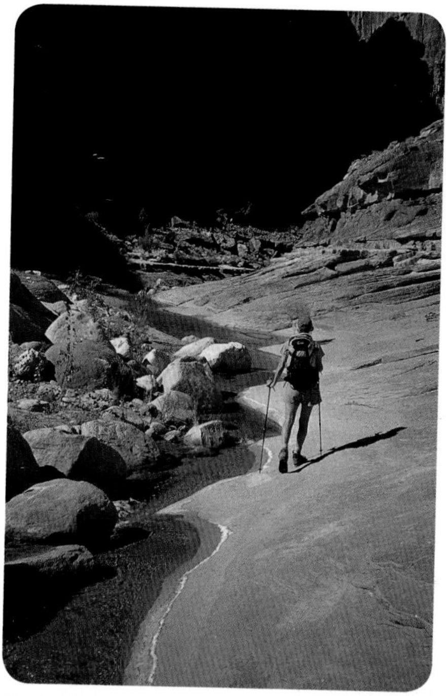

Dark Canyon

Nearly an hour from the trailhead, arrive at a startling viewpoint. The heart of Dark Canyon is visible southeast. Five minutes farther, reach the **canyon rim** at 2.2 mi (3.5 km), 5280 ft (1609 m), atop a point jutting into the void. Take a break here. Sit. Admire the scenery. Steel yourself before plummeting generally south-southeast into the abyss via the **steep rubble slope** that drops sharply from the rim.

Initially descend left of the point, through a draw, among P-J and boulders. Then curve right and drop through talus. Stay focused, move cautiously, follow the cairns. Where paths diverge, go whichever way appears most accommodating. Just 20 minutes below the rim, the route is more clearly defined.

Bottom-out in a **tributary drainage** at 3 mi (4.8 km), 4160 ft (1268 m). Strong, experienced hikers will arrive here about 40 minutes after departing the rim. Others might take a full hour to complete the descent.

Go left (east), down the rocky, brushy drainage, gradually curving left (northeast). At 3.4 mi (5.5 mi), 4000 ft (1219 m), intersect **Dark Canyon** on a bench above the perennial creek.

If dayhiking, explore upstream or down from where you first intersect Dark Canyon. Both options are rewarding.

If backpacking, follow the creek upstream (right / southeast). Before reaching **Lost Canyon** (right / south-southwest) at 4.2 mi (6.8 km), you'll cross the stream repeatedly and pass several viable campsites on low benches. Most are shadeless. A few are near sheltering cottonwoods.

Upstream from Lost Canyon, Dark Canyon constricts. The route follows limestone ledges above the wash until **Youngs Canyon** (left / northeast) at 10.2 mi (16.4 km). Between Lost and Youngs, the creek flows over blue-grey limestone speckled with intrusions of red chert. Occasionally visible above that is another layer of limestone rife with marine fossils. Youngs Canyon bears a perennial stream and has a cascade at its mouth. Water is scarce in Dark Canyon beyond 11.2 mi (18 km).

Downstream from where you first intersect Dark Canyon, curve right (east) to reach the mouth of **Lean-To Canyon** (right / east) at 3.6 mi (5.8 km). From Lean-To, Dark Canyon trends north-northwest, reaching Lake Powell (depending on the fluctuating water level) at about 9.6 mi (15.5 km), 3600 ft (1097 m). Shortly beyond is where the Colorado River flows through Cataract Canyon into the lake.

The first half hour past Lean-To Canyon necessitates a few stream crossings but is relatively easy, along the canyon floor. Upon reaching a series of pouroffs, ascend ledges on the right (east-northeast) wall. The **ledge route** affords secure footing but is narrow, awkwardly overhung in places, eventually contours 150 ft (46 m) above the canyon floor, and will give acrophobes an unnerving sense of exposure.

Within two hours of Lean-To, the route finally drops to the mouth of the **first tributary drainage** (right / east). This is a logical turnaround point unless you're intent on dipping your toe in either **Lake Powell** or the **Colorado River**. If the lake is high, it will be impossible to hike all the way to the river. If the lake is low, you'll encounter mud flats well before arriving at the river.

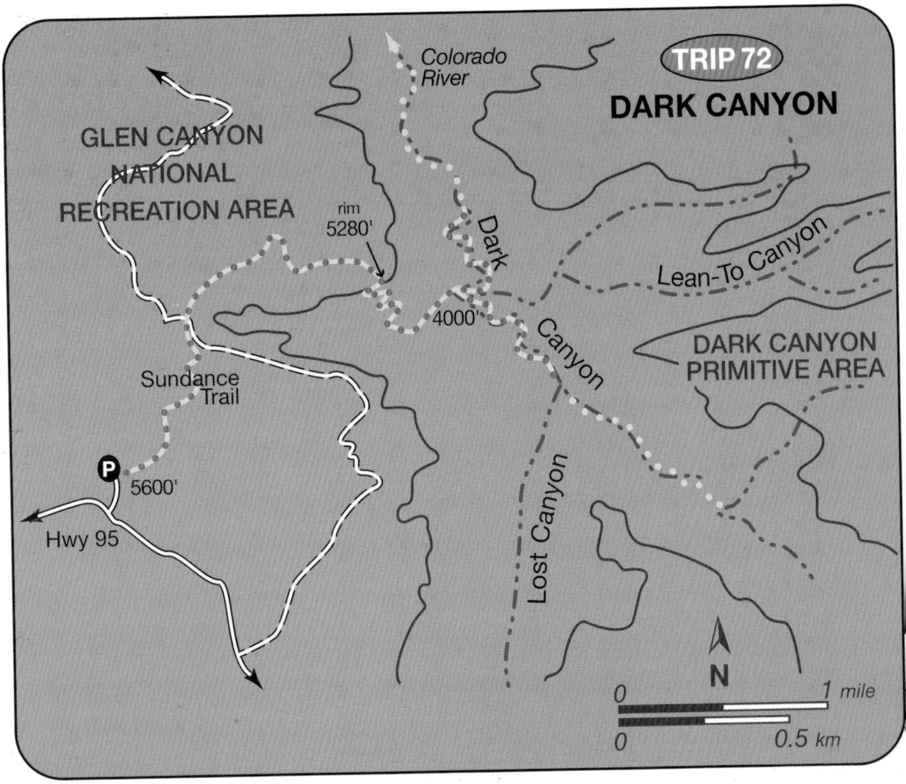

TRIP 73

SANDTHRAX SLICKROCK

LOCATION	North Wash, northwest of Lake Powell
ROUND TRIP	3 mi (4.8 km)
ELEVATION GAIN	520 ft (159 m)
KEY ELEVATIONS	trailhead 4450 ft (1356 m), saddle 4970 ft (1515 m)
HIKING TIME	1¼ to 3 hours
DIFFICULTY	moderate
MAP	Trails Illustrated *Glen Canyon, Lake Powell & Capitol Reef* USGS *Turkey Knob*

OPINION

There are 45 muscles in the human face. Most have only one purpose: to express nuances of emotion. Give them all a vigorous workout. Go hiking on a great expanse of slickrock.

We call it *slickwalking*. It inspires a rapturous sense of freedom. With no vegetation to shunt you this way or that, you can follow your bliss. The rock's gritty surface ("slick" is actually a misnomer) grants extraordinary traction, enabling you to negotiate steep pitches with gravity-defying impudence. And the colorful, sensuous, monolithic terrain underfoot, coupled with the constant, unhindered views, make it a beautiful experience.

The name of this slickwalk is one we've given it because our suggested route ascends above the northwest rim of Sandthrax Canyon—a dangerously technical slot. Nearby are the three Irish Canyons, which are popular, technical slots. Hikers can probe Blarney, Shillelagh and Leprechaun canyons about 0.5 mile (0.8 km) before climbing equipment, skill and experience are necessary. If you're a hiker, however, not a climber, we recommend cruising over the domes high above Sandthrax.

There's no trail up there. You won't find cairns, nor should you build any. This is improv hiking. Our suggested destination—a panoramic vantage on the crest of the sandstone reef—is but one possibility. Ignore our *On Foot* directions altogether if you like. Once you're on the rock, just go: up, around, over, wherever. On slickrock, the joy is in the approach, not the arrival. Further intrigue awaits around every sensuous curve.

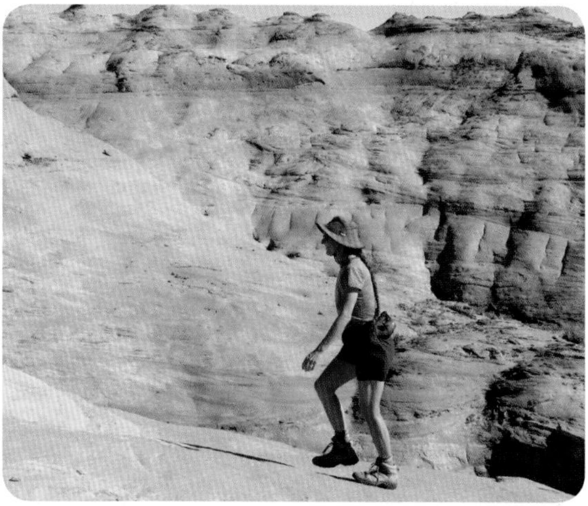

Sandthrax slickrock

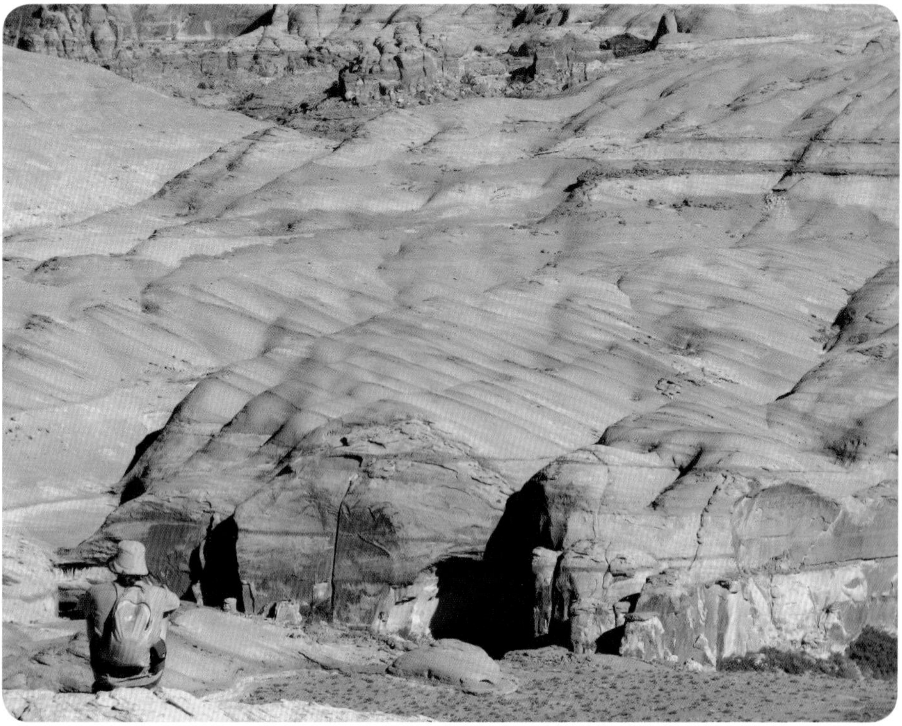

Overlooking North Fork Butler Canyon

If you're new to slickwalking, be sure you can descend whatever you ascend, because steep terrain is always more challenging on the way down. Frequently look back and remember what you see, so you can easily retrace your steps. Stay within your comfort zone. If you're deeply hesitant, trust your instinct: find another way forward, or turn back.

Though it's possible to follow our suggested round trip in 1¼ hours, allow more. Give your face muscles the full drill: surprise, wonder, excitement, enthusiasm, happiness, humor, disbelief, and fascination.

FACT

BY VEHICLE

From Hanksville, drive Hwy 95 south 26 mi (42 km) to the junction with Hwy 276. Reset your trip odometer to 0, bear left on Hwy 95, and proceed east-southeast. At 1.2 mi (2 km) the sandstone walls on both sides of North Wash rise steeply. At 2.2 mi (3.5 km) turn left (east) onto the unpaved spur paralleling the highway.

From Lake Powell, just north of the Hite Marina turnoff, set your trip odometer to 0 in the middle of the bridge spanning the Colorado River. Drive Hwy 95 northwest. Soon cross the bridge over the Dirty Devil River. After

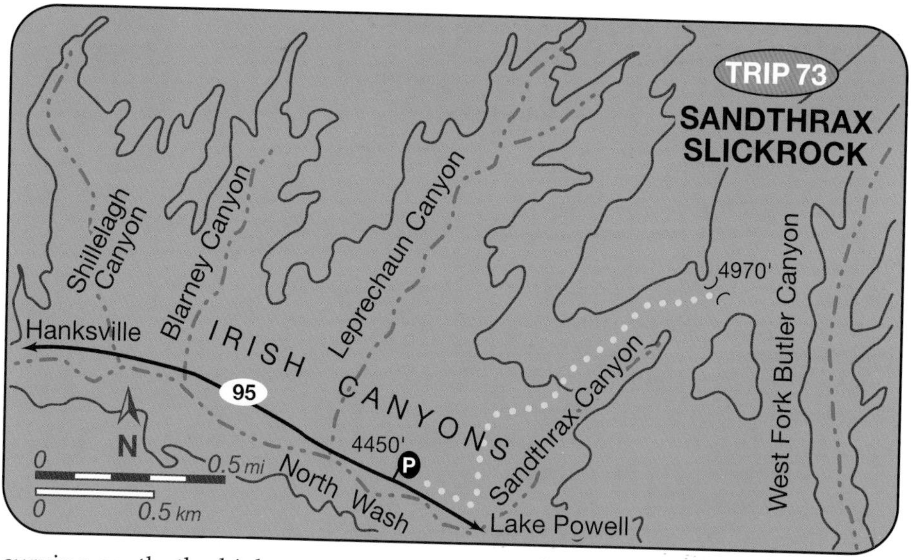

curving south, the highway again turns northwest and enters North Wash. At 14 mi (22.6 km), near milepost 29, pass Hog Springs rest area (left / southwest). At 18.9 mi (30.5 km) turn right (east) onto the unpaved spur.

From either approach, bear right at the Irish Canyons trailhead sign. Follow the sandy spur east-southeast, paralleling the highway. Before the sand deepens, park among the cottonwoods at 4450 ft (1356 m).

ON FOOT

Follow the sandy spur east-southeast about 220 ft (200 m). Observe the sandstone to your left. You're looking for an easy place to mount it. Just past a small bay is a low **finger of pink sandstone**. Clamber onto it. Follow the crest of the finger left (northwest). Soon curve right (east).

Continue working your way northeast. With variations to find the easiest way onward and upward, this will remain your general direction of travel all the way to a 4970-ft (1515-m) **saddle** on the crest of the sandstone reef, about 1.5 mi (2.4 km) from your vehicle.

The pass itself is white stone. The higher, rounded stone on both sides is pink. The gorge immediately below the far (east) side of the saddle is the left (west) fork of Butler Canyon. The vast slickrock wilderness beyond is an engaging sight.

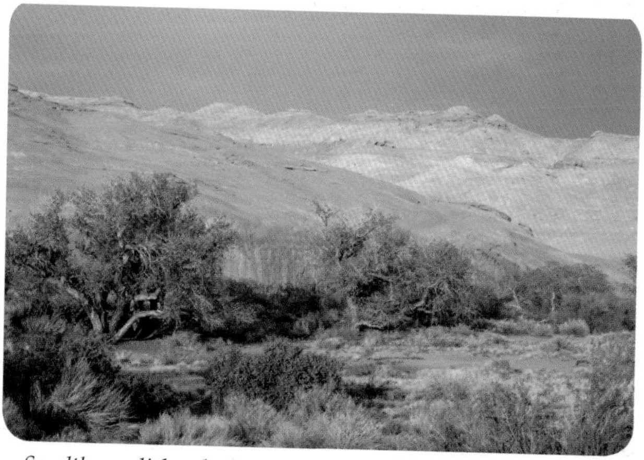

Sandthrax slickrock ascent route

CEDAR MESA

OPINION

Like fracture lines writhing across bone after a traumatic impact, the canyons of Cedar Mesa veer in every direction. The place is cracked open. Shot full of fissures.

Among them are Mule, Slickhorn, Road, Lime, Fish, Owl, and Bullet canyons. The longest, of course, is Grand Gulch. Within each are countless south-facing walls with sheltering, sun-baked alcoves. That's what drew the original inhabitants: abundant accommodation.

If ghosts exist, you'll be bumping into them constantly on Cedar Mesa. The Ancestral Puebloans were remarkably successful at wresting a living from this harsh land. They thrived here. And evidence of their tenure is more prevalent than most hikers have the patience and skill to recognize. Yet every hiker who visits Cedar Mesa is soon aware they've entered a venerable outdoor museum where the number and quality of relics within dayhiking range is astonishing.

Where no pictograph, petroglyph, granary, kiva or cliffhouse is visible, the canyons themselves—deep, narrow, colorful, convoluted—keep hikers entranced. So perhaps it's wrong to assume the ancient ones were survivalists who settled here only because it was practical to do so. Theirs was obviously a culture that valued art. Maybe what they appreciated most was Cedar Mesa's pervasive, voluptuous beauty.

Even if they didn't, you should. Make artistic appreciation the essence of your Cedar Mesa experience. With an open mind, the bare walls of this gallery can be more compelling than anything adorning the halls of the Louvre.

FACT

BEFORE YOUR TRIP

It's wise to restock your provisions, fill your vehicle's gas tank, and top-up all your water containers before driving to Cedar Mesa. There are no convenient grocery stores or gas stations, and Kane Gulch Ranger Station has no public water supply. The nearest towns are Hanksville, Blanding, Bluff, and Mexican Hat.

Backcountry permits are required in the following Cedar Mesa canyons: Mule (north and south forks), Grand Gulch, Fish, Owl, Slickhorn (all forks), Road, and Lime.

A day-use permit costs $2 per person, per day. A seven-consecutive-day pass costs $5 per person. An overnight permit costs $8 per person, per trip. Pay for and obtain your day-use permit at the iron rangers located near the trailheads.

Reserve your overnight permit up to 90 days in advance by phoning the BLM Field Office in Monticello: (435) 587-1500. Obtain your permit in person, the morning your trip begins, at the Kane Gulch Ranger Station. It's open daily, 8 a.m. to noon.

Visit www.blm.gov/ut/st/en/fo/monticello/recreation/grand_gulch_and_cedar.3.html for complete details regarding Cedar Mesa backcountry permits.

Car camping (primitive, random) is possible along the Cedar Mesa trailhead access roads. Follow Leave No Trace principles. The nearest, official, front-country campground is at Natural Bridges National Monument (Trip 76).

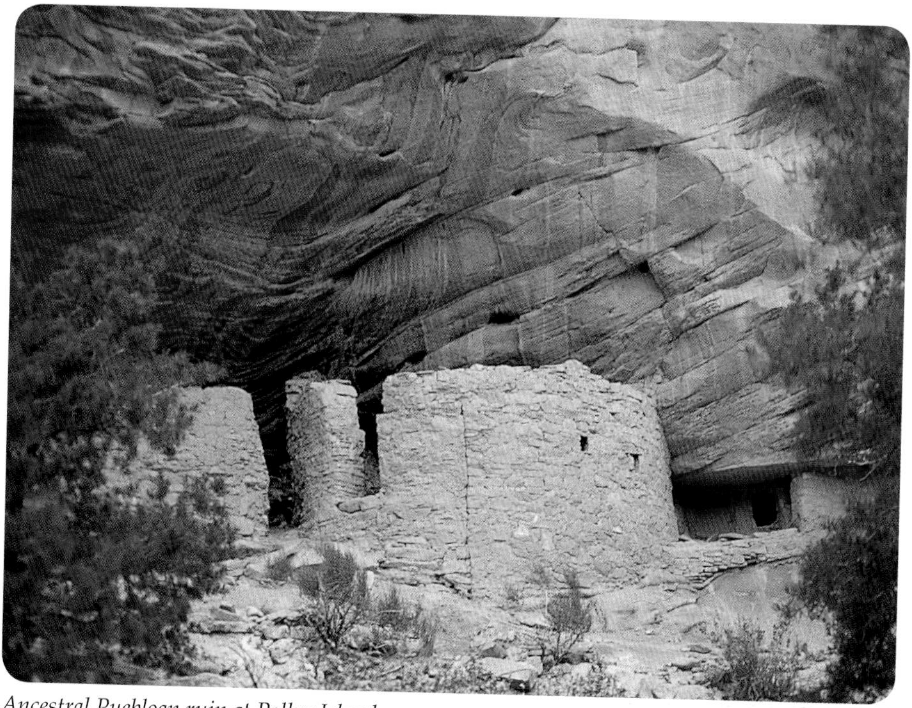

Ancestral Puebloan ruin at Pollys Island

You're dayhiking? Carry a full day's water: at least three quarts (liters) per person. It will save you from searching for scarce, unreliable water sources and will prevent you from having to spend time filtering or purifying.

You're backpacking? You'll have to find water sources en route, you should top-up your supply at every opportunity, and you'll need to filter or purify whatever you consume. Ask at the Kane Gulch Ranger Station how much water to expect en route and where you'll likely find it. Carry a couple extra water bottles, or a large-but-lightweight collapsible water jug, so you can haul water from its source to your camp.

BY VEHICLE

The unpaved roads accessing Cedar Mesa trailheads off Hwy 261 should, when dry, be passable in a 2WD car. High clearance is preferable, however, and 4WD is ideal.

From Hanksville drive Hwy 95 south, gradually curving southeast. Cross the northeast arm of Lake Powell, near Hite Marina. From the junction with Hwy 275 (Natural Bridges National Park), proceed east on Hwy 95. Just 1.8 mi (2.9 km) farther, turn right (south) onto Hwy 261.

From Hwy 191, just south of Blanding, turn west onto Hwy 95 and reset your trip odometer to 0. At 28.5 mi (45.9 km) turn left (south) onto Hwy 261.

From either approach, drive south 3.8 mi (6.2 km) to Kane Gulch Ranger Station, on the left (east).

To reach the trailheads for Trips 74 through 84, follow the *By Vehicle* directions in each trip, starting at either the ranger station or the Hwy 261 junction, whichever is most convenient for you.

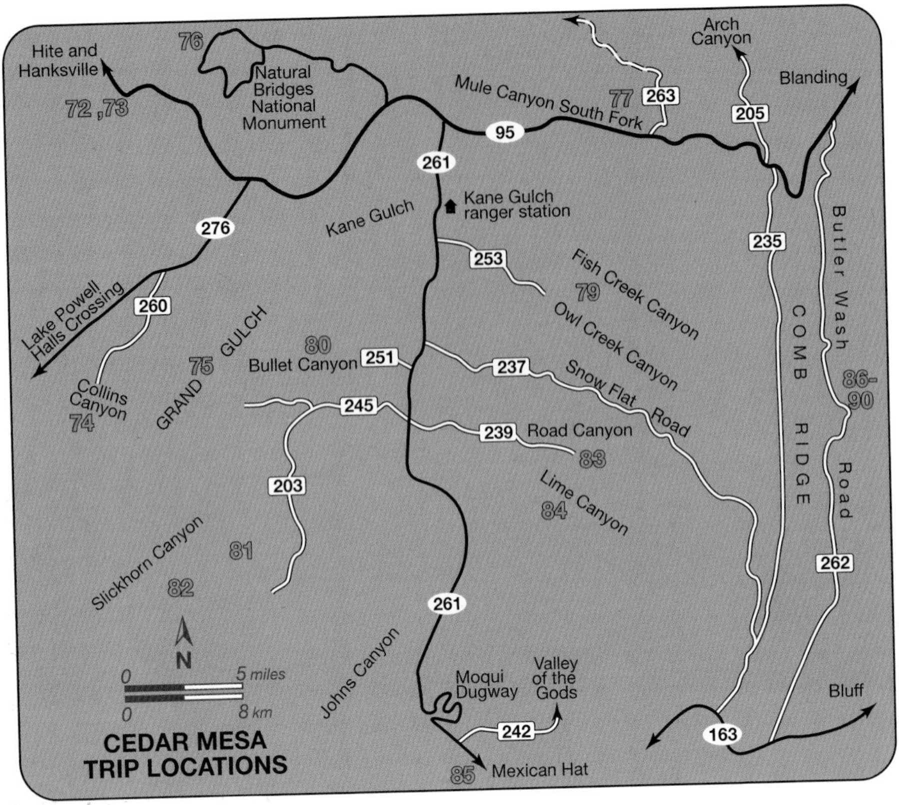

HISTORY

Richard Wetherill

Pothunter is a euphemism for *greedy bastard*. Specifically, the term refers to someone seeking ancient artifacts for personal gain, often illegally, while disregarding archaeological protocol.

Richard Wetherill, the first person to thoroughly investigate the remains of Ancestral Puebloan culture in Grand Gulch, is often called a pothunter. But if those who so casually toss him into the midden[1] of history knew more about him, they might be less harshly judgmental.

Born into a Quaker ranching family in 1858, Wetherill lived in Bluff, Utah, then Mancos, Colorado, near Mesa Verde. His honest relationship with the local Utes earned him permission to freely range the canyons, where his fascination with ruins and artifacts drew him to a career as explorer, guide, excavator, and trading post proprietor.

Wetherill is credited with the discovery of Cliff Palace, now within Mesa Verde National Park, and the discovery of Keet Seel, now within Navajo National Monument. He also initiated excavation of Pueblo Bonito, the largest prehistoric ruin in the U.S., now within Chaco Culture National Historical Park. He devoted his life to searching for the remains of the vanished culture known as the *Anasazi*[2]. He was the most dedicated and prolific archaeological explorer on the Colorado Plateau.

In the winter of 1894, Wetherill probed every ledge and alcove in Grand Gulch. He returned in the winter of 1897, which was much colder. One bitter, snowy night, worried about the mummies he'd found in a cave and that were now exposed at camp, Wetherill and his wife slept with them in their tent.

Today, archaeologists are rightly appalled at the damage done by Wetherill. He was initially unconcerned about site preservation. But archaeology was in its infancy. Wetherill was among its pioneers. He learned in the field, not in the classroom. He sold what he found, but much of it went to The American Museum of Natural History. Some was displayed at the St. Louis World's Fair.

Wetherill never became rich. His intense curiosity about Anasazi culture was a door to a more ardent life, but it was not a huge financial step beyond the hardscrabble ranch where he eked out a living with his extended family. He excavated first for his own edification, later for commercial ends. Soon he was working systematically, digging carefully with trowel and brush, taking meticulous notes, categorizing each artifact and describing where he found it in situ.

He appreciated stratigraphy (the study of layers within an archaeological site) before it was embraced by mainstream archaeology. As a result, he was the first to identify that Basketmaker culture was distinct from, and much older than, Anasazi culture.

The brutality of these people was another Wetherill discovery. He reported finding projectile points mingled with skeletal remains. It's now well documented that violent massacres including torture and mutilation were common in ancient times on the Colorado Plateau. But Wetherill was the first to arrive at this startling, chilling conclusion.

Wetherill's short life would make a gripping, epic movie right to the end: he was murdered in 1910 at the age of 52. To learn more about him, read *Richard Wetherill: Anasazi*, by Frank McNitt.

McNitt describes an intelligent, independent, stubborn iconoclast who cultivated humanistic relationships but whose very nature threatened others less talented or secure. The book persuasively argues that Wetherill's reputation was subverted by ambitious Eastern academics, envious of his discoveries, and government Indian agents, jealous of his influence among the Navajo.

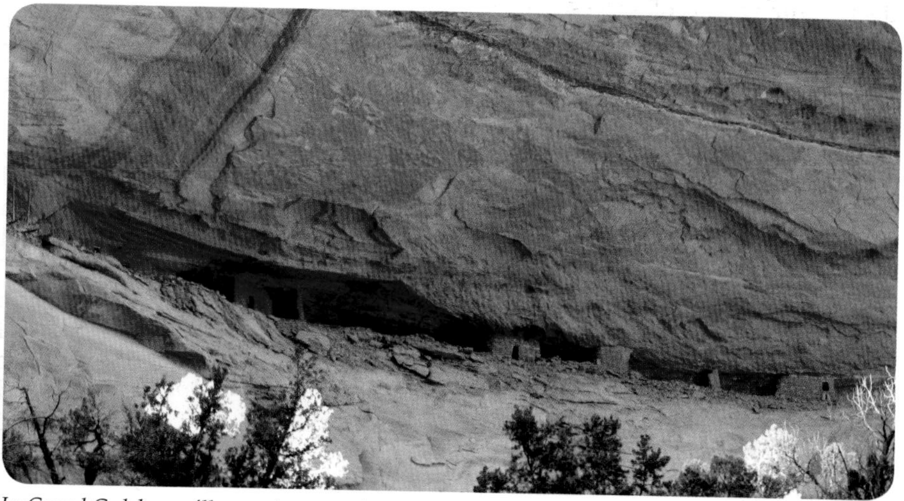

In Grand Gulch, you'll see ruins or rock art at least every 2 mi (3.2 km).

[1]A mound or deposit containing waste from daily human life. Middens below archaeological ruins in southern Utah were designated communal dumps that accumulated over generations and are thus invaluable sources of archaeological evidence. To set foot on a midden is to diminish its value to researchers.

[2]*Anasazi* is a Navajo word meaning *ancestral enemies*. In 1936 archaeologist Alfred Kidder began using it in reference to the prehistoric culture that thrived on the Colorado Plateau. The Hopi, however, object to the term. Instead, they call their ancestors *Hisatsinom*, which means *Old Ones*. Other tribes also object but each uses a different substitute word. In response, many archaeologists dropped *Anasazi* from their professional vocabulary and replaced it with the much broader *Ancestral Puebloans*. Others still prefer *Anasazi*, arguing that *puebloan*, a Spanish term meaning *inhabitant of a town*, is itself a misnomer. A few remain open to the possibility that *Anasazi* is historically accurate. Many old Navajo tales describe interaction with "ancient enemies." Some even describe watching these enemies abandon the Colorado Plateau. No archaeological evidence suggests the Navajo and Anasazi cultures actually overlapped, yet it's conceivable they did. So the debate continues, and both *Anasazi* and *Ancestral Puebloan* still appear in literature.

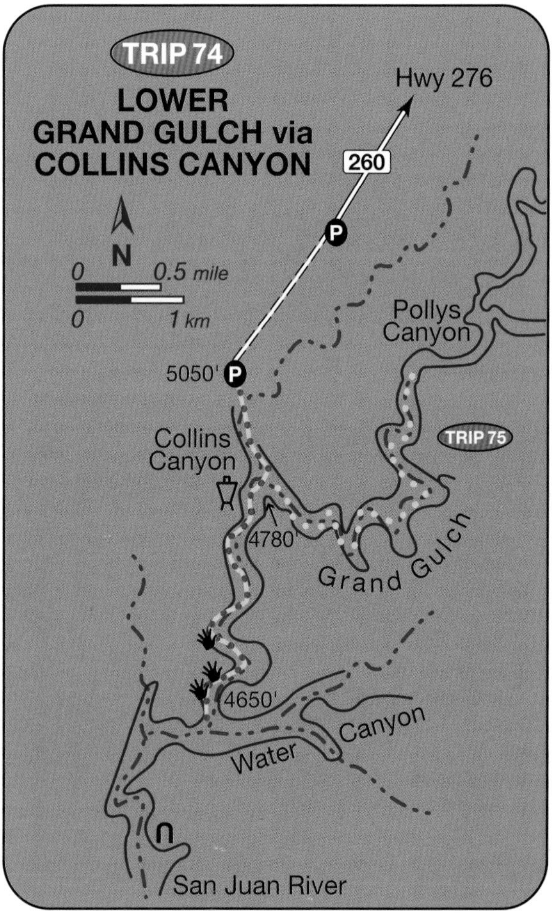

TRIP 74

LOWER GRAND GULCH via COLLINS CANYON

LOCATION	Cedar Mesa, Grand Gulch Primitive Area south of Hwy 276
ROUND TRIP	13.6 mi (22 km) to 4th pictograph panel
ELEVATION CHANGE	400-ft (122-m) loss and gain
KEY ELEVATIONS	trailhead 5050 ft (1540 m), confluence of Collins Canyon and Grand Gulch 4780 ft (1457 m) Water Canyon 4650 ft (1418 m)
HIKING TIME	6 to 8 hours
DIFFICULTY	easy
MAPS	Trails Illustrated *Grand Gulch Plateau* USGS *Red House Spring*

OPINION

Rock art is maddeningly difficult to decipher. But the ancient ones occasionally left what seems to be a lucent message.

They sipped pigment, held a hollow reed to their mouth, placed their other hand against stone, and spat, creating a handprint silhouette. Or they simply dipped a hand in colorful mud and pressed it on a canyon wall.

Surely what they were saying is "I am!"

It's a spontaneous surge of wonder at the miracle of life. A joyful burst of self recognition. An exuberant "thank you great spirit for manifesting in me." A plea to eternity not to forget "I was here."

They all did it. Men, women, children. Sometimes they did it en masse, as if shouting in one booming voice, "We are!"

Handprint pictographs and petroglyphs, more than any other form of rock art, enable us to feel the vitality of the former canyon residents. So you should certainly feel it when you witness the hundred hands panel in lower Grand Gulch.

It's a mere two-hour hike from Collins Spring trailhead. And within another hour you'll see two more significant panels. One is 100 ft (305 m) long. The other comprises more than 100 animals and anthropomorphs (square-shouldered human figures with triangular torsos and miniature arms and legs).

Collins Canyon affords easy access to the outdoor museum of lower Grand Gulch. Though you should first check at Kane Gulch Ranger Station, you'll likely find Collins Spring trailhead accessible when foul weather has rendered other Cedar Mesa roads impassable. And ranchers used to herd cattle off the mesa-top into Grand Gulch via Collins, which assures you the hiking poses no difficulty. You'll initially descend ledges dynamited out of the canyon wall: a bovine boulevard.

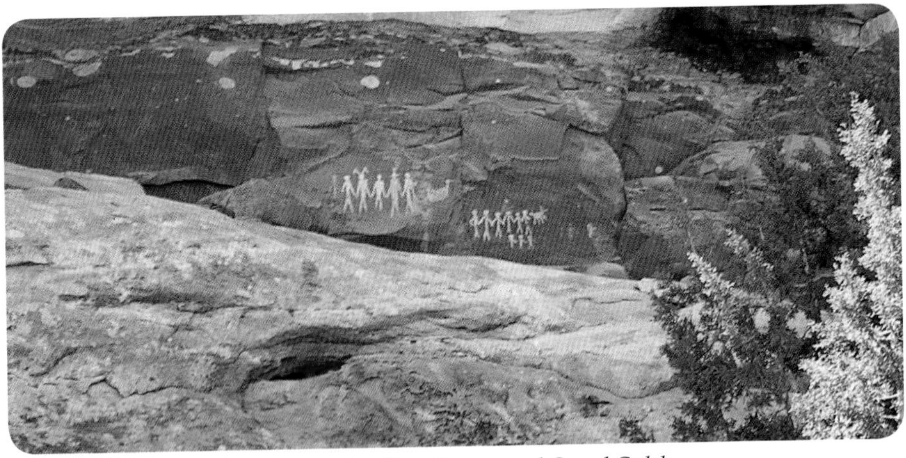

Family pictograph near confluence of Collins Canyon and Grand Gulch

FACT

BY VEHICLE

It's about a 40-minute drive to Collins Spring trailhead from Kane Gulch Ranger Station. Car camping is possible several places beside unpaved road 260, between Hwy 276 and the trailhead.

From the junction of Hwys 261 and 95, just north of Kane Gulch Ranger Station, drive Hwy 95 generally west 9.5 mi (15.3 km). Turn left onto Hwy 276 and proceed southwest 6.6 mi (10.6 mi). Turn left (east) onto unpaved road 260 signed for Collins Spring trailhead and reset your trip odometer to 0.

At 2.4 mi (3.9 km) proceed straight, ignoring the left spur. After 4.5 mi (7.2 km) the road crosses slickrock slabs. At 6 mi (9.7 km) the road is narrower and rougher. Reach Collins Spring trailhead parking area at 6.5 mi (10.5 km), 5050 ft (1540 m).

ON FOOT

The trail departs the south end of the parking area, near the trail register. It initially heads south, soon curves left (east), drops across slickrock, and switchbacks into Collins Canyon.

Descend along the left (northeast) side of the drainage. Within 15 minutes proceed through a gate. In the sandy wash, pass a **cowboy camp** beneath a west-facing alcove at 4800 ft (1463 m). Ahead, upon reaching slickrock again, bear right onto a trail and bypass a 40-ft (12-m) pouroff.

About 40 minutes along, pass a tributary drainage (left / north-northeast) at 4840 ft (1476 m). Curve right (southeast) to follow the trail onto a sandy bank.

At 2 mi (3.2 km), 4780 ft (1457 m), after hiking nearly an hour, reach the **confluence of Collins Canyon and Grand Gulch**. Pause here. Memorize what you see, so you'll know where to exit upon your return.

Left (northeast) leads up-canyon through Grand Gulch (Trip 75) 36 mi (58 km) to Kane Gulch Ranger Station. Just five minutes in that direction is a campsite where you could base yourself for your down-canyon excursion.

Turn right (south) to hike down-canyon through **lower Grand Gulch**. The San Juan River is 15.7 mi (25.3 km) ahead. In a couple minutes pass through a short **narrows**.

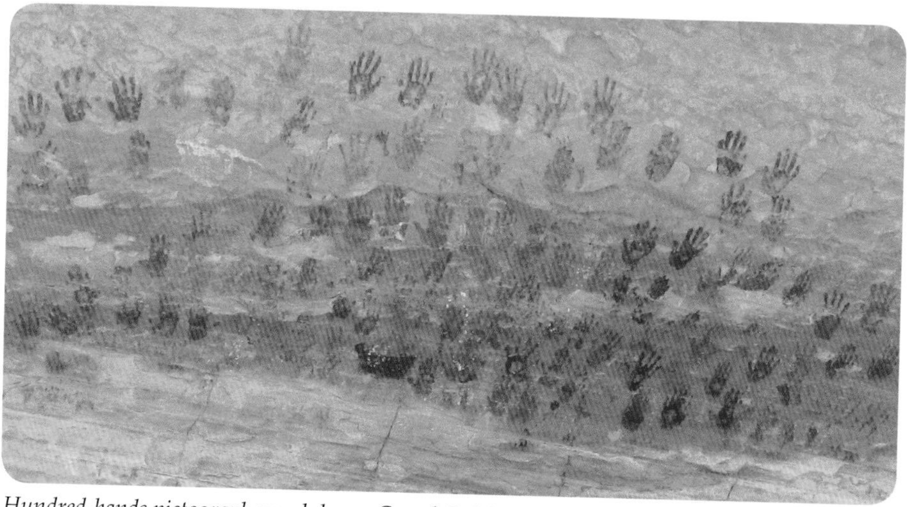

Hundred-hands pictograph panel, lower Grand Gulch

Immediately past a keyhole-shaped slot, detour right (south) up a steep, sandy trail about 50 yd/m to a shallow overhang. Here, about 2.3 mi (3.7 km) from the trailhead, is an impressive **pictograph panel** featuring a family holding hands. It's on pink-brown rock, left of a broad, desert-varnish-streaked wall, between two juniper trees. A second panel and the remains of at least two structures are nearby.

About 40 minutes down-canyon from the confluence, the main wash swings 0.25 mi (0.4 km) east, then doubles back west. Beyond that curve, look for a **pictograph panel** featuring 100 handprints. It's on the right (north) wall, above a bench, in a prominent south-facing alcove. You've now hiked 3.5 mi (5.6 km) from the trailhead, in about one hour and 40 minutes.

Resuming down-canyon (west), curve left (south) in 0.3 mi (0.5 km). At 4.1 mi (6.6 km), bear right (south), ignoring a tributary drainage (left / east). After meandering farther west, curve left (south) again, ignoring another tributary drainage (right / north).

At 6.5 mi (10.5 km), 4820 ft (1470 m), look right (west) for a 100-ft (30.5-m) long **pictograph panel** featuring red, white, and green anthropomorphic figures.

Just five minutes farther down-canyon (south), about three hours from the trailhead, look up (right / west) at the base of a huge, slightly overhanging wall without desert varnish. A **pictograph panel** features 100 animals, snakes, ravens, and friendly, waving humanoids in grey, red, white, and yellow.

Another 15 minutes down-canyon will bring you to **Water Canyon** (left / east)—a multi-fingered tributary drainage at 7.6 mi (12.1 km), 4650 ft (1418 m). True to its name, running water is likely to be present near the confluence.

You've now hiked the stretch of lower Grand Gulch richest in rock art. So Water Canyon is a satisfactory turnaround point for a dayhiking excursion.

If you continue down-canyon, expect to reach **Shaw Arch** (left / east) in perhaps one hour and 15 minutes. The abutment walls feature red, green and yellow handprint pictographs, and nearby boulders bear several dozen petroglyphs.

TRIP 75

GRAND GULCH: COLLINS TO KANE

LOCATION	Cedar Mesa, Grand Gulch Primitive Area south of Hwy 276, west of Hwy 261
DISTANCE	38 mi (61.2 km) one way
ELEVATION CHANGE	270-ft (82-m) loss, 1660-ft (506-m) gain
KEY ELEVATIONS	Collins Canyon trailhead 5050 ft (1540 m), confluence of Collins Canyon and Grand Gulch 4780 ft (1457 m), Bannister Ruin 4854 ft (1480 m), Step Canyon 5240 ft (1598 m), Bullet Canyon 5340 ft (1628 m), Split Level Ruin 5860 ft (1787 m), Kane Gulch trailhead 6440 ft (1963 m)
HIKING TIME	3 to 5 days
DIFFICULTY	moderate
MAPS	Trails Illustrated *Grand Gulch Plateau*, USGS *Red House Spring, Pollys Pasture, Cedar Mesa North, Kane Gulch*

OPINION

Grand Gulch is big. It's 50 mi (81 km) long and drains about 1000 sq mi (1610 sq m).

Grand Gulch is deep. The walls rise 300 to 700 ft (91 to 213 m) above the canyon floor.

Grand Gulch is tortuous. It bends roughly every 200 to 600 yd (183 to 549 m).

Grand Gulch is remote. It's so far from any large city that the night sky is among the darkest and starriest in the U.S.

Grand Gulch is archaeologically rich. Around nearly every bend is a cave or sheltering cliff. Many face south. And most of those harbor Ancestral Puebloan rock art or ruins including granaries, dwellings, kivas, and burial sites.

Grand Gulch is sublimely beautiful. Hiking here is a master class in sculpture taught by the greatest artist of all: Erosion. Her work beggars the human imagination. Yes, *she*. Art this sensuous surely required a female touch.

While Grand Gulch has several entry and exit points affording numerous hiking options, the three- or four-night backpack trip described here—entering via Collins Canyon, exiting via Kane Gulch—is the supreme, one-way journey.

Supreme, however, does not preclude *arduous*. And what primarily makes Grand Gulch an arduous trek are lengthy, dense, unavoidable thickets of riparian vegetation that have colonized the canyon floor.

If you've never encountered tamarisk (also called *saltcedar*), you'll soon know it intimately and hate it vehemently. It's a water-hogging, hiker-vexing, non-native shrub as aggressively invasive as Genghis Khan's Mongol hordes. Each flower produces thousands of tiny seeds. Tamarisk quickly grows deep taproots, greedily sucks up water, and routs other, less combative vegetation by depositing salt on the surrounding soil.

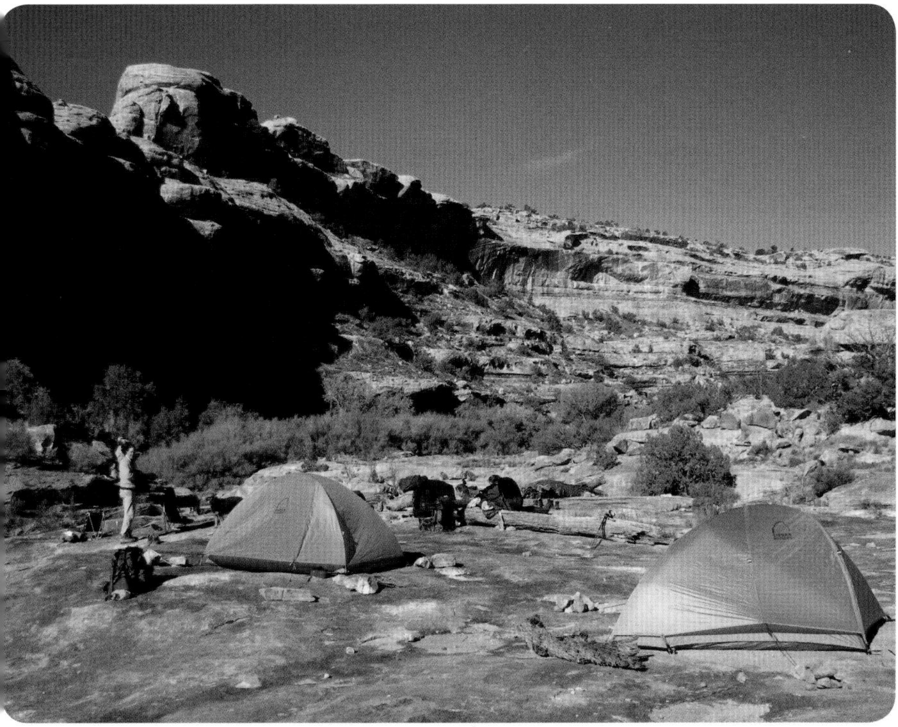

Grand Gulch, near Big Pouroff

Trail crews continue battling tamarisk in Grand Gulch, slashing hikeable tunnels through much of it. But the BLM lacks the funds to win this war. So you'll often have to hold your arms out like a cowcatcher, put your head down, and plow into it. Weeks after our last Grand Gulch trip, we were still finding tamarisk leaves in the crevices of our packs.

Occasionally, you *will* stride unhindered through Grand Gulch. Segments of the main channel are firm, dry gravel. Slickrock is easy and fun to walk on, and you'll find plenty here. In its upper reaches, the canyon widens, so you'll be shortcutting meanders via paths across benches. Just don't expect to keep your boots dry without great effort, because much of the main channel is wet. Pools, mud and quicksand are frequent obstacles.

As for camping in Grand Gulch, there are far more options than the few we've mentioned in our *On Foot* description. Many are excellent. In late spring and early fall—prime canyon-country hiking season—Grand Gulch is busy, and your competitors will snatch the most obvious, accessible campsites by early afternoon. To find an acceptable, Leave No Trace site, you might have to hike longer and be more creative than you'd prefer. The wickedly dominant tamarisk compounds this challenge, rarely granting enough bare, level ground for a single tent.

Four days (three nights) is the minimum time necessary for strong hikers to start at Collins Canyon, finish at Kane Gulch Ranger Station, and appreciate the scenic wonders and cultural treasures en route. Bannister Ruin, Big Man Panel, Jailhouse Ruin, Perfect Kiva, Green Mask pictograph, Split Level Ruin, Turkey Pen Ruin, and Junction Ruin are but a few of the celebrated archaeological sites.

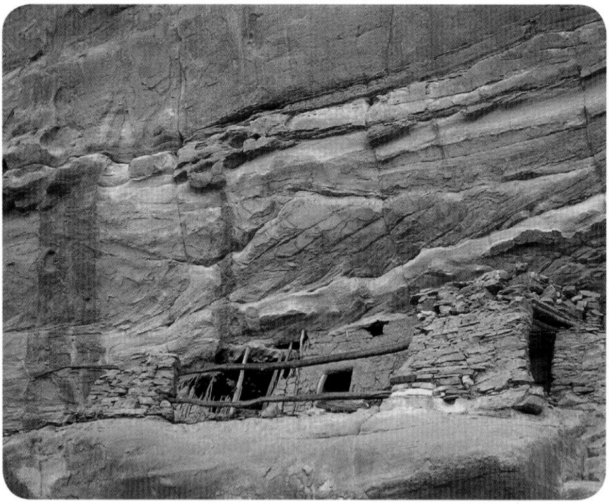

Bannister ruin, Grand Gulch

There are dozens more. Some are obvious. Others require a sharp eye to detect and patience to investigate.

Though we've hiked Grand Gulch several times, we can't yet claim to know it intimately. Our next trip will be longer, more deliberate, and richer. Ideally, approach Grand Gulch at what musicians call the *tempo giusto*: the right pace. Be fast only when speed is appropriate. Be slow when restraint enhances the experience.

FACT

BEFORE YOUR TRIP

Water should be available at sufficiently frequent intervals throughout Grand Gulch that you don't have to plan your journey around particular springs, though you should top-up your supply at every opportunity. Ask at the Kane Gulch Ranger Station how much water to expect en route and where you'll likely find it.

BY VEHICLE

Kane Gulch trailhead

From the junction of Hwys 95 and 261, drive Hwy 261 south 3.8 mi (6.2 km) to Kane Gulch Ranger Station. Turn left (east) into the parking lot. Elevation 6440 ft (1963 m). Leave your shuttle vehicle here, where the one-way trip ends.

Collins Canyon trailhead

It's about a 40-minute drive from Kane Gulch Ranger Station to Collins Spring trailhead, where the one-way trip begins. Car camping is possible several places beside unpaved road 260, between Hwy 276 and the trailhead.

From the junction of Hwys 261 and 95, just north of Kane Gulch Ranger Station, drive Hwy 95 generally west 9.5 mi (15.3 km). Turn left onto Hwy 276 and proceed southwest 6.6 mi (10.6 mi). Turn left (east) onto unpaved road 260 signed for Collins Spring trailhead and reset your trip odometer to 0.

At 2.4 mi (3.9 km) proceed straight, ignoring the left spur. After 4.5 mi (7.2 km) the road crosses slickrock slabs. At 6 mi (9.7 km) the road is narrower and rougher. Reach Collins Spring trailhead parking area at 6.5 mi (10.5 km), 5050 ft (1540 m). Start hiking here.

ON FOOT

The trail departs the south end of the parking area, near the trail register. It initially heads south, soon curves left (east), drops across slickrock, and switchbacks into **Collins Canyon**.

Descend along the left (northeast) side of the drainage. Within 15 minutes proceed through a gate. In the sandy wash, pass a **cowboy camp** beneath a west-facing alcove at 4800 ft (1463 m). Ahead, upon reaching slickrock again, bear right onto a trail and bypass a 40-ft (12-m) pouroff.

About 40 minutes along, pass a tributary drainage (left / north-northeast) at 4840 ft (1476 m). Curve right (southeast) to follow the trail onto a sandy bank. At 2 mi (3.2 km), 4780 ft (1457 m), after hiking nearly an hour, reach the **confluence of Collins Canyon and Grand Gulch**.

Right (south) is lower Grand Gulch (Trip 74), which leads 15.7 mi (25.3 km) to the San Juan River. Begin hiking up-canyon by turning left (northeast) and curving right (south-southeast). Kane Gulch Ranger Station is 36 mi (58 km) distant. Just five minutes in that direction is a viable campsite.

At 5 mi (8.1 km), 4854 ft (1480 m) pass **Bannister Ruin**. It's high on the left (northwest) wall. Ahead, Grand Gulch begins meandering generally northeast.

Reach possible campsites just before two-tiered, 25-ft (7.6-m) **Big Pouroff** at 8.7 mi (14 km), 5000 ft (1524 m). Bypass it on the left (north).

Up-canyon, the smooth, gravel wash allows easy walking for the next 3 mi (4.8 km). Look for a ruin (left / northwest) about 30 minutes beyond Big Pouroff. About 30 minutes farther is another ruin visible from a bench above the tamarisk.

About 1½ hours from Big Pouroff, look left (northwest) for a high ruin beneath a thin overhang. It's across from where Government trail descends off the right (southeast) rim.

Just ten minutes farther, reach **Polly's Canyon** (right / east) at 11.8 mi (19 km), 5080 ft (1550 m). There are several campsites here. Polly's Spring is 0.1 mi (0.2 km) up the wash. Polly's Island, in the middle of the main canyon, is the result of an abandoned meander.

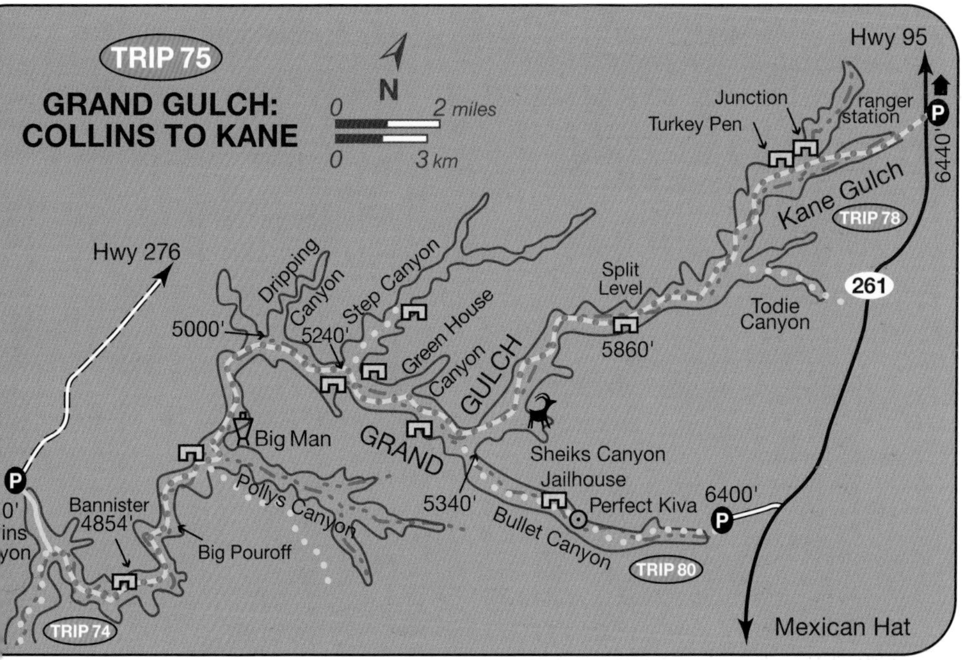

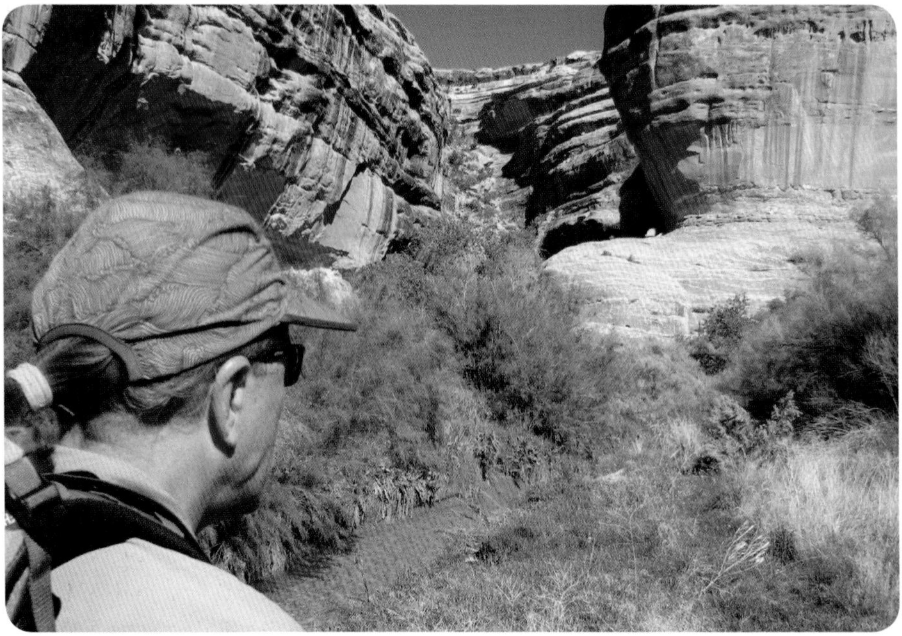

Grand Gulch, near Bullet Canyon confluence

At 13.3 mi (21.4 km), about 25 minutes north of Polly's Canyon, watch right for a steep, cairned, bootbeaten path ascending 200 ft (61 m) to **Big Man Panel**. The pictographs are just above a narrow bench, high on a northwest-facing wall, beneath an overhanging rim. The primary anthropomorphic figures are 6 ft (1.8 m) tall. A more apt name would be *Big Couple Panel*.

On the canyon floor, just above the opposite side of the wash from Big Man, is a campsite beneath cottonwoods. About 20 minutes north of Big Man, look left for a ruin. It's on an accessible, south-facing ledge.

Pass **Dripping Canyon** (left / north) at 15.7 mi (25.3 km), 5000 ft (1524 m). A couple minutes farther, just past a slickrock ledge, a bootbeaten path ascends steeply left to a high bench affording a couple tentsites among sage and grass. The path immediately returns to the canyon floor.

Grand Gulch begins meandering generally southeast. Between here and the Totem Pole, at 20 mi (32 km), there are few viable campsites. Riparian vegetation remains dense until beyond Sheik's Canyon, at 23.8 mi (38.3 km).

At 18.5 mi (29.8 km), 5240 ft (1598 m) pass **Step Canyon** (left / north). Camping is possible near the mouth. Necklace Spring is 0.8 mi (1.3 km) up Step Canyon. Impressive ruins are 20 minutes up. Camping is possible about 30 minutes up.

Grand Gulch again meanders generally southeast. After crossing the inner channel about ten minutes beyond Step Canyon, look up left for a ruin in a southeast-facing alcove. It's a square, two-story tower with a wood-frame door. The rock art right of it includes numerous handprints and a zigzag snake.

Pass **Totem Pole**, a slickrock spire, at 20 mi (32.2 km). It's near the mouth of **Green House Canyon** (left / north). There's a reliable spring 0.2 mi (0.3 km) up this tributary.

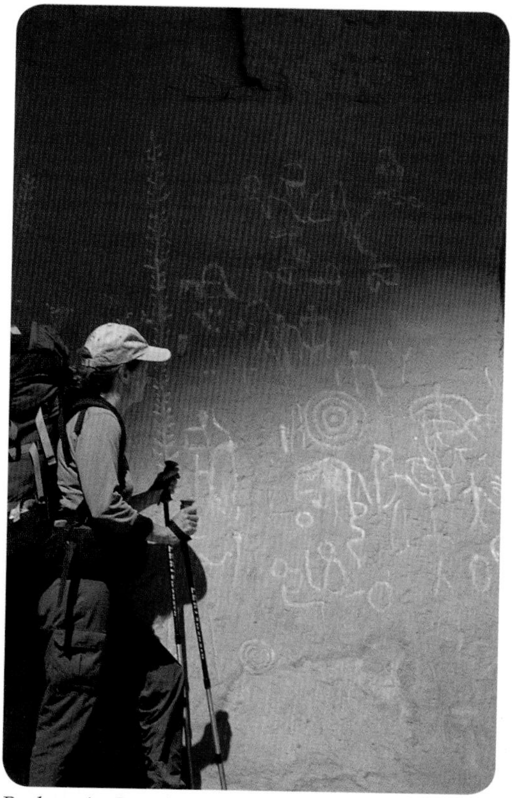

Rock art in Grand Gulch

Reach **Bullet Canyon** (right / southeast) at 22.4 mi (36.1 km), 5340 ft (1628 m). The mouth harbors several campsites. Just 330 yd (300 m) up this major tributary is a tower ruin on a shallow ledge in the left (northeast) wall. Detour up Bullet 2.5 mi (4 km) to **Jailhouse Ruin** and 0.25 mi (0.4 km) farther to **Perfect Kiva** at 5630 ft (1716 m).

Grand Gulch trends northeast from Bullet Canyon all the way to Kane Gulch. From here on, the canyon is wider, allowing you to hike outside the confines of the main channel. The deepest section of the Gulch, where the walls rise 650 to 700 ft (198 to 213 m), is between Bullet and Todie canyons.

Resume up Grand Gulch from Bullet. Within eight minutes, look left for an accessible ruin in the first bay (left / north). A couple minutes farther, at 22.7 mi (36.5 km), the second bay (left / north) affords campsites on slickrock and harbors minor ruins at the base of the canyon wall.

About fifteen minutes farther, obscured by trees and brush, is **Sheik's Canyon** (right / east-southeast) at 23.8 mi (38.3 km), 5440 ft (1660 m). Camping is viable near the canyon mouth. Detour 0.2 mi (0.3 km) up the narrow drainage to a small alcove (left / north). It contains abundant rock art, including the **Green Mask** pictograph. There's a spring nearby.

Continuing up Grand Gulch from Sheik's, pass **The Thumb**, a 40-ft (12-m) sandstone pinnacle, at 24.3 mi (39.1 km). About one hour from Sheik's, pass **Shelf Ruin** in a large, south-facing alcove at 26.3 mi (42.3 km). It has three, cascading levels. Look for more ruins on a high ledge at 27.3 mi (44 km).

Split Level Ruin, nearly two hours from Sheik's, is left (north) at 28 mi (45.1 km), 5860 ft (1787 m). It's in Grand Gulch's deepest alcove, where the canyon meanders north-northwest. Five minutes beyond it is another structure in a high alcove.

Shortcut a meander by following a bootbeaten path onto a bench about 45 minutes from Split Level Ruin. Pass a level campsite among juniper. Enter a mile-long **burn** where an idiot set fire to toilet paper and cremated a once-elegant cottonwood groove at the mouth of Todie Canyon.

At 30.8 mi (49.6 km), 5750 ft (1753 m) pass **Todie Canyon** (right / northeast). About 12 minutes up Todie is a reliable spring. At 32.4 mi (52.2 km) pass Fortress Canyon (left / north-northwest). At 33 mi (53.1 km) pass a pictograph panel

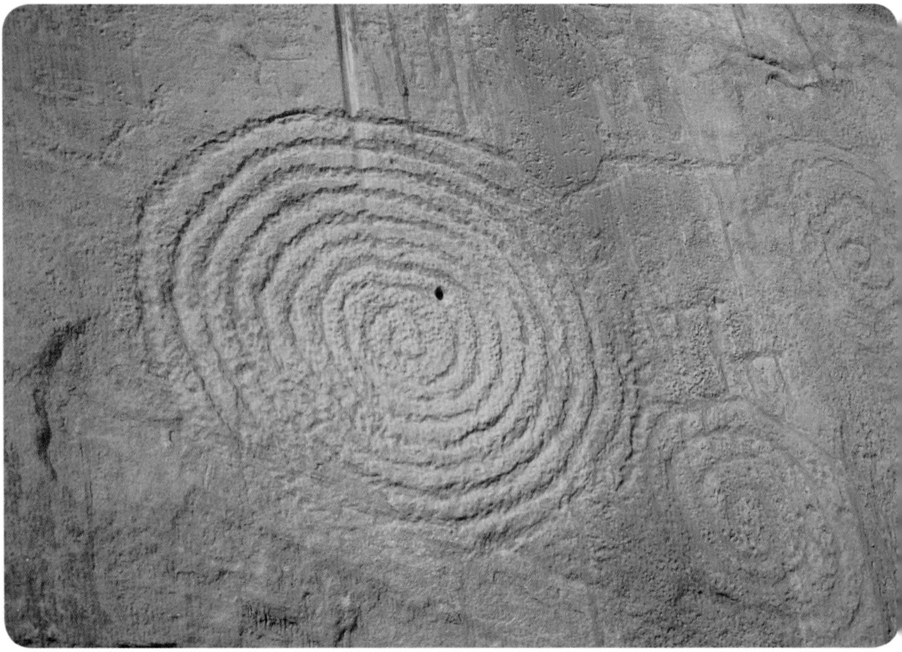

comprising swirls, squares, hands, and an antelope. Four minutes farther, Stimper Arch is visible above the north rim.

Turkey Pen Ruin is in a deep, sandy alcove (left / north) at 33.3 mi (53.6 km), 5900 ft (1799 m). Dwellings, granaries, and a kiva are evident. You'll also see pictographs and petroglyphs. Turkey Pen is not a whimsical name. The Ancestral Puebloans domesticated turkeys. They ate them, of course, but also wove turkey feathers into blankets.

After Grand Gulch bends right (east), reach the broad confluence with **Kane Gulch** (right / southeast) at 34 mi (54.7 km) 5920 ft (1805 m). There are several campsites here shaded by cottonwoods. **Junction Ruin** is prominently visible in an accessible alcove on the west wall. It comprises the foundations of about 14 structures. Originally there were several more. Though severely degraded, this is one of Cedar Mesa's largest archaeological sites and remains impressive.

Bear right, enter Kane Gulch, and begin a generally northeast ascent. Cross Hwy 261 and reach Kane Gulch Ranger Station at 38 mi (61.2 km), 6440 ft (1963 m).

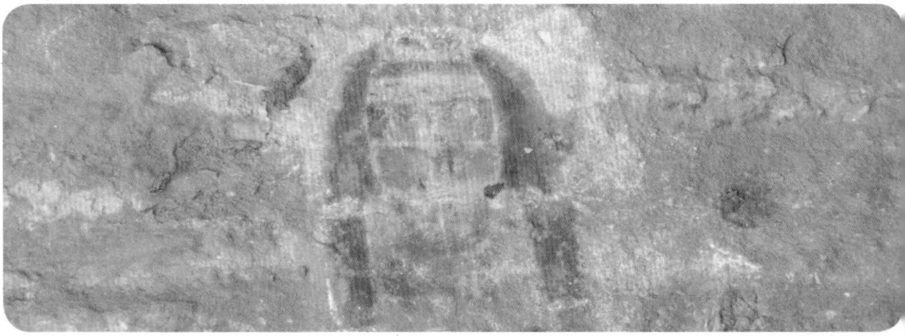

Green Mask pictograph, Sheik's Canyon

TRIP 76

NATURAL BRIDGES NATIONAL MONUMENT

LOCATION	Cedar Mesa, Hwy 95 between Lake Powell and Blanding
LOOP	8.6 mi (13.8 km)
ELEVATION CHANGE	640-ft (195-m) loss and gain
KEY ELEVATIONS	trailhead 6200 ft (1890 m) Sipapu Bridge 5740 ft (1750 m) Kachina Bridge 5710 ft (1740 m) Owachomo Bridge 5950 ft (1814 m)
HIKING TIME	3½ to 4½ hours
DIFFICULTY	moderate
MAP	Trails Illustrated *Manti-La Sal National Forest*

OPINION

Skyglow is the glow visible in the sky over most cities and towns. Astronomers measure it according to the Bortle Dark-Sky Scale. One = an absolutely dark sky. Ten = maximum light pollution. And Natural Bridges National Park is the only place in the U.S. to earn a Bortle-class-two rating, which is why it's now an International Dark Sky Park (www.darksky.org).

So when you come to Natural Bridges, stick around. Not so long as the park's first custodian (22 years in a tent), but at least overnight. It's a small, remote park that most visitors, en route to someplace else, pop into for only an hour. They drive to the overlooks, admire the bridges, then scram. But there's a superb, half-day loop hike here: through White and Armstrong canyons, beneath the bridges. And if you settle into the park's excellent frontcountry campground, you'll get to admire the darkest, starriest sky in the nation.

The hike would be worthwhile even without the bridges. The canyons are deep enough that periodically, during the span of 1,000 years, they served as a secluded, protective home for Ancestral Puebloans. A few of their rock-art panels and the remains of a couple dwellings attest to this. Horsecollar Ruin, named for the unusual shape of its doors, is visible from an overlook along the park road.

But the bridges are tremendous. That's why the park was established more than a century ago, in 1908 by President Teddy Roosevelt, making it the first national-park service area in Utah. And approaching the bridges on foot, from below, via the Cedar Mesa sandstone canyons, is exciting. They are, after all, enormous: 180 to 268 ft (55 to 82 m) long, 106 to 220 ft (32 to 67 m) high.

All natural bridges are the result of running water. That's why they're usually within canyons and often difficult to see. Compared to natural arches (shaped by a variety of erosional forces, typically in high, exposed locations), bridges are rare and secretive. Arches National Park, for example, contains more than 2000 arches, whereas this park has but three bridges.

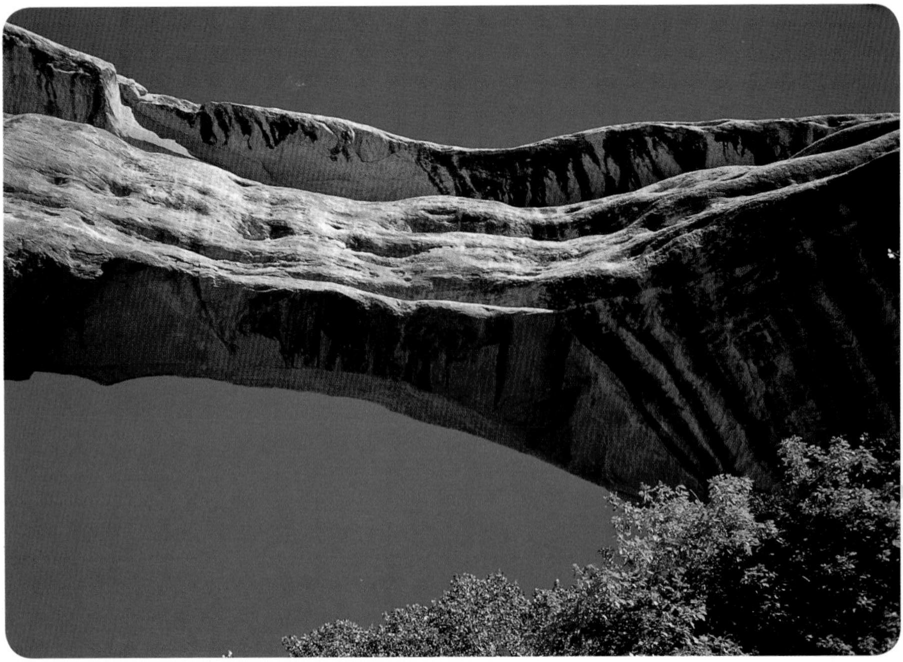

Sipapu Bridge

Sipapu is the world's second largest natural bridge and the highest and longest in the park. The name is a Hopi term referring to the small hole or depression in the floors of subterranean ceremonial chambers known as *kivas*. Kivas have been central to Native spiritual traditions since ancient times. A sipapu symbolizes the portal through which the original humans first entered the world. It also serves as a reminder of our earthly origins.

Kachina is the world's third largest natural bridge and the youngest in the park. Though difficult to spot from the park road, the bridge will dominate your life while you're hiking the trail below it. Luckily no one was there when 4,000 tons of rock fell from Kachina's north side in June, 1992. Petroglyphs near the bridge resemble symbols painted on Hopi Kachina dolls, hence the name.

Owachomo is one of the world's oldest and thinnest natural bridges and as such is the park's most spectacular. Given that it's made of stone, it's a mere thread: just 9 ft (2.7 m) thick. *Owachomo* is a Hopi word meaning "rock mound." There *is* such a feature on the bridge's east abutment, but it's really the gracefully long sound of the word *O-wa-cho-mo* that's evocative of the incredibly sinuous span.

If you camp at Natural Bridges National Monument, notice how the light fixtures have been modified. They're as dim as possible, they point down, and they're shielded to prevent the light from spilling beyond its required focus. It's a reminder how common and unnecessary light pollution is, and how easy it is to curb.

Gazing up at an inky, starry sky, you're admiring the universe. It puts your earthly existence into perspective. It lifts your thoughts from the mundane to the profound. And it links you with all the people who've previously occupied this planet: every culture, clan, tribe, going back to the dawn of humankind. We've all stared into the heavens at night, marveled at what we saw, and wondered…

FACT

BEFORE YOUR TRIP

Bring more water than you think you'll need for your entire stay. The park's only public source of potable water is a faucet at the visitor center. The water comes from an 800-ft (244-m) well, which is extraordinarily deep even for canyon country. The well pumps are powered by the park's enormous array of solar panels. You might or might not encounter water on the hike, so assume you won't. Carry more than you'll need: at least three quarts (liters) per person.

BY VEHICLE

From the northeast arm of Lake Powell, near Hite Marina, drive Hwy 95 generally southeast. Pass the junction with Hwy 276 (right / southwest), reset your trip odometer to 0, and proceed east. At 7.7 mi (12.4 km) turn left (north) onto Hwy 275.

From Hwy 191, just south of Blanding, drive Hwy 95 generally west. Pass the junction with Hwy 261 (left / south), reset your trip odometer to 0, and proceed west. At 1.8 mi (2.9 km) turn right (north) onto Hwy 275.

From either approach, reach the National Bridges National Park visitor center at 4.6 mi (7.4 km), 6505 ft (1983 m). The campground is at 5 mi (8 km). Pass the Sipapu Bridge overlook at 7.1 mi (11.5 km) and a picnic area just beyond. Reach the Sipapu Bridge trailhead at 7.6 mi (12.2 km), 6200 ft (1890 m).

Continuing on Bridge View Drive (a paved, one-way loop), Kachina Bridge overlook is at 9.5 mi (15.4 km) and Owachomo Bridge overlook at 11.4 mi (8.4 km). Complete the loop at 14 mi (22.5 km).

ON FOOT

Begin a counter-clockwise loop to all three bridges by following the cairned path across slickrock. It descends generally west-northwest over the rim of **White Canyon**. Carved steps and handrails offer assistance on steep pitches. Stairways and ladders enable you to negotiate cliffbands.

About halfway down, a left spur leads to a fine view of Sipapu Bridge. After this short detour, resume descending generally north-northeast on the main trail. About 30 minutes from the trailhead, bottom-out in White Canyon wash beneath **Sipapu Bridge** at 0.6 mi (1 km), 5740 ft (1750 m).

From the trail register under the bridge, go left (west). Follow the trail down-canyon. Pass the confluence with **Deer Canyon** (right / north) at 1.4 mi (2.3 km). Bear left (west-southwest) in White Canyon.

Five minutes farther is **Horsecollar Ruin** (right / north), opposite a small arch. It's an unusual collection of dwellings and granaries in a deep alcove. Reaching it requires only a quick detour but entails a steep slickrock scramble.

Resume hiking down-canyon: generally southwest. At 2.5 mi (4 km), look for a small granary (left / south) just above the wash. Reach **Kachina Bridge** at 3 mi (4.8 km), 5710 ft (1740 m), near the confluence of White and Armstrong canyons. Look for pictographs on both bridge abutments, and 100 ft (30 m) south of the bridge, on the right (west).

White Canyon proceeds right (southwest). Enter **Armstrong Canyon** by bearing left (south). A couple minutes beyond Kachina Bridge, the main trail

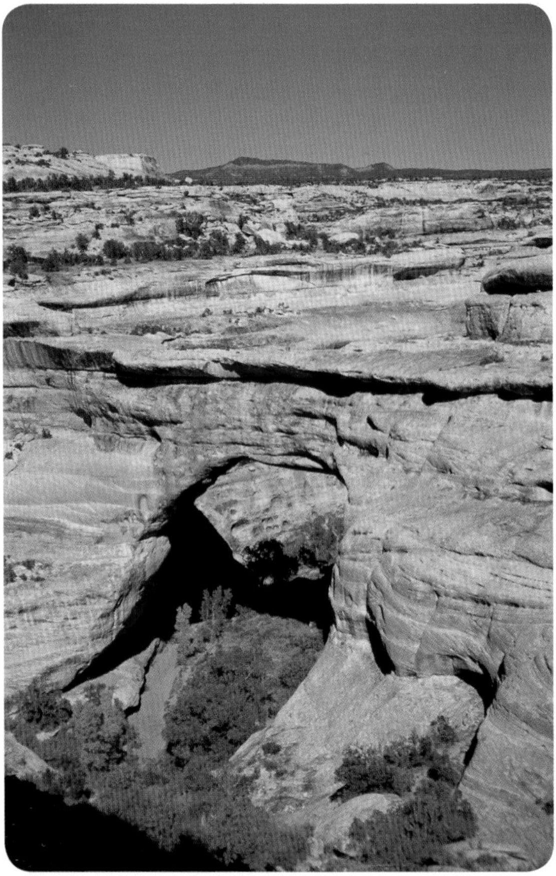
Sipapu Bridge, White Canyon

avoids a pouroff in the wash bottom ahead by ascending slickrock (steps, hand rails) to a **junction** on a bench. Left continues ascending to the park road. Go right, gradually curving west, to follow Armstrong up-canyon. Soon overlook the pouroff below, then drop into the wash.

Ignoring tributary drainages, keep following Armstrong Canyon. It meanders generally southeast. The main trail crosses a sandy bench to avoid brush and minor obstacles. About an hour from Kachina Bridge, look for petroglyphs (right / north). They're on a buttress, at a curve, above the limb of a sprawling cottonwood.

Two minutes farther, bypass boulders by ascending briefly left. Within another 15 minutes, watch for a sign indicating where the trail ascends left to a slickrock ledge midway up the wall. Just ten minutes farther, reach **Owachomo Bridge** at 6.2 mi (10 km), 5950 ft (1814 m). It parallels the canyon instead of crossing it.

Ascend a slickrock cascade beneath the bridge. Go left, up stone steps near the west abutment. A fence-lined trail then leads generally north. Reach the paved overlook and intersect the **park road** about 15 minutes above the bridge.

Bear left (north). On the far side of the road, pick up the signed trail leading generally north, across the **mesa**, through pygmy P-J forest (piñon and juniper). Cross the road twice more.

At 7.7 mi (12.4 km) reach a **junction**. Left leads west-southwest to the Kachina Bridge overlook. Proceed straight (north). Reach the **Sipapu Bridge trailhead** at 8.6 mi (13.8 km), 6200 ft (1890 m).

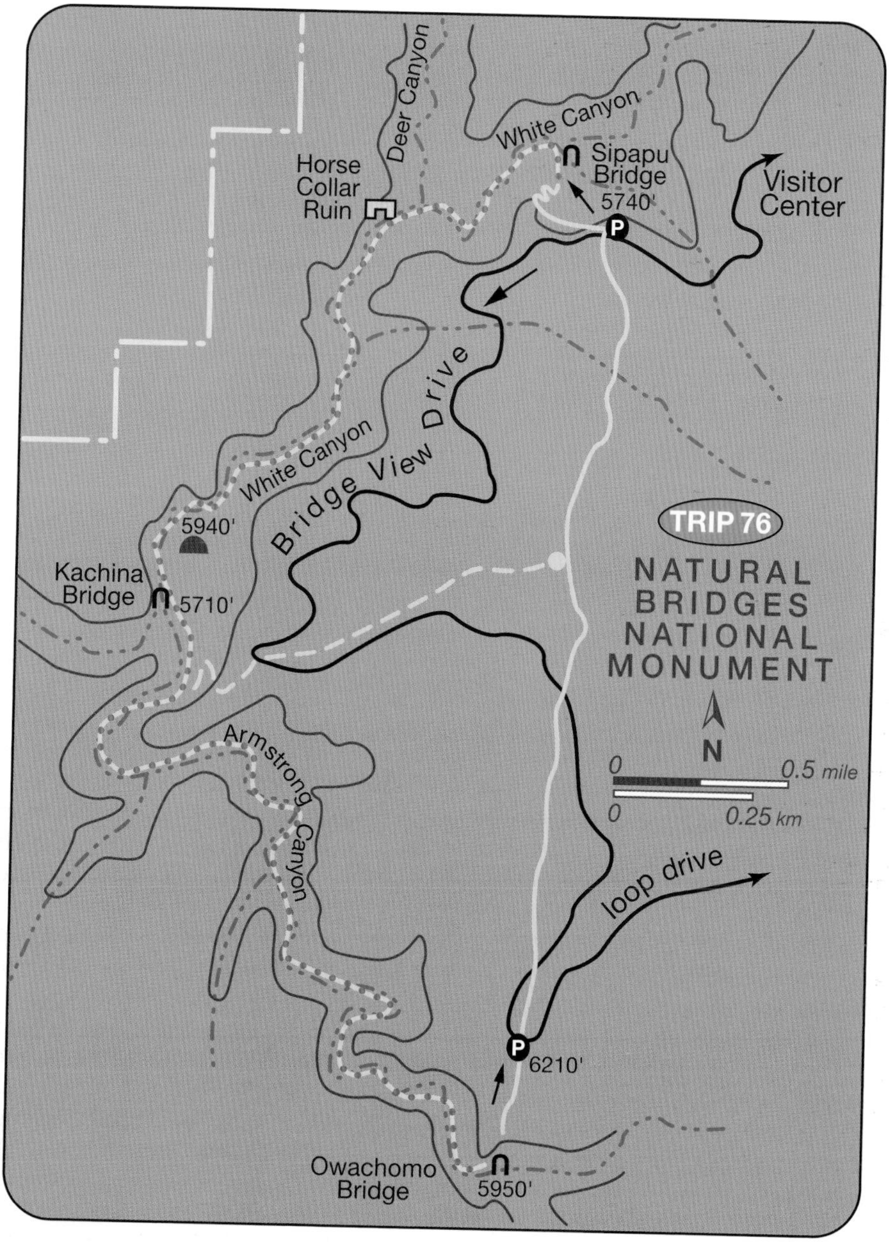
Deer Canyon
White Canyon
Horse Collar Ruin
Sipapu Bridge
5740'
Visitor Center
Bridge View Drive
White Canyon
5940'
Kachina Bridge
5710'
TRIP 76
NATURAL BRIDGES NATIONAL MONUMENT
N
0
0.5 mile
0
0.25 km
Armstrong Canyon
loop drive
6210'
Owachomo Bridge
5950'

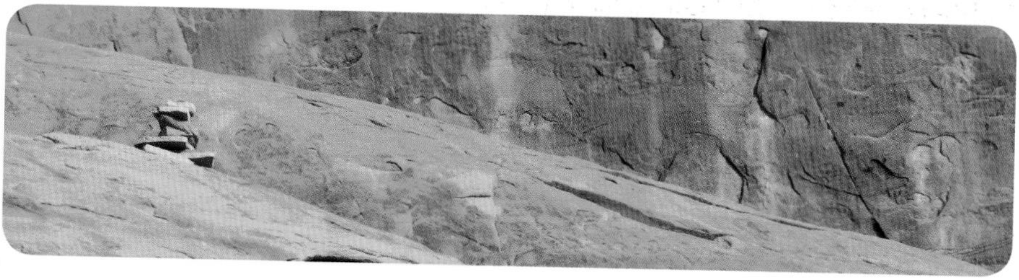

TRIP 77

MULE CANYON SOUTH FORK

LOCATION	Cedar Mesa, west of Comb Ridge east of Natural Bridges National Monument
ROUND TRIP	7.5 mi (12.1 km)
ELEVATION GAIN	400 ft (122 m)
KEY ELEVATIONS	trailhead 5900 ft (1800 m), highpoint 6260 ft (1909 m)
HIKING TIME	3½ to 4 hours
DIFFICULTY	easy
MAP	Trails Illustrated *Grand Gulch Plateau*

OPINION

Look at a 1960s USGS 1:24 000 topographical map of southern Utah, and you'll see something that, from today's perspective, is shocking: the ancestral puebloan archaeological sites are labeled. The words "Cliff Dwelling" and "Ruins" appear frequently on many quadrangles. But you'll find that information absent on a 1980s version of the same map.

What happened in the intervening years that caused government maps to become less informative? Land-management officials realized publicizing the locations of historical treasures was a sure way to lose them. There were just too many pot-hunting greedheads, destructive ORVers, and insensitive oafs who couldn't be trusted with such precious data.

Since then, not only have maps become mute with regard to archaeology, so have the men and women behind the desks at "information centers" purporting to serve visitors seeking to appreciate the wonders of canyon country.

They can't protect native cultural heritage and serve the public at the same time. So they protect rather than serve. It's sad, frustrating, and completely understandable.

Land-management officials hope you'll do the hard work of discovery yourself and en route develop a more reverent attitude and enjoy a more rewarding experience. We support that ethic. But we recognize you'll need motivation, which is why this book points the way (without using GPS coordinates) to numerous well-documented archaeological sites. None are secrets revealed, but all will pique your interest and deepen your appreciation while sharpening your ability to further investigate the canyon-country outdoor museum on your own, with only a compass and topo map for guidance. An up-to-date, eviscerated topo, that is.

Until then, you'll find Mule Canyon's south fork a motivating hike. It's well known, easy to reach, close to a paved highway. Yet it abounds with south-facing alcoves where the ancient ones built homes that have endured—due to their structural integrity, sheltered perches, and the arid climate—seven to nine hundred years without restoration.

Geologically, the south fork is unremarkable. It's not deep. The walls are not sheer. It's merely pretty. What distinguishes the canyon is the number and accessibility of the archaeological sites, including one that looks as if it could have inspired Frank Lloyd Wright.

Our *On Foot* directions describe where to look for five ancestral puebloan dwellings. But you can ignore our guidance if you think it will diminish your sense of exploration. Getting lost in this straightforward, easy-to-walk corridor should be impossible. While heading up-canyon (generally northwest), just keep scanning the south-facing overhangs for evidence of human construction.

Because the south fork is just 0.3 mi (0.5 km) from Hwy 95, it doesn't require a lengthy drive on an unpaved road. That means it's available to hikers year round. It also means you can expect to occasionally hear passing vehicles. Mule Canyon's north fork runs parallel to the south fork, is equally intriguing, and is just beyond earshot of vehicle noise.

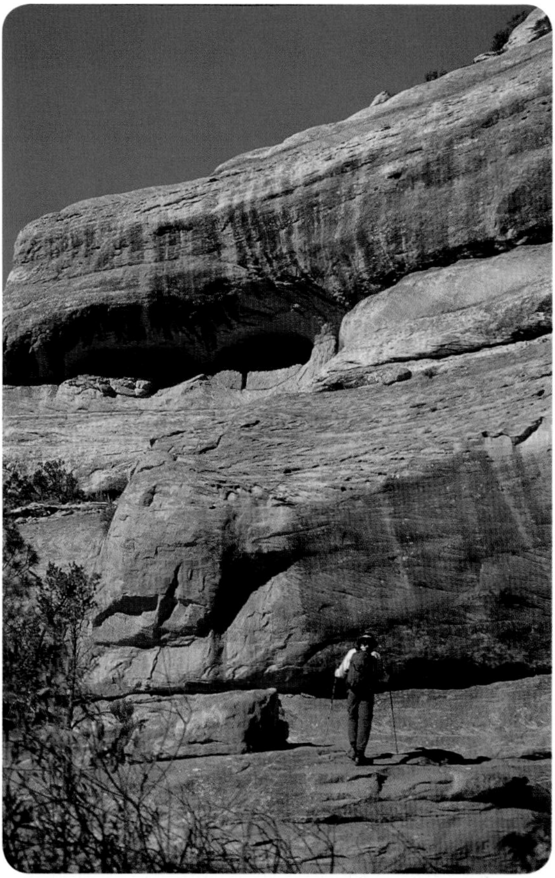

Mule Canyon South Fork

FACT

BY VEHICLE

From the junction of Hwys 261 and 95, just east of Natural Bridges National Monument, reset your trip odometer to 0 and drive Hwy 95 southeast. At 8.4 mi (13.6 km) pass the Mule Canyon roadside ruin (left / north). At 8.9 mi (14.3 km) turn left (northeast) onto unsigned, unpaved Texas Flat Road 263.

From the junction of Hwys 191 and 95, just south of Blanding, reset your trip odometer to 0 and drive Hwy 95 west. Soon cross Comb Ridge. At 19.5 mi (31.4 km) turn right (northeast) onto unsigned, unpaved Texas Flat Road 263. Just 0.5 mi (0.8 km) farther west is the Mule Canyon roadside ruin (right / north).

From either approach, cross the cattleguard and proceed east 0.3 mi (0.5 km) to where the road, on a causeway, crosses the shallow south fork of Mule Canyon. Just beyond, the road widens sufficiently to allow a couple vehicles to park on the right, at 5900 ft (1800 m).

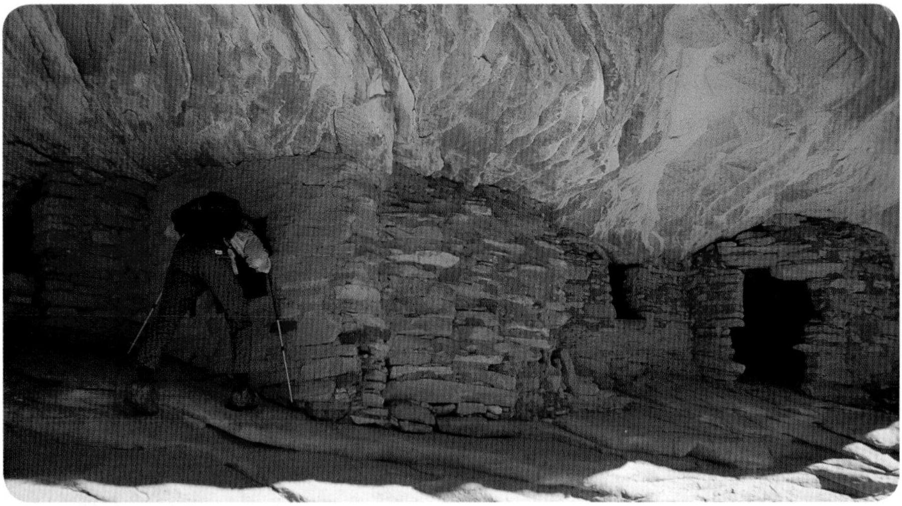
Many ruins in Mule Canyon are accessible.

ON FOOT

Drop into the canyon on the north side of the causeway. There's a **BLM fee box** in the wash. Follow the wash up-canyon, initially north, soon curving left (west).

Overall, your general direction of travel will be northwest until you return down-canyon. Make forward progress wherever it's easiest: mostly in the wash, sometimes on benches above it, often on a bootbeaten path among cottonwoods, piñon pine, juniper, tumbleweed, and sage.

The canyon walls are only about 70 ft (21 m) high at this lower end. Ahead, as the canyon deepens and the walls solidify, continually glance right (north). The ancestral puebloans favored south-facing alcoves for their dwellings.

At 1.25 mi (2 km), 6000 ft (1829 m), about 25 minutes along, look for the **first ruin**. Just 35 ft (11 m) above the wash, it faces west. The walls' complexity and durability attest to the skill of the native stonemasons.

Pass a tributary drainage (right) at 2.5 mi (4 km), about one hour along. Seven minutes farther, where the canyon briefly runs east-west, look right (north) for a **second ruin** in a shallow depression high above. A 6080-ft (1854-m) bench on the left affords a good vantage. Just beyond is a boggy, grassy area rife with manzanita and piñon.

About one hour and 20 minutes along, at 6120 ft (1866 m), pass the first **giant ponderosa** in the canyon. More are visible on the rim above. The canyon walls here are more monolithic. Follow a path on the left side of the wash to a small pouroff pool. Three minutes past the giant ponderosa, look right about 60 ft (18 m) above the wash for a **third ruin** with vertical structures.

There are two ways to reach this third ruin. Scramblers can friction-walk up slickrock to the bulging ledge where the ruin is located. Or you can continue 110 yd (100 m) farther up the canyon and turn right into a gully. Two minutes past a huge, balancing boulder, look north. Right of and beyond the cottonwoods and ponderosas in the wash, the small alcove is visible. Proceed north up the slickrock, then turn right (southeast) on the ledge where the ruin is located.

Back in the wash, continue up-canyon. Near 6180 ft (1884 m), about 1¾ hours from the trailhead, reach a substantial **pouroff**. Backtrack 20 yd/m to bypass it

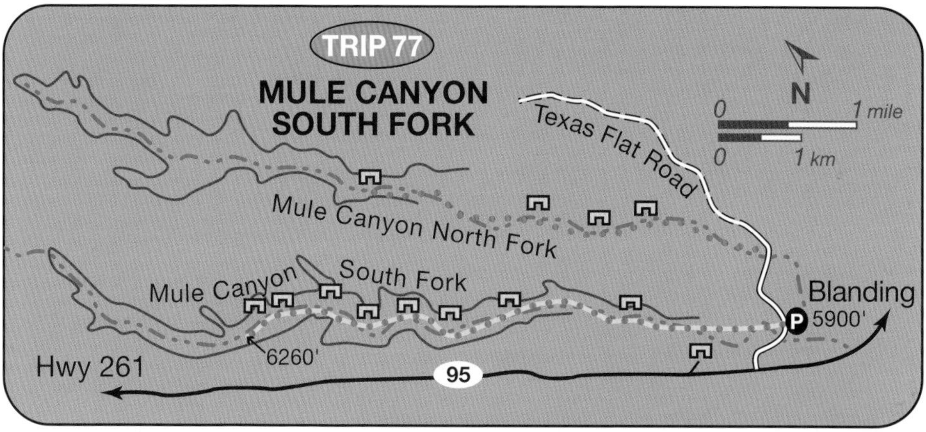

on a sandy path. Skirt left of a second, smaller pouroff. Pass beneath a giant ponderosa. The main canyon continues north. Ignore the tributary drainage (left / west).

The canyon is now thickly wooded with ponderosa, piñon and oak. A couple minutes past the tributary, look east for **small ruins** facing west. They're about 100 ft (30 m) above the wash, at the base of a heavily desert-varnished wall. Ascend left (west) for a better view.

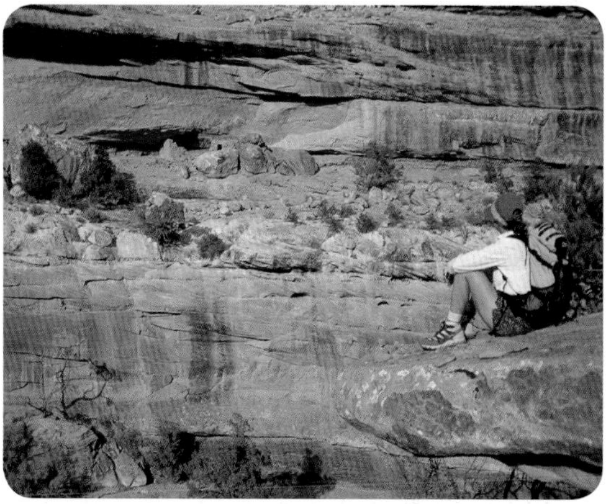

Look in south-facing alcoves for ruins.

Near 3.75 mi (6 km), 6260 ft (1909 m), about 2 hours along, reach another **pouroff**. Bypass it via the right ledge, then drop back into the wash. About 20 yd/m beyond a short stretch of dark-grey bedrock, look up right. Two **minor ruins** are barely visible. They're on the north wall, facing south, beneath a scant overhang. Improve your view by clambering up the ledges.

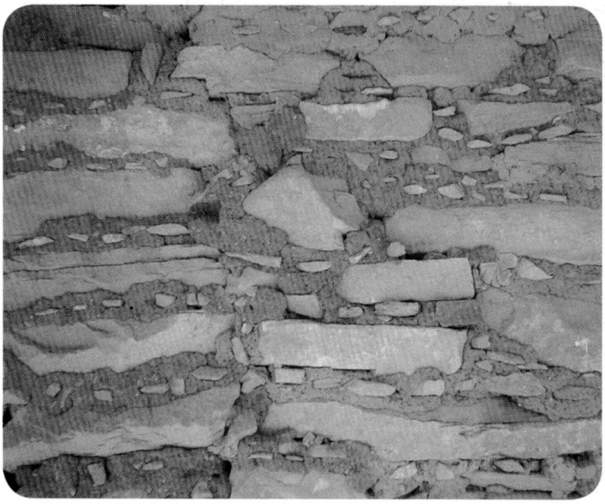

Ancestral Puebloan stonework

This is an agreeable turnaround point. Simply retrace your steps down-canyon, generally southeast. Without slowing to look for ruins, expect to arrive at your vehicle in about 1½ hours.

TRIP 78

KANE GULCH

LOCATION	Cedar Mesa, Grand Gulch Primitive Area west of Hwy 261 at Kane Gulch Ranger Station
ROUND TRIP	8 mi (12.9 km) to confluence beneath Junction Ruin 9.4 mi (15.1 km) to Turkey Pen Ruin
ELEVATION CHANGE	520-ft (159-m) loss and gain to confluence beneath Junction Ruin, additional 70-ft (21-m) loss and gain to Turkey Pen Ruin
KEY ELEVATIONS	trailhead 6440 ft (1963 m), confluence beneath Junction Ruin 5920 ft (1805 m), Turkey Pen Ruin 5850 ft (1784 m)
HIKING TIME	4 to 5 hours for confluence beneath Junction Ruin 5 to 6 hours for Turkey Pen Ruin
DIFFICULTY	easy
MAPS	Trails Illustrated *Grand Gulch Plateau*, USGS *Kane Gulch*

OPINION

Grand Gulch for dummies.

If you're new to canyon country, where hiking often entails freelancing—finding your own way over ledges, around pouroffs, through complex, untracked slickrock terrain—this is an ideal introductory trip.

The trailhead is beside the paved highway, within shouting distance of the ranger station. The trail's convenience and popularity ensures you won't be alone. The route is dead easy to follow yet imparts the sense that you're navigating. Within two hours it leads to Junction Ruin—an impressively large archaeological site. En route, the scenery is typical of Cedar Mesa canyons: an intimate overture leads to an intriguing ostinato that builds to a dramatic crescendo.

Hiking in Kane Gulch is so engaging that a destination is unnecessary. If you turned around just before reaching the confluence with Grand Gulch, this would still be a premier albeit short dayhike. But the confluence is climactic. The cottonwood grove, with its park-like ambience, invites you to rest after admiring Junction Ruin and before returning to the trailhead.

Preferably, don't stop at the confluence. Sample Grand Gulch—the mother of all Cedar Mesa canyons—by continuing to Turkey Pen Ruin, which is enhanced by a flourish of ancient rock art. A few minutes farther is Stimper Arch. Most dayhikers should turn around at Turkey Pen or Stimper.

Experienced canyon-counry hikers can opt for a more adventurous one-way trip described below, which entails exiting via rugged Todie Canyon then hitchhiking back to the Kane Gulch trailhead.

Though camping is allowed at the confluence of Kane and Grand gulches, we don't recommend it. Too close to the trailhead. Too busy. Too noisy. Canyon walls amplify sound—the chatter of other campers as well as the roar of passing jets. Seriously. Grand Gulch is directly beneath a flight path that remains surprisingly busy until late each night. Camping atop Cedar Mesa is actually quieter, because the sound doesn't reverberate.

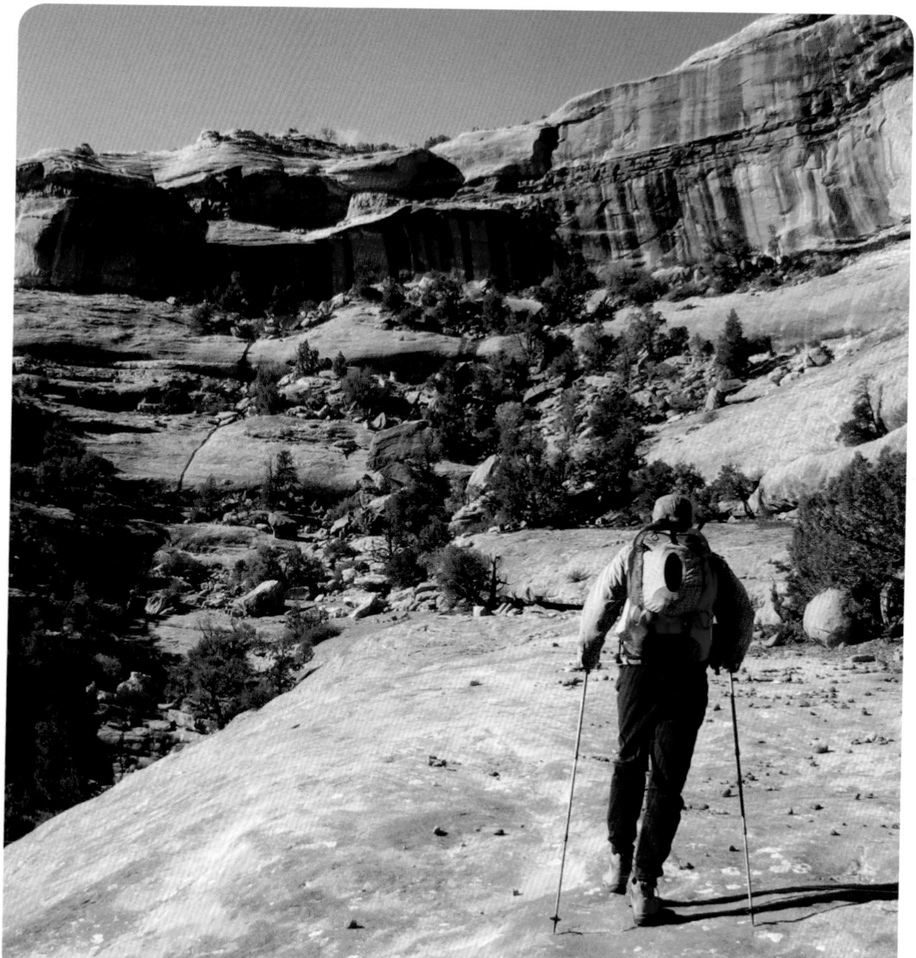

Kane Gulch

FACT

BY VEHICLE

From the junction of Hwys 95 and 261, drive Hwy 261 south 3.8 mi (6.2 km) to Kane Gulch Ranger Station. Turn left (east) into the parking lot. Elevation: 6440 ft (1963 m).

ON FOOT

From the signed trailhead on the west side Hwy 261, head southwest across the sagebrush flat.

In about 250 yd (230 m) drop into the shallow tail of **Kane Gulch**. Pass through a gate. The draw, initially bordered by willows, soon deepens into an incipient sandstone canyon. Keep following it generally southwest.

Within 30 minutes, proceed down cascading slickrock. In spring, or after recent rain, you'll follow a small stream. Ahead, you'll be hiking in the sandy,

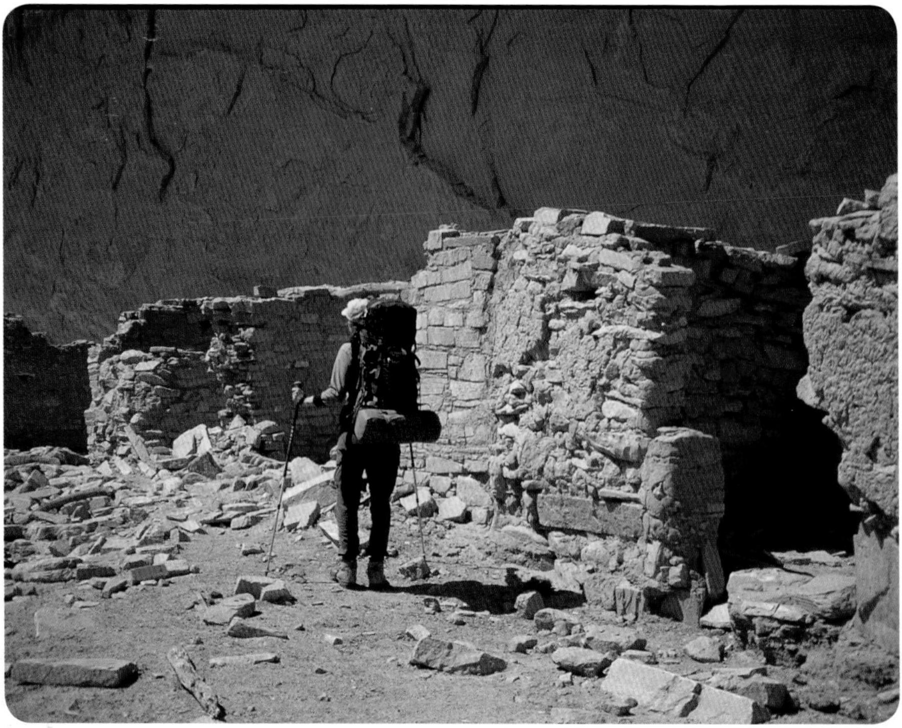

Turkey Pen ruin, Grand Gulch

brushy wash bottom, across more slickrock, through bouldery pockets, along sandstone ledges, beside shallow pools, and among cottonwoods.

Near 1 mi (1.6 km) note the aspen trees. This is about 2000 ft (610 m) lower than their typical habitat. The forebears of the trees you see today were transported here by glaciers 11,000 years ago.

At 2 mi (3.2 km) skirt right of a major pouroff. Descend to the canyon floor, which is now about 350 ft (107 m) below the canyon rim. A short stretch of trail along the right (north) wall spares you from negotiating a boulder jam and minor pouroffs. After dropping steeply down to the wash again, proceed on bootbeaten path and slickrock.

Enter the broad **confluence of Kane Gulch and Grand Gulch** at 4 mi (6.4 km), 5920 ft (1805 m). There are several campsites here shaded by cottonwoods.

Junction Ruin is prominently visible in an accessible alcove on the west wall of Grand Gulch. It comprises the foundations of about 14 structures. Originally there were several more. Though severely degraded, this is one of Cedar Mesa's largest archaeological sites and remains impressive.

To follow Grand Gulch down-canyon, proceed straight (west). It soon curves left (south). You'll be hiking in sand and gravel on the canyon floor, occasionally crossing grassy benches.

At 4.7 mi (7.6 km), 5850 ft (1784 m), reach **Turkey Pen Ruin** in a deep, sandy alcove in the right (north) wall. Dwellings, granaries, and a kiva are evident. You'll also see pictographs and petroglyphs. *Turkey Pen* is not a whimsical name. The Ancestral Puebloans domesticated turkeys. They ate them, of course, but also wove turkey feathers into blankets.

A couple minutes farther, the canyon curves left (east) at 5 mi (8.1 km), and **Stimper Arch** is visible above the left (north) rim. Most dayhikers should turn around at Turkey Pen or Stimper and retrace their steps through Kane Gulch.

After turning right (west) again, the canyon soon bends left, passes **Fortress Canyon** (right / north-northwest) at 5.6 mi (9 km), then continues generally south-southwest.

At 6.1 mi (9.8 km) in Grand Gulch is a mile-long **burn** where an idiot set fire to toilet paper and cremated a once-elegant cottonwood groove at the mouth of Todie Canyon.

Keen, strong hikers—undeterred by the burn, eager for a little more challenge and solitude—can turn left (northeast) into **Todie Canyon** at 7.2 mi (11.6 km), 5750 ft (1753 m), follow it generally east-southeast 2.1 mi (3.4 km) to Todie Flat trailhead at 6400 ft (1951 m), then march 1.2 mi (1.9 km) on level, dirt road to **Hwy 261**.

A one-way, 10.5-mi (16.9-km) dayhike—in Kane, down Grand, out Todie—though only slightly longer than a round trip to Turkey Pen via Kane, is much more demanding. Todie is rough. Attaining the rim above Todie requires a short, steep scramble. Plus you'd have to hitchhike 3.7 mi (6 km) north to Kane Gulch Ranger Station.

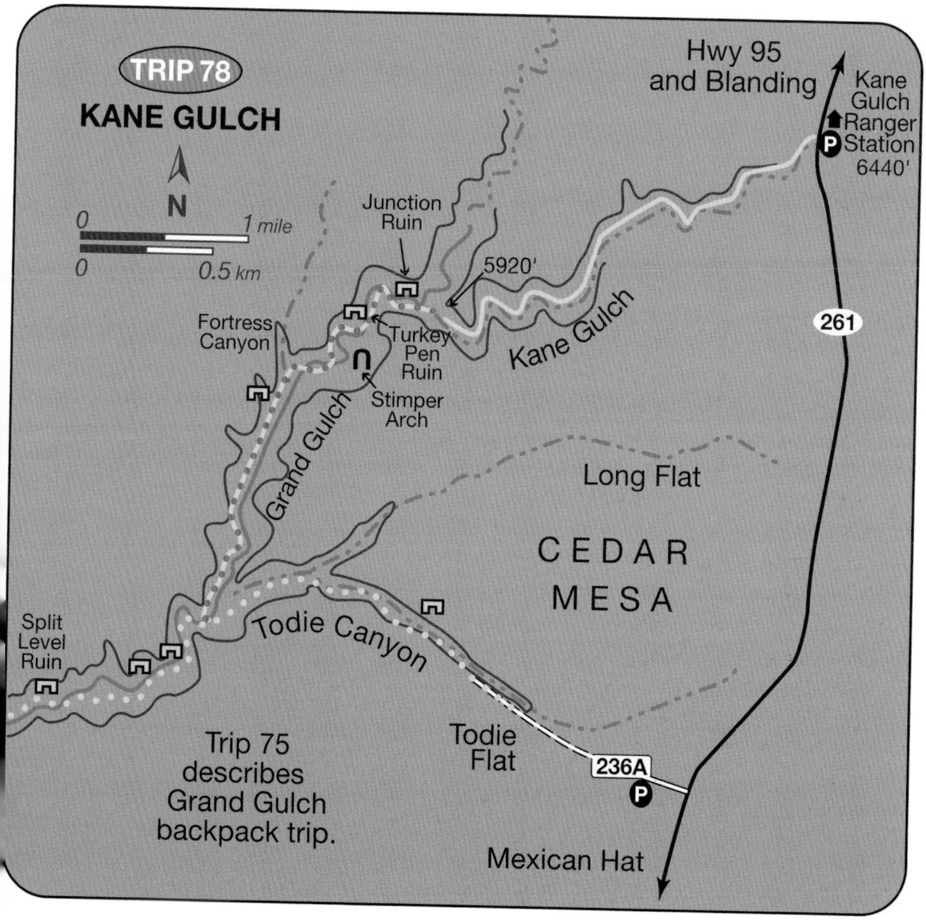

TRIP 79

FISH & OWL CREEK CANYONS

LOCATION	Cedar Mesa, east side of Hwy 261
LOOP	17 mi (27.4 km)
ELEVATION CHANGE	1360-ft (415-m) loss and gain
KEY ELEVATIONS	trailhead 6200 ft (1890 m)
	Fish & Owl confluence 4840 ft (1476 m)
HIKING TIME	8 to 10 hours, or overnight
DIFFICULTY	challenging dayhike, moderate backpack
MAP	Trails Illustrated *Grand Gulch Plateau*

OPINION

Clear skies are silent. Cloudy skies are strident. The noise is visual but can be distracting almost as if it were audible. That's why a still firmament, like a hushed library, is conducive to concentration and allows deeper appreciation. So here's hoping you hike Fish and Owl canyons beneath a calm, shatterproof-blue sky, because this loop offers more visual stimuli than most of us are normally capable of appreciating.

The lava-lamp textures of the 500-ft (152-m) walls are psychotropic, plus they're embellished with eccentric pinnacles, sensuous pouroffs, three arches, and numerous Ancestral Puebloan structures. Inviting campsites are abundant in the lower reaches of both canyons. To find yet more ruins, detour below the Fish-and-Owl confluence to McCloyd Canyon.

Following our *On Foot* directions, you'll hike the Fish-and-Owl loop clockwise: down Fish, up Owl. Both the Fish entry and Owl exit are steep, requiring athletic agility and balance. You'll plunge sharply into Fish. Departing Owl, the route wriggles, writhes and squirms long enough to tax your patience. Still, it's easier to descend into Fish and ascend out of Owl.

What's *not* easy—though worth considering if you're swift and strong—is flashing the entire loop in a single, long, challenging day. It's possible. We've done it. The accomplishment was exhilarating. But we found backpacking Fish and Owl more satisfying because it enabled us to appreciate marvels we previously raced past without even noticing.

The ruins here are small and obscure. Bring a monocular or ultralight binoculars. Observe frequently and patiently. Study the walls intently where the canyon floor provided an expanse of arable land. The Natives also farmed atop the mesa, so some structures are just beneath the rim.

FACT

BEFORE YOUR TRIP

Yes, they're named Fish *Creek* Canyon and Owl *Creek* Canyon, and you might find ample water flowing in both, but they can also be parched for long periods. If dayhiking, pack all the water you'll need for the entire trip: at least

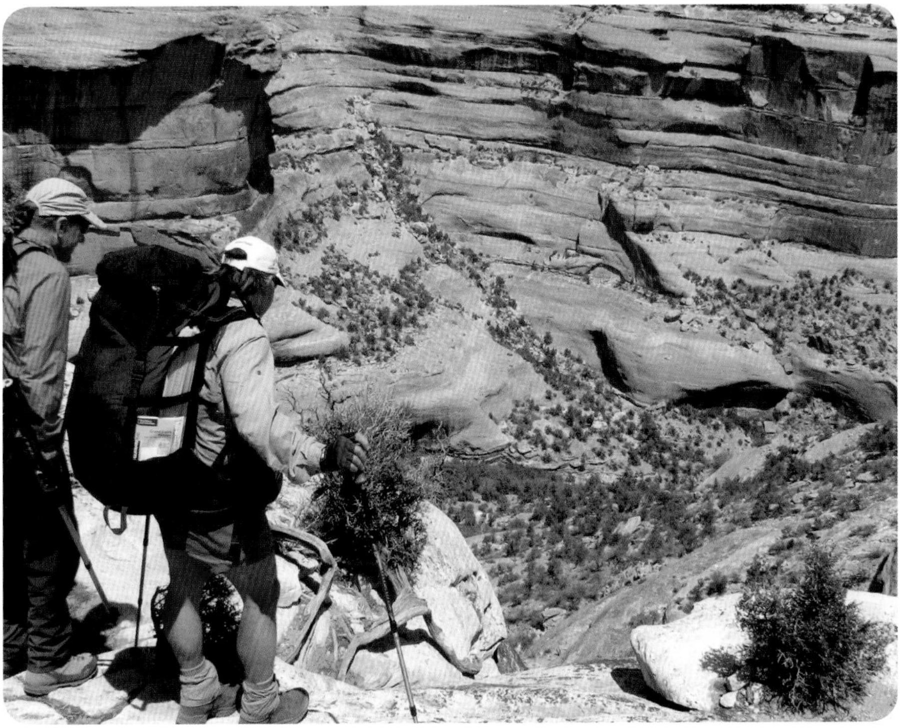

Starting the descent into Fish Creek Canyon

three quarts (liters) per person. If backpacking, stop at Kane Gulch Ranger Station before driving to the trailhead. Ask how much water to expect and where you'll likely find it.

Bring a 30-ft (10-m) length of ultralight climbing rope to lower packs over the 12-ft (4-m) down-climb necessary to enter Fish Canyon. This shouldn't be necessary with daypacks but can be helpful with hefty backpacks.

BY VEHICLE

From the junction of Hwys 95 and 261, drive Hwy 261 south 3.8 mi (6.2 km) to Kane Gulch Ranger Station. Reset your trip odometer to 0 and continue south. At 1.1 mi (1.8 km) turn left (east) onto Road 253. Again reset your trip odometer to 0. Proceed straight at 0.4 mi (0.7 km), ignoring the left (northeast) fork. The road curves right (southeast). Reach the road's end trailhead parking area for Fish and Owl canyons at 5.2 mi (8.4 km), 6200 ft (1890 m).

ON FOOT

From the sign near the north end of the parking area, follow the sandy trail generally north among P-J (piñon pine and juniper). It soon bends right (north-northeast).

Within 45 minutes, at 1.7 mi (2.7 km), 6140 ft (1872 m), reach the rim of a **Fish Creek Canyon tributary** and attain an exciting view into the abyss. A small dwelling is visible on the opposite cliff.

An abrupt drop ensues. Competent scramblers carrying only daypacks find the initial 12-ft (4-m) down-climb poses neither difficulty nor danger. Backpackers

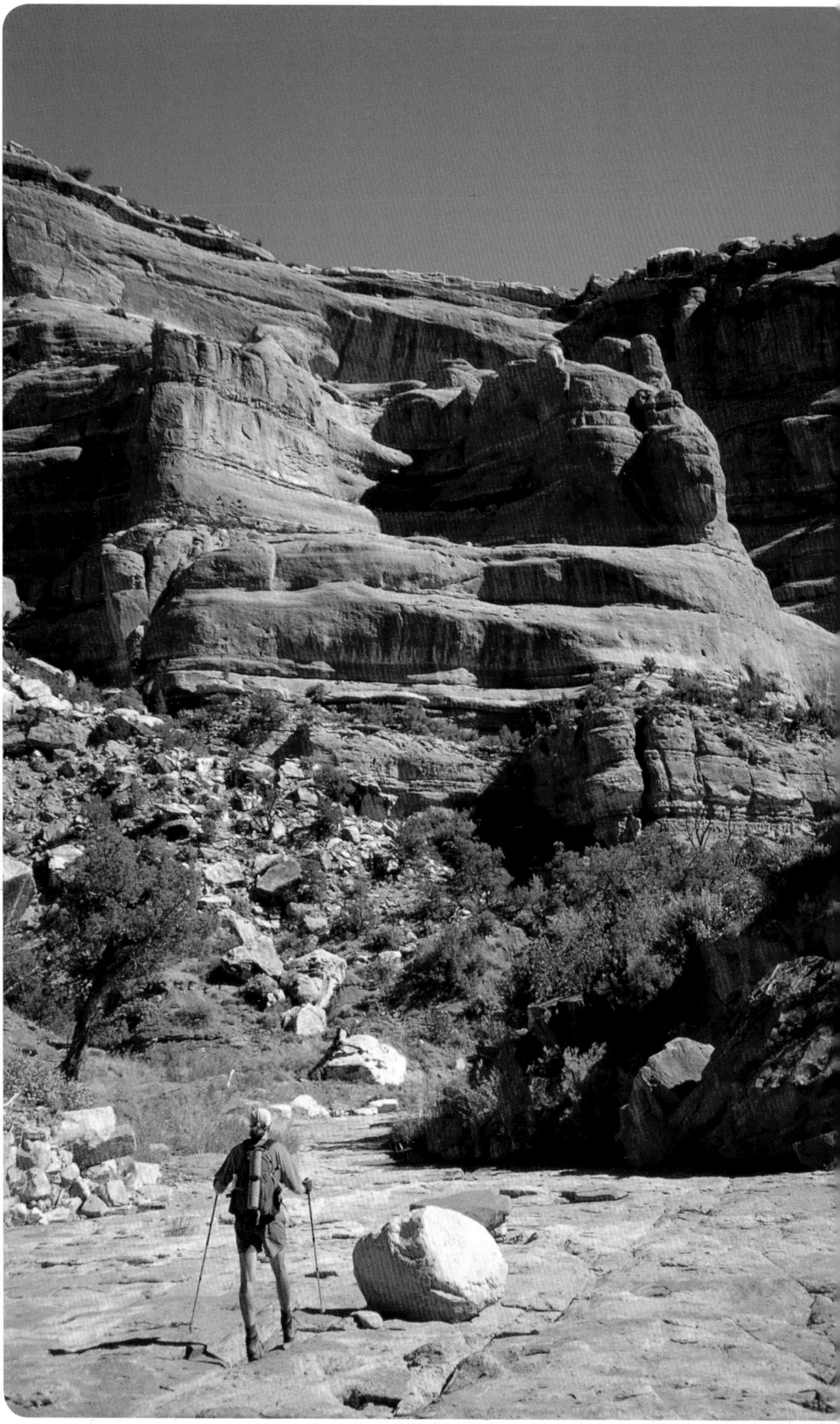

Fish Creek Canyon

might rope their packs down, so they can scramble unburdened. Below, there are no obstacles of note though the descent remains steep.

Reach the **tributary floor** at 5500 ft (1677 m). Total hiking time: about 1¼ hours. Turn right and proceed down-canyon, generally east. Find the path of least resistance through a chaotic jumble of slabs, boulders, benches and brush. Pass a weeping wall and a minor pouroff.

At 3 mi (4.8 km), 5400 ft (1646 m), 1¾ hours, intersect **Fish Creek Canyon**. Ponderosa pines thrive here. Continue down-canyon by bearing right, gradually curving east-southeast.

About 2½ hours along, at 5250 ft (1601 m), the canyon floor is largely mauve bedrock that allows easy walking for the next 15 minutes. The canyon walls comprise interesting minarets and fins. Stately cottonwoods contrast vividly with the reddish walls.

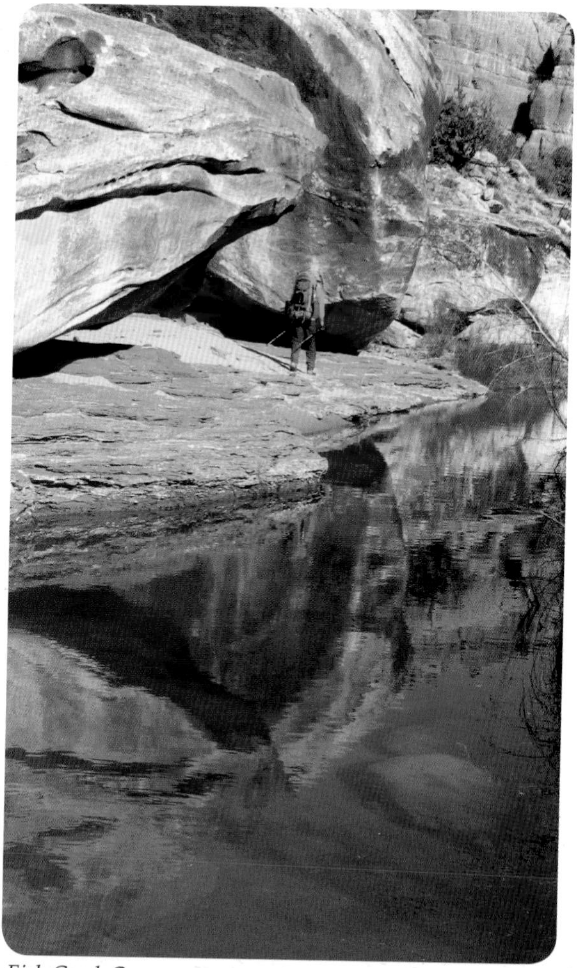
Fish Creek Canyon

Near 4.75 mi (7.6 km), about 3½ hours from the trailhead, look for an arch in the left (east) wall. At 3¾ hours, 5100 ft (1555 m), watch for a viable campsite among P-J on a bench (right / west). Continue down-canyon, generally southeast.

Nearing the confluence, the canyon bends right (south) and the walls diminish. About four hours along, an arch is visible in the right (west) wall. Reach the **confluence of Fish and Owl creek canyons** at 10 mi (16 km), 4840 ft (1476). Total hiking time: about 4¼ hours. Potential campsites are shaded by cottonwoods.

If you camp near the confluence, you should have time to detour 1.5 mi (2.4 km) farther down Fish Creek Canyon (easy, level) to see several ruins near the mouth of **McCloyd Canyon**, a right (northwest trending) tributary.

From the Fish-and-Owl confluence, resume the loop by curving right (north-northwest) into **Owl Creek Canyon**. Hike in the wash or on the benches for the next 30 minutes.

About 4¾ hours along, glimpse Nevills Arch to the north. It's right of three pinnacles. The cobblestone wash here slows progress. Opt for the benches.

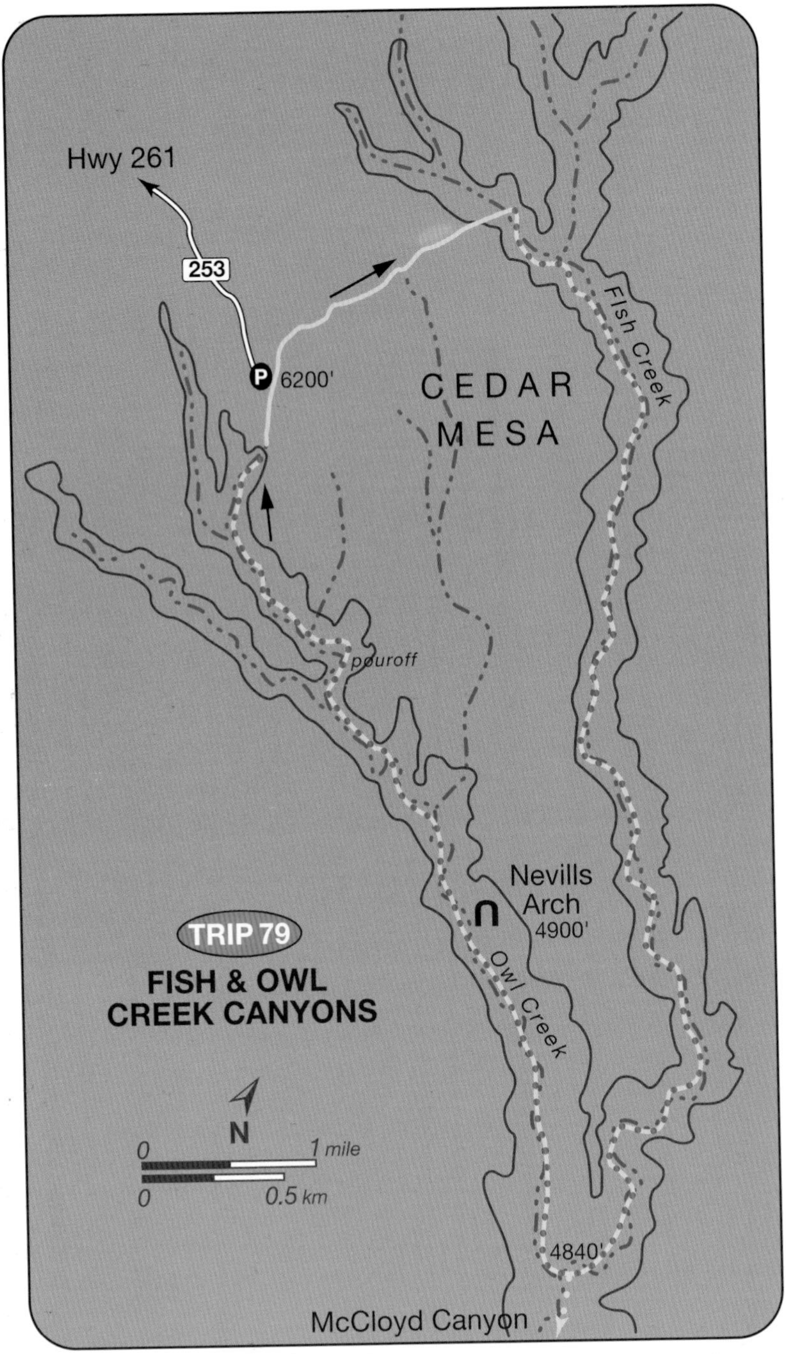
Hwy 261
253
P 6200'
CEDAR
MESA
Fish Creek
pouroff
Nevills
Arch
4900'
Owl Creek
TRIP 79
FISH & OWL
CREEK CANYONS
N
0
1 mile
0
0.5 km
4840'
McCloyd Canyon

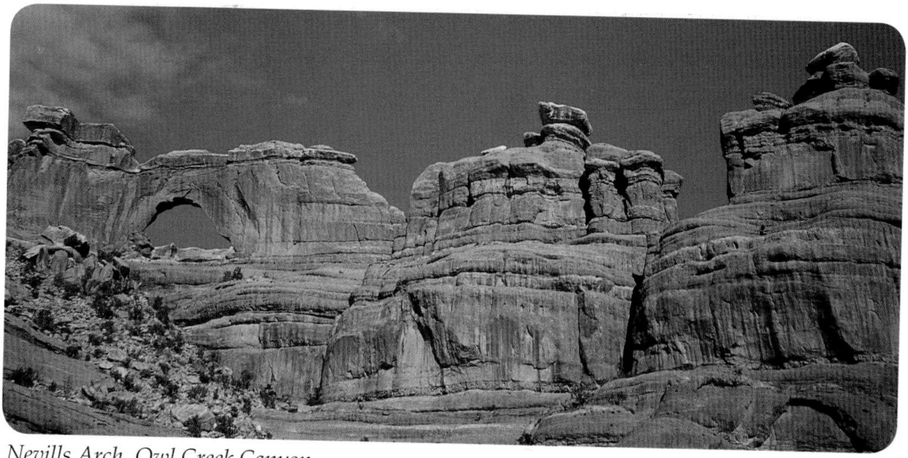

Nevills Arch, Owl Creek Canyon

At 12 mi (19.3 km), 4900 ft (1494 m), pass **Nevills Arch**. It's in a fin, high on the right (north) wall. Three ancient dwellings are also visible within 0.5 mi (0.8 km) of the arch.

Ahead the canyon floor is rockier, brushier, thickly strewn with flashflood debris. Near 13 mi (20.9 km) bypass a **low pouroff** via the left (south) bench. Then work your way along whichever side of the wash is easiest.

Soon follow a cairned, bootbeaten route ascending the right (north) wall. It's rough, narrow, and seems unnecessary until it bypasses a **huge pouroff** and deep plunge pool far below.

At 15 mi (2.4 km), 5240 ft (1598 m), about seven hours along, bear right (north) into the **north fork of Owl Creek**. Left (west) is the south fork. Be alert for cairns. They offer invaluable guidance from here on.

Go right (north) into a tributary drainage, then curve west above another **pouroff**. Ascend steep slickrock on the right, above a rugged narrows. Follow cairns back into the wash.

Arrive at a magnificent, **sculpted pouroff**. Ascend the path (right / north). Follow cairns on an increasingly technical ascent among imposing boulders. Contour south along a ledge, then proceed up-canyon, generally west-northwest.

Curve right (north) up the **east arm** of Owl Creek Canyon's north fork. Keep following the cairns. Negotiate yet more boulders and slickrock friction pitches. Watch for a kiva in an alcove. Finally ascend through bushes and trees to crest the **canyon rim** at 16.7 mi (26.9 km), 6180 ft (1884 m). Total hiking time: nearly eight hours.

Follow cairns left (north-northwest) across slickrock and among P-J. Within five minutes, reach the **trailhead** at 17 mi (27.4 km), 6200 ft (1890 m).

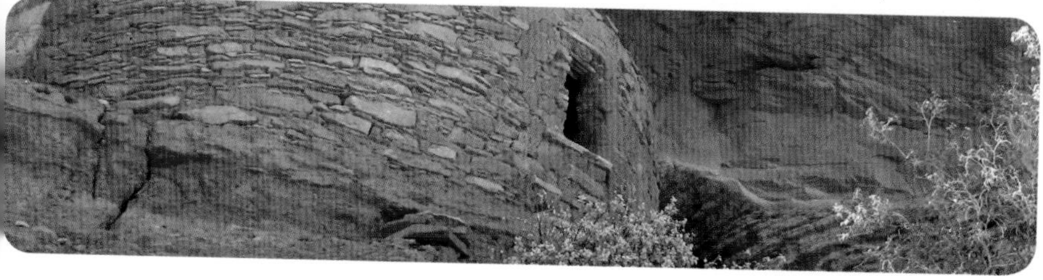

TRIP 80

BULLET CANYON

LOCATION	Cedar Mesa, west of Hwy 261
ROUND TRIP	9.5 mi (15.3 km) to Jailhouse Ruin
ELEVATION CHANGE	770-ft (235-m) loss and gain to Jailhouse Ruin
KEY ELEVATIONS	trailhead 6400 ft (1951 m) Perfect Kiva and Jailhouse Ruin 5630 ft (1716 m) Grand Gulch confluence 5340 ft (1628 m)
HIKING TIME	4 to 5 hours for Perfect Kiva and Jailhouse Ruin
DIFFICULTY	moderate
MAPS	Trails Illustrated *Grand Gulch Plateau* USGS *Cedar Mesa North, Pollys Pasture*

OPINION

You will not pierce this canyon like a bullet. Brush, trees, boulders—all seen to have amassed here with the mischievous intent of forestalling your progres But if you persist down this Grand Gulch tributary, as it deepens you'll se numerous ancient dwellings and granaries. Ultimately, you'll witness two c Cedar Mesa's celebrated archaeological sites: Perfect Kiva and Jailhouse Ruin.

Perfect Kiva, true to its name, is magnificent. It will likely be the be preserved kiva you'll ever have the privilege of visiting in the backcountry. you're lucky, the juniper ladder will still be in place, allowing you to descen beneath the reconstructed roof so you can hunker in the subterranean chamb and imagine the ancient ones' pagan rituals.

The white, moonlike pictographs above nearby Jailhouse Ruin are uniqu striking, visible from a distance. But the site is named after a small, barre window that gives the initi false impression that one the structures had been prison cell. Remembe Jailhouse Ruin and Perfe Kiva are immeasurab valuable and extreme fragile. Approach them wi reverence.

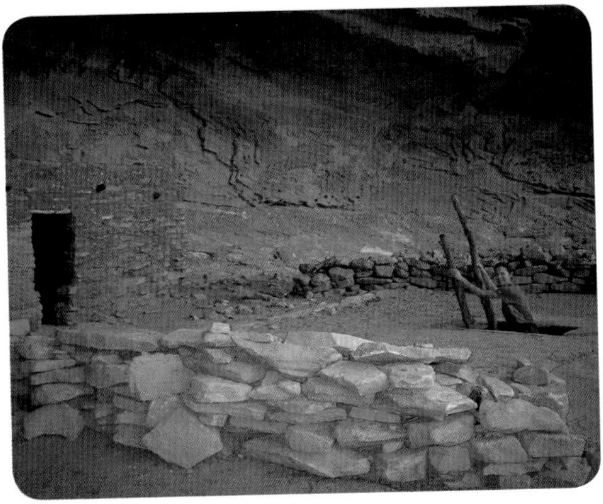

Perfect Kiva, Bullet Canyon

Backpacking into Bul is an option we do recommend. The canyon heavily visited. Oth campers nearby will alm certainly shatter any sense wilderness. Besides, y won't be—or should

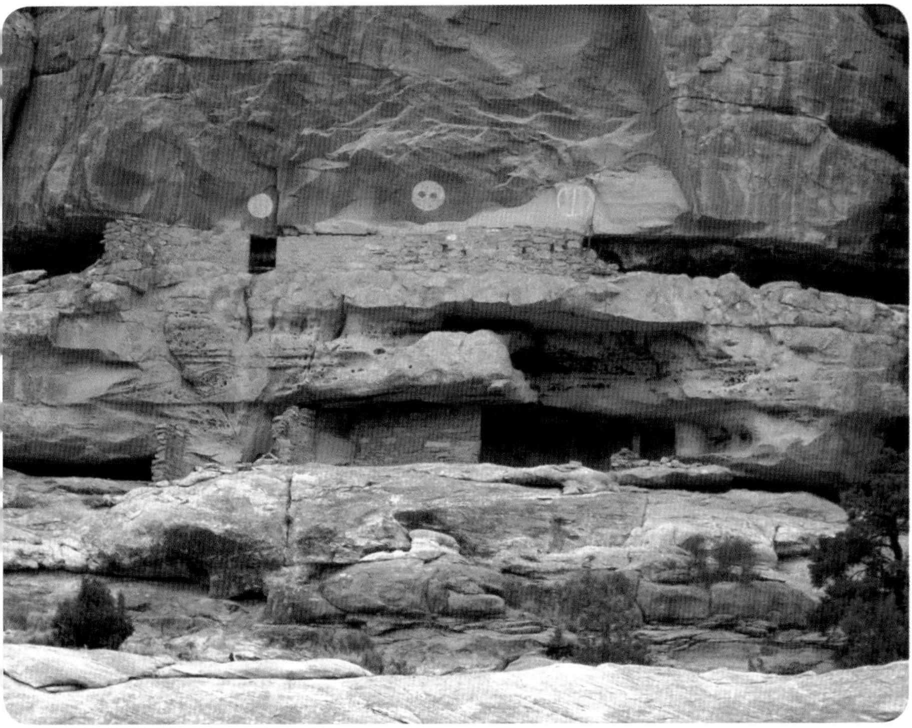

Approaching Jailhouse Ruin

be—poking around the ruins at night. So you might as well backpack into other, lonelier Cedar Mesa canyons where serenity prevails. Superior options include Lower Grand Gulch (south of Collins Canyon), Fish and Owl canyons, and the Slickhorn Canyon complex.

FACT

BY VEHICLE

From the junction of Hwys 95 and 261, drive Hwy 261 south 3.8 mi (6.2 km) to Kane Gulch Ranger Station. Reset your trip odometer to 0 at the ranger station and drive south on Hwy 261.

At 7.1 mi (11.4 km) turn right (west) onto Road 251. Proceed 1.1 mi (1.8 km) to the Bullet Canyon trailhead parking area. Elevation: 6400 ft (1951 m).

ON FOOT

Follow the path west about four minutes to the mesa rim, then descend a cairned slickrock route. Soon reach the wash bottom. Bear right (west) into the canyon: over ledges, among boulders, around pouroffs.

About 30 minutes along, just after a prominent overhang, pass a **tributary drainage** (left / southeast). The canyon is now impressively deep. Continue

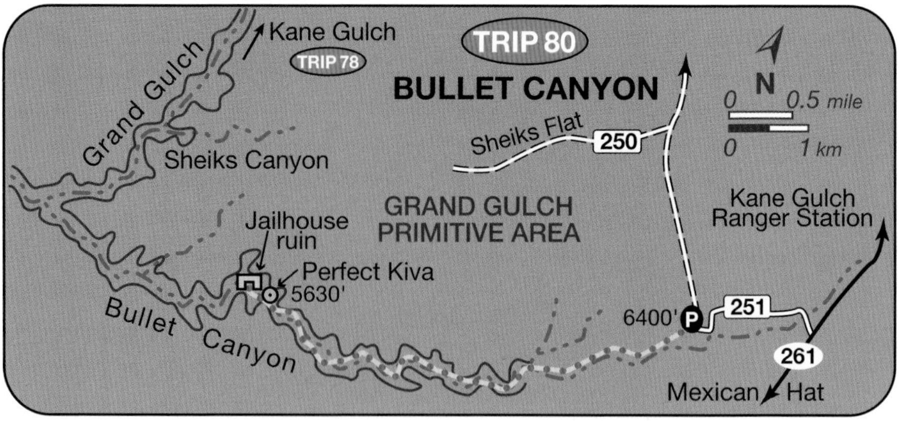

right (west). Follow cairns down a slickrock cascade. Bypass a small pouroff via the right (north) wall.

Below the pouroff, about 45 minutes from the trailhead, avoid the boulder-choked wash by contouring along a high ledge (right / north). Beyond, you must negotiate the wash—a maelstrom of boulders and cobblestones. You can sometimes avoid the chaotic inner channel by ascending the dirt slope (right / north).

The way forward, still generally west, remains challenging for about 35 minutes. You then get a reprieve but must tunnel through riparian thickets (reeds, horsetail, etc.)

At 6000 ft (1829 m), after hiking about 1¼ hours, pass another **tributary drainage** (left / southeast). Bear right (west) to proceed down-canyon. Seven minutes farther, at 5660 ft (1726 m), the wash is smooth, firm sand. Finally, the hiking is easy. The canyon curves right (northwest).

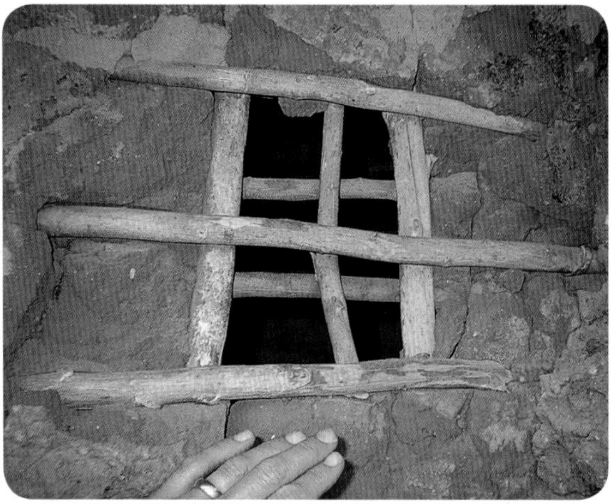
Juniper window in Jailhouse Ruin

About two hours along, look right (north-northeast) for the south-facing alcove protecting **Perfect Kiva** at 4.5 mi (7.2 km), 5630 ft (1716 m). Ten minutes farther, at 4.75 mi (7.6 km), **Jailhouse Ruin** is built into small ledges on the canyon's right (north) wall.

Ahead, the canyon jogs left (south) then curves right and continues generally northwest to intersect **Grand Gulch** at 7.25 mi (11.7 km), 5340 ft (1628 m).

TRIP 81

FIRST FORK SLICKHORN CANYON

LOCATION	Cedar Mesa, west of Hwy 261
LOOP	8.8 mi (14.2 km) to Third Fork
ELEVATION CHANGE	670-ft (204-m) loss and gain
KEY ELEVATIONS	First Fork trailhead 6100 ft (1860 m) Third Fork confluence 5430 ft (1655 m)
HIKING TIME	3½ to 4½ hours
DIFFICULTY	moderate
MAPS	Trails Illustrated *Grand Gulch Plateau* USGS *Pollys Pasture, Slickhorn Canyon East*

OPINION

Throw yourself into a canyon.

It sounds ominous. And 45 minutes beyond First Fork trailhead, it looks as ominous as it sounds. You arrive at a pouroff, and the shallow wash you've been walking suddenly falls away into the abyss of Slickhorn Canyon.

The view is dizzying—well worth the walk even if you don't continue into the canyon. But equally startling is the fact that you *can* continue into the depths without it being your final, fatal leap.

The Slickhorn Canyon complex rivals nearby Grand Gulch for beauty and intrigue. The dreamscape walls of Slickhorn could have inspired Andreas Vollenweider's seminal recording *Caverna Magica*. And the ancient ones left much for us to discover and admire here. Dwellings and rock art are abundant. Below the First Fork pouroff, for example, is a pristine kiva.

But Slickhorn is smaller than Grand Gulch and poses more challenge to hikers, so it's neither as famous nor as popular and thus offers more solitude.

Of the many ways to explore Slickhorn, a simple in-and-out round trip starting at First Fork trailhead is the easiest. Bear in mind, however, the entire Slickhorn complex is rugged and largely trail-less.

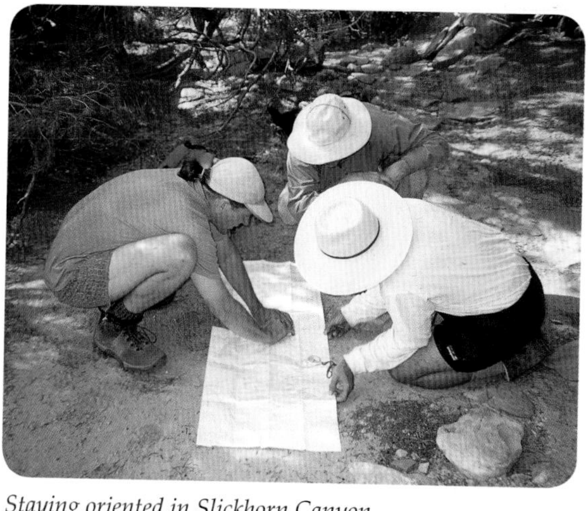

Staying oriented in Slickhorn Canyon

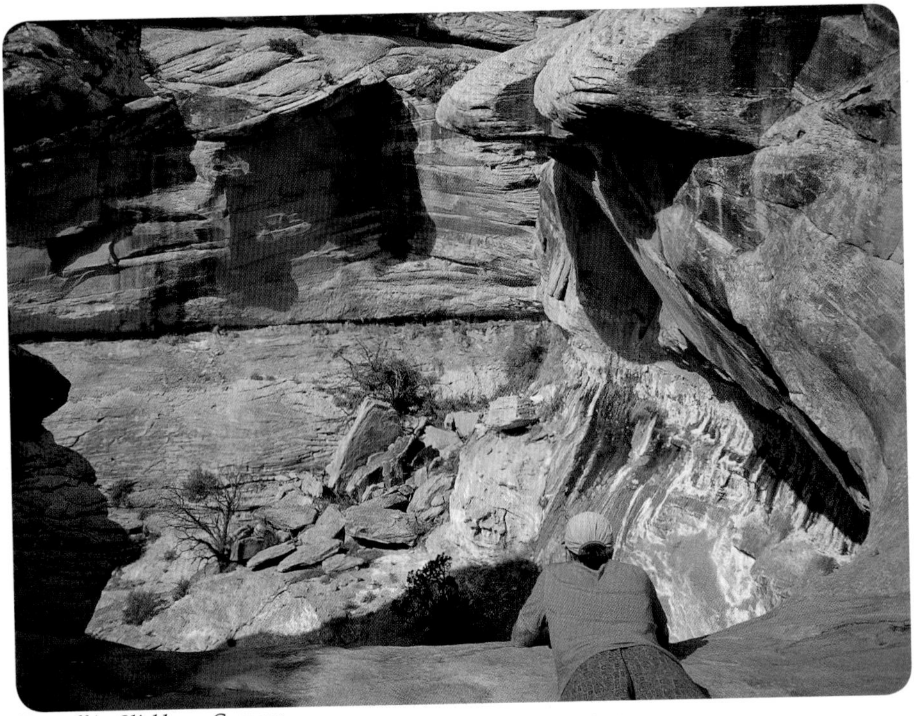
Pouroff in Slickhorn Canyon

Entering via First Fork, you'll encounter steep terrain, slickrock friction pitches, and vertiginous ledges. You'll simply face less routefinding than is necessary elsewhere in Slickhorn, for example along the loop comprising Third and Trail forks (Trip 82). A half-day Slickhorn sampler appeals to you? Over the edge you go at First Fork.

FACT

BY VEHICLE

From the junction of Hwys 95 and 261, drive Hwy 261 south 3.8 mi (6.2 km) to Kane Gulch Ranger Station. Reset your trip odometer to 0. Continue south. At 9.7 mi (15.6 km), just north of milepost 19, turn right (west) onto Road 245. Again reset your trip odometer to 0. At 0.4 mi (0.6 km) pass the BLM iron ranger and proceed through a gate. At 2.6 mi (4.2 km) fork left (southwest) onto Road 203. At 4.3 mi (6.9 km) fork right (west). Reach the First Fork Slickhorn trailhead at 4.7 mi (7.6 km), 6100 ft (1860 m).

ON FOOT

From the trail register at the top of First Fork, follow the shallow, sand-and-slickrock drainage southwest. In about 15 minutes, hop down a 4-ft (1.2-m) pouroff or bypass it on the left. Pass a tributary drainage (left / east). Continue down the wash, gradually curving right (west).

The next mile is easy walking over gentle sandstone cascades and slickrock slabs. About 20 minutes along, pass a small ruin beneath an overhang (right / north).

At 1.7 mi (2.7 km), 5860 ft (1787 m), about 45 minutes from the trailhead, reach a major **pouroff**. Visible below is the bona fide canyon: 300 to 400 ft (91 to 122 m) deep. Pick up the path starting above the pouroff. It ascends left (south). Proceed up two, short, slickrock friction pitches to a prominent **ledge**. Follow the ledge south.

While on the ledge, note the sandstone monolith on the opposite wall, about 0.3 mi (0.5 km) down-canyon from the pouroff. The descent route ahead reaches the canyon floor in that vicinity. The ledge also grants you a view of (a) a small ruin near the rim of the tributary drainage north of the pouroff, and (b) an alcove harboring a well-preserved kiva halfway up the opposite wall, 220 yd / 200 m down-canyon from the monolith. Identifying that alcove now will help you reach the kiva later.

Resume south along the ledge into a **cove**. Curving right (southwest) out of the cove, be alert for cairns and bootbeaten path. The sharp descent route into the canyon begins here, at 2 mi (3.2 km).

Navigate the ledges and steep slickrock with the aid of cairns and snippets of bootbeaten path. If safe passage appears to end, retreat and observe until the way forward is apparent. After working your way down the first two obvious ledges, the route contours left (south) to a discreet break in the cliff band below. Continue descending cautiously.

Bottom-out in **Slickhorn Canyon** at 2.3 mi (3.7 km), 5600 ft (1707 m). Turn left and follow the bouldery wash down-canyon, generally southwest.

Within seven minutes, look for a path ascending right (north) to the aforementioned **alcove** harboring a well-preserved, 700-year-old kiva. It's fragile and invaluable. Treat it reverently. Leave no trace of your visit.

Beyond the alcove, Slickhorn Canyon becomes less rocky. A path soon appears and progress is easier. After curving left (south) pass **Second Fork** (left / east) at 4 mi (6.4 km). Look for ruins on opposite sides of the main canyon here. You'll also find viable campsites at this confluence.

Where the main canyon veers right (west) at 4.4 mi (7.1 km), 5430 ft (1655 m), reach **Third Fork** (left / east). Retrace your steps back to First Fork trailhead. Trip 82 describes a loop comprising Third and Trail forks.

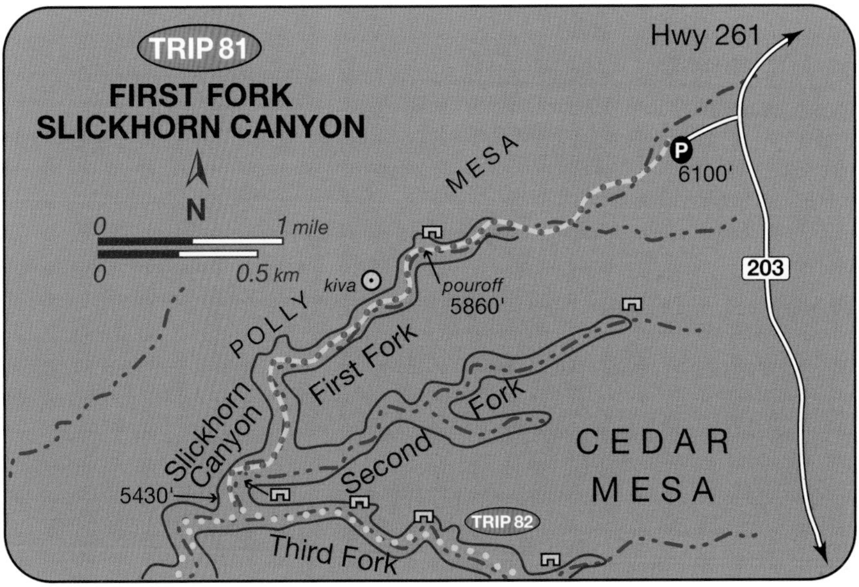

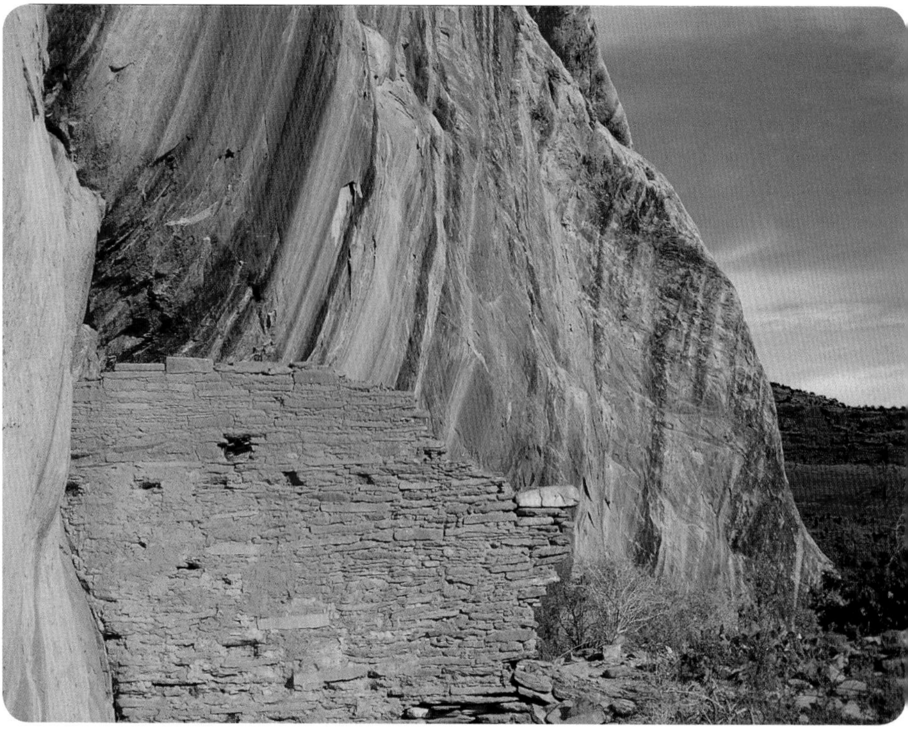

Ruins in Slickhorn Canyon

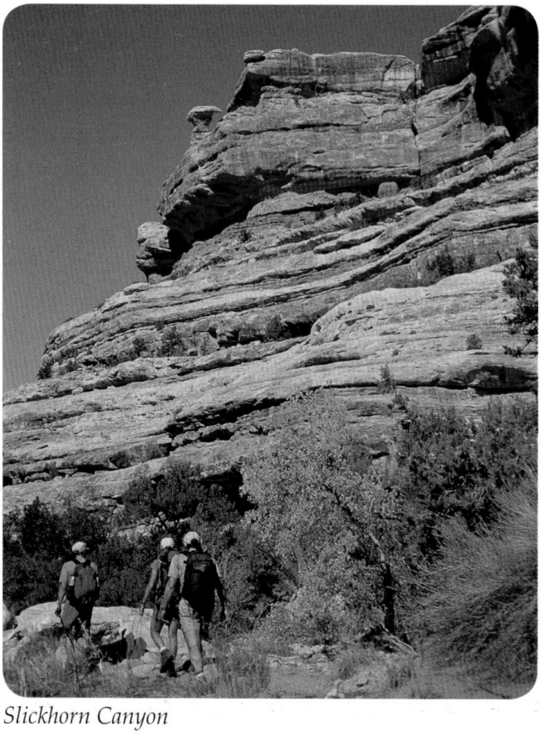

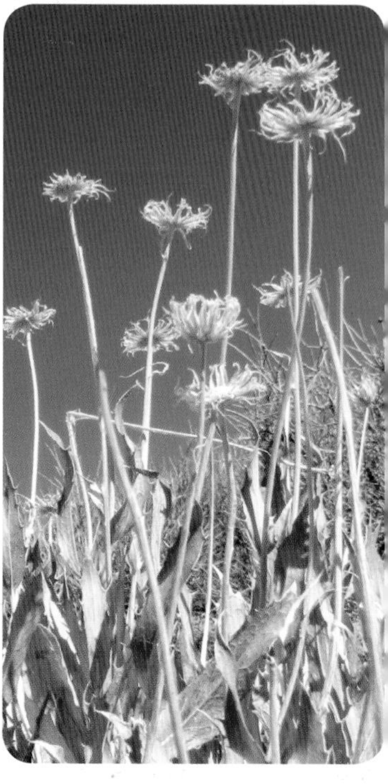

Slickhorn Canyon

TRIP 83

ROAD CANYON

LOCATION	Cedar Mesa, east of Hwy 261
ROUND TRIP	8 mi (12.9 km), or 3 mi (4.8 km) for Seven Kivas shortcut
ELEVATION CHANGE	800-ft (244-m) loss and gain, or 400-ft (122-m) loss and gain for Seven Kivas shortcut
KEY ELEVATIONS	trailhead 6400 ft (1951 m), Seven Kivas shortcut traihead 6000 ft (1829 m), Seven Kivas 5600 ft (1707 m)
HIKING TIME	6 hours, or 1½ hours for Seven Kivas shortcut
DIFFICULTY	moderate
MAPS	Trails Illustrated *Grand Gulch Plateau* USGS *Snow Flat Spring Cave, Cigarette Spring Cave*

OPINION

Road Canyon, like neighboring Lime Canyon, invites you to romp. Come here to sample Cedar Mesa on a short, fun, athletic dayhike.

Access is quick and easy. The canyon is trail-less but allows you to contour long distances on scenic ledges well above the canyon floor. It's a refreshing change from nearby Grand Gulch, where backpackers follow the wash-bottom most of the way, often thrashing through riparian thickets.

The primary difference between Road and Lime is that Road offers a specific, compelling destination: Seven Kivas ruin.

A kiva, of course, is a subterranean ceremonial chamber. Kivas have been central to Native spiritual tradition since ancient times. But a single kiva served several families. So a group of seven kivas suggests Road Canyon was distinctly sacred.

The absence of large dwelling sites in Road Canyon, and the lack of dwellings adjacent to Seven Kivas, suggest Natives residing elsewhere on Cedar Mesa gathered here for momentous ritual ceremonies. It's intriguing to imagine. Unfortunately, you'll also have to use your imagination when admiring the kivas.

The structures are perhaps eight centuries old, and they look it. This is literally an archaeological *ruin*. That's because, oddly, it's located in a very shallow alcove, thus

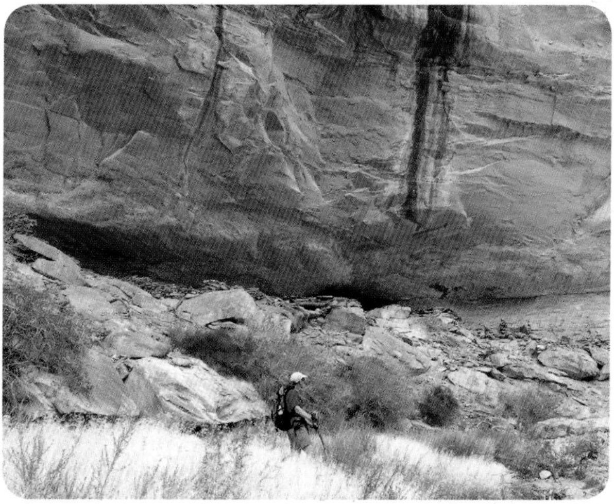

Beneath Seven Kivas, Road Canyon

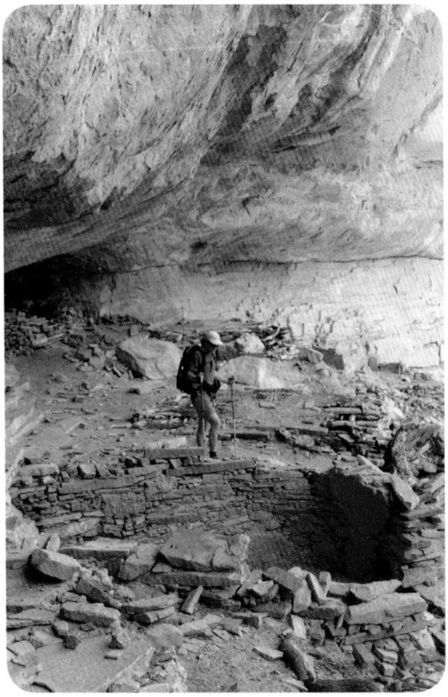
The best preserved of the Seven Kivas

exposed to the full brunt of the weather. Maybe the clustered kivas represent a hasty, last-ditch effort to elicit divine intervention in whatever calamity soon forced the ancient ones to abandon Cedar Mesa and all of the Colorado Plateau.

But hiking Road Canyon would be worthwhile even without the kivas. Granaries and small ruins are visible en route. The deep canyon itself is engaging, and finding your way around the pouroffs and along the ledges makes it more so. Anyone accustomed to defined trails, however, might be unnerved by the freelance nature of this trip.

Ideally, don't fixate on Seven Kivas ruin. Shoot for it, but appreciate the canyon along the way. Or, if your tractor beam is locked onto the famous ruin, and you want to get there fast, opt for the shortcut route described below. You'll miss most of Road Canyon, but you'll reach the kivas in about 45 minutes. Make that just over an hour if you lack a vehicle with sufficient clearance to drive the final, rough section of road to the shortcut trailhead.

Whichever way you arrive at Seven Kivas ruin, allow time to sit and ponder its significance. Ancestral Puebloan spirituality is a mystery, but here's a solid fact that might serve as a mental foothold. In the floor of every kiva is a small hole or depression. The Hopis call it a *sipapu*. It symbolizes the portal through which the original humans first entered the world. It also serves as a reminder of our earthly origins.

FACT

BY VEHICLE

From the junction of Hwys 95 and 261, drive Hwy 261 south 3.8 mi (6.2 km) to Kane Gulch Ranger Station. Reset your trip odometer to 0 at the ranger station and drive south on Hwy 261.

At 9.7 mi (15.6 km), just north of milepost 19, turn left (east) onto Cigarette Spring Road 239. Again reset your trip odometer to 0.

At 0.9 mi (1.5 km) pass the BLM iron ranger. At 1.3 mi (2.1 km) proceed straight, ignoring a left (north) fork. At 3.3 mi (5.4 km) proceed straight, ignoring the right (south) fork to Lime Canyon. At 3.4 mi (5.5 km), go left to reach the Road Canyon trailhead parking area. Elevation: 6400 ft (1951 m).

For the Seven Kivas shortcut, continue driving the main road east. Cross a wash at 5.6 mi (9 km). Just 30 yd/m ahead is a left (north) spur. Park there unless you have a high-clearance vehicle. Follow the main road 330 yd (300 m) farther—about a six-minute walk—then fork left (north). In another 0.8 mi (1.3 km)—

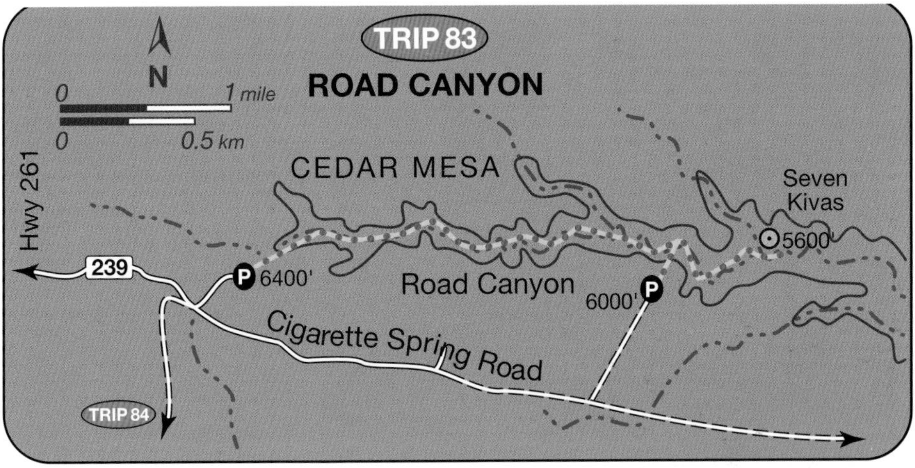

about a 13-minute walk—reach the road's end trailhead at the edge of an east-west draw. Total distance from Hwy 261: 6.5 mi (10.5 km). Elevation: 6000 ft (1829 m). Skip below for the Seven Kivas shortcut *On Foot* directions.

ON FOOT

The trail descends northeast through P-J forest (piñon and juniper). In about eight minutes, reach the **rim of Road Canyon** at 6320 ft (1927 m). Drop into the dry wash, following cairns.

Hiking down-canyon, your general direction of travel will remain east all the way to the Seven Kivas. About 15 minutes along, proceed across slickrock slabs. Soon step down through willows at a minor **pouroff**. The wash is sandy and brushy.

About 25 minutes from the trailhead, encounter a cottonwood in the wash. Look ahead (east). A ruin is visible midway up the far canyon wall. A few minutes farther, at 6150 ft (1875 m), go left up the slickrock to another ruin.

Where the canyon bends left (northeast), about 45 minutes along, a trail is evident. Two minutes farther, ruins are visible two-thirds of the way up the wall.

At one hour, near 6020 ft (1835 m), study the northeast wall for a granary in a shallow depression. Seven minutes farther, bear right, ignoring a tributary drainage on the left.

The canyon is now much deeper. About 1¾ hours along, at 5830 ft (1777 m), stay on the right (south) bench to bypass a **pouroff**. Several minutes farther, bypass a **pouroff** via the second ledge above its left side.

Pass a tributary drainage, then reach another **pouroff** nearly two hours from the trailhead. Bypass it via the ledge on the right, contouring about 100 ft (30 m) above the canyon floor. A ruin is visible north, across the canyon, at nearly the same height as your ledge.

About 2½ hours along, descend to the slickrock below at 5700 ft (1738 m). Pass a tributary drainage (left / northwest). A large alcove here harbors no ruins. Round a point distinguished by a bulbous pillar. Directly ahead (north), just above head height, are the disheveled circles of the **Seven Kivas** in a shallow alcove at 4 mi (6.4 km), 5600 ft (1707 m), about three hours from the trailhead.

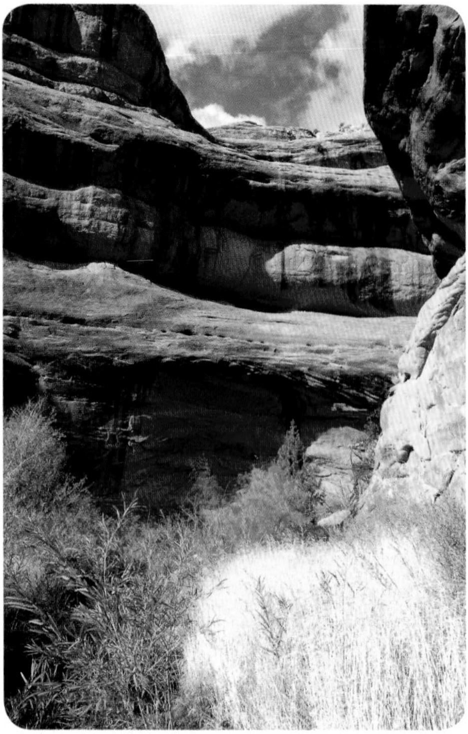

Road Canyon

About ten minutes farther down-canyon is a pouroff. Look right, above the nearby boulders, for a petroglyph panel on a black-stained rock. It bears a dozen figures. To continue exploring Road Canyon, bypass the pouroff via the ledge on the right (south) wall.

Seven Kivas Shortcut

From the shortcut trailhead, at 6000 ft (1829 m), a cairned route departs the south side of the east-west draw. Follow cairns north, dropping 20 ft (6 m) into the draw.

Cross above a pouroff, head east, and round the point. Work your way down slickrock. Resume on bootbeaten path. Watch for cairns. Ledges allow a reasonably comfortable descent. About 20 minutes from the shortcut trailhead, bottom-out in **Road Canyon wash** at 5650 ft (1722 m). Bear right to proceed down-canyon, generally east.

Pass a tributary drainage (left / northwest). A large alcove here harbors no ruins. Round a point distinguished by a bulbous pillar. Directly ahead (north), just above head height, are the disheveled circles of the **Seven Kivas** in a shallow alcove at 5600 ft (1707 m), about 45 minutes from the shortcut trailhead.

About ten minutes farther down-canyon is a pouroff. Look right, above the nearby boulders, for a petroglyph panel on a black-stained rock. It bears a dozen figures. To continue exploring Road Canyon, bypass the pouroff via the ledge on the right (south) wall.

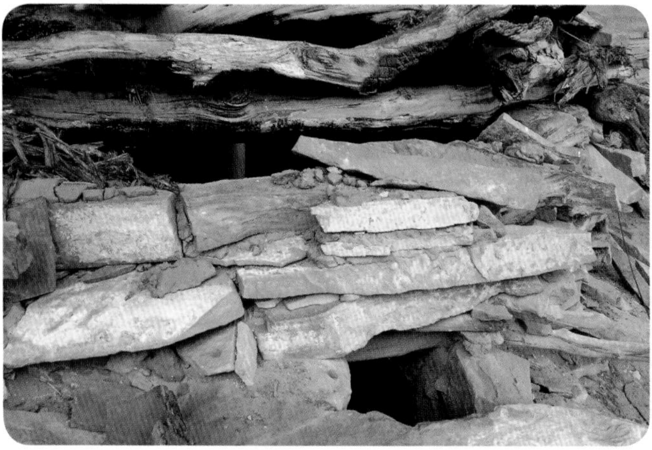

TRIP 84

LIME CANYON

LOCATION	Cedar Mesa, east of Hwy 261
ROUND TRIP	4 mi (6.4 km) for ledge route or up to 15 mi (24 km) for wash route
ELEVATION CHANGE	500-ft (152-m) loss and gain for ledge route or up to 1200-ft (366-m) loss and gain for wash route
KEY ELEVATIONS	trailhead 6400 ft (1951 m) north-wall ledges 6000 ft (1829 m) four alcoves 5900 ft (1799 m) impassable pouroff 5200 ft (1585 m)
HIKING TIME	2 hours for ledge route, or up to 7 hours for wash route
DIFFICULTY	easy ledge route, moderate wash route
MAPS	Trails Illustrated *Grand Gulch Plateau*, USGS *Snow Flat Spring Cave, Cigarette Spring Cave*

OPINION

After washing a down sleeping bag (an arduous task best avoided as long as possible), you should put it in a clothes dryer on low heat. When the bag's no longer sodden, it helps to add several clean tennis balls to the dryer. The balls jostle apart the clumps of wet down and fluff them up.

Walking serves the same purpose for people that tennis balls do for wet down bags. When our thoughts lie heavy in our brains like sodden clumps, walking jostles them apart and fluffs them up. That's because walking quickly exposes us to the accidental, unexpected, random, unfiltered.

But it helps to walk in new, strange places. And when you're walking without a destination, all the better.

For most of us, canyon country is as new and strange as it gets. And on Cedar Mesa, Lime Canyon offers no destination of note.

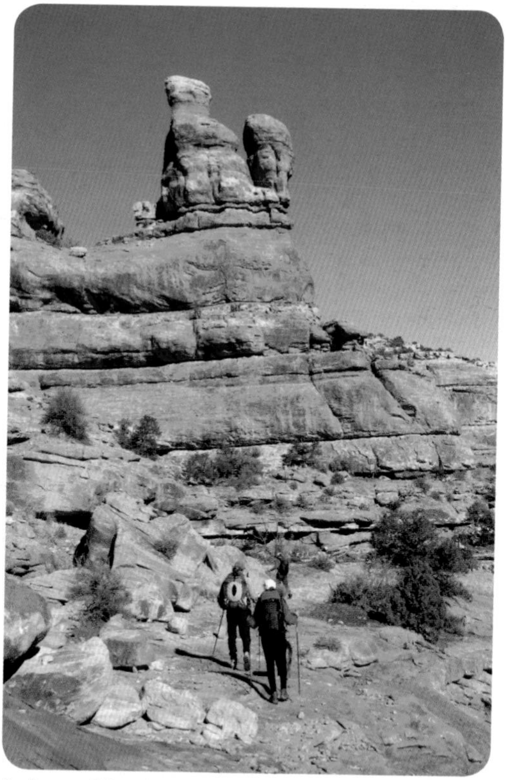

Ledge walking in Lime Canyon

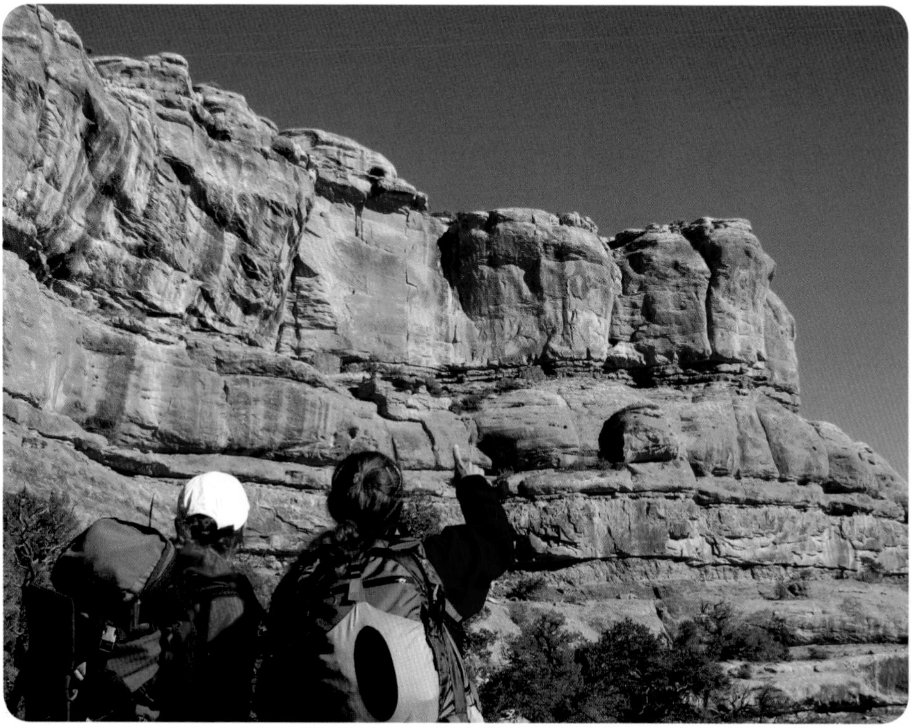

Locating ruins, Lime Canyon

It's simply a wild, lonely, beautiful, stimulating place to enjoy a walk that will jostle and fluff up your thoughts.

As in nearby Road Canyon, there's no trail here. You'll be freelancing, either along ledges or down the wash. The ledge route is shorter and less strenuous—a good choice for a couple-hour ramble. The wash route can keep you entertained for most of a day, or less.

Stay on the ledges if you've had your fill of the riparian jungles that flourish in many canyons, like Grand Gulch. Lime isn't that shaggy, however, so follow the wash if you're keen to go long and deep. Numerous small, Ancestral Puebloan ruins are visible on both routes.

Either way, you can see most of Lime Canyon before sunset, which is great, because you really don't want to get your down bag dirty.

FACT

BY VEHICLE

From the junction of Hwys 95 and 261, drive Hwy 261 south 3.8 mi (6.2 km) to Kane Gulch Ranger Station. Reset your trip odometer to 0 at the ranger station and drive south on Hwy 261.

At 9.7 mi (15.6 km), just north of milepost 19, turn left (east) onto Cigarette Spring Road 239. Again reset your trip odometer to 0.

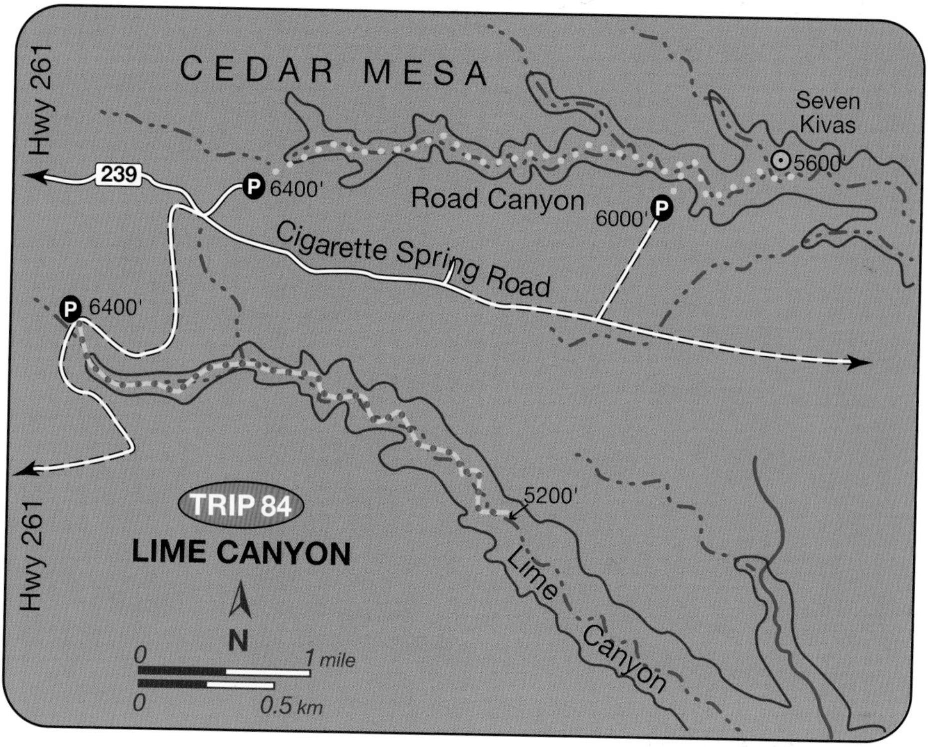

At 0.9 mi (1.5 km) pass the BLM iron ranger. At 1.3 mi (2.1 km) proceed straight, ignoring a left (north) fork. At 3.3 mi (5.4 km), the right (south) fork leads to Lime Canyon but requires a high-clearance vehicle. If you prefer to walk this final approach, drive a minute farther on the main road, then go left and park at the trailhead for Road Canyon (Trip 83).

Continuing the drive? At 5.1 mi (8.2 km), 6400 ft (1951 m), the road abruptly curves left (south) and crosses a small, rough wash. This is the tail of Lime Canyon. Park near here, wherever there's room to tuck your vehicle off the road.

ON FOOT

Enter the wash, turn left (east), and gradually drop into the canyon.

Ledge Route

After the initial descent into Lime Canyon, it becomes evident that you can, by bearing left, opt to hike along the left (north) wall, above the wash. Just keep contouring generally southeast, mostly on slickrock, following a surprisingly long, very accommodating system of ledges. Watch for south-facing ruins. About an hour along, attain a distant view down-canyon. Ahead, the ledge walking becomes more challenging, but it's possible to carry on.

Wash Route

Keep descending into Lime Canyon via the wash. Head generally southeast. Encounter several pouroffs that pose no difficulty. Pass a tributary drainage (left / north) about 45 minutes along. After hiking 1½ hours, pass a tributary drainage (left / north) opposite an amphitheater (right / south). A double hoodoo pinnacle is visible here, at 5900 ft (1799 m). Proceed five minutes farther down-canyon to where four, inaccessible alcoves are within view. Each harbors ancient structures. Explorers can keep following Lime Canyon until reaching an impassable, 30-ft (9-m) pouroff at 5200 ft (1585 m), about 3½ hours from the trailhead.

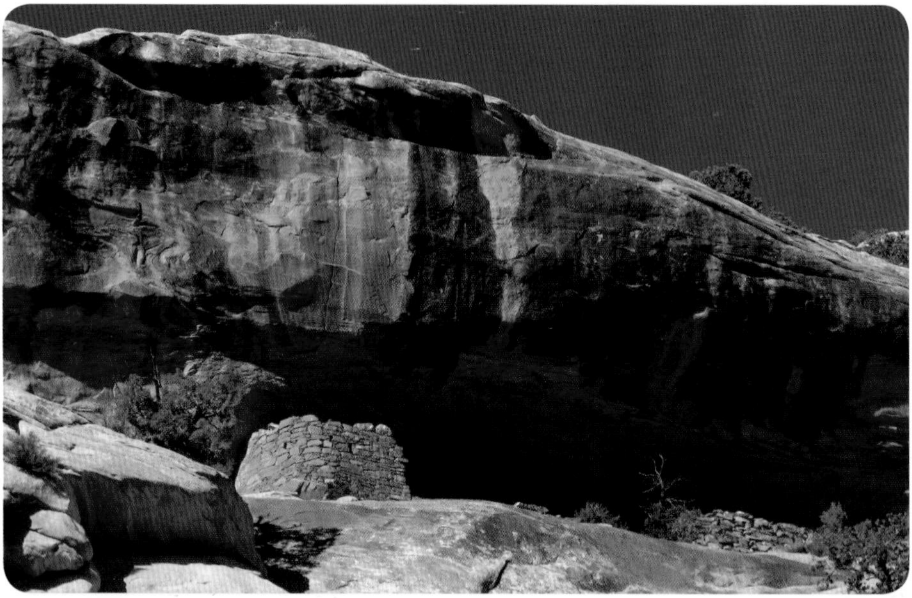

Lime Canyon ruins

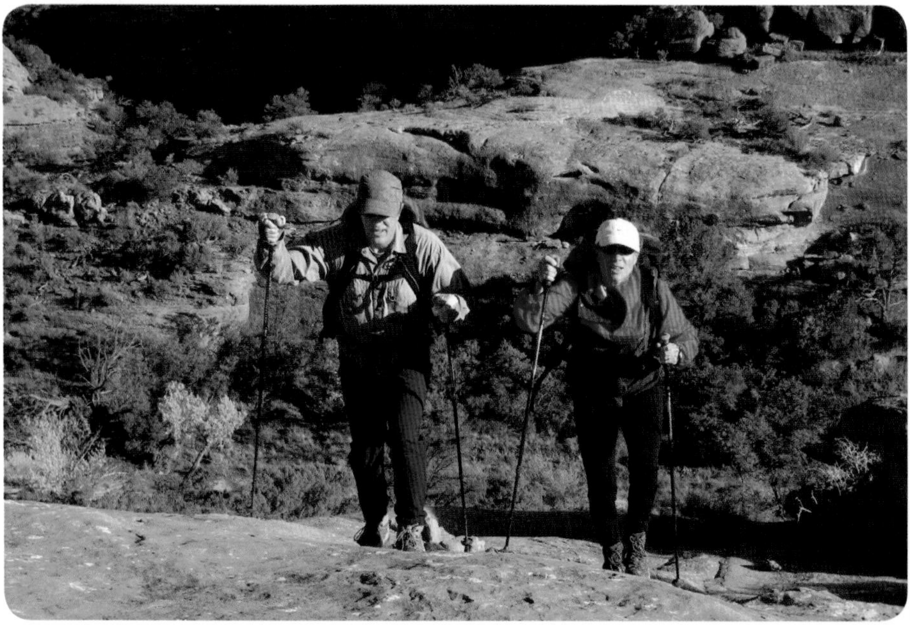

TRIP 85

HONAKER TRAIL

LOCATION	northwest of Mexican Hat
ROUND TRIP	8 mi (12.9 km) from water-tank trailhead
ELEVATION CHANGE	1244-ft (379-m) loss and gain
KEY ELEVATIONS	water-tank trailhead 5126 ft (1563 m) canyon-rim trailhead 5160 ft (1573 m) Horn Point 4520 ft (1378 m) San Juan River 3950 ft (1204 m)
HIKING TIME	3½ to 4 hours
DIFFICULTY	moderate
MAP	USGS *The Goosenecks*

OPINION

We're drawn to mystery. Forging into terra incognita titillates us. That's one of the appeals of hiking. It's full-body contact with the unknown.

That's also why the view from the Honaker trailhead might compel you *not* to hike: there appears to be no mystery ahead.

You can see your destination—the San Juan River—in the canyon bottom far below. You can see both walls of the canyon, upstream and down.

But what you cannot see—and this is the mystery that, should you step off the canyon rim and begin the descent, will likely compel you to keep hiking to the very nadir—is the miraculous trail itself.

Built to service gold placer claims on the San Juan River, the trail was a one-year construction project supervised by stage coach owner Henry Honaker and completed in June 1894.

The first horse to set hoof on the trail, however, fell to its death near Horn Point. No pack animal every completed the round trip, and the mines proved unprofitable.

Don't let that scare you. Despite the precipitous topography, hiking here is surprisingly safe. The trail is excellent: distinct and comfortably broad all the way to the river. Stay en route, and you'll face no exposure.

Expect to complete the descent in about one hour, all the while enjoying the unfolding mystery of just how in the hell Honaker's gonna get you down to the river. Ascending back to the canyon rim also takes about an hour.

Deep in the abyss, the silence is exquisite. Quickly putting what feels like a great distance between you and any sign of civilization is soothing. Though the trip requires only half a day, camping beside the river at trail's end is an inviting possibility.

The Honaker trail is near the bottom of the Moqui Dugway—the graded, unpaved stretch of Hwy 261 sinuously climbing 1200 ft (366 m) in 3 mi (4.8 m) to the top of Cedar Mesa. So consider hiking here on your way to or from the mesa.

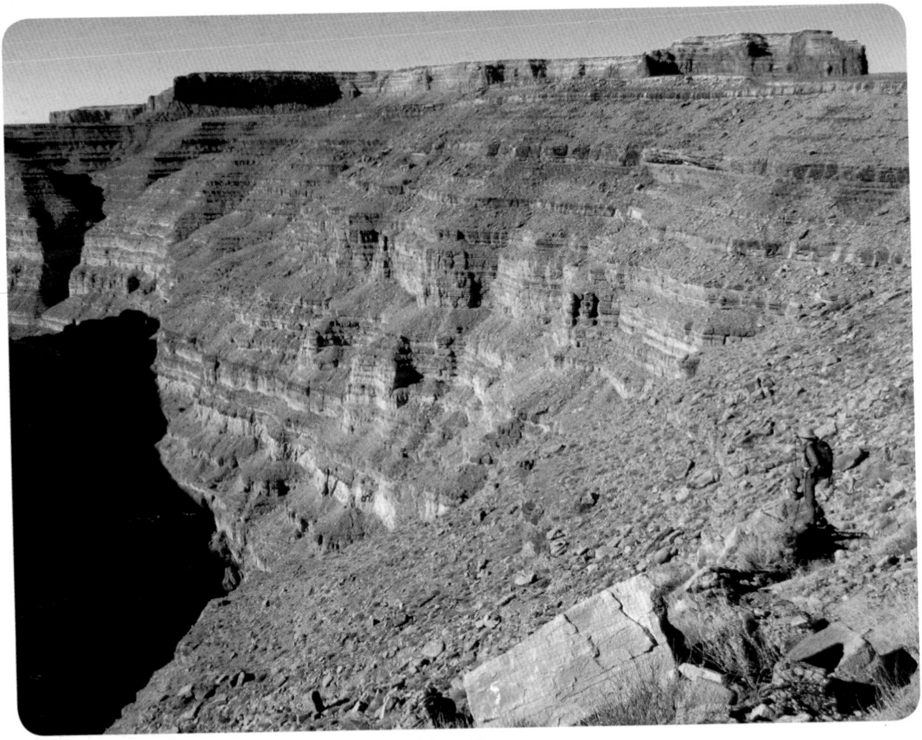

The Honaker trail descends into San Juan River Canyon.

Also nearby is Goosenecks State Park, where you can drive to the edge of the San Juan River Canyon. At the overlook, you'll see the river, 1500 ft (457 m) below, traveling six, serpentine miles to proceed just 1 mi (1.6 km) west. But there's no trail there. The state park is for peepers; the Honaker trail is for leapers.

FACT

BY VEHICLE

From Cedar Mesa, drive Hwy 261 south. Reset your trip odometer to 0 at the Muley Point turnoff, then begin a steep, switchbacking descent of the unpaved Moqui Dugway. Pavement resumes below. At 8.7 mi (14 km) turn right (southwest) for Goosenecks State Park.

From the junction of Hwys 163 and 261 (4 mi / 6.4 km north of Mexican Hat, or 19 mi / 30.6 km southwest of Bluff), turn west onto Hwy 261. Proceed 0.9 mi (1.4 km) then turn left (southwest) for Goosenecks State Park.

From either approach, continue only 0.5 mi (0.8 km), then turn right (northwest) onto an unpaved spur. The paved road quickly leads southwest to the state park (camping, toilets, no water, no fee), on a promontory overlooking the San Juan River Canyon Goosenecks.

Follow the unpaved spur generally west another 2.5 mi (4 km) to a fork near a water tank. Park here, at 5126 ft (1563 m). Left (west) leads to the canyon rim, but is passable only in a high-clearance 4WD vehicle. Better to walk. It takes just 35 minutes at a brisk pace.

ON FOOT

Starting at the water-tank trailhead, you'll hike 2 mi (3.2 km) on the 4WD road to the canyon-rim trailhead, then 2 mi (3.2 km) down to the river.

Follow the 4WD road left (west). Cedar Mesa is prominently visible right (north). In about five minutes, at 0.6 mi (1 km), the road curves left (south).

Within 20 minutes, at 5230 ft (1595 m), where a flat area allows parking or camping, the road veers right (west). It drops sharply into a draw and is briefly rock strewn before curving south.

About 30 minutes along, at 5210 ft (1588 m), reach a T-junction near the canyon rim. Go left (south-southwest). The buttes and pinnacles of Monument Valley punctuate the western horizon.

A minute or so farther, abandon the road, step down a low slickrock ledge, and angle right (southwest) across gravel. Soon intersect a spur, turn right, and follow it right (west).

About 35 minutes from the water-tank trailhead, reach the **canyon-rim trailhead** at 2 mi (3.2 km), 5160 ft (1573 m). The trail descends left (south-southwest) from the large cairn.

From here on, precise directions are unnecessary and would only be confusing. There are no junctions. Just keep following the trail.

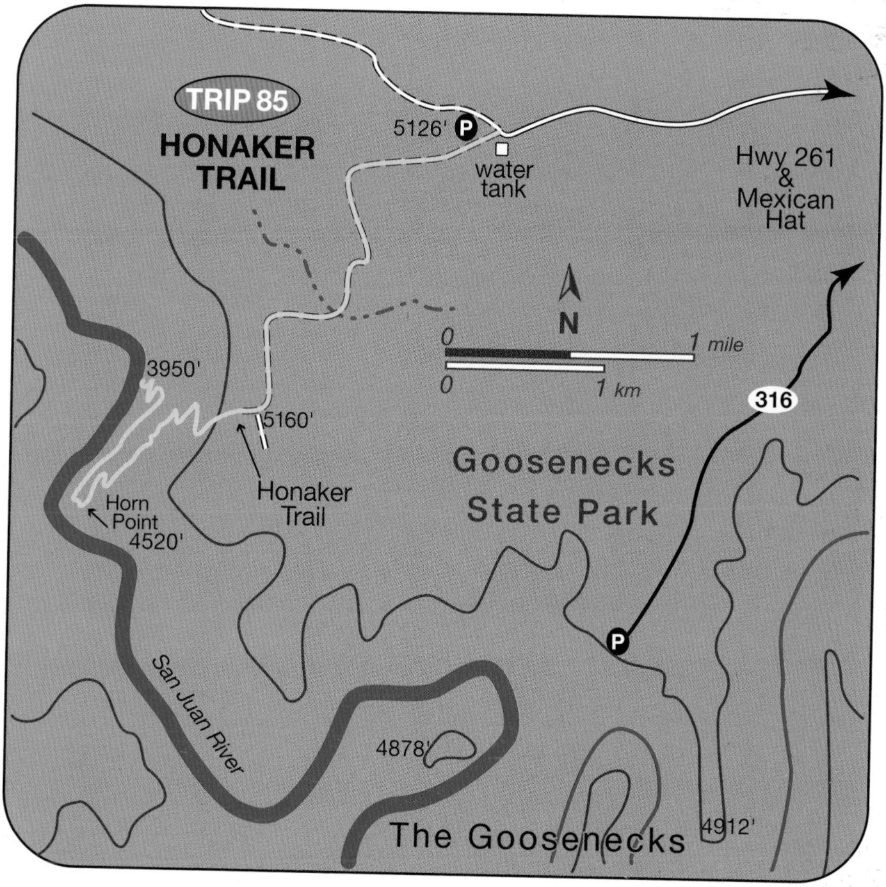

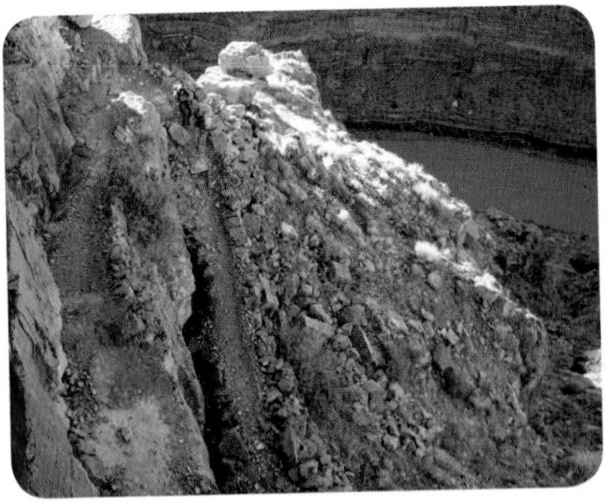

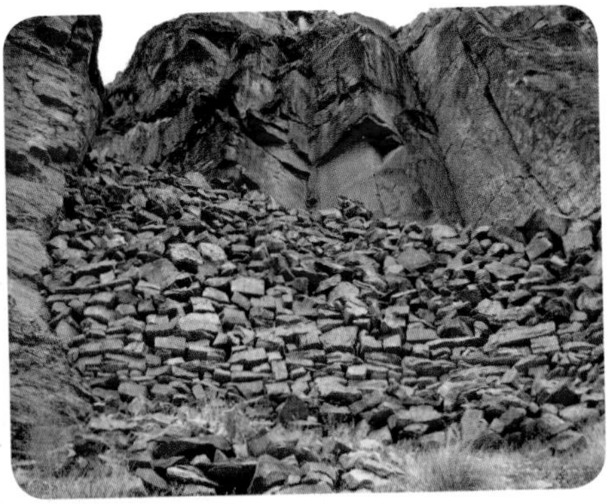

The ingeniously-constructed trail descends to the San Juan River.

The descent is steep and rocky only occasionally and briefly. Rarely is gymnastic effort required. Most of the way, you'll lose elevation very gradually, on long, sweeping switchbacks.

A little more than halfway down, at 4520 ft (1378 m), reach **Horn Point**—a flat-topped peninsula jutting into the canyon. The river is now audible.

At Horn Point, the trail drops suddenly but—thanks to marvelous trail construction—gently. For a short stretch, the trail is a mini **causeway** beside sheer rock.

On the switchbacks below, look up at the point. This was the crux of Honaker's enterprise. You'll see how he created an unlikely passage by meticulously stacking hundreds of boulders.

Above the point, the canyon walls were more gradually sloped and the sedimentary layers thinner. Beneath the point, you'll hike beside a much thicker layer of solid, vertical stone.

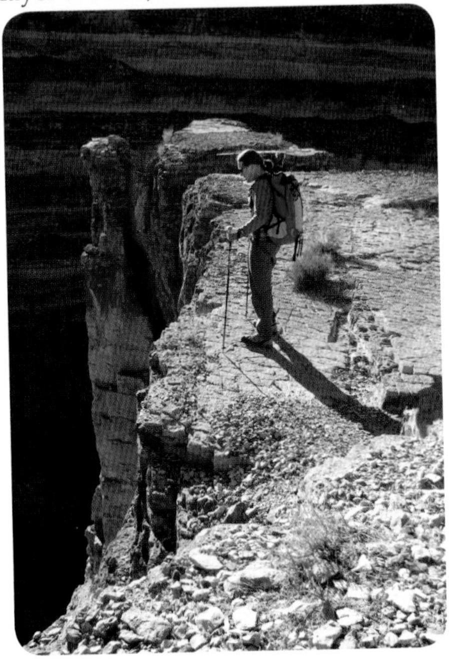

Horn Point

Resume on a lengthy switchback, contouring north at 4200 ft (1280 m). A broad stretch of sandy riverbank is visible below, up-canyon (south). After a long switchback in that direction, the terrain still doesn't allow a quick, direct descent. Several more long switchbacks remain.

Within one hour of departing the canyon rim, or about 1½ hours after departing the water tank, reach the **San Juan River** at 4 mi (6.4 km), 3950 ft (1204 m).

There's abundant flat ground for pitching a tent here. Willows and tamarisk flourish at the water's edge. Far down-river (north) is Lake Powell.

Strong dayhikers will complete the ascent to the canyon rim in one hour.

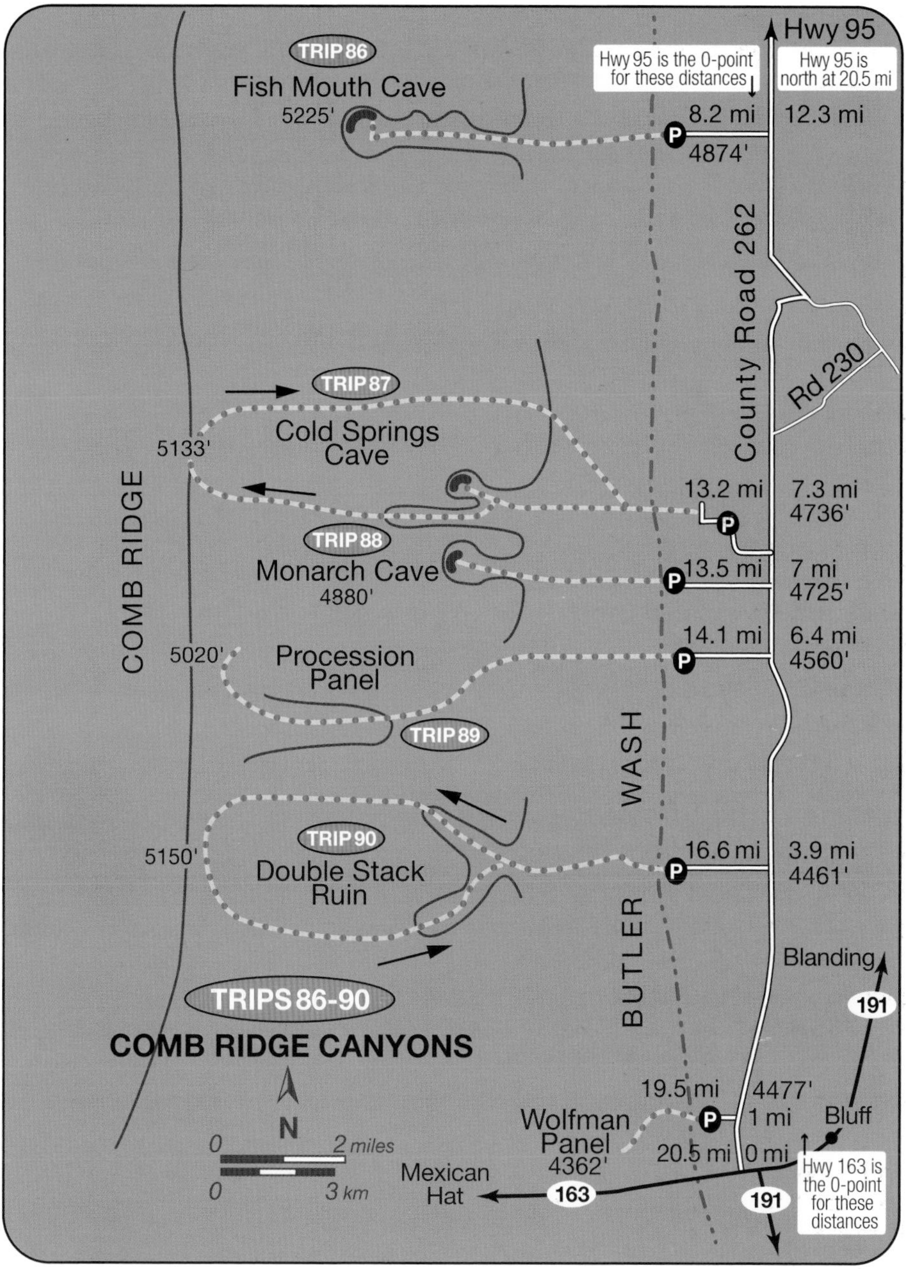

3.9 mi (6.3 km)
Left (west) are three forks. Of those, the two forks to the right (northwest) loop through the **Double Stack Ruin trailhead**, 30 yd/m distant, at 4461 ft (1360 m).

6.4 mi (10.3 km)
The left (west) fork leads 30 yd/m to **Procession Panel trailhead**, at 4560 ft (1390 m).

7 mi (11.3 km)
The left (west) fork leads 110 yd/100 m to **Monarch Cave** trailhead, beside cottonwoods, at 4725 ft (1440 m).

7.3 mi (11.8 km)
The left (west) fork leads a short distance to **Cold Springs Cave trailhead**, at 4736 ft (1444 m). Directly east is a brown-orange, white-topped promontory.

8.1 mi (13 km)
Proceed through a fence. Bear left on Road 262 where Road 230 forks right.

9.7 mi (15.6 km)
Reach a junction. Road 230 rejoins from the right. Proceed left on Road 262 and continue north.

12.3 mi (19.8 km)
Shortly before a fence are two left (west) forks that join and lead a short distance to **Fish Mouth Cave trailhead**, at 4874 ft (1486 m). Between the Fish Mouth forks and the fence, ignore the next pair of forks (left and right).

20.5 mi (33 km)
Intersect **Hwy 95**. The elevation here is 5335 ft (1626 m). Left ascends over Comb Ridge and continues west across Cedar Mesa. Right (east) intersects Hwy 191, just south of Blanding, in 9.5 mi (15.3 km).

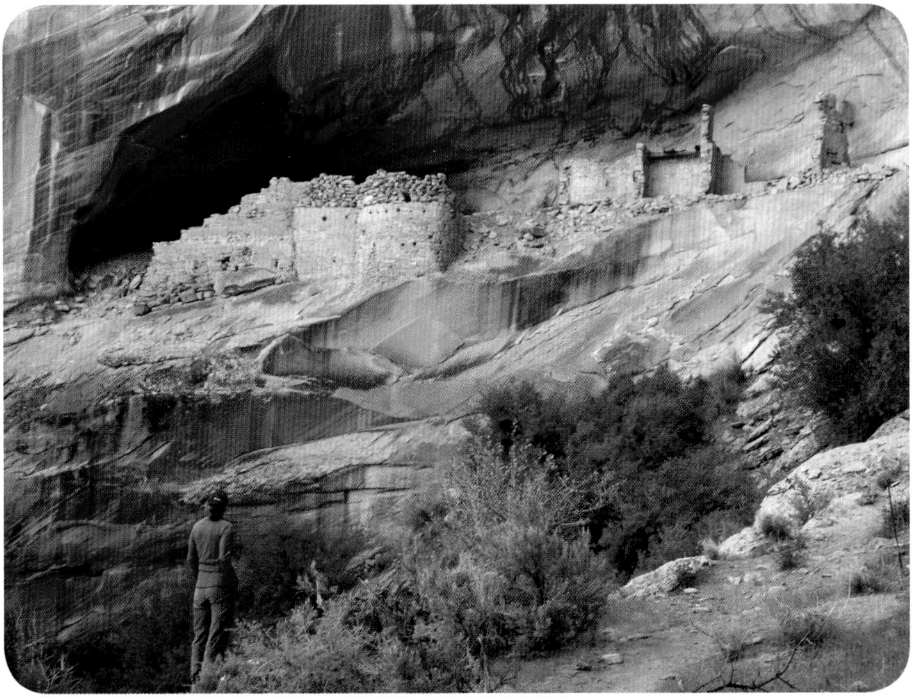

Monarch Cave

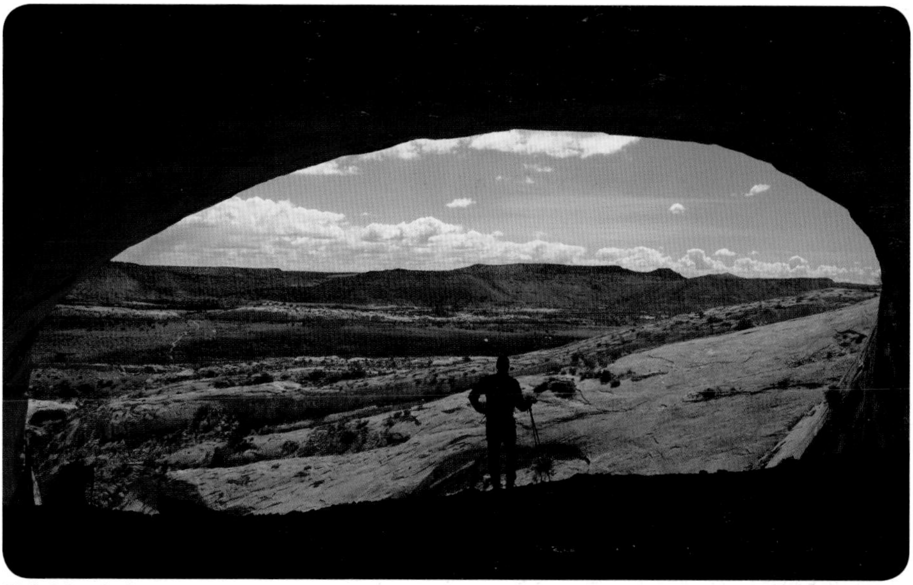

Fish Mouth Cave

ON FOOT

trip 86 Fish Mouth Cave hiking time 1½ hours
round trip 2 mi (3.2 km) elevation gain 351 ft (107 m)

From the parking area, Fish Mouth Cave is visible left (west). Follow the sandy road in that direction, beside the fence. Go left, past the "no vehicles" sign, but 10 yd/m farther abandon the road by turning right (west-northwest) onto a trail into the wash.

Soon opt for the trail on the right bank, along the broken rock. Pass a crumbling, **minor ruin** (right). Two minutes farther, cross bedrock. Follow the trail left (west) back into the wash and among cottonwoods.

Stay on the most prominent, boot-beaten trail—sometimes in the wash, other times along one of the banks. Keep hiking generally west.

One minute after the trail ascends between **slickrock arms** (about 20 minutes from the trailhead), ascend right (north) to a **minor ruin** under a deep overhang.

After resuming in the wash for a couple minutes, pass another minor ruin beneath an overhang. Two minutes farther, ascend a **slickrock crescent**. The small cave above (right) contains a minor ruin.

Your destination is visible at the head of the canyon. The final ascent is steep—first on slickrock, then on a sandy trail among boulders and talus. Favor the right (north) side of the draw.

Enter **Fish Mouth Cave** at 1 mi (1.6 km), 5225 ft (1593 m). The impressive grotto harbors little evidence of the ancient ones. Look for handprints (deep in, far right), tiny ruins, metates, corn cobs. What's spectacular here is the stupidity and irreverence of recent visitors who've desecrated the cave with graffiti.

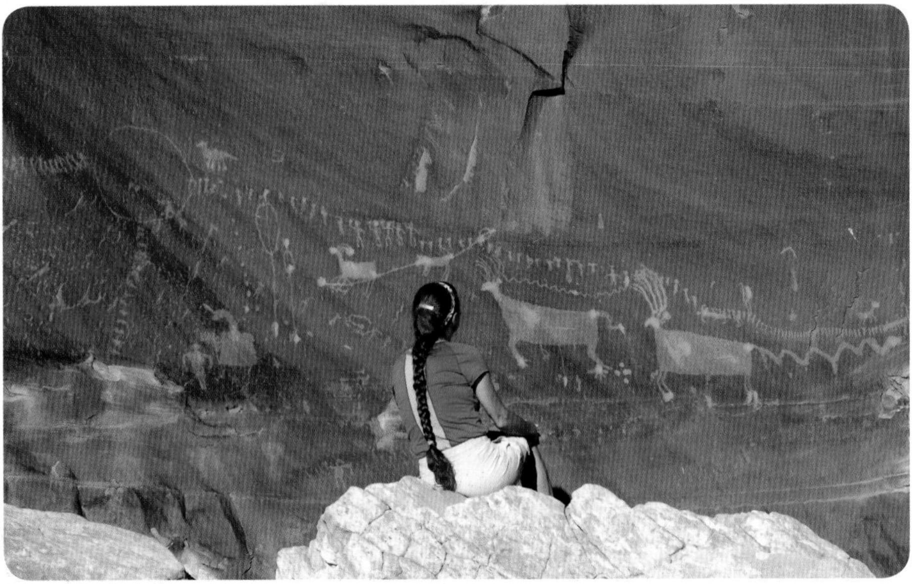

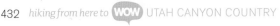

Procession Panel

trip 87 Cold Springs Cave hiking time 2 hours
circuit 3 mi (4.8 km) elevation gain 397 ft (121 m)

Your immediate destination is the low, prominent cave visible west. After probing the basin harboring the cave, you'll complete a clockwise circuit: hiking up the canyon immediately left (south) of the basin, surmounting the crest of Comb Ridge, then descending the canyon immediately right (north) of the basin.

The trailhead-access here is rough, perhaps requiring you to park shy of where the **spur road** now ends at a washout. After crossing the washout on foot, proceed west on what used to be the remainder of the spur. In another minute, the spur curves right (north). Just before the spur ends, go left onto trail.

The trail drops into a **double-channeled arroyo**, tunnels through tight vegetation, then surmounts the far bank. Continue directly west toward the dirt trail visible above the nearest slickrock outcrop. Beyond, the path continues in a wash.

About 15 minutes from the trailhead, reach a **small confluence** at 4790 ft (1460 m). Right (northwest) quickly enters Cold Springs basin. Left (west) is a narrow, sandstone defile through which you'll begin a clockwise circuit after returning from the cave.

For now, go right (northwest). Immediately ahead is a **minor pouroff**. Bypass it via the left (west) wall. Enter a slickrock basin and see **Cold Springs Cave** ahead. A spring drips in the recesses of the cave. Look for artistic and architectural evidence of the ancient ones along the upper, right wall of the basin.

Back at the **small confluence**, turn right (west). Hike through the **defile**. About six minutes along, a cairn guides you right, onto level slickrock. Where it peters in about four minutes, follow a faint path just left of the drainage, then resume on slickrock.

Right (northeast) are sheer, rose-and-buff walls. Aim for the gap visible north-northwest. About 20 minutes from the small confluence, top out near 5133 ft (1565 m) on the **crest of Comb Ridge**.

Descend right (east-southeast) into the **next canyon**. Bypass boulders via the left side of the drainage. A trail is soon evident. About one hour after leaving the small confluence, approach the **canyon mouth**. Just east of (beyond) a stand of cottonwoods, follow the trail right (southeast).

Hike east-southeast about 220 yd (200 m) to drop into the **double-channeled arroyo**. You're now on familiar ground. Upon emerging from the arroyo, go right on the spur road. The brown-orange, white-topped promontory directly east of the trailhead is a helpful landmark.

trip 88 Monarch Cave
round trip 2 mi (3.2 km)
hiking time 1 hour
elevation gain 157 ft (48 m)

From the south edge of the parking lot, the trail descends southwest into an **arroyo**. Hike west, beneath cottonwoods, across the broad wash. In a couple minutes, the trail surmounts the far bank and rises onto slickrock.

The trail is on the left (west) side of the **slickrock**, then drops left (south) into a wash. Proceed up-canyon: right (northwest).

At 20 minutes, 4829 ft (1472 m), ascend onto a slickrock bench. **Monarch Cave**, and the ruin it shelters, are visible west-southwest, about 165 yd (150 m) ahead. The structure is perched on a ledge at 4882 ft (1488 m). Below is a pool shrouded by vegetation. Above is a grand pouroff.

trip 89 Procession Panel
round trip 4 mi (6.4 km)
hiking time 3 hours
elevation gain 590 ft (180 m)

From the parking loop, the trail departs southwest. It quickly descends into a tamarisk-filled **arroyo**. Ascend the far bank, follow the briefly-level trail left (south-southwest), then drop into a **second arroyo**. At the bottom, go right for 30 seconds before angling left: up and out.

Follow the trail northwest across **sage flats** for about a minute, then drop into a **third arroyo**. This one has a small, exposed, slickrock reef in it. Go directly across this arroyo, ascend out, then ascend the sandy trail southwest.

Reach **slickrock** about 10 minutes from the trailhead. The trail remains evident—either boot-beaten into sand among scrub, or cairned across slickrock. It continues a gentle, westward ascent.

After hiking about 30 minutes, three distinct drainages are visible ahead. Proceed directly west, toward the middle one. Cairns should lead in that direction.

Ascend a **long, slickrock ramp**. To your right (north) the slope falls sharply to an impressive, sandstone bowl. At the top of the bowl is a great pouroff.

Continue the ramping ascent until, about 50 minutes from the trailhead, a steep-but-safe descending friction-walk is possible right (northwest). Bottom-out well above the lip of the great pouroff. You're now in the **middle drainage** you observed earlier.

Proceed generally west, following scraps of boot-beaten route through the **sandy wash**. Soon access an ascending, **slickrock ramp** on the right (north) side of the canyon. It leads north-northwest, past the pink and black, desert-varnished wall, to the farthest, west-facing prow.

That's where you'll find **Procession Panel**: on the right, at 2 mi (3.2 km), 5020 ft (1530 m), slightly more than an hour from the trailhead. It comprises 179 petroglyph figures. The site also affords a grand view. And if you ascend slightly higher, you'll attain a climactic panorama from the crest of **Comb Ridge**.

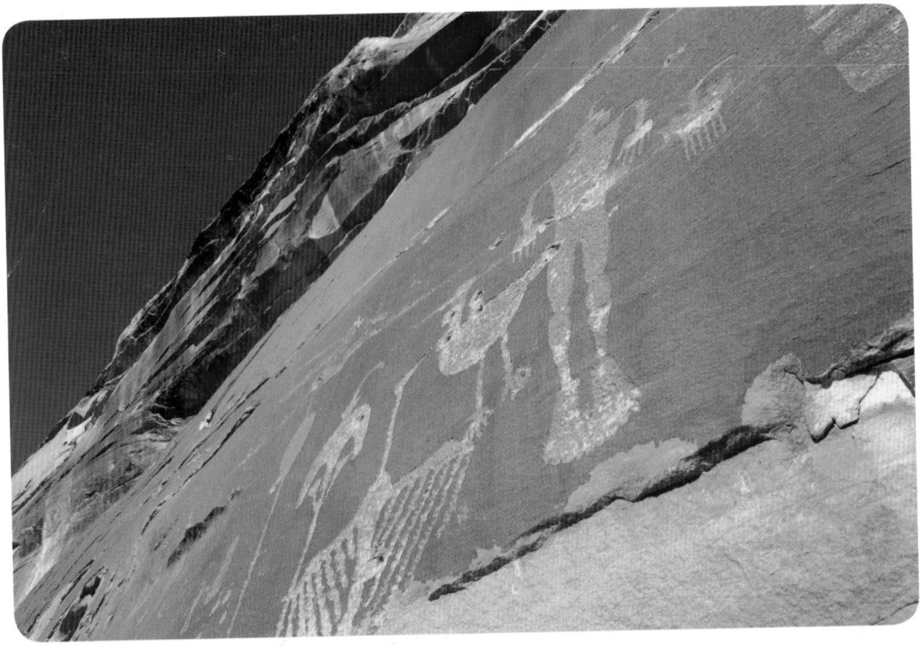

Wolfman Panel, Butler Wash

When you leave, initially vary your descent by staying left, high, along the base of the cliff. Close observation of the walls will reveal many more petroglyphs. Soon drop right and return the way you came.

trip 90 Double Stack Ruin
circuit 5 mi (8 km)
hiking time 4 hours
elevation gain 690 ft (210 m)

The trail immediately drops northwest into an **arroyo**, then ascends the far bank. Proceed northwest through sage about one minute, then cross another deep **arroyo**. About a minute farther, cross a **shallow wash**, then ascend a sandy path. Reach **slickrock** about five minutes from the trailhead.

Cairns lead north-northwest. Pass a series of small, descending depressions (tinajas). One minute farther, at the edge of slickrock, follow a sandy path into the **wash**. Go left (west-northwest) up the vegetated drainage, sometimes on a bench among sage.

Pass a crude, teepee-shaped structure. One minute beyond it, about 12 minutes from the trailhead, ignore a right (north) drainage. (The path in that direction quickly ends at a pouroff.) Bear left (west). Proceed up the **main wash**. The easiest path is on the right (north) bank.

About 18 minutes from the trailhead, arrive at a **confluence**. The canyon forks here, at 4485 ft (1367 m). Following the directions below, **begin a counterclockwise loop** that returns to this point.

Go right, into the north fork. A big alcove is visible ahead. Pass the remains of a second, crude, teepee-shaped structure. From the wash, a well-preserved ruin is now visible on a high ledge, on the canyon's right wall. This is the upper portion of **Double Stack Ruin**.

About 15 yd/m farther are the remains of the accessible, lower portion of Double Stack. Note the kiva (a huge log still spans it), a spiral pictograph numerous handprints (white, red), and a metate (stone with a concave surface) used to grind corn into flour).

Continue west, beyond Double Stack, up the north fork. Pass a shallow alcove (left). Walk into a **long, deep alcove** (right). It contains no obvious rock art or ruins. Near the far end of the alcove is a **pouroff**. So, about two-thirds of the way through the alcove, go left, out of the alcove, then proceed up-canyon on the left side of the wash to skirt the pouroff.

Above the pouroff, the wash is briefly rougher, bouldery, choked with vegetation. Work though it, probably by ascending the right slope then dropping back in. Where grey bedrock spans the floor, pick up a dirt path on the left (south). Your immediate goal—the ridgecrest—is visible ahead.

Having overcome the obstacles—about a 15-minute task—arrive at a **slickrock ramp** rising northwest. Though steep, it grants a fun, 15 minute, final ascent. Reach the **crest of Comb Ridge** at 5150 ft (1570 m). Total hiking time: one hour and 40 minutes. Looking east-southeast, over the canyon you just ascended, you'll see cottonwoods in Butler Wash. A panoramic view extends to the western horizon. Monument Valley is visible southwest.

Turn left and hike south along the crest. In a couple minutes, angle left (southeast). Descend through broken rock, then on slickrock, then among trees and boulders in the drainage. You're aiming for the canyon parallel to (immediately south of) the one you ascended to the crest.

Bypass a **small pouroff** by traversing slickrock about 10 ft (3 m) above its right side. About 30 minutes below the crest, bypass a **big pouroff** by descending the trail on its right side.

Reach yet another **big pouroff**. Just above its lip, cross to the left side of the drainage. Then descend ledges along the canyon wall. Soon reach the wash bottom. Proceed down-canyon.

Nearly an hour below the crest, reach the **confluence near Double Stack Ruin**. You're now on familiar ground. Bear right and retrace your steps to reach the trailhead in about 18 minutes.

Wolfman Panel hiking time 30 minutes
round trip 1 mi (0.6 km)
elevation gain 115 ft (35 m)

From the slickrock bench, follow the tiny drainage west. Soon reach the **canyon rim** at 4435 ft (1352 m). Butler Wash is visible below. Cairns indicate the descent route. Go left (south-southwest) on the ledge. Immediately past the small alcove, look left (east), above you. The **Wolfman Panel** is on the west-facing wall, at 4362 ft (1330 m), 15 minutes from the upper parking area. On the return, after ascending to the slickrock bench, go left (northeast) a couple minutes along the canyon rim. Look left (north) to see a couple ruins on the far canyon wall.

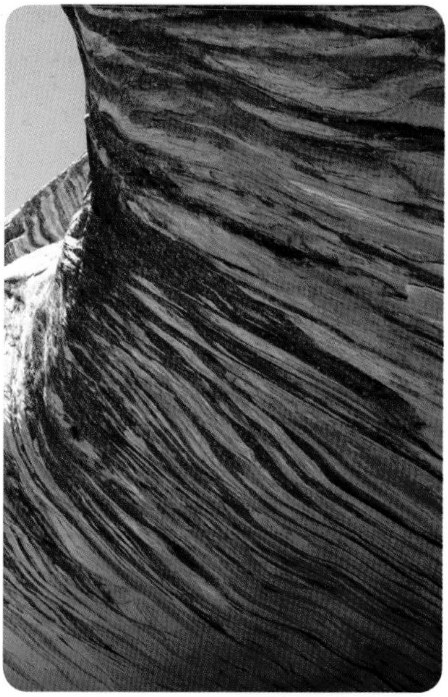
Alcove near Double Stack Ruin

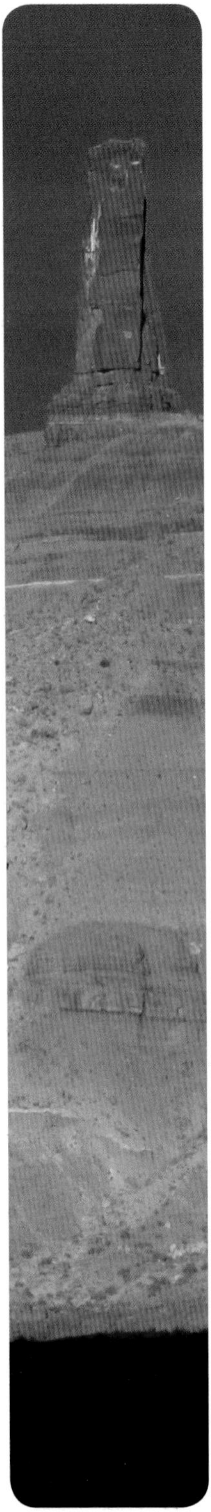

INFORMATION SOURCES

NATIONAL PARKS

Arches National Park
(435) 719-2299
www.nps.gov/arch

Bryce Canyon National Park
(435) 834-5322
www.nps.gov/brca

Canyonlands National Park
(435) 719-2313 general info
(435) 719-4351 backcountry info
(435) 259-4712 Island in the Sky District
(435) 259-4711 Needles District
www.nps.gov/cany

Capitol Reef National Park
(801) 425-3791 ext 111
www.nps.gov/care

Glen Canyon National Recreation Area
(520) 608-6404
www.nps.gov/glca

Zion National Park
(435) 772-3256 Springdale
(435) 586-9548 Kolob Canyons (I-15, Exit 40)
www.nps.gov/zion

STATE PARKS

Anasazi State Park Museum (Boulder)
(435) 335-7308
http://stateparks.utah.gov/parks/anasazi/

Dead Horse Point State Park (Moab)
(435) 259-2614
http://stateparks.utah.gov/parks/dead-horse/

Edge of the Cedars State Park (Blanding)
(435) 678-2238
http://stateparks.utah.gov/parks/edge-of-the-cedars/

Snow Canyon State Park (St. George)
(435) 628-2255
http://stateparks.utah.gov/parks/snow-canyon/

Castle Rock, from Castle Valley

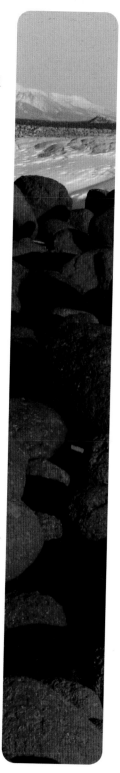

GRAND STAIRCASE - ESCALANTE NATIONAL MONUMENT
www.blm.gov/ut/st/en/fo/grand_staircase-escalante.html
utgsmail@blm.gov

Big Water Visitor Center
(435) 675-3200

Cannonville Visitor Center
(435) 826-5640

Escalante Interagency Visitor Center
(435) 826-5499

Kanab Visitor Center
(435) 644-1300

BUREAU OF LAND MANAGEMENT
www.blm.gov/ut/st/en.html

Moab Field Office
(435) 259-2100
82 East Dogwood

Monticello Field Office
(435) 587-1500
435 North Main Street

CONSERVATION

Glen Canyon Institute
(801) 363-4450
www.glencanyon.org

Southern Utah Wilderness Alliance
(801) 486-3161
www.suwa.org

Utah Open Lands
(801) 463-6156
www.utahopenlands.org

The Henry Mountains, from near Boulder

INDEX

Abyss Canyon 280
All American Man 350
Amasa Back 293
America's Wild Legacy 9
Ancestral Puebloans 11, 368, 425
Angel Arch 350
Angels Landing 51
Arches NP 10, 17, 260, 266, 269
Armstrong Canyon 385
Averett Canyon 135

Bannister Ruin 378
Barrier-Canyon style 14, 314
Beartrap Canyon 39
Behind the Rocks 286
Bell Canyon 240
Bement Arch 170
Big Ledge Ruins 409
Big Man Panel 380
Big Pocket 350
Big Spring 71, 334
Black Dragon 256
Bluff 143, 425
Boulder 185, 188, 192
Boulder Mail Trail 192
Bowtie Arch 272
Box-Death Hollow 136
Bridge Canyon 110
Brimstone Gulch 154
Broken Bow Arch 144, 166
Bryce Canyon NP 117, 121, 126
Bryce Point 124

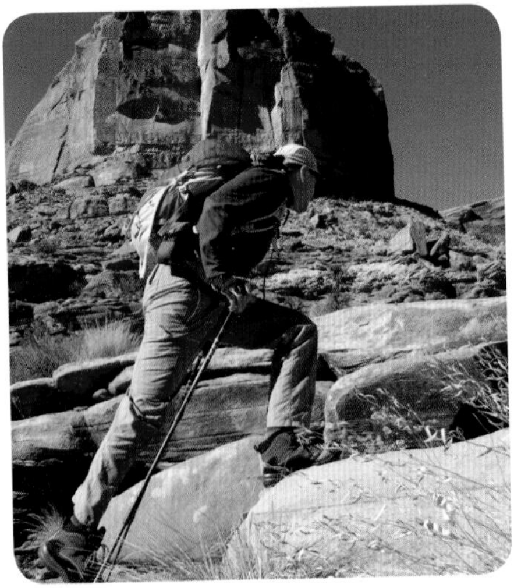

Buckskin Gulch 81, 84, 94
Bullet Canyon 381, 402
Burr Trail Road 199, 203, 207
Bush Head Canyon 94
Butler Canyon, N Fork 366
Butler Wash 425

Cable Mtn 61
Calf Creek 174, 183, 188
Cannonville 104, 130
Canyonlands NP 13, 27, 314, 322, 325, 329, 334, 338, 343, 350
Capitol Reef NP 207, 212, 216, 221, 227, 231
Cassidy Arch 221
Cassidy trail (Red Canyon) 127
Cathedral Butte 350
Cedar City 41, 140
Cedar Mesa 143, 368
Chesler Park 343
Chimney Canyon 250
Chimney Rock 212
Chute Canyon 247
Chute of Muddy Creek 250
Civilian Conservation Corps 56
Cliff Canyon 115
Cockscomb, The 81
Cohab Canyon 221
Cold Springs Cave 432
Collins Canyon 373, 376
Colorado Plateau 12, 15
Colorado River 15, 91, 141, 303, 320
Comb Ridge 425
Corona Arch 272
Cottonwood Canyon Road 100, 105
Coyote Buttes 76
Coyote Gulch 158, 162
Crack Canyon 244
Crack in the Wall 162
Culvert Canyon 275
Curtis Bench 235
cryptogamic soil 21

Dark Canyon 360
Davis Gulch 170
Dead Horse Point State Park 319
Death Hollow 177, 192
Deertrap Mtn 67
Delicate Arch 269
Devils Garden 260
Devils Kitchen 343

Dirty Devil River 16
Double-O Arch 261
Double Stack Ruin 434
Dragonfly Canyon 275
Druid Arch 343
Dry Fork Coyote 156

Early Weed Bench 150
East Rim Zion Canyon 69
Echo Canyon 61
Elephant Canyon 344
Elephant Hill 343
Escalante 176, 181, 185, 188, 192
Escalante River 146, 150, 158, 163, 174, 203

Fairyland 117
Fence Canyon 148
Fiery Furnace 266
Fin Canyon 260
Fish Creek Canyon 396
Fish Mouth Cave 431
Fisher Towers 32, 310
Five Fingers Canyon 358
flashflood 28
Fortymile Gulch 166
Four Faces 350
Fox Canyon 150
Fremont River 212
Fruita 218
Frying Pan trail 221

Glen Canyon NRA 145, 360
Goblin Valley 234, 241, 244, 247
Gold Bar Rim 275
Golden Cathedral 146
Golden Throne 227
Goosenecks State Park 422
Grand Canyon 89
Grand Gulch 143, 370, 373, 376, 392
Grand Staircase-Escalante NM 18, 79, 85, 100, 104, 130, 145, 174, 179, 183, 188, 199, 203
Grand Wash 221
Great Gallery 9, 314
Green River 15, 256

Hackberry Canyon 100
Hanksville 16, 236, 240, 244, 247, 314
heat exhaustion 30

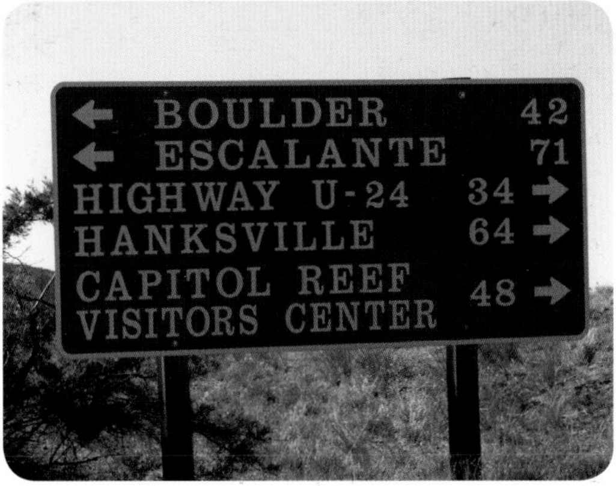

heatstroke 31
Hells Backbone Road 137
Hickman Bridge 217
Hidden Canyon 67
Hidden Splendor Mine 251
Hidden Valley 286
Hite 365
Hole-in-the-Rock Road 140, 148, 151, 155, 159, 164, 168, 172, 174
Honaker Trail 421
Hop Valley 39
Horse Canyon 199
Horseshoe Canyon 314
House Rock Valley Road 79, 86
Hurricane Wash 158

Island in the Sky 322, 325, 329

Jackass Canyon 303
Jackson Hole 296
Jacob Hamblin Arch 158
Jailhouse Ruin 381, 402
Jeep Arch 275
Junction Ruin 392

Kachina Bridge 383
Kanab 76, 81, 84, 89, 100, 104, 130
Kane Creek Road 293
Kane Gulch 376, 392
Kane Gulch Ranger Station 368, 378, 397, 403, 406, 410, 418
Kolob Arch 39
Kolob Canyons 39, 48

La Sal Mtns 279, 295
La Verkin Creek 39
Lake Powell 110
Landscape Arch 260
Lathrop Canyon 322
Lean-To Canyon 361
Lee Pass 39
Lee's Ferry 89
Left Fork North Creek 46
Lick Wash 104, 130
Little Death Hollow 199
Little Wild Horse Canyon 240
Lime Canyon 417
Losee Canyon trail 127
Lower Black Box 259
Lower Calf Creek Falls 183

Mamie Creek 192
Mary Jane Canyon 306
McCloyd Canyon 396
Mill Creek Canyon 282
Moab 13, 262, 267, 269, 272, 275, 278, 282, 286, 293, 298, 303, 306, 310, 319, 330
Moab Rim 286
Molly's Castle 235
Monarch Cave 430, 433
Monticello 335, 339
Mormon pioneers 9, 61, 92, 140
Morning Glory Canyon 298
Muddy Creek 250
Mule Canyon South Fork 388
Murphy Hogback 325

Natural Bridges NM 383
Navajo Knobs 216

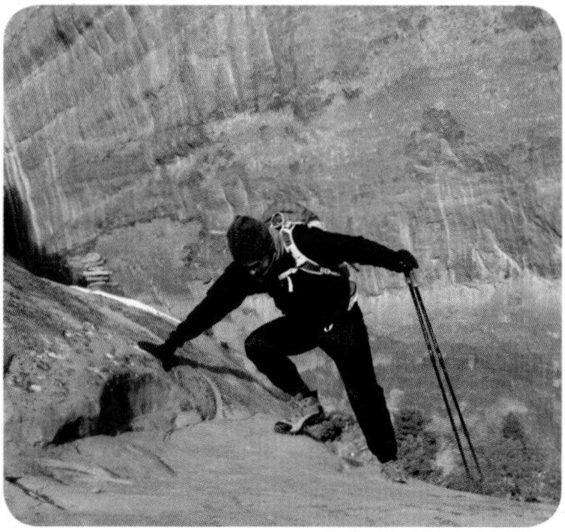

Primitive loop, Arches National Park

Navajo loop 121
Navajo sandstone 18, 61, 80
Needles, The 343
Needles District 13, 334, 338, 350
Negro Bill Canyon 298
Neon Canyon 146
Newspaper Rock 13, 335, 339
North Fork Virgin River 71
North Wash 365
Notom Road 208, 231

Oak Creek Canyon 110
Observation Point 61
Orderville Canyon 71
Owachomo Bridge 383
Owl Creek Canyon 396

Page, Arizona 89
Paleo-Indians 9
Paria Canyon 84, 89
Paria Canyon-Vermilion Cliffs Wilderness 76, 81, 84, 89
Peekaboo (Bryce) 121
Peekaboo (Canyonlands) 338, 350
Peek-a-boo Gulch (Escalante) 154
Perfect Kiva 381, 402
petroglyphs 13
Phipps Arch 179
pictographs 13
Pine Creek 136, 178, 192
Polly's Canyon 379
Porcupine Rim trail 303
Procession Panel 425, 432
Professor Creek 306
Queens Garden 121

Rainbow Bridge 110
Red Canyon 126
Red Cliffs Desert Reserve 34
Redbud Creek Canyon 110
Redrock Heritage 8
Rill Creek Canyon 282
Road Canyon 413
rock art 12, 285, 287

Saddle Arch 211
St. George 34
Salt Creek Canyon 340, 350
San Juan River 15, 421
San Rafael Reef 26, 240, 244, 247, 251, 256

San Rafael River 258
Sand Creek 177, 192
Sandthrax Canyon 365
Sego Canyon 13
Seven Kivas 413
Sheets Gulch 231
Sheik's Canyon 381
Silver Falls Creek Canyon 203
Sipapu 414
Sipapu Bridge 383
Skull Arch 267
Skutumpah Road 104, 130
Slickhorn Canyon 405, 409
Slickrock Trail (Moab) 278
Snow Canyon 34
Sooner Bench 168
Spanish explorers 9, 91
Split Level Ruin 11, 377, 381
Spooky Gulch 154
Spotted Wolf Canyon 26
Spring Canyon 212
Squaw Canyon 334, 340
Step Canyon 380
Stevens Arch 164
Strike Valley 209
Subway, The 46
Sunrise Point 117
Southern Utah Wilderness Alliance 8
Syncline Valley 329

Telephone Canyon 56
Temple of Sinawava 55, 71
Timber Creek 44
Titan Tower 313
Todie Canyon 381, 395
Tomsich Butte 250
Torrey 217, 223, 228
Turkey Pen Ruin 392
Twentyfive Mile Wash 150

Upheaval Canyon 329
Upheaval Dome 332
Upper Calf Creek Falls 188
Upper Jump 350
Upper Muley Twist 207

Virgin River 51, 61, 71

Wall of Windows 125
Wall Street 122
Walter's Wiggles 51, 58
Waterpocket Fold 211, 216, 221
Wave, The 76
West Rim (Zion Canyon) 51, 56
Wetherill, Richard 370
White Canyon 10, 385
White House trailhead 84, 89
White Rim Road 322, 325
Willis Creek Canyon 44, 104, 130
Willow Gulch 166
Wire Pass 79, 81, 84
Wolfman Panel 434
Wolverine Canyon 199
Wolverine Loop Road 200, 205
Wrather Arch 98

Yabut Pass 116
Yellow Rock 100

Zion Canyon 54, 62, 71
Zion Narrows 71
Zion NP 27, 39, 46, 51, 56, 61, 71

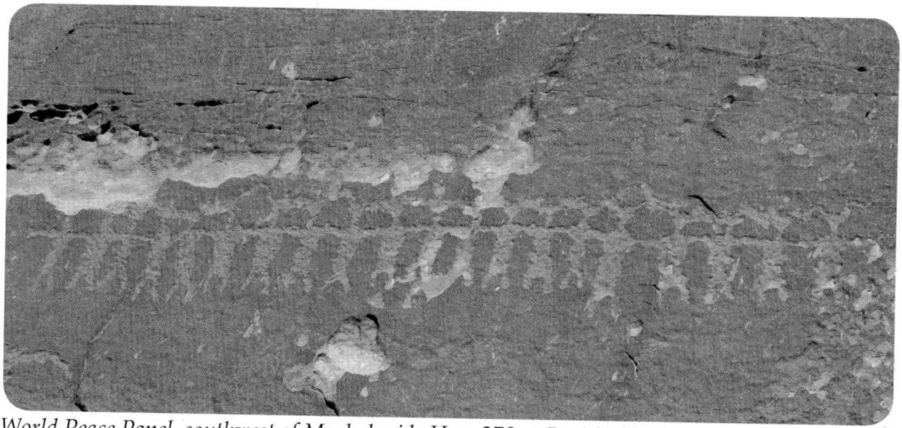

World Peace Panel, southwest of Moab, beside Hwy 279 at 5 mi (7.8 km)

THE AUTHORS

Kathy and Craig are dedicated to each other and to hiking, in that order. Their second date was a 20-mi (32-km) dayhike in Arizona. Since then they haven't stopped for long.

They've trekked through much of the world's vertical topography, including the Nepalese Himalaya, Patagonian Andes, and New Zealand Alps. In Europe, they've hiked throughout Spain's Costa Blanca Mountains, Mallorca's Serra de Tramuntana, the Alpes Maritimes and Hautes Alpes in France, and Italy's Monti Liguri. In North America, they've explored the B.C. Coast, Selkirk and Purcell ranges, Montana's Beartooth Wilderness, Wyoming's Grand Tetons, the Colorado Rockies, the California Sierra, and Arizona's Grand Canyon and Superstition Wilderness. Visit Kathy and Craig's website: www.hikingcamping.com. You'll find their blog posts are often mini-guidebooks, and their photo gallery is constantly growing.

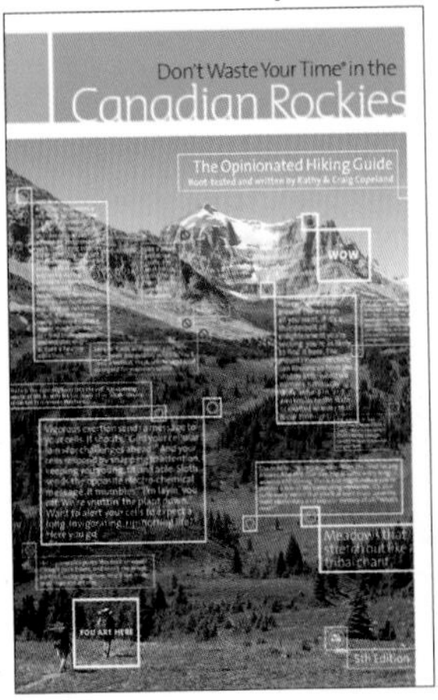

In 1989, they moved from the U.S. to Canada, so they could live near the range that inspired the first of their refreshingly unconventional books: *Don't Waste Your Time in the Canadian Rockies, The Opinionated Hiking Guide*. Its popularity encouraged them to abandon their careers—Kathy as an ESL teacher, Craig as an ad-agency creative director—and start their own guidebook publishing company: hikingcamping.com. Kathy and Craig's other books include *Where Locals Hike in the Canadian Rockies, Where Locals Hike in the West Kootenay, Camp Free in B.C.*, and a *Done in a Day* series featuring the ten premier hikes near Moab, Whistler, Jasper, Banff, and other adventure gateways.

To create the book you now hold in your hands—*Hiking From Here To Wow: Utah Canyon Country*—Kathy and Craig hiked more than 2,000 mi (3,220 km). They shot nearly 3,000 photos. They recorded hundreds of pages of field notes. And they continue to return to southern Utah frequently. "It has a firm grip on our souls," Kathy says.

Though the distances they hike are epic, Kathy and Craig agree that hiking, no matter how far, is the easiest of the many tasks necessary to create a guidebook. What they find most challenging is sitting at their Canmore, Alberta home, with the Canadian Rockies visible out the window, and spending twice as much time at their computers—writing, organizing, editing, checking facts—as they do on the trail.

The result is worth it. Kathy and Craig's colorful writing, opinionated commentary, and enthusiasm for the joys of hiking make their guidebooks uniquely helpful and compelling.

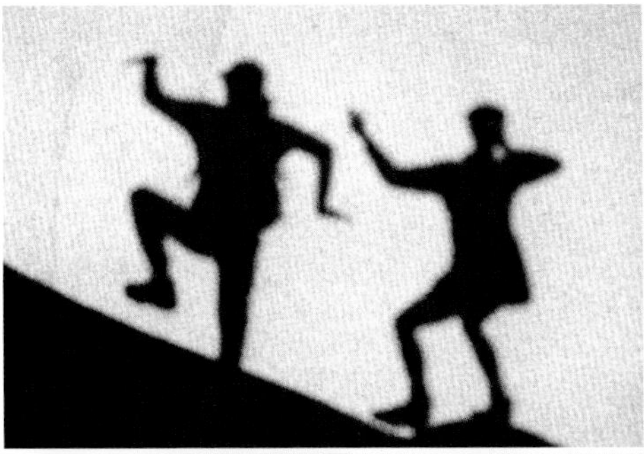

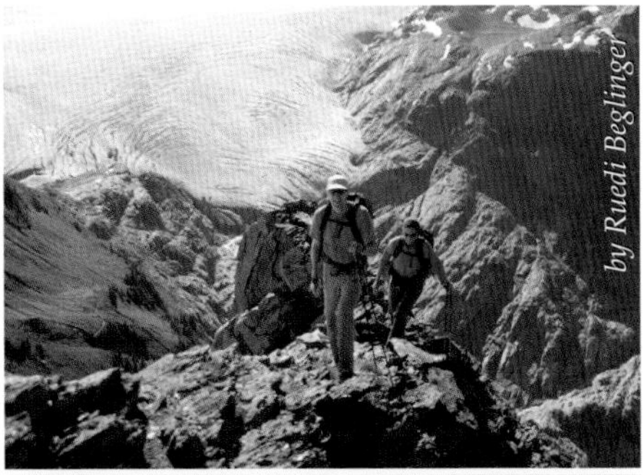

by Ruedi Beglinger

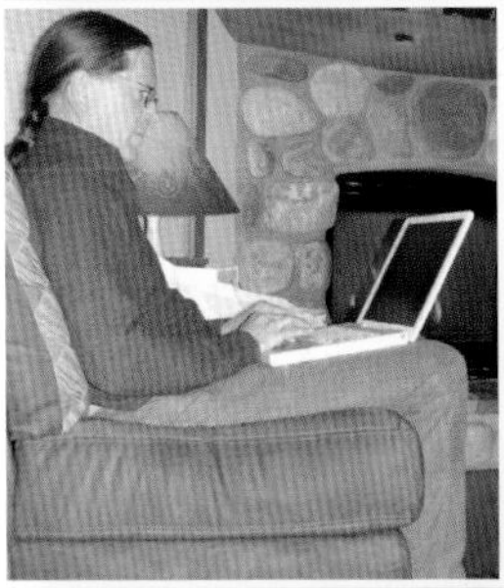

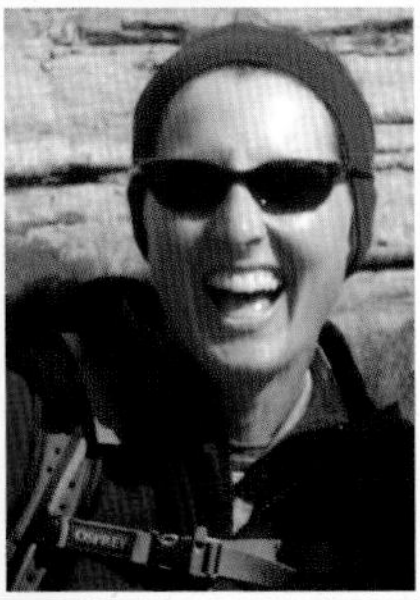

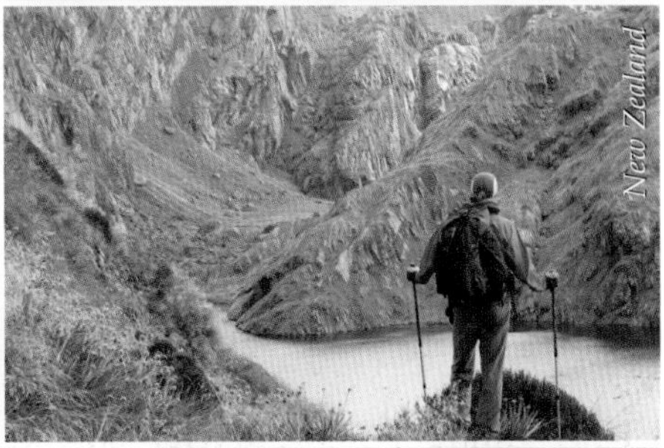

New Zealand

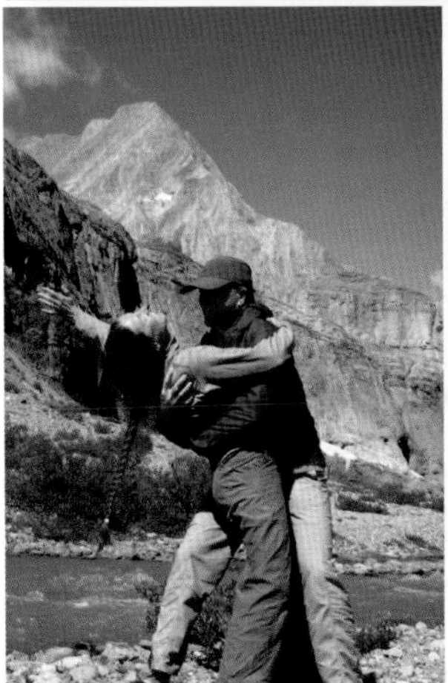

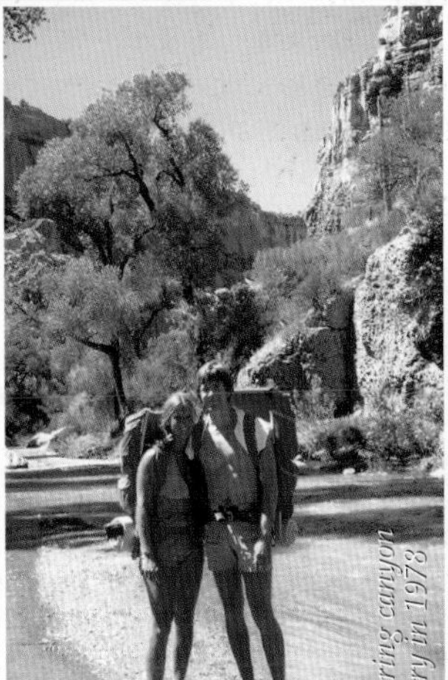

Exploring canyon country in 1978

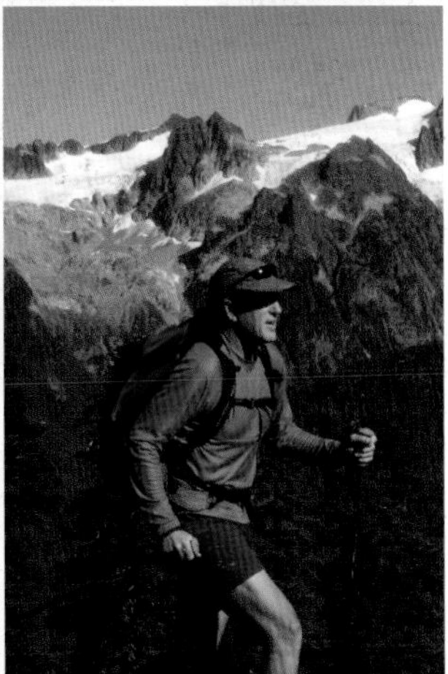

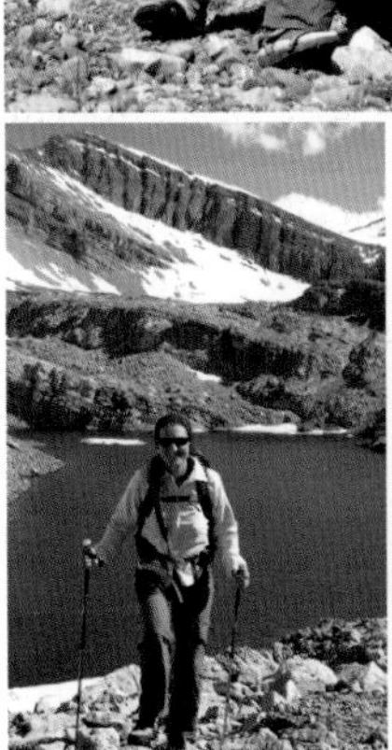

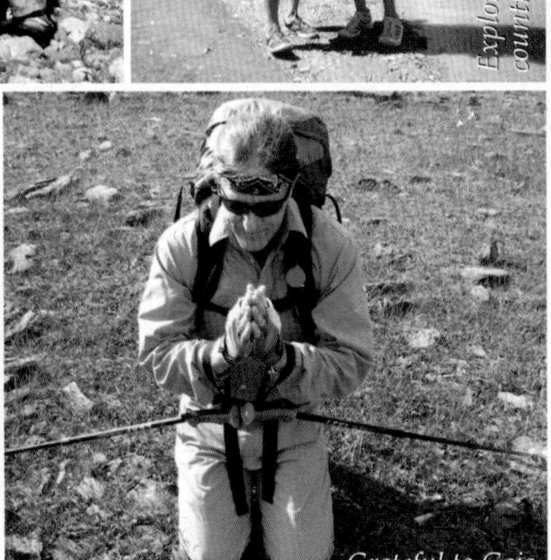

Grateful to Gaia

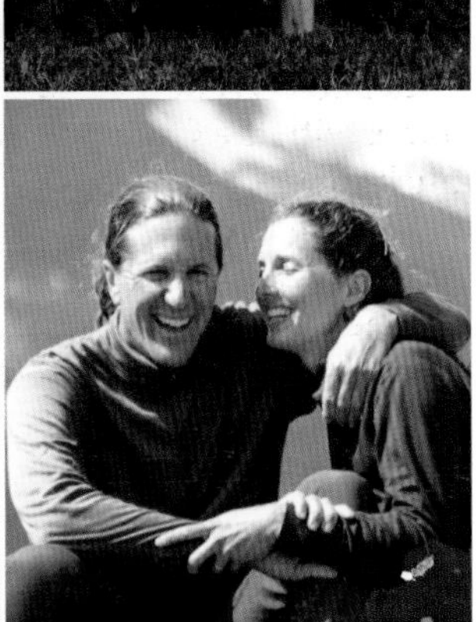

The Authors

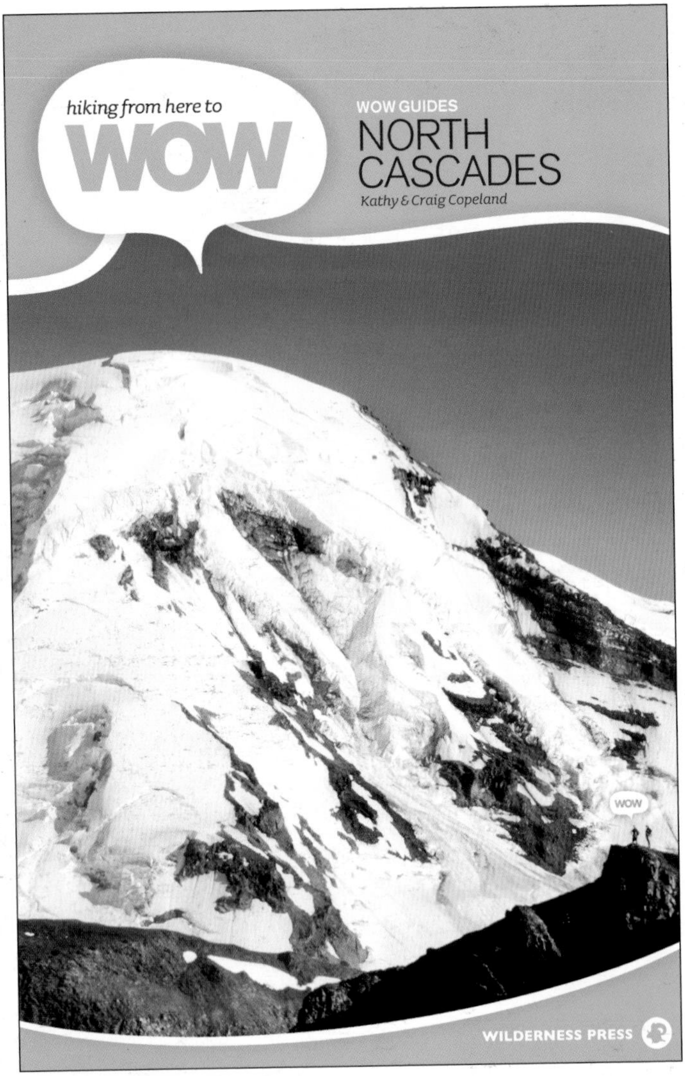

Hiking from here to WOW: North Cascades

50 Trails to the Wonder Of Wilderness

ISBN 978-0-89997-444-6 The authors hiked more than 2,000 mi (3,220 km) through North Cascades National Park plus the surrounding wilderness areas, including Glacier Peak, Mt. Baker, and the Pasayten. Then they culled their list of favorite trips down to 50—each selected for its power to incite awe. Their 262-page book describes where to find the cathedral forests, psychedelic meadows, spiky summits, and colossal glaciers that distinguish the American Alps. And it does so in refreshing style: honest, literate, entertaining, inspiring. Like all *WOW Guides*, this one is full color throughout, with a trail map for each dayhike and backpack trip. First edition, May 2007.

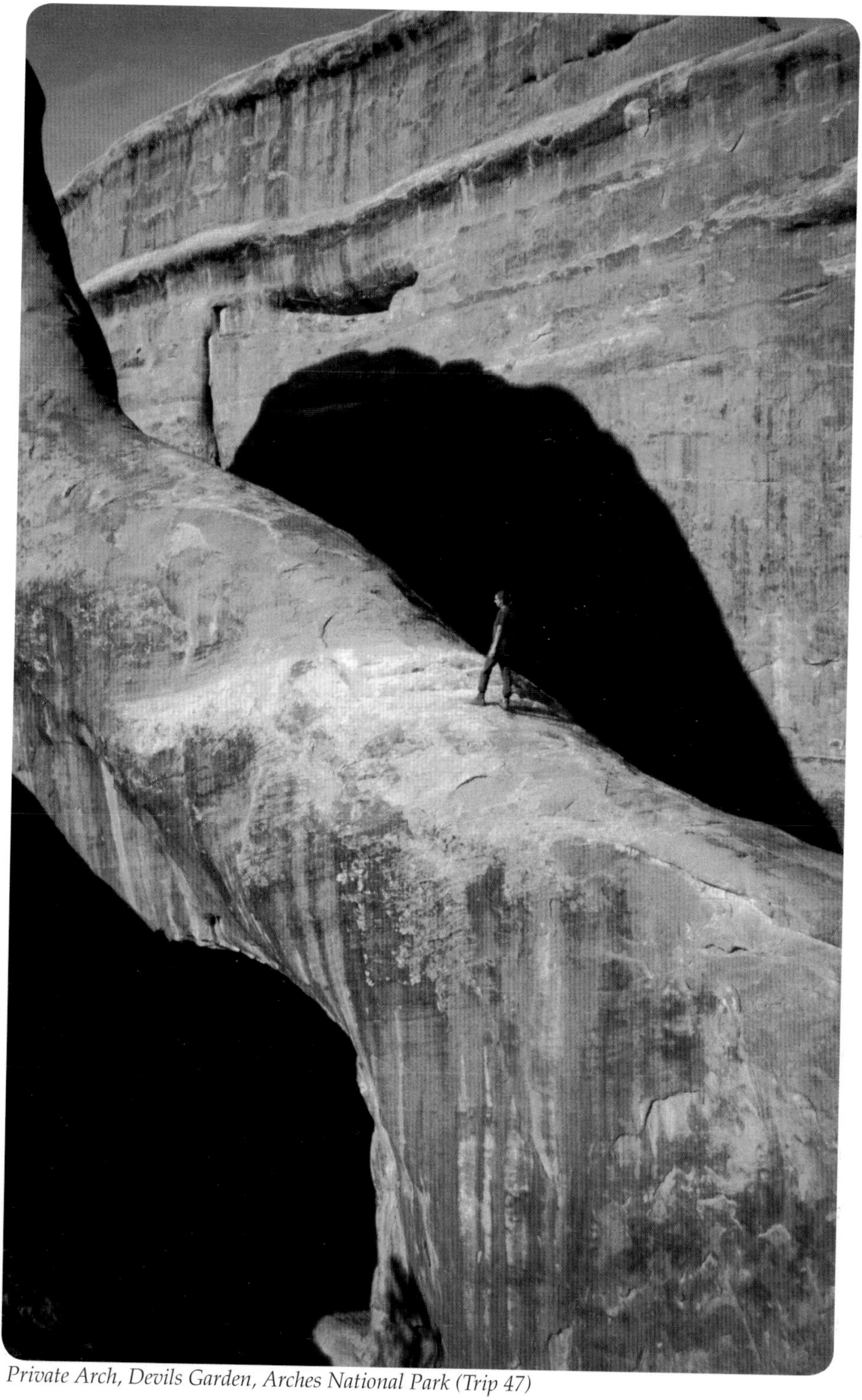

Private Arch, Devils Garden, Arches National Park (Trip 47)

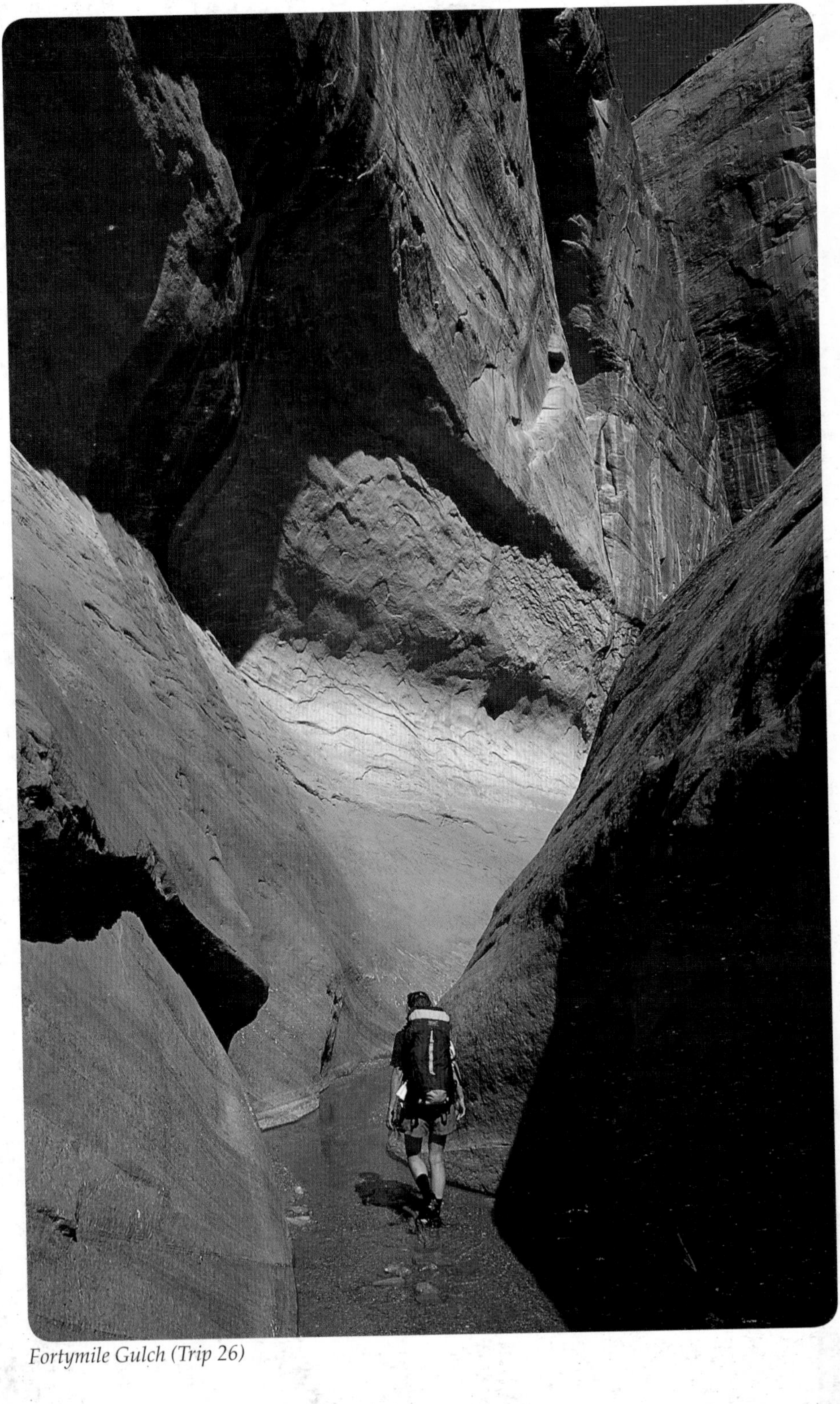

Fortymile Gulch (Trip 26)